The Fieldwork Anthology: A Classic Research and Practice Collection

Christine R. Privott, MA, OTR/L

Editor

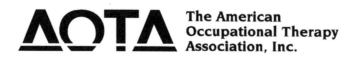 **The American Occupational Therapy Association, Inc.**

The American Occupational Therapy Association, Inc. Mission Statement

The mission of the American Occupational Therapy Association is to support a professional community for members, and to develop and preserve the viability and relevance of the profession. The organization serves the interest of its members, represents the profession to the public, and promotes access to occupational therapy services.

Disclaimers

"This publication is designed to provide accurate and authoritative information in regard to the subject matter covered. It is sold or distributed with the understanding that the publisher is not engaged in rendering legal, accounting, or other professional services. If legal advice or other expert assistance is required, the services of a competent professional should be sought."

—*From the Declaration of Principles jointly adopted by the American Bar Association and a Committee of Publishers and Associations*

It is the objective of the American Occupational Therapy Association to be a forum for free expression and interchange of ideas. The opinions expressed by the contributors to this work are their own and not necessarily those of either the editors or the American Occupational Therapy Association.

AOTA Director of Nonperiodical Publications: Frances E. McCarrey
AOTA Managing Editor of Nonperiodical Publications: Mary C. Fisk
Text design by World Composition Services, Inc.
Cover design and photography by Paul A. Platosh

ISBN 1-56900-092-1

Printed in the United States of America

Table of Contents

Preface

Welcome to the world of clinical education. If you are a practitioner, student, or educator exploring occupational therapy clinical education for the first time, then you will find this anthology critical to your development. If clinical education is already your role and responsibility in OT, then this resource will enhance performance and instill value in clinical education and help you to continue to spread the good news about fieldwork.

For purposes of this anthology, the words *clinical education, fieldwork,* and *fieldwork education* are used interchangeably. All these concepts refer to clinical practice outside the classroom. A student makes the gradual transition from classroom to clinic by applying recently-learned theory and technique. Similarly, the words *clinical educator, fieldwork educator, clinical supervisor,* and *fieldwork supervisor* are used interchangeably here. These refer to an occupational therapy practitioner who learns to *teach* students the principles of practice and clinical applications needed for successful occupational therapy practice. We must always keep in mind that clinical education encompasses both the student *and* the occupational therapist, who receive guidance from education programs.

Before we explore and understand the structure of this anthology, we must define the meaning of fieldwork education. In 1995, the American Occupational Therapy Association's Representative Assembly charged the Intercommission Council to prepare a position statement on fieldwork. In April 1996, the Representative Assembly approved the following statement titled, *Purpose and Value of Occupational Therapy Fieldwork Education.*

The purpose of fieldwork experience is to provide occupational therapy students with the opportunity to integrate academic knowledge with the application of skills at progressively higher levels of performance and responsibility. The academic setting emphasizes the acquisition of knowledge and the cognitive growth of the student. The clinical setting emphasizes the direct application of this knowledge through supervised intervention with patients and clients. The unique contributions of fieldwork experience include the opportunity to test first hand the theories and facts learned in academic study and to refine skills through client intervention under the supervision of qualified practitioners.

Supervised fieldwork experience in occupational therapy is an integral part of both the educational process and professional preparation. It is intended to complement academic preparation by offering additional opportunities for growth, application of knowledge, development and testing of clinical skills, and validation and consolidation of those functions that comprise professional competence.

The goal of the educational process is to produce competent occupational therapy practitioners. Upon completion of Level II fieldwork education, the student is expected to function at or above the minimum entry level of competence. Therefore, fieldwork experiences should be structured to offer opportunities for development of the necessary skills and abilities expected of entry-level practitioners.

While general objectives for fieldwork education have been identified by fieldwork and academic educators in occupational therapy, it is important to recognize that each fieldwork placement has its own unique characteristics. The philosophy of the placement and its organization and environment directly affect the fieldwork education program. Thus, each fieldwork placement must establish its own educational objectives in collaboration with the educational institution to reflect learning outcomes that are realistic and feasible given the types of learning experiences available.

Effective clinical practice requires not only a solid knowledge base, but also effective interpersonal behavioral characteristics. The value of both the academic and clinical components of the educational process must be acknowledged. If there is to be a productive interaction between the two settings, there must be mutual respect for the contributions of each.

(*AJOT,* November/December 1996, Volume 50, Number 10)

This AOTA statement amply clarifies the purpose and value of fieldwork education and urges the profession to remain invested in clinical education.

Abiding by principles found in the study of occupational behavior, we have roles and responsibilities as in clinical educators. Whenever we discuss outcomes and learning, we must also be alert to the fact that a changing healthcare environment may require us to develop different learning strategies in order to adequately prepare students for what the future may hold for occupational therapy.

There are 12 occupational therapy roles identified and two of these roles reflect the area of clinical education and the other 10 could not exist without clinical education as a foundation defined by AOTA in *Occupational Therapy Roles Document* (AOTA, 1994). The role of *Fieldwork Educator* is defined as an individual who manages Level I or II fieldwork in a practice setting, and provides students with opportunities to achieve practitioner competencies. The Fieldwork Educator may rise to the role of *Fieldwork Coordinator, Academic Setting,* who is responsible for managing the student fieldwork program within the academic setting. This individual now has a greater sense of the bridge between practice and education and therefore prepare students for the role of Practitioner, OTR or Practitioner, COTA. These occupational therapy roles, which integrate the classroom and the clinic, enable our profession to remain dynamic and competitive.

Part of the challenge of fieldwork is the ever-changing healthcare environment. Throughout this anthology you will see references to "innovative fieldwork." What may not seem innovative to one therapist, may appear just that to another. "Innovative fieldwork" here simply refers to a model of fieldwork which is different from traditional one-to-one supervision, medical model of student fieldwork. We must be able to increase our awareness and comfort levels when confronting what some might consider newfangled approaches to fieldwork. The views and practices of academicians and clinicians in fieldwork need to meet those of consumers, agencies, regulators, and other practitioners.

Fieldwork educators and other practitioners appear to adhere to rigid fieldwork laws. OT clinical education should, in reality, provide us with the basic tools to solve problems. Certainly, problem solving and learning occurs in such areas as clinical reasoning, professional competence, and clinical competencies. Are these experiences 'operationalized' during fieldwork? We must remember that

we have a unified system of occupational therapy principles that help us explain our profession; we have evaluations, treatment interventions, and functional outcomes studies that explain the what, why, where, and how of OT service delivery. It is possible to use these to simplify and interpret the seeming laws of fieldwork in order to evolve new philosophies of fieldwork education. As you use this anthology, keep in mind how we 'operationalize' fieldwork according to traditional views, Some of the variables affecting traditional fieldwork are

- consumer-driven healthcare
- healthcare changes that affect the scope of fieldwork
- changes in scope of occupational therapy supervision
- the freedom to expand occupational therapy services.

Clearly, innovation will be needed in the face of the changes that are now sweeping the entire healthcare industry. The rate of these changes is suggested by the 1996 AOTA survey of members concerning changes in employment settings and client populations (*OT Week,* November 14, 1996). According to the survey, the greatest change occurred in employment settings: therapists moved from inpatient care to outpatient clinics, ambulatory care facilities, skilled nursing homes, and home health agencies—especially over the last five years. Thus, the occupational therapy profession mirrors the overall healthcare industry trend toward mergers, rationalization, home care, etc. These data illustrate the rapid transformation of health care that we might expect to see in the 21st century and underscore the importance of responsive and creative clinical education.

AOTA has provided us with an enormously useful document, *The Essentials for the Accreditation of an Occupational Therapy or Occupational Therapy Assistant Program* (AOTA, 1995), which sets the standards for all facets of our profession. Perceived obstacles in implementing innovative fieldwork are often centered around this document. The standards that relate to fieldwork education can be summarized and interpreted in Table 1.

The Essentials challenges us to grasp the significant concepts of a successful education program. This anthology is designed to help us meet that challenge.

Table 1

From *Essentials*	Comment
1. Fieldwork must subscribe to the standards of the profession and the Code of Ethics.	1. This is the foundation of occupational therapy fundamental to any fieldwork experience. The Code of Ethics guides us.
2. Fieldwork objectives should be collaboratively developed between the school, site, and student.	2. Collaboration is the key to success in innovative settings. The Fieldwork Evaluation Form should be utilized.
3. There should be regular communication with the fieldwork site, school, and student.	3. Routine feedback about objectives should occur prior to and during fieldwork. This process is a continuous cycle of feedback/prevention that should accompany fieldwork.
4. Fieldwork is designed to promote clinical reasoning, reflect current practice, develop professional competence, apply ethics, and expand clinical competencies related to human performance.	4. Any and all settings with OTR with at least one year experience and NBCOT certified. Individual judgement on legal, ethical, professional ramifications of innovative settings.
5. The ratio of fieldwork educators to students shall be appropriate for proper supervision and frequent assessment in achieving the fieldwork objectives.	5. The quantity and quality of supervision is subject to interpretation by each clinical program, by state regulations, standards of practice, ethical responsibilities, and the student's learning needs. Some models of supervision may require more effort to develop.
6. Fieldwork can be provided with various groups across the lifespan, people with psychosocial and physical performance deficits and various service delivery models.	6. Fieldwork must remain reflective of ever-changing current practice. Minimum number of hours only and flexibility with placements.

How to Use This Anthology

The present volume was conceived to offer students, faculty, and practitioners (including fieldwork educators) the opportunity to study the significant fieldwork education literature in one convenient location. Included are journal articles, both domestic and international, plus AOTA documents on fieldwork committee reports, projects, and position statements.

The anthology is divided into seven sections to be user-friendly to the student doing a research project or dissertation, to the faculty member searching for assignments or lecture content, or to the practitioner who is a new fieldwork supervisor or needs a refresher course on supervision. The seven sections are:

1. Cognitive learning styles and clinical reasoning

2. Research on educational outcomes related to fieldwork

3. Research on fieldwork supervisor learning and training

4. Research on students' perceptions and attitudes related to fieldwork

5. Models of fieldwork

6. International occupational therapy articles

7. AOTA fieldwork task force and committee reports and references

Each section is preceded by an introduction and a Table of Contents which provides an alphabetical listing by author of the articles in that section. We also include a bibliography of books and manuals on the subject of occupational therapy fieldwork.

The original concept of the anthology was to include related clinical education topics from other professions such as nursing, speech and language pathology, and physical therapy; this quickly became unwieldy and was abandoned. However, we intend to update this anthology at regular intervals (every three to five years) so that the profession has a comprehensive resource of clinical education materials.

As a member of AOTA, the reader also has access to the full resources and consultation from the various departments at the national association and the American Occupational Therapy Foundation (AOTF), which houses an excellent library.

This anthology has been supported by the combined efforts of many AOTA volunteers and staff. The idea was initially discussed during the Fieldwork For The Future Task Force meetings during 1994–1996, and the recommendation for this anthology was included in the Task Force's final report approved by the Representative Assembly in 1996. The members of the Fieldwork For The Future Task Force included:

Robin Bowen, EdD, OTR
Carole Hays, MA, OTRK, FAOTA
Elizabeth Maruyama, MPH, OTR
Barbara Townsend, MPH, OTR/L
Paula Young, BAS, COTA
Mary Ann Curtis, MBA, MA, OTR/L
(National Office Staff Liaison).

Acknowledgments

The entire staff of AOTA's Education Department has been, as usual, exemplary of AOTA's commitment to serve its members. Warm thanks to Bunny Lanahan for helping me to gather AOTA fieldwork documents and to Rhona Zukas and Mary Ann Curtis for providing me with an historical perspective on fieldwork.

Special thanks to Mary Binderman, the Director of the AOTF Library, and her staff for the tedious task of locating the articles—even over the holidays.

Finally, thanks to my husband Daryl for his encouragement and loyalty. It's true that one works better as a part of a team.

SECTION ONE | Cognitive Learning Styles and Clinical Reasoning

A clinical education document would not be complete without a section devoted to clinical reasoning and adult cognitive learning styles. These concepts are fundamental to providing appropriate occupational therapy services based on the client's needs and life story.

Occupational therapy clinical reasoning refers to the way therapists work and think in the practice arena. It is the ability of the therapist to "provide insights into the complexities of understanding the patient's story, and in doing so, make clear the immense importance of narrative to the clinical reasoning process" (Mattingly and Fleming, 1994). Therapists in a typically complex practice setting are required to communicate in a noncomplex manner their client's story and make certain aspects of practice more understandable to those around them. Clinical reasoning principles "reassure therapists who have experienced the difficulties and frustrations of entering the personal world of the patient within the structure of a biomechanical environment that the inevitable tensions that result can be reconciled. Therapists are encouraged to recognize and respect that multiple types of considerations both characterize and are important to daily practice" (Mattingly and Fleming, 1994).

Clinical reasoning enables us to cross the bridge from mediocre technique to a refined working model of human occupation. That bridge to practice and the ability to communicate clinical reasoning is formed in part by the observation and acknowledgment of various adult learning styles. The clinical supervisor and the student each have their own preferred learning style, which are acquired through a history of life experiences and combined with daily life pressures and demands. Some adults learn best through modelling based on direct observation. Some adults learn by assimilating the information passively and contributing only when they feel comfortable. Some adults prefer to learn and work independently in their own space, and some adults learn best in collaboration in a group atmosphere.

Barbara Gaiptman and Arlene Anthony (1993) state that it is:

> important for us to take a minute to distinguish the concept of learning styles from the concept of abilities. Abilities refer to qualities such as athletic ability. When we use athletic ability as an example, it becomes obvious that more is better. Learning styles are different however; learning styles are valued according to circumstances or context. No individual style is better or worse than any other. (p. 4–4)

Knowing and accepting different learning styles allows both therapist and student the freedom to expand in thought and action and makes clinical education that much easier.

The articles in this section will hopefully provide the impetus to acquire new learning skills and apply clinical reasoning in your environment. Special attention should be paid to the bibliography at the end of the anthology for a listing of more comprehensive sources on this topic.

Fieldwork Education: Shaping a Foundation for Clinical Reasoning

Ellen S. Cohn

Key Words: clinical competence • education, occupational therapy • fieldwork education, occupational therapy

The need to teach fieldwork students to critically examine practice has been a recurrent theme in recent occupational therapy literature; however, students need to learn routines and standard clinical skills before they can reflect on their practice. This article proposes a variety of strategies to teach technical skills while simultaneously providing a foundation for clinical reasoning.

Ellen S. Cohn, EdM, OTR/L, is Academic Fieldwork Coordinator, Tufts University–Boston School of Occupational Therapy, Medford, Massachusetts 02155.

This article was accepted for publication July 13, 1988.

The value of fieldwork education in our profession has never been questioned (Presseller, 1983). Historically, fieldwork education has represented a commitment to the philosophical notion that education for professionals is both theoretical and practical (Nystrom, 1986). The justification for practical fieldwork education is rooted in the work of the philosopher John Dewey (1904), who claimed the actions professionals take in the real world depend on a unique mental analysis and interpretation of each new situation encountered. This understanding of professional practice provides the rationale for placing the novice in the situation of practice, so that the novice may comprehend the unique mental analysis of the seasoned professional. Dewey outlined two methods for the practice phase of professional education: (a) the apprenticeship method, which emphasizes the development of skills, and (b) the laboratory method, which emphasizes the development of reflective intelligence or the complex reasoning process that underlies our practice. Dewey said that the novice cannot attend to both concrete skills and abstract analyses, but will focus on one or the other in the practice situation. If the two methods of designing the practice phase of professional education, each with a different purpose, have value, then we are faced with the challenge of designing our fieldwork programs to teach technical skills and simultaneously provide a foundation for clinical reasoning.

Technique Versus Critical Analysis

The *Guide to Fieldwork Education* (AOTA, 1985) states, "The purpose of fieldwork is to provide occupational therapy students with the opportunity to integrate academic knowledge with application skills at progressively higher levels of performance and responsibility" (p. 1). Furthermore, "the unique contributions of the fieldwork experience include the opportunity to test, first-hand, the theories and facts learned in academic study and to refine skills through client interaction" (p. 1). In other words, Level II fieldwork programs should help students develop clinical techniques and analyze or reflect on their practice.

Research has illustrated that students value clinical techniques and applications (Barris & Kielhofner, 1985). Although fieldwork and academic educators may not want to spend all of their time teaching specific techniques, this is what entry level baccalaureate students perceive themselves as needing. Developmental theorists tell us that students need to learn routines and standards before they develop creative alternatives (Loganbill, Hardy, & Delworth, 1982; Perry, 1979). For example, students need to learn how to assess range of motion in a standardized way before they can elaborate on that foundation and assess range from a functional perspective. Experience also tells us that students are searching for the "right way" to think and perform and that their tolerance for ambiguity is relatively low. Hence, we are caught between two fundamentally different agendas for fieldwork students: (a) an initial focus on technical skills and students' need to learn the routine application of treatment modalities and (b) the development of effective clinical reasoning. Meeting both of these agendas is a tremendous challenge. This paper proposes strategies that will help students first to develop technical skills and then to move to a more analytical approach to practice. These strategies serve as a foundation for shaping clinical reasoning in fieldwork students.

Strategies for Meeting the Challenge

A Reflective Stance Toward Practice

A reflective stance toward practice was advanced by Rogers (1983) and supported by the Entry-Level Study Committee report (AOTA, 1987), which repeatedly emphasized the need for critical thinkers. Thinking like professionals will help us become recognized in the health care system and in our larger society (Parham, 1987). Schön (1987) argued that skillful practice often depends less on factual knowledge or rigid decision-making models than on the capacity to reflect before taking actions in cases where established theories do not apply. However, most professional programs, including occupational therapy, teach students only standard theories and how to apply them to straightforward cases. Our schools fail to equip future professionals with the skills they need to deal with the difficult problems confronted in practice. When theories are applied in a standardized and mechanistic manner, we run the risk of missing our patients' views of their functional problems. Parham (1987) shared various examples in which the patient and the therapist had different constructions of the situations and focus of therapy because the therapist routinely selected standard technical solutions, whereas the patient had concerns that were not addressed by routine solutions. Parham illustrated this problem in the story of a talented and intelligent woman who had cerebral palsy and was asked to put beads in a jar during her occupational therapy (p. 556). Schön suggested that in order to move professionals beyond techniques, professional education should be centered on enhancing practitioners' ability to reflect on their practice. We must creatively design our fieldwork programs to move students beyond standard technical solutions and acquaint them with the complexities of clinical reasoning.

Over the years of working with occupational therapy students, I have observed many fieldwork educators struggling with the expectation that in a mere 3 months we could actually teach clinical reasoning. A recent fieldwork survey (Cohn & Frum, 1988) provided evidence that students are not prepared for the thinking challenges inherent in clinical practice and that fieldwork educators are searching for support in their efforts to help students develop clinical reasoning. When fieldwork educators were asked to identify their needs for continuing education, the top priorities were "bridging the gap between classroom and clinic" and "linking theory to practice." "Students lacking integration of knowledge and skills" was identified as one of the three major problems currently facing fieldwork educators (Cohn & Frum, 1988, p. 326). Furthermore, the new AOTA Fieldwork Evaluation requires us to provide feedback on students' performance in the judgment domain. With the advent of the new evaluation and the addition of the judgment section, I fear that clinical reasoning has become yet another "skill" to be taught. Clinical reasoning has been interpreted as having a reason for connecting a particular treatment decision to a particular frame of reference. Although theory helps us to make this connection, it is insufficient, by itself, to address the problems that occupational therapists encounter in practice. There is more to clinical reasoning than translating academic theory into practice. Clinical reasoning is based on our knowledge of procedures, interactions with patients, and interpretation and analysis of the evolving situation. It is a complex process dependent upon years of experience. The clinician's ability to create an original response to the patient's unique condition moves beyond the knowledge base (Mattingly, 1987). It may be unrealistic to expect students to emerge from a 3-month fieldwork experience with clinical reasoning firmly established; more realistically, we can expect that the fieldwork experience will serve as a foundation or preparation for clinical reasoning.

Consistent Patient Population

To develop technical skills and confront the complexities inherent in carrying out the standard treatment plan, students must repeat interactions with the same patients over an extended period of time so that patterns can be discerned. Students must work with a variety of patients with a similar diagnosis so they can learn when routine treatment approaches are appropriate and when they are not. When clinicians confront obstacles to their initial formulations of patients' treatment needs, they must reformulate their plans and reason in a new way. Thus, problems in practice facilitate the clinical reasoning process. A reasoning process that moves from the routine to the nonroutine is based on the need to modify the treatment program.

4 | Cognitive Learning Styles and Clinical Reasoning

Students must establish routines to reassure their technical skills before they can begin to reflect on their practice.

Currently, some Level II fieldwork programs are split into two 6-week segments with the intention of providing a broad exposure to a variety of diagnoses. Perhaps a 12-week program with a consistent patient population would enhance students' opportunities to reflect on their practice and evaluate the effectiveness of their treatment. One of the major challenges of occupational therapy is finding the delicate balance between support and challenge for patients. Clinical reasoning includes thinking about how to structure activities so that we can meet the patients' needs without pushing them too far. Without repeated exposure to the same patients, students will not have the opportunity to search for this delicate balance between support and challenge or to confront situations where the routine does not fit. If the fieldwork center is unable to provide a 12-week affiliation with a consistent patient population, perhaps students could, at the least, treat two patients with a similar diagnosis so that they can compare and contrast patients, thereby moving beyond the technical skill level to a more analytical and adaptive response to individual patients' needs and goals.

Questions

As students develop technique with a consistent patient population, educators may begin to relate theory and technique by asking probing questions at certain points in the clinical reasoning process. When routine approaches do not meet patients' needs and students are at a loss for ideas, educators can ask them to develop a range of strategies and to provide their rationale for choosing them. The first question, "What will you do?" relates to technique, and the second question, "Why are you doing it?" relates to theory. Questions such as "What do you see as this patient's possibilities?" focus students' attention on the patient. Questions may elicit a factual or an interpretive response: for example, "What kinds of splints are used for ulnar deviation?" requires a straightforward answer, and "What kind of splint do you recommend for this particular patient?" requires an arguable one. Factual questions have an important function, because they clarify what the starting point of any interpretation must be—facts. Interpretive questions require students to go beyond the facts to relate, criticize, clarify, justify, and apply the ideas being discussed. They require the evaluation and synthesis necessary for effective clinical reasoning. The fieldwork educator's task is to ask questions related to both ends of the continuum between technique and critical analysis.

Observing the Patient–Therapist Dyad

Traditionally, students shadow or observe therapists treating patients during the first week of fieldwork. In some settings, this observation period is open ended, and fieldwork educators ask students what they have observed. In other settings, the observations are structured, and students are directed to observe specific things such as the treatment activities or patients' performance. Rarely are students invited to focus on the patient–therapist dyad. Since clinical reasoning emerges in the process of interaction between therapist and patient, we should encourage students to question the reasoning embedded in the therapist's actions in the very first weeks. One of the most difficult reasoning tasks a therapist faces is designing and revising his or her approach to a particular patient. Therefore, it would be helpful to ask students to construct a hypothetical treatment story of the patient on the basis of the referral information. This story would include students' expectations of patients' clinical pictures and functional prognoses. Once students have observed patients, they can reconstruct their hypothetical treatment story to include patients' constructions of their problems and student's own observations of the clinical pictures. This approach to the initial observation of the patient may indeed teach students the technical skill of observation and help them build the foundation for testing their assumptions. From an educational perspective, the fieldwork educator can also use this experience to begin to assess students' knowledge. Do students know enough about the condition diagnosed to formulate realistic assumptions? If the diagnosis is a right cerebrovascular accident, do students mention muscle tone in their initial story construction? Why not encourage students to begin to revise their initial stories with feedback from patients? When students and patients create a shared story, students learn to collaborate with patients and are made aware early on that their interpretation of patients' needs must be constantly modified.

Role Modeling

Christie, Joyce, and Moeller (1985), in their study of fieldwork supervision, found that competent clinicians served as good role models. The role model, or mentor, is widely recognized as playing a critical role in shaping, teaching, coaching, and assisting future practitioners. As role models, fieldwork educators teach technical skills and a respect for and application of theory. We must recognize that the valuing of theory is a developmental process. Initially we need to model technical application. However, if our intention is to encourage students to value the critical examination of our practice, then we must simultaneously model reflection on our own practice. This we do by involving our students in the questioning of the effectiveness of our practice.

Telling Stories

Experience, captured in the form of stories remembered, influences therapists' treatment decisions. These stories provide a repertoire of expectations that therapists can apply to new situations. Experienced therapists have a library full of stories—students do not. From an educational perspective, the role of fieldwork educators is that of a continuous storyteller. Through stories, fieldwork educators begin to share their reasoning process and the belief system that guides their practice. Students cannot learn clinical reasoning by watching our actions, because the thought behind the action is not self-evident. We must delineate why we responded to a patient in a particular way and share our continuous revision of our approach to a particular patient. We design our treatment plans with the assumption that the plan will be constantly modified. Students are often unaware of this assumption. Students frequently design treatment plans and wait for the supervisor to suggest reevaluation of the treatment. Fieldwork educators must make their initial reasoning process explicit and then share their reformulations as therapy progresses.

Chunking Information

There is evidence that expert and novice problem solvers differ in their use of problem-solving strategies (Dreyfuss & Dreyfuss, 1986). One difference is the use of a cognitive strategy known as *chunking,* which refers to a way of organizing and categorizing information into units. Experts chunk, or cluster, data into larger information units than do novices. In clinical practice, experienced therapists create memory structures that reflect their clinical priorities. Therapists choose and name the things they notice. Depending on our theoretical frames of reference, clinical experiences, and clinical roles, we organize information differently. In the clinical situation, we may choose to organize patient data either around the patient's functional strengths or around the patient's symptoms. In this example, the clinical priority, function, serves as the framework for organizing patient data. Both of these frameworks are examples of categorizing data, but the functional status framework offers a broader perspective. For example, we can organize our observations of a child with cerebral palsy around the child's spastic muscle tone, primitive postural reflexes, and poorly controlled purposeful movement, or we can organize observations of the same child around the child's ability to use reflex patterns to eat and dress. Thus, we see that the ways in which we choose to categorize information influences the clinical choices we make. By asking students to chunk their treatment sessions, we gain a greater understanding of how they organize their reasoning process. We can also share our perspectives and organizing frameworks to share our treatment priorities.

Case Studies

Many fieldwork education programs require students to complete a case study. How often do educators model this case study or its revision? We could model the value of reflecting on practice by presenting a case study early in the fieldwork experience. Students will then observe that we are willing to risk sharing our thought processes. Instead of thinking of case studies as a review of textbook descriptions of patients' clinical conditions and listing long- and short-term goals, we need to present case studies in a process-oriented format. If we build the case presentation around the process of therapy, the constant revision of the treatment plan over time, the obstacles presented, or how patients and therapy changed, we are sharing our knowledge, experience, and thought processes. Moreover, we are modeling the critical professional ethos of reflection on practice.

Videotapes

A powerful tool for encouraging reflection on practice is the use of the video camera. Some students have reported that just knowing the camera is on forces them to think about their practice more carefully. Videotapes help students clarify their assumptions regarding their own behavior and the impact of their own behavior on patients. For example, one student reported that, while viewing a videotape following a particularly difficult group session, she realized that her body language, facial expressions, and irritated tone of voice contributed to the difficulty within the session. Before viewing the videotape, the student was able to articulate to the fieldwork educator that she was having a hard time. The videotape helped to clarify the contributing factors.

Reviewing videotapes of treatment sessions also helps students and fieldwork educators identify the various critical moments in the treatment session. Throughout the treatment sessions, experienced therapists make judgments or choices regarding which action to take at a given moment. This action is in response to the patient's performance. If experienced therapists shared videotapes of their own treatment sessions, they would be able to stop the action, discuss the reasoning behind their actions, and teach theoretical concepts. Together, students and field-work educators could evaluate the efficacy of the therapy session. Perhaps alternative strategies based on different frames of reference could be introduced.

Conclusion

No one can reason for or make judgments for another person, but we can provide models of our reasoning. Some of the strategies for teaching clinical techniques and shaping clinical reasoning are working with a consistent patient population to discern patterns, focusing on the patient–therapist interaction to observe how experienced clinicians solve problems, and using videotapes, case studies, and questions to help students internalize the value of clinical reasoning. The example we provide of reflecting on our own practice can model the clinical reasoning foundation that students will continue to build through reflecting on their own practice.

Acknowledgments

I thank Cheryl Mattingly, Project Director of the AOTA/AOTF Clinical Reasoning study, and the occupational therapy staff at University Hospital, Boston, for their support in the development of these ideas. This article is based on a keynote presentation to the New England Occupational Therapy Education Council, June 1987.

References

American Occupational Therapy Association. (1985). *Guide to fieldwork education*. Rockville, MD: Author.

American Occupational Therapy Association. (1987). *Occupational therapy: Directions for the future* (A report of the Entry-Level Study Committee, an ad-hoc committee of the Executive Board of the American Occupational Therapy Association, Inc.). Rockville, MD: Author.

Barris, R., & Kielhofner, G. (1985). Generating and using knowledge in occupational therapy: Implications for professional education. *Occupational Therapy Journal of Research, 5*, 113–124.

Christie, B. A., Joyce, P. C., & Moeller, P. L. (1985). Fieldwork experience, part I: Impact on practice preference. *American Journal of Occupational Therapy, 10*, 671–674.

Cohn, E. S., & Frum, D. C. (1988). Fieldwork supervision: More education is warranted. *American Journal of Occupational Therapy, 5*, 325–327.

Dewey, J. (1904). The relation of theory to practice in education. In *The third yearbook of the National Society for the Scientific Study of Education. Part I. The relation of theory to practice in education of teachers* (pp. 9–30). Chicago: University of Chicago Press.

Dreyfuss, H. L., & Dreyfuss, S. E. (1986). *Mind over machine*. New York: The Free Press, Macmillan.

Loganbill, C., Hardy, E., & Delworth, U. (1982). Supervision: A conceptual model. *Counseling Psychologist, 10*, 1.

Mattingly, C. (1987). [Clinical Reasoning Study]. Unpublished raw data.

Nystrom, E. P. (1986). The differentiation between academic and fieldwork education. In *Occupational Therapy Education: Target 2000 Proceedings* (pp. 90–94). Rockville, MD: American Occupational Therapy Association.

Parham, D. (1987). Toward professionalism: The reflective therapist. *American Journal of Occupational Therapy, 41*, 555–561.

Perry, W. (1979). *Forms of intellectual and ethical development in the college years*. New York: Holt, Rinehart & Winston.

Presseller, S. (1983). Fieldwork education: The proving ground of the profession. *American Journal of Occupational Therapy, 3*, 163–165.

Rogers, J. C. (1983). Eleanor Clarke Slagle Lectureship—1983; Clinical reasoning: The ethics, science, and art. *American Journal of Occupational Therapy, 9*, 601–616.

Schön, D. (1987). *Educating the reflective practitioner: How professionals think in action*. New York: Basic Books.

The Correlation Of Learning Styles With Student Performance In Academic And Clinical Course Work

M. Jo Cunningham
Becki A. Trickey

The purpose of this preliminary study was to determine any correlation between learning styles and performance in the academic and clinical course work of occupational therapy students at the Medical University of South Carolina. The Learning Styles Inventory (LSI) by Kolb is a simple self-description test. designed to determine the student's learning style preference. The specific aims of the project are:

1. To determine any correlation between the learning styles of the occupational therapy students and their performance in their academic course work.

2. To determine any correlation between the learning styles of the occupational therapy students and their performance on their psychosocial field work experience.

M. Jo Cunningham, MEd, OTR, is assistant professor and program director, Occupational Therapy, Medical University of South Carolina, Charleston 29425.

Becki A. Trickey, MHS, OTR, is an associate in the occupational therapy program, Medical University of South Carolina, Charleston.

3. To determine any correlation between the learning styles of the occupational therapy students and their performance on their physical dysfunction field work experience.

Thirteen members of the senior occupational therapy class, between the ages of 21 and 27 years, were selected to participate in the study. Among the subjects were 11 females and two males.

APPARATUS

The LSI is designed to measure individual learning styles by asking the subject to rank groups of four words that describe different learning modes. These learning modes are identified as: Concrete Experience (CE), Reflective Observation (RO), Abstract Conceptualization (AC), and Active Experimentation (AE). Once determined, these modes are computed, using a predesigned grid, to determine the four possible learning styles: Converger, whose dominant learning abilities are AC and AE; Assimilator, whose learning abilities are AC and RO; Accommodator, whose abilities are CE and AE; and Diverger, whose abilities are CE and RO.

Results of the study showed there was no significant correlation between any of the four learning styles and the academic course work or the psychosocial field work. While three of the learning styles displayed similar scores, the Converger presented a lower score on the physical dysfunction clinical area. A one-way analysis of variance was computed for the variables academic course work, psychosocial field work, and physical dysfunction field work. A significance level of .05 was established. The physical dysfunction field work showed a significance level of .056. While this does not fall in the significant range, its nearness warrants further investigation.

Data will continue to be gathered and computed to determine whether a larger sample size will substantiate the original findings.

Clinical Reasoning in Medicine Compared With Clinical Reasoning in Occupational Therapy

Maureen Hayes Fleming

Key Words: clinical competence • problem solving

This article highlights some observations made in the American Occupational Therapy Association/American Occupational Therapy Foundation Clinical Reasoning Study, an ethnographic study of 14 occupational therapists working in a large teaching hospital. Concepts and premises that frequently appear in the clinical reasoning in medicine literature are discussed and compared and contrasted to observations and interpretations made of the practice and reasoning strategies of the occupational therapists who were participants in the Clinical Reasoning Study. It is postulated that similarities in the reasoning strategies of the members of the two professions are a result of use of the scientific model that calls for hypothetical reasoning. Differences, it is proposed, are accounted for by the difference in the particular focus, goals, and tasks of the two professions and the nature of the practice in those arenas. Five hypotheses are proposed as questions for further research in clinical reasoning in occupational therapy.

Maureen Hayes Fleming, EdD, OTR, FAOTA, is Associate Professor, Department of Occupational Therapy, Graduate School of Arts and Sciences, Tufts University–Boston School of Occupational Therapy, 26 Winthrop Street, Medford, Massachusetts 02155.

This article was accepted for publication July 1, 1991.

The purpose of the Clinical Reasoning Study, sponsored by the American Occupational Therapy Association and the American Occupational Therapy Foundation, was to identify the clinical reasoning processes of occupational therapists (Gillette & Mattingly, 1987). Most of the literature on clinical reasoning reports studies of problem solving and decision making by physicians and medical students. The literature on clinical reasoning by physicians contains many findings, interpretations, assumptions, and recommendations that differ from reasoning among occupational therapists. These differences seem to be great enough to warrant discussion.

The first reason for such a discussion is that if one assumes that occupational therapists use reasoning strategies that are the same as those of physicians, then one would miss some salient aspects of therapists' reasoning. Therefore, the prevention of inappropriate assumptions at the outset of an understanding of the clinical reasoning processes of occupational therapists is a central purpose of this article. Second, an understanding of the reasoning processes gives additional insight into the nature and purpose of the practice. Third, some characteristics of clinical reasoning in occupational therapy are highlighted, many of which are explored in greater depth in other articles in this issue. Fourth, this article raises questions and offers hypotheses regarding potential relationships between the nature of the practice and the reasoning strategies employed by occupational therapists.

Purpose and Method

The aim of the Clinical Reasoning Study was to examine the reasoning strategies of occupational therapists in their day-to-day practice, and ethnographic methodology was used (see the Method section in the Mattingly and Gillette [1991] article in this issue). Therefore, the results of this study are descriptive. These results are interpretations of our observations and interactions with the therapists and of extensive analysis of the videotaped and transcribed treatment sessions and individual and group interviews with therapists. Thus, the results of the research are both descriptive and interpretive, as is the goal of phenomenological research (Karlsson, 1988). We sought to understand the reasoning of therapists who were participants in the Clinical Reasoning Study, based on their own perceptions of their experience of thinking as clinicians. Our interpretations are primarily an attempt to provide a language for understanding the day-to-day experience of thinking in practice.

Terminology

The terminology used in the literature in the general area of clinical reasoning is inconsistent, and some terms overlap or have different meanings. In this article, some terms are used to refer to specific, distinctive concepts. For some of these terms, whole bodies of literature argue the nature of the phenomena and its lexical denotation. I do not address these arguments here; instead, I offer definitions for the terms that I have used.

Reasoning. This refers to the many ways in which a person may think about and interpret an idea or phenomenon. This may range from a simple perception to a complex abstract construction and includes many forms of inquiry and interpretation. In this article, the term *reasoning* is used as an umbrella term to cover all aspects of thinking.

Judgment. This refers to the process by which a person appraises a situation and determines the best course of action to take. Clinical judgment is a somewhat old-fashioned but useful term to refer to a still unspecified but likely complex phenomenon thought to characterize the reasoning of experienced thinkers and workers of many types. It is often associated with the art of practice.

Problem solving. This refers to the mental process by which one sequentially identifies a problem, interprets aspects of the situation, and selects a method to alleviate the problem.

Decision making. This refers to the process by which one makes a choice among two or more alternatives. In the present article, this term refers to formal, professional decision making and is associated with the science of practice.

Expert systems. This refers to computerized systems that use artificial intelligence methods to model problem solving and decision making in medicine.

Reasoning strategies. This refers to methods or approaches to reasoning or the selection of a structure or organization for one's reasoning process. Examples are the deductive method, the intuitive method, and the heuristic method.

Features of reasoning. This refers to particular aspects of a reasoning process, such as cue identification and pattern matching.

Goals and Traditions of Research in Clinical Reasoning

In the early work on physicians' reasoning, the primary goal was to improve the clinical judgment of practicing clinicians. Meehl (1954) enjoined psychiatrists and psychologists to use statistics to improve their ability to predict the behavior of their patients. Feinstein (1967) encouraged a systematic analysis of clinical judgment to improve physicians' judgments and to make them more scientific. Improvement of the effectiveness of clinical practice, both for the profession and the individual practitioner, remains the overall goal of research in clinical reasoning in medicine. In the early clinical reasoning research, it was often assumed that this research would result in the identification of the particular or best reasoning strategy or style for physicians. It seems that as the work on medical decision making and problem solving expands, identification of the only or the best or even the typical strategy becomes less likely. Many researchers have commented on the complexity and possibly elusive character of medical reasoning (Hammrick & Garfunkel, 1991).

Research in clinical reasoning has expanded rapidly in the past 10 years. Several different types of research are currently being conducted. Three somewhat different traditions in clinical reasoning research are defined below. One should be aware that I am creating a bit of an artificial separation here, and many of the research projects reported may have used more than one of these types of research styles and goals employed in the same or related studies (Hershey & Baron, 1987).

Medical problem solving seeks to describe the cognitive processes that physicians employ in identifying and solving patient's medical problems. Perhaps the most widely known work in this area is that of Elstein, Schulman, and Sprafka (1978). Recent research in medical problem solving seems to focus on the goal of highlighting particular features of reasoning. Some of this research correlates particular features with specific skills, such as diagnostic accuracy. *Medical decision making* focuses on the application and development of sophisticated statistical methods to guide or model medical decisions. Lusted (1968, 1983) is generally considered the seminal theorist in this endeavor. Most of his work focuses on making decisions about choice of treatment for particular diseases or conditions in high-risk situations (Kassirer, Kuipers, & Gory, 1982). *Expert systems,* or the use of artificial intelligence, are used to model or evaluate physicians' identification of a clinical condition and treatment selection. Most of this work focuses on diagnostic skill (Kleinmuntz, 1963, 1984). I reviewed some literature in this area and found that its potential applicability to occupational therapy does not appear to be great. I therefore do not discuss the results of this research in the present article.

The goals of this Clinical Reasoning Study were to try to understand and describe reasoning processes and to identify general strategies and particular features of reasoning that therapists use to guide their practice. Some of the reasoning processes and features identified are discussed below.

Statistical Analysis Versus Clinical Prediction

Much of the current work on clinical reasoning in medicine relies on, and even seeks to develop, statistical methods for the determination of the diagnosis, prognosis, and treatment of diseases and medical conditions (Mancuso & Rose, 1987; Patten, 1978). Statistical measures are used in at least three ways. One use of statistics is the application of statistical analysis to the study of physicians' problem-solving strategies (Kassirer, 1976). The two purposes of the statistical analysis are to study medical problem solving in itself (Johnson, Duran, Hassebrook, Moller, & Prietula, 1981) and to develop models for expert decision making (Doubilet & McNeil, 1985; Fox, 1984). A third purpose, which is typical of medical decision-making research, is to develop a body of knowledge regarding probabilities of disease entities occurring in members of a given population, the likelihood of an individual acquiring a particular disease given several physiological and demographic characteristics, or the probability of success of a particular treatment given various considerations (Pauker, 1976) and the prognosis given the various individual characteristics and the treatment options (Cutter, 1979). These probability assessments can then be used by physicians as a referent by which to make decisions regarding diagnosis, prognosis, and treatment. Authors also use statistics to enjoin physicians to make more and better use of statistics as a basis for their reasoning in daily practice (Haynes, Sackett, & Tugwell, 1983; Meehl, 1954). Proponents of the use of statistical reasoning claim that this will reduce uncertainty in medical decision making and problem solving (Raiffa, 1970).

In the Clinical Reasoning Study, we saw no formal use of statistics in everyday practice. However, therapists did often predict the likely outcome of treatment. These predictions were made in linguistic, not statistical, terms. This is a form of reasoning that Meehl (1954) referred to as *clinical prediction,* which he saw as inferior to statistical prediction. The clinical prediction is a type of assessment based on the therapists' clinical experience with similar patients in combination with formal knowledge acquired in their academic education. The following statements from therapists are typical of their clinical predictions.

> You don't usually see this much spasticity in the lower extremities with kids with this type of cerebral palsy. So, I'm not sure if he will ever ambulate independently. He will be a mobile child though. I can't say right now if that will mean crutches or a wheelchair. But he will be mobile.

> A really strong and motivated [person with paraplegia] could probably get [rehabilitated] in 6 weeks.

> She will probably be discharged to a nursing home because even though she can do a lot of activities independently, her judgment is so poor that it is really unsafe for her to live alone.

Therapists, especially experienced ones, used these informal predictions and estimates often. They had considerable trust in these clinical judgments. They appeared to be satisfied with the clinical method, relying on their knowledge and experience to identify clinical conditions and assess current functional performance and predict outcome. The occupational therapists seemed to have little interest in using statistics in their day-to-day prac-

tice. For this and other reasons, it seems safe to say that there are few similarities between the occupational therapy and medical decision-making literature. However, occupational therapists did demonstrate reasoning strategies and features similar to those in the medical problem-solving literature.

Reasoning Strategies

Hypothetical Reasoning

Newell and Simon (1972) proposed that physicians and other experts, such as chess players, employ three strategies to solve problems: recognition, hypothesis testing, and heuristic search. Many researchers since then have observed these strategies in physicians and medical students (Elstein & Bordage, 1979). Research in medical problem solving, medical decision making, and expert systems is based on this work by Newell and Simon and subsequent theorists and investigators. Most current research tends to focus on the hypothesis-testing method.

Newell and Simon (1972) also identified a sequence of events in thinking that take place with the use of the hypothesis-testing strategy. They proposed that the person first seeks cues; then searches for the appropriate problem space (e.g., body system or disease process); then generates hypotheses regarding the potential relation of the cues given the proposed problem space; then tests the hypothesis against other information, cues, or hypotheses. This sequence is still thought to be a common one and continues to influence research in medical decision making and problem solving. Feinstein (1973a, 1973b, 1974) developed and proposed a more careful search of problem space and suggested that physicians should think first about more broadly defined spaces and then systematically narrow the search through ever-smaller subsystems. Elstein et al. (1978) also observed instances of recognition, hypothesis testing, and heuristic search. Their work will be discussed in the section on features of reasoning.

An analysis of the videotapes and transcripts that constitute the raw data of the Clinical Reasoning Study revealed that the therapists who participated in this study used the three problem-solving strategies proposed by Newell and Simon (1972). These therapists often used hypothesis testing, sometimes called *propositional reasoning,* but the ways in which they used this method may be different from the usual ways that hypothesis testing is used by physicians. For example, physicians make a diagnosis of the disease or clinical condition, so the initial mystery is already solved when the patient comes to occupational therapy. The occupational therapists' task is to know generally how that disease or disability will affect the person's functional performance and to evaluate specific details of that performance. Therefore, when the diagnosis was a fairly common one, the experienced therapists easily recalled what the problems might be and

990

what the evaluation and treatment sessions should be like. Hypothesis generation and testing commonly came into play in five types of instances: (a) when there was no diagnosis (either because the physician had not made one, it was unknown, or the therapist had not been told what it was), (b) when the therapist was unfamiliar with the diagnosis, (c) when the therapist wanted to know more details of the problem or the person, (d) when the therapy was not going as smoothly as expected, and (e) when the therapist noticed something atypical about the patient.

There is some indication that therapists' use of these strategies is influenced by their experience and how they frame the problem. Regarding experience, there was a tendency for new therapists to generate fewer hypotheses and to rely more heavily on the recognition method. Conversely, the more experienced therapists tended to generate more hypotheses and use the heuristic search method. The experienced therapists recognized the patient's clinical conditions readily and used hypothesis testing, heuristic search, or both to discover the details of that particular patient's limitations, given the generalities for patients with that condition. The novice clinicians used heuristic search when they did not recognize what the condition was and were searching for a category or problem space. Regarding framing of the problem, newer therapists tended to see the whole problem as the medical condition and think that all of the patient's behavior was related to the disease. Experienced therapists had a more dynamic view and wondered about the interplay of such factors as the medical condition and the person's original personality and other events in his or her life. The novice therapists seemed to frame the problem as follows: This is a condition that I am supposed to treat. Conversely, the experienced therapists seemed to frame the problem as follows: This is a person who has to face a lot of problems, and I have to figure out the best way for me to help this patient figure out what he or she wants to work on and how.

Occupational therapists used hypothesis generation and testing in many instances. Sometimes this was used in the diagnostic sense, as in the case of experienced therapists trying to identify the cause of a person's functional problems when the diagnosis was unknown. More frequently, hypothesis testing was used to figure out why an aspect of therapy was not working. Hypothesis testing was also used to generate ideas about which activities within a given treatment category would be most effective. In general, it appeared that therapists used the hypothetical strategy more when thinking about treatment than when thinking about diagnosis. Therefore, occupational therapists, like physicians, use the hypothetical method, but its place in the reasoning sequence may differ, that is, the use of the method itself may be prompted by different events in occupational therapy than in medicine.

Linear Progression Versus Discontinuous Search

It is generally assumed that persons using the hypothetical approach think in an orderly, linear progression (Hoffman, 1960). The person focuses on the problem and proceeds in a focused manner to gather data, generate and test hypotheses, and decide on the most likely possibility (Fulop, 1985). Physicians are expected to follow a sequential line of inquiry that includes gathering such data as medical history, current ailment, clinical observations, and laboratory test results. After gathering these data, they generate hypotheses about the possible cause of the ailment and logically test those hypotheses to determine which hypothesized cause of the ailment is most likely. This results in a diagnosis (Balla, Elstein, & Gates, 1983). One line of research in medical decision making produced branching programs, or decision trees, which improve the physician's decision-making power. These trees inform the physician of the percentage value of two or more possible diagnoses given various conditions or the percentage survival rates of patients with a particular clinical condition undergoing various treatments. So, for example, the physician can choose between pharmacological or surgical intervention for a patient based on the percentage survival rates of groups of persons with the same condition who were given one of those two treatments. Although the greatest advantage of these trees is the statistical data that they provide, they also serve to keep the physician focused on the decision-making task and to assist in excluding irrelevant data.

Therapists in the Clinical Reasoning Study did not appear to use a linear form of logic all of the time. They often seemed to begin a particular line of inquiry in a hypothetical mode and then shift out of a propositional style of reasoning to ask questions or answer patients' questions in a more social, rather than focused or professional, style. Similarly, Rogers and Masagatani (1982) found that during an evaluation procedure, occupational therapists often moved out of a strictly problem-solving mode to address the immediate concerns of the patient. Later, they resumed their logical thinking pattern in a search for definition or resolution of the clinical problem. The same pattern was often seen among therapists in the Clinical Reasoning Study during evaluation sessions and even more frequently during treatment sessions. Typically, therapists would be engaged in a line of hypothetical reasoning concerning the details of the patient's physical or performance problem. Then they would interrupt that stream of thought when the patient said or did something that caused the therapist to temporarily abandon the focus on the physical problem. A moment or so later, they would return to the evaluation procedure. Examples of this shift were (a) a patient asking a question about something, commenting on what was happening, or noting a similarity of a particular activity to one that he or she enjoyed and (b) therapists complimenting patients on their hair, dress, or room decorations or asking about their weekend activities. Therapists often responded to a patient with informal comments or requests for the person to extend the conversation. At such times, the therapist did not seem to be engaging in conversation to gather data, but rather, to engage in conversation as an equal, not as a professional to a patient.

Initially, this shift seemed to be a shift from therapy to socializing and back to therapy. Soon we realized that therapists considered both working on the person's body and interacting with the person as a person to be part of therapy. Therefore, the shift was not into and out of therapy, but rather, from one aspect of therapy to another. (For an example of such a shift, see the Appendix.)

The therapist was concerned about the patient and his progress in therapy. The patient had stayed in his apartment for the weekend in order to test out his ability to function there. The therapist was also concerned about the patient's ability to adjust to the situation and how much of an emotional impact the visit would have on him. She and other therapists often commented that when patients first go back to "the real world," the full impact of their disability and its permanence hits them, and the emotional impact is often great. Therefore, rather than demonstrating a disrupted train of thought, the therapist was simply shifting from one line of inquiry to the other. She and other experienced therapists often seemed to carefully tack a difficult course between the procedural aspects of treatment and the social-emotional concerns of the patient. The notion that occupational therapists work with both the physical and emotional aspects of the person is not a new one. It is part of the long-standing philosophy of the profession (Fidler & Fidler, 1963). What does seem to be a new observation is that the therapists' reasoning is greatly influenced by these two concerns and that these dual concerns are interwoven in practice. I believe that therapists' thinking about the patient's physical-medical problem may be guided by hypothetical reasoning, whereas thinking about the person's social-emotional condition may be guided by another type of reasoning.

Sequential Versus Continuous Reasoning

Clinical decision-making research usually focuses on the formulation of a hypothesis of the diagnosis, prediction of prognosis, and assessment of the probable outcome of available treatments (Lusted, 1983). Each is considered an important decision point (Cutter, 1979), and often they are considered to be separate intellectual operations. Further, each of these thinking tasks is thought of as separate from the taking of any action, such as conducting treatment.

These therapists' clinical reasoning did not take the form of fairly clear-cut decision points or events. It was not time-delineated with decisions following in an orderly sequence, nor were diagnosis, prognosis, and treatment selection considered only once. There were few one-time decision-making points or events. Thinking about problems and possible solutions seemed to be more of a continuous stream of small decisions or temporary hypotheses.

In addition, thinking was not considered to be a function necessarily separate from action. Thinking was often tested in action. The results of the action or the patient's reaction often prompted the therapist to think differently or act differently in the immediate situation. This interchange of thought and action and the quick revision of hypotheses and action plan occurred so rapidly that we often commented that all of these processes were conducted simultaneously. Experienced therapists seemed to be constantly revising their plans, not because they did not get it right the first time, but rather, to fine-tune their plans in accordance with the patient's needs, wishes, body, abilities, and limitations. Therapists who were confident about their skills trusted themselves to know generally what the goals and treatment for the patient should be and could therefore both attend to the smaller details and be more responsive to the particular patient. For example, unlike novices, the experienced therapists did not make up treatment plans ahead of time, which would involve spending hours figuring out goals and recalling theories and therapeutic principles and techniques. Instead, they usually knew what they wanted as an overall goal and had a list of possible treatment strategies but did not select a particular treatment activity until the treatment session began, at which time interaction with the patient might lead them to try various techniques until the right one was found. Therapists typically say, "Try this for me," "Let's see if this works," "What do you think?" or "What do you want to try?" Therapists frequently said that diagnosis is not separate from treatment. They used phrases like "You are always evaluating" or "Treatment and evaluation go hand in hand" to express what seemed to them to be a continuous process of evaluation—and not necessarily diagnosis—of the patient. This included the person's abilities, physical and emotional status, preferences, degree of change, and progress. What therapists seemed to be referring to when they said that evaluation and treatment go together was a process of almost continuous hypothesis generation, evaluation, and revision. Therapists were attentive to many cues in several categories of problems that might affect functional performance. They recognized cues as patterns or potential parts of patterns. These, in turn, prompted hypotheses about the patient's physical or emotional condition. These hypotheses were then evaluated against further observation or subjected to further inquiry. After this evaluation, the dominant hypothesis may be substantiated, negated, revised, or modified.

The therapists often used the general strategy of diagnosis, prognosis, and treatment selection, but not in the linear progression that physicians use to make major decisions about diagnosis and treatment. Instead, they seemed to use the sequence rapidly and in many instances to ferret out the smaller details of the person's functioning and determine actions that the therapist or the patient might take to improve that function. Perhaps because part of the essence of the practice is action, thinking may be influenced by action. Certainly, the way they practiced and described their practice made their reasoning strategies look more like what Buchler (1955) called *active judgment*. Perhaps in practice occupational therapists use a form of clinical judgment that is enhanced by having taken similar actions in the past and applying those strategies to the new situation.

Features of Problem Solving

Elstein et al. (1978) identified four features important to medical problem solving: cue identification, multiple hypothesis generation, cue interpretation, and hypothesis evaluation. These researchers found that the most successful diagnosticians among the physicians in their studies acquired a greater number of cues and interpreted them more accurately than did the least successful diagnosticians. A study conducted by Allal (as cited by Elstein et. al., 1978) identified that

> The physician's information processing activity. . .is not a unidimensional list of problem formulations. Rather it is a structured set of formulations that may be described in terms of four features: hierarchical organization, competing formulations, multiple subspaces and functional relationships. (p. 176)

Allal noted that, of these, the only feature that was 100% consistent across physicians and across cases was competing formulations. Of the other three features, multiple subspaces was the next most common feature; functional relationships, the least common.

The researchers in the Elstein group (Elstein et al., 1978) explored other features of medical problem solving and concluded that clinical judgment is complex and multifaceted, stating, "We may speculate that different problems require different medical paradigms and that no single theoretical model is sufficient for so complex an activity as clinical medicine" (p. 288). Recent studies also indicate that medical problem solving is multifaceted, and researchers continue to identify features of the process. Pattern recognition seems to play an important part in the reasoning of medical students and physicians (Coughlin & Patel, 1987).

Pattern discrimination, the ability to correctly discriminate between two or more similar patterns, is another important feature in medical decision making. Papa, Shores, and Meyer (1990) found that pattern discrimination abilities bore a high relationship to diagnostic accuracy in medical students and practicing physicians.

Some researchers (Bordage & Zacks, 1984; Grant & Marsden, 1987) argued that the manner in which knowledge is structured or organized in one's mind significantly influences the physician's ability to make decisions. They implied that facility in pattern discrimination is a function of this structure. Coughlin and Patel (1987) also identified inference making as a critical skill and found that experienced physicians use inference making less frequently than do medical students. They hypothesized that this is because they readily recognize more conditions than do the medical students.

Occupational therapists demonstrated use of the four characteristics identified by Elstein et al. (1978). Most displayed many of the characteristics identified by Allal (as cited by Elstein et al., 1978). One novice therapist did not seem to generate competing formulations. She dropped out of the study and the profession early in the year that we began to study novices, so little analysis has been given to this phenomenon. One experienced therapist seemed to generate only one or very few hypotheses or formulations of the problem and often seemed reluctant or slow to give up on an assumption, even in the face of cues from the patient that the therapy was not proceeding smoothly. All the other experienced therapists tended to generate several hypotheses, which they often arranged as competing formulations. Of the three experienced therapists whom we studied most intensively, all searched multiple subspaces and sought functional relationships. Two had a clear hierarchical structure to their knowledge.

Pattern recognition was a common occurrence in experienced therapists and a much desired goal among novices. Pattern discrimination seemed to be the central focus of the experienced therapists' early evaluations of patients' performance and again later as they determined what sort of progress the person was or was not making. They also employed the pattern discrimination and heuristic search when inquiring about aspects of the patient's behavior, which seemed to be different from what is usually expected in that diagnosis.

There seem to be many similarities between the features of reasoning that Elstein et al. (1978) and others identified in physicians and medical students and those observed in occupational therapists.

Focus of the Clinical Reasoning Study

Origin Versus Future Function

Most studies of clinical reasoning in medicine focus on diagnosis. Diagnosis is often seen as the most critical aspect of decision making and practice. Critical to the diagnostic reasoning process is history taking. The person's birth, development, habits, environment, and other factors that might contribute to the acquisition of a disease or condition are important considerations in medical diagnosis. The history of the disease itself is a central concern and helps the therapist in diagnosis and prognosis. Diagnosis and history taking were not a central focus for the occupational therapists in the Clinical Reasoning Study. Diagnosis occupied very little of the therapists' reasoning time. Patients came to therapy with a medical diagnosis, and the therapist's task was to know how that diagnostic condition would influence present and future function. The therapist was primarily concerned with what a person could do now and might be able to do in the future. The therapists considered etiology important but not most important. They conducted careful evaluations and made fine-grained observations of current functional performance. They made accurate predictions of possible gains in functional levels and were concerned about what those gains would mean to the patient's eventual performance level and what that would mean to his or her future. Most therapists considered the patient's history when imagining a person's possible future, and then considered whether aspects of his or her past might influence the potential for actualizing that future. For example, if a person had a history of substance abuse, the therapist often thought that the person's ability to live in an independent living situation would depend on the physical gains that the therapist expected the person to make and the support that the therapist hoped the patient would get from his family to join Alcoholics Anonymous. The prognosis was considered a relatively likely outcome, but not a fact or fate. Possibilities for the future and progress toward it were the therapists' main concerns. In other words, the primary focus of the therapists' thinking was not on the current disability and its treatment, but rather, on the functional possibilities in the future.

Possibly, if the therapist's primary task is to help the person function in the future, then the visualization of future possibilities is an important aspect of occupational therapists' clinical reasoning. Because the occupational therapist does not make a definitive diagnosis as a part of his or her task, history is not as critical a piece of the puzzle as it is for the physician. Conversely, the ability to imagine new ways that this person could function in the future may be essential to occupational therapy practice. If so, a very different kind of reasoning is indicated.

Generalization Versus Individualization

A primary aim of scientific medicine is identification of how the processes of the human body interact with each other and other elements and organisms to result in illness and disability. As such, scientific medical research, like all of science, seeks to identify that which is generally true. Science tests theories until general law statements can be made (Bunge, 1967). Medicine, like all applied scientific practices, employs these laws to solve classes of problems.

The therapists in the Clinical Reasoning Study had an appreciation for science and medicine, and the experienced therapists were quite familiar with the manifesta-

tions, course, and usual outcome of a wide range of diseases and disabilities. They worked with people with disabilities and knew the limitations that these disabilities caused. However, they were more often interested in the particulars of the person and the slight variations in the manifestation of the disability or the resulting limitations than they were in the general condition. They were always saying that one must individualize treatment for each patient.

Individualization refers to the tailoring of treatment to the particular skills, needs, and interests of each patient. The notion that a treatment is specific to a particular patient contradicts the common assumption that all people with a given disease or disability can be treated with the same remedy. These therapists seemed to take both the scientific approach and the individual approach, trying to meld them together. They had many procedures, treatment modalities, and strategies that were frequently used with most persons who had the same sort of injury. What they seemed to enjoy most, however, was not the precise application of the correct procedure, but rather, the search for the best way for this person. This meant that they wanted to find activities that would motivate the patient to try something new but that would also allow this patient some well-earned success.

The integration of concern for the patient with concern for problem resolution seemed to be a common but not always harmonious way of thinking about and conducting therapy. This interest in the individual would naturally lead therapists away from the medical decision-making approach, in which the norm and statistical probabilities are central and individual variations are peripheral. It seems that if effective occupational therapy includes or is primarily focused on the understanding of particulars about the patient and the condition, then a reasoning strategy that is sensitive to particulars rather than to general characteristics and laws must be brought into play.

Discussion

Occupational therapists, physicians, and other health care professionals work with people who have medical problems and conditions. Because scientific medicine requires the use of the hypothetical or propositional form of reasoning, it makes sense that all practitioners employ that form of reasoning when applying medical knowledge to address health problems. When occupational therapists were reasoning about the person's physical disability, the reasoning strategies they employed were most like the reasoning strategies of physicians, as reported in the medical clinical reasoning literature. However, when therapists thought about other aspects of the person and his or her situation, they used other forms of reasoning.

Although occupational therapists work with persons with physical disabilities, the nature and goals of the practice differ from the goals of physicians. It therefore makes sense that therapists' knowledge, interests, and reasoning strategies would also differ. Concerns for individualizing treatment, facilitating independent functional performance, and creating a future new life for the person lead the occupational therapist to emphasize some aspects of the person and his or her situation more than the medical condition. Mostofsky and Piedmont (1985) posited that physicians address three aspects: the disease, the person, and the predicament. The physician's primary task is to address the disease first. In other words, the physician attends to the disease so as to alleviate or reduce the person's predicament. Conversely, the occupational therapist's role is to address the predicament and reduce its effect on the person's future life, given the consequences of his or her disease or disability. Both professions, therefore, are concerned with all three aspects, but in a different sequence and with different aims and expertise.

It appears that the nature and goals of occupational therapy practice and the philosophy of the profession have influenced the development and use of particular reasoning strategies. The influence of the scientific model and medical knowledge have contributed to the ability to use other reasoning strategies, particularly hypothetical, or propositional, reasoning. Therapists seem to shift their focus to various aspects of the person, disease, or predicament that demands their attention. It appeared to the various members of the Clinical Reasoning Study research team that therapists employed different reasoning strategies in order to focus their inquiry in each of these areas.

Conclusion

Two of the primary goals of qualitative research are to observe and interpret a phenomenon and to raise hypotheses for future study. Five hypotheses are offered here:

1. Occupational therapists use several types of reasoning strategies in the course of their clinical practice.
2. The nature and goals of the practice influence the development and use of various reasoning strategies.
3. In the practice situation, a particular aspect of the whole problem will prompt therapists to select a reasoning strategy that is well suited to guide inquiry into that aspect of the problem.
4. When thinking about the patient's medical problem, therapists often use hypothetical reasoning.
5. When thinking about the patient's psychological, social, or interpersonal aspects, therapists often use strategies other than the hypothetical method.

Further qualitative research is necessary to elucidate the nature and structure of these reasoning strategies and the situations that prompt their use. Quantitative research is necessary to determine the degree to which therapists employ the hypothetical and other reasoning strategies. ▲

Appendix

Interaction Between an Occupational Therapist and a Patient as a Part of Therapy

Therapist: What are you doing this weekend?
Patient: Probably staying in my air-conditioned house.
Therapist: Are you going to stay in Charlestown?
Patient: Yeah.
Therapist: So you're not going to use the bathroom?
Patient: Obviously not. I can't get in it.
Therapist: But you wouldn't have been able to anyway, right?
Patient: No.
Therapist: It would be nice just to be in a place though. The doors are not wide enough to get in? What did you say you can't get into?
Patient: The hallway's too narrow. I can't make the turn.
Therapist: Is it like a right turn like that?
Patient: Yeah.
Therapist: You might be surprised though what Karen might be able to just up and turn your chair.
Patient: If I took the legs off I could probably turn it in backwards.
Therapist: You'd be surprised.
Patient: [Inaudible.]
Therapist: No, but sometimes you can. Sometimes you're surprised at maneuverability. Can I see that right hand one more time? Okay. Put your fingers down. Come down. Come all the way up. You know, it's funny. Where your thumb comes in that's a hard place. Can you try to . . . any motion to do that? Yeah, you do. You have a little of that. If you can . . . I think part of what happens is because the muscle that you have in your thumb [inaudible] this way, naturally if you had no active motion in your thumb, your thumb would come out a little bit more possibly. But because this is where it's strong, it wants to go in like that.
Patient: Well, I can get down there, but . . .
Therapist: Yeah, except what happens when you come up?
Patient: The pressure on this falls off. There's pressure up here but not down there.
Therapist: Yeah, so that's when it's hard to pick things up.

References

Balla, J. I., Elstein, A. S., & Gates, P. (1983). Effects of prevalence and test diagnosticity upon clinical judgments of probability. *Methods of Information in Medicine, 22,* 25–28.

Bordage, G., & Zacks, R. (1984). The structure of medical knowledge in the memories of medical students and general practitioners: Categories and prototypes. *Medical Education, 18,* 406–416.

Buchler, J. (1955). *Nature and judgment.* New York: Columbia University Press.

Bunge, M. (1967). *Scientific research I: The search system.* New York: Springer Verlag.

Coughlin, L. D., & Patel, V. L. (1987). Processing of critical information by physicians and medical students. *Journal of Medical Education, 62,* 818–828.

Cutter, P. (1979). *Problem solving in clinical medicine*. Baltimore: Williams & Wilkins.

Doubilet, P., & McNeil, B. J. (1985). Clinical decision making. *Medical Care, 23*, 648–662.

Elstein, A. S., & Bordage, G. (1979). Psychology of clinical reasoning. In G. Stone, F. Cohen, & N. Adler (Eds.), *Health psychology: A handbook*. San Francisco: Jossey-Bass.

Elstein, A. S., Schulman, L. S., & Sprafraka, S. A. (1978). *Medical problem solving: An analysis of clinical reasoning*. Cambridge, MA: Harvard University Press.

Feinstein, A. R. (1967). *Clinical judgment*. Baltimore: Williams & Wilkins.

Feinstein, A. R. (1973a). An analysis of diagnostic reasoning I. The domains and disorders of clinical macrobiology. *Yale Journal of Biology & Medicine, 46*, 212–232.

Feinstein, A. R. (1973b). An analysis of diagnostic reasoning II. The strategy of intermediate decisions. *Yale Journal of Biology and Medicine, 46*, 264–283.

Feinstein, A. R. (1974). An analysis of diagnostic reasoning III. The construction of clinical algorithms. *Yale Journal of Biology and Medicine, 47*, 5–32.

Fidler, G., & Fidler, J. (1963). *Occupational therapy: A communication process in psychiatry*. New York: Macmillan.

Fox, J. (1984). Formal and knowledge-based methods in decision technology. *Acta Psychologica, 56*, 303–331.

Fulop, M. (1985). Teaching differential diagnosis to beginning clinical students. *American Journal of Medicine, 79*, 745–749.

Gillette, N. P., & Mattingly, C. (1987). The Foundation—Clinical reasoning in occupational therapy. *American Journal of Occupational Therapy, 41*, 399–400.

Grant, J., & Marsden, P. (1987). The structure of memorized knowledge in students and clinicians: An explanation for diagnostic expertise. *Medical Education, 18*, 406–416.

Hammrick, H. J., & Garfunkel, J. M. (1991). Editor's Column—Clinical decisions: How much analysis and how much judgment? *Journal of Pediatrics, 118*, 67.

Haynes, R. B., Sackett, D. L., & Tugwell, P. (1983). Problems in the handling of clinical and research evidence by medical practitioners. *Archives of Internal Medicine, 143*, 1971–1975.

Hershey, J. C., & Baron, J. (1987). Clinical reasoning and cognitive processes. *Medical Decision Making, 7*, 203–211.

Hoffman, P. J. (1960). The paramorphic representation of clinical judgment. *Psychological Bulletin, 57*, 116–131.

Johnson, P. E., Duran, A. S., Hassebrook, F., Moller, J., & Prietula, M. (1981). Expertise and error in diagnostic reasoning. *Cognitive Science, 5*, 235–283.

Karlsson, G. (1988). A phenomenological study of decision and choice. *Acta Psychologica, 68*, 7–25.

Kassirer, J. P. (1976). The principles of clinical decision making: An introduction to decision analysis. *Yale Journal of Biology and Medicine, 49*, 149–164.

Kassirer, J. P., Kuipers, B. J., & Gory, G. A. (1982). Toward a theory of clinical expertise. *American Journal of Medicine, 73*, 251–259.

Kleinmuntz, B. (1963). Computers in behavioral science. *Behavioral Science, 8*, 154–156.

Kleinmuntz, B. (1984). Diagnostic problem solving by computer: A historical review and current state of the science. *Computers in Biology and Medicine, 14*, 255–270.

Lusted, L. B. (1968). *Introduction to medical decision making*. Springfield, IL: Charles C Thomas.

Lusted, L. B. (1983). Medical decision making: Analyzing options in the face of uncertainty. *Journal of the American Medical Association, 249*, 2133–2142.

Mancuso, C. A., & Rose, D. N. (1987). A model for physicians' therapeutic decision making. *Archives of Internal Medicine, 147*, 1281–1285.

Mattingly, C., & Gillette, N. (1991). Anthropology, occupational therapy, and action research. *American Journal of Occupational Therapy, 45*, 972–978.

Meehl, P. E. (1954). *Clinical vs. statistical prediction*. Minneapolis: University of Minnesota Press.

Mostofsky, D. I., & Piedmont, R. L. (1985). *Therapeutic practice in behavioral medicine*. San Francisco: Jossey-Bass.

Newell, A., & Simon, H. (1972). *Human problem solving*. Englewood Cliffs, NJ: Prentice Hall.

Papa, F. J., Shores, J. H., & Meyer, S. (1990). Effects of pattern matching, pattern discrimination and experience on diagnostic expertise. *Academic Medicine, 65*, s21–s22.

Patten, D. D. (1978). Introduction to clinical decision making. *Seminars in Nuclear Medicine, 8*, 273–282.

Pauker, S. G. (1976). Coronary artery surgery: The use of decision analysis. *Annals of Internal Medicine, 85*, 8–18.

Raiffa, H. (1970). *Decision analysis*. Reading, MA: Addison–Wesley.

Rogers, J. C., & Masagatani, G. (1982). Clinical reasoning of occupational therapists during the initial assessment of physically disabled patients. *Occupational Therapy Journal of Research, 2*, 195–219.

Clinical Reasoning Process for Service Provision in the Public School

Laura Hall, Wendy Robertson, Mary Ann Turner

Key Words: decision making • delivery of health care • pediatrics

This paper outlines the clinical reasoning process used to guide decisions on the provision of occupational therapy services in the Wake County Public School System in North Carolina. The process is based on a theoretical framework derived from occupational therapy theory and public law. Benefits of using the clinical reasoning process include (a) increased consistency of decision making among therapists; (b) increased appropriateness of decisions regarding whether a student needs educationally based occupational therapy services, what type of occupational therapy service would meet the student's need, and how often this service should be provided; and (c) improved ability of therapists to articulate to all those involved with a student the reasoning behind decisions to provide educationally based occupational therapy services. The schematic diagrams that depict this process provide a useful tool for therapists with varied work experiences entering school-based practice.

Laura Hall, OTR/L, is a Staff Occupational Therapist, Wake County Public School System, 3600 Wake Forest Road, Raleigh, North Carolina 27611.

Wendy Robertson, MS, OTR/L, is a Staff Occupational Therapist, Wake County Public School System, Raleigh, North Carolina.

Mary Ann Turner, MS, OTR/L, is a Staff Occupational Therapist, Wake County Public School System, Raleigh, North Carolina.

This article was accepted for publication May 1, 1992.

The practice of occupational therapy in the public school setting presents a number of unique challenges, including the establishment of a standard to determine which students need services and which type of service is most appropriate. Although the American Occupational Therapy Association (AOTA) provides guidelines for service decisions based on an interpretation of the Education for All Handicapped Children Act of 1975 (Public Law 94–142), therapists must "rely on their own understanding of these written interpretations and on their professional judgement to determine whether a student needs occupational therapy" (Carr, 1989, p. 503). Particular states can also expand the services mandated by the federal law. Carr (1989) presented criteria used in Louisiana to give therapists "standards by which to make clear-cut decisions" (p. 506). Although Carr (1989) reported numerous benefits from using the Louisiana criteria, other therapists claimed that the criteria discriminated against students with severe disabilities (Giangreco, 1990; Rainforth, 1990; Spencer, 1990). In our experience, therapists in public school systems still disagree on how to make decisions about service provision.

In struggling to develop justifiable, objective, and ethical eligibility criteria, occupational therapists in North Carolina's Wake County Public School System (WCPSS) realized that they had to focus on clearly articulating the clinical reasoning process used to make decisions about service provision. The purpose of articulating this process was to make the most appropriate decision about service provision for a particular student regardless of the pressures of practical considerations such as staff availability and district resources. Before any reasonable eligibility criteria can be effectively developed, the clinical reasoning process employed to make decisions must be examined, articulated, and agreed on. Decisions about occupational therapy treatment and service provision are the outcome of the clinical reasoning process (Rogers, 1983).

Since 1986, AOTA and the American Occupational Therapy Foundation (AOTF) have funded research to study clinical reasoning in occupational therapy (Gillette & Mattingly, 1987). This research, known as the Clinical Reasoning Study, was initiated to examine the reasons behind occupational therapy clinical decisions and thus to facilitate training of occupational therapy students in clinical reasoning. An initial impetus for this ongoing research was the realization that fieldwork clinicians teach more by action and frequently have difficulty articulating the reasoning behind these actions (Saltz, 1991). Rogers and Masagatani (1982) reached the same conclusion about the 10 therapists in their descriptive study of the clinical reasoning process in occupational therapy. As Rogers (1983) pointed out, clinical judgments or decisions are not made on the basis of one or two test scores or an isolated observation, but are determined through the complex process of clinical reasoning.

Clinical Reasoning

The clinical reasoning process is the problem-solving strategy used under conditions of uncertainty. The uncertainty can arise from an ill-defined problem that requires more information than is available at the outset to reach a solution. The nature of the problem changes over time as information defined by the practitioner's underlying philosophy and frame of reference is gathered. Rogers (1982) perceived functional independence, which is achieved through an interaction of personal and environmental factors, to be the philosophy that drives occupational therapy practice.

For occupational therapists in the schools, an ill-defined problem often faced is poor handwriting. To clarify the problem and to determine an intervention strategy, the therapist must investigate the student's skills and environmental expectations and the interaction between these variables. The investigation or information collection process is structured and organized by multiple hypotheses beginning with broad, nonspecific hypotheses that are refined, supported, or not supported as information is gathered (Barrows & Feltovich, 1987). Barrows and Feltovich (1987) stated that "reasoning guided by multiple hypotheses is the appropriate and effective way to approach the resolution of poorly understood situations that require resolution" (p. 90). Some hypotheses related to poor handwriting are as follows: (a) student has inadequate visual-motor skills to meet classroom expectations, (b) environmental expectations are not appropriate for this student's developmental level, or (c) poor handwriting is due to poor tactile and kinesthetic processing. Through the clinical reasoning process, therapists construct a picture of the student within the educational environment that decreases enough of the uncertainty surrounding the problem to enable them to formulate "prudent decisions" (Rogers, 1983, p. 614).

Methods to enhance the efficacy of the clinical reasoning process have been offered in the literature (Barrows & Feltovich, 1987; Mattingly & Gillette, 1991; Rogers, 1983; Rogers & Masagatani, 1982). One of these methods is a fixed or routinized approach to data collection to prevent a premature end to information gathering. The medical review of systems used by physicians is an example of a routinized approach (Barrows & Feltovich, 1987). The use of the Occupational Therapy Uniform Evaluation Checklist as recommended by Rogers (1983) and the Uniform Terminology Grid presented by Dunn and McGourty (1989) are examples specific to occupational therapy. Another strategy is to continually reassess all information collected in light of each additional piece of information so that data are not forced to fit a preset idea. Pelland's (1987) Conceptual Model of Treatment Planning reflected this need for continual adjustment. A third strategy suggested in the literature is the use of peer and professional consultation (Rogers, 1983).

By sharing information and eliciting possible competing hypotheses, therapists can formulate a clearer and more complete picture of the problem. Mattingly and Gillette (1991) reported that the therapists involved in the clinical reasoning study found group viewing sessions that generated various interpretations of the same information beneficial to problem solving. These three methods were advocated to ensure that the outcome of the reasoning process, a clinical judgment, would be the most appropriate decision for the specific problem addressed.

Although the results of the clinical reasoning process (a particular treatment recommendation) are not generalizable, the process itself can be generalized and taught. At Wake County Public School System, through open discussion of each occupational therapist's clinical reasoning, the therapists developed a schematic guide to provide structure for the clinical reasoning process used to make treatment and service determinations within the educational environment.

Frame of Reference

The nature and scope of questions posed during the data collection phase of the clinical reasoning process are defined by the underlying philosophy and frames of reference. The philosophy driving the clinical reasoning process presented is reflected in the *Uniform Terminology for Occupational Therapy — Second Edition* (AOTA, 1989b). Occupational therapy practice is defined in terms of occupational performance areas and occupational performance components. Occupational performance areas were activities of daily living, work activities, and play and leisure activities. Performance components are those abilities required for occupational performance and include sensorimotor, cognitive, and psychosocial and psychological components (AOTA, 1989b). Frames of reference consistent with the philosophy supporting the clinical reasoning guide include the occupational behavior model (Reilly, 1969) and the Model of Human Occupation (Kielhofner & Burke, 1980). The occupational behavior model describes children as "individuals who occupy particular life roles in their families, school and communities" (Takata, 1980, p. 11). Occupational therapy clients in the school system are therefore not observed solely in terms of their disability, but as persons who are experiencing difficulty with their life roles, primarily with the student role. This view involves the total child as he or she functions within the context of the school environment. The view that students cannot be observed in isolation from their school environment comes from the Model of Human Occupation, in which human beings are open systems that interact with their environments (Kielhofner & Burke, 1980). Occupational therapy in the public school works to establish or reestablish an occupational role for identified students within the school environment that includes work, play, self-care, and the underlying performance components.

Several assumptions underlie the clinical reasoning process used by occupational therapists in the Wake County Public School System. One of those assumptions is that occupational therapy services provided in the school environment differ from occupational therapy services provided in a clinical or medical setting. The medical model identifies dysfunction or disease and develops strategies to increase function or decrease dysfunction (Stephens, 1989). The underlying cause of the dysfunction is the focus of treatment (Ottenbacher, 1982). The educational model begins with a nondysfunctional person who is expected to gain skills and knowledge (Stephens, 1989). The cause of dysfunction is not of direct concern to educators (Ottenbacher, 1982). School-based occupational therapists are concerned with dysfunction and disease only in the context of their effect on the student's capacity to meet educational goals.

Another assumption is that occupational therapy differs philosophically from special education. Occupational therapy uses a developmental approach targeting sensorimotor development "within the context of the overall maturation of the central nervous system" (Royeen & Marsh, 1988, p. 714). Education tends to be more oriented toward skills acquisition with the emphasis on content, not on the underlying causes and processes. Occupational therapists working within the school system "must be able to explain how the occupational therapy services they recommend for a particular child are consistent with the intent of EHA" (Coutinho & Hunter, 1988, p. 711). Using an articulated clinical reasoning process, these therapists should be able to explain that educationally related occupational therapy services are not clinical services placed in a school building. It would then be clearer that "a student may need occupational therapy in the clinical setting (medical model), but would not be eligible for services in the educational setting" (Stephens, 1989, p. 597) if the dysfunction does not directly affect educational progress.

The mandates of Public Law 94–142 form another set of assumptions that guides this clinical reasoning process. Those mandates state that

> the term "related services" means transportation and such developmental, corrective, and other supportive services as are required to assist a child to benefit from special education, and includes . . . occupational therapy (Reg. 300.13, p. 102:53). The definition of "special education" is a particularly important one under these regulations, . . . a child is not handicapped unless he or she needs special education. Therefore, if a child does not need special education, there can be no "related services," and the child (because not "handicapped") is not covered under the Act. (Comment 1 following Reg. 300.14, p. 102:54)

Public Law 94–142 has been amended and retitled Individuals With Disabilities Education Act (Public Law 101–476). All students are eligible for occupational therapy as a related service if they are identified as being in need of special education. This identification as needing special education does not mean that the student needs occupational therapy to function independently in the educational environment. Occupational therapy as a related service is provided only in cases when the student is not able to benefit from special education already provided for his or her specific educational disability. Occupational therapy as a related service "includes (1) Improving, developing or restoring functions impaired or lost through illness, injury, or deprivation; (2) Improving ability to perform tasks for independent functioning when functions are impaired or lost; and (3) Preventing through early intervention initial or further impairment of loss of function" (Gilfoyle & Farace, 1981, p. 811).

Public Law 94–142 describes educational environments as existing on a continuum from *least restrictive* (i.e., regular education classroom with consultative services) to *most restrictive* (i.e., residential placement) and mandates that students be served in the least restrictive environment. Occupational therapy services must be provided in a manner consistent with this mandate. Using three types of service (direct, monitoring, and consultation) and adjusting the frequency of service allows occupational therapy services to be provided along a continuum to best meet the student's educational needs.

The need to define educationally relevant occupational therapy services and methods of providing these services is critical to the practice of school-based occupational therapy. In this paper we present not eligibility criteria but the reasoning process behind these service provision decisions. The term *eligibility* itself is misleading because, as explained above, any student identified as a special education student is eligible for occupational therapy as a related service. The issues are whether a student needs occupational therapy to function effectively in the school environment and what type of service best meets that student's needs. The phrase *type of,* as opposed to *level of,* service shifts the focus away from an implied differential value placed on direct, monitoring, and consultation services.

A Schematic Guide for the Clinical Reasoning Process

Determination of the Need for Service

According to Mattingly (1991), clinical reasoning in occupational therapy results in action. "It involves deliberation about what an appropriate action is in this particular case, with this particular patient, at this particular time" (Mattingly, 1991, p. 981). Determining a particular student's need for occupational therapy service is a complex, nonlinear process in which many factors are considered. Rogers and Holm (1991) stated that "diagnostic reasoning is the component of clinical reasoning that results in the occupational therapy diagnosis" (p. 1053). Through this reasoning the problem is defined, an explanation of the problem is provided, and signs and symptoms indicative of the problem are outlined.

Stage 1: Referral. The initial contact or referral may be initiated by parents or school personnel as per state guidelines. As mandated by Public Law 94–142, a child must be identified as having a disability requiring special education to be eligible for special programs and thereby to receive occupational therapy as a related service. Should the child not be identified as a special education student, the referral process ends with possible programmatic consultation or referral for private occupational therapy evaluation and services (see Figure 1). *Programmatic consultation,* also referred to as colleague consultation, "addresses the needs of other professionals in the educational environment" (AOTA,1989a, p. 20) to increase the skills and knowledge of other professionals. If the student is in the process of being identified or is already identified as a special programs student, the referral continues to the next stage.

Stage 2: Screening. Screening is an informal assessment of a student's functioning based on observation,

record review, and teacher and parent interviews. As defined by AOTA, this is a Type II screening (AOTA, 1989a). At this stage, three questions of equal importance are posed (see Figure 2). The first question is whether the referring problem seems to affect school performance. The teacher may be asked to fill out a functional performance questionnaire that was developed by occupational therapists in the Wake County Public School System to assess the student's performance in the classroom in areas related to occupational therapy practice. This allows for a systematic review of students' performance as previously discussed to enhance the efficacy of the clinical reasoning process.

The second question is whether the referring problem seems to be within the area of occupational therapy practice. Occupational therapists in the Wake County Public School System address visual motor, fine motor, gross motor, sensory processing, sensory perception, and neuromuscular components of the performance areas of school and work, play and leisure, and daily living skills as appropriate for that student's functioning within the school environment. Usually the referring problem is affecting school performance; however, a child may be experiencing a clinical problem but be able to function in the classroom. For example, a child with cerebral palsy may benefit from clinical intervention to enhance the

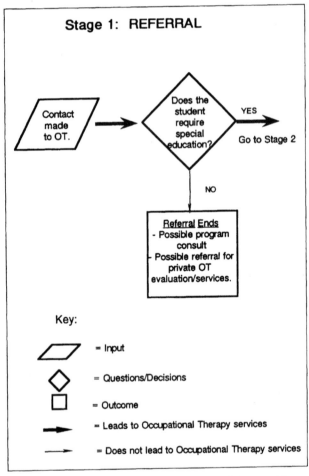

Figure 1. First stage of the determination of the need for occupational therapy. *Note.* OT = occupational therapy.

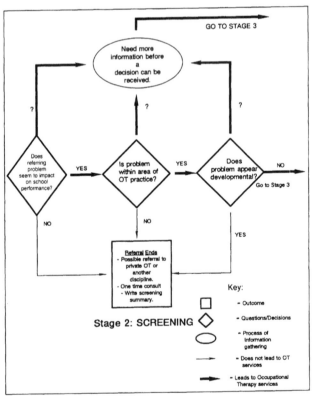

Figure 2. Second stage of the determination of the need for occupational therapy. *Note.* OT = occupational therapy.

quality of his or her movement but may be functioning effectively in the school environment.

The third question addresses the issue of developmental problems. A problem is considered developmental if the student's assessed abilities in the three performance areas are commensurate with the student's cognitive functioning and the student is following a typical and predictable developmental sequence of skill acquisition. This situation allows for the continuation of the information collection and referral process for the student with multiple disabilities who may exhibit fine motor skills commensurate with mental ability, but whose skill acquisition cannot follow a typical developmental sequence. For example, a student with cerebral palsy who is functioning in the profound range of mental retardation in cognitive, language, and fine motor areas may continue to benefit from occupational therapy intervention to develop fine motor or oral motor skills needed to meet the demands of the educational curriculum. If the information gathered in the screening stage is considered adequate to answer all three questions, then a decision can be made to end the referral process or to continue to Stage 3, full evaluation. If more information is needed to answer any of the questions, Stage 3 is necessary.

Stage 3: Evaluation. Evaluation continues the process of collecting information with a variety of testing tools, including criteria-referenced nonstandardized and standardized tests, clinical observations of neuromuscular and sensory functioning based on Ayres's (1976) clinical observations, and observations of functional skills (see Figure 3).

Stage 4: Outcome. The outcome is a judgment reached through the synthesis of all the information collected during the first three stages. The presence or absence of a discrepancy between tested skills and cognitive ability and the presence or absence of clinical issues determine whether the referring problem falls within the scope of occupational therapy practice. In a medical set-

ting, the diagnosis is used as a prognosticator for current and future functioning. In an educational setting, IQ or mental age as determined by psychological testing is used to predict a student's potential for academic and vocational success and his or her rate of learning. To attempt to habilitate a child's fine motor or visual-perceptual skills beyond his or her ability to comprehend and conceptualize may be nonproductive and misleading because success in higher academic and skilled tasks depends heavily on cognitive skills such as symbolic reasoning, discrimination, analysis, memory, and the ability to make references (see Figure 4).

In the Wake County Public School System, the therapists have decided to use a psychometric approach in determining significant deviation. A significant discrepancy is thought to exist when a student scores lower than one standard deviation below his or her measured IQ or more than 12 months below his or her mental age on standardized testing tools measuring gross motor, fine motor, visual perception, perceptual motor, and sensory integrative functioning. A need for occupational therapy is determined when any area of occupational performance is significantly discrepant from a student's IQ and thereby prevents the student from accessing his or her

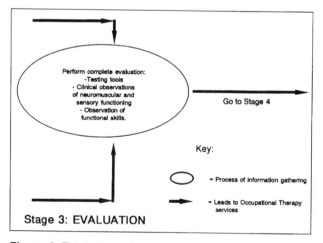

Figure 3. Third stage of the determination of the need for occupational therapy.

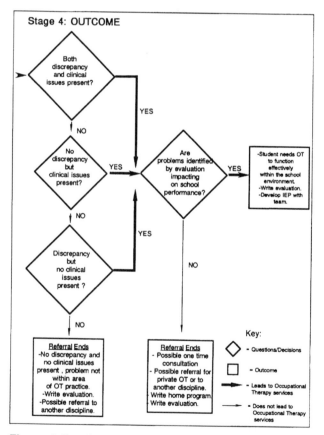

Figure 4. Fourth stage of the determination of the need for occupational therapy. *Note.* OT = occupational therapy; IEP = individualized education program.

education. The presence of clinical issues is determined by a cluster of behaviors or soft signs of neurological dysfunction, not by a single or isolated observation. For example, a child with Down syndrome who shows global delays in all areas tested and has skills commensurate with cognitive functioning may be unable to meet the fine motor demands of the classroom because his or her muscle tone is severely hypotonic, which interferes with the ability to develop fine motor skills in a normal and predictable sequence. This child would benefit from occupational therapy service to address the underlying neuromuscular dysfunction that is affecting classroom performance and contributing to abnormal developmental patterns. If no discrepancy exists and there are no clinical issues, the problem is not considered to be within the scope of occupational therapy practice and the student would not require occupational therapy as a related service. If there is a discrepancy or clinical issues and if the problems identified are affecting school performance, the student needs occupational therapy as a related service.

Determination of Type of Service

Once it has been determined that the student needs occupational therapy to function in the classroom, the type of service to meet the student's needs must be chosen (see Figure 5). As advocated by AOTA (1989a), the occupational therapy department of the Wake County Public School System is committed to offering a multiservice approach to occupational therapy service provision, including direct service, monitoring, and consultation. *Direct service* uses therapeutic techniques to remediate problems identified through the evaluation process and is carried out at least once weekly by an occupational therapist or certified occupational therapy assistant (AOTA, 1989a). *Monitoring* involves "teaching and direct supervision of other professionals or paraprofessionals who are involved with the implementation of intervention procedures" (AOTA, 1989a, p. 19), whereby the occupational therapist sets up the program but someone else carries it out. *Case consultation* is used "to develop the most effective educational environment for children with special needs" (AOTA, 1989a, p. 20). Research on the efficacy of different service types is very limited. When Dunn (1990) compared consultation and direct service in a pilot study, her results indicated that consultation services were as effective as direct services in meeting the student's educational goals when the same amount of time was spent in consultation as in direct treatment.

If the individualized education program (IEP) goals

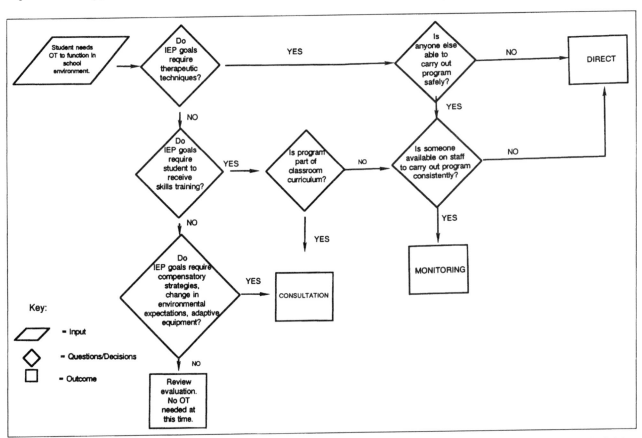

Figure 5. Determination of type of occupational therapy service needed. *Note.* OT = occupational therapy; IEP = individualized education program.

require use of purposeful activities and other therapeutic techniques and there is no one else who can carry out the program safely, direct service is indicated. If purposeful activities and other therapeutic techniques are not required to meet the IEP goals, but the student needs skills training (i.e., a specific handwriting program) that is not part of the classroom's regular curriculum and someone other than the occupational therapist is available to safely and consistently carry out the skills training program, then monitoring is indicated. If no one is available to safely and consistently carry out the program, then direct service is again the most appropriate. If the IEP goals require skills training that is part of the curriculum but some adaptations are needed, then case consultation would be provided. Additionally, if compensation strategies, changes in environmental expectations, or adaptive equipment is the only intervention required to meet the IEP goals, then case consultation would be indicated. Although the primary factor in determining service type is the treatment strategy employed, there is always an ebb and flow between service types with continual review of progress toward meeting the student's IEP goals. This allows for flexibility in adjusting service type as the student improves or as more intensive intervention is needed. The ultimate goal is for the student to gain functional independence and graduate from occupational therapy services.

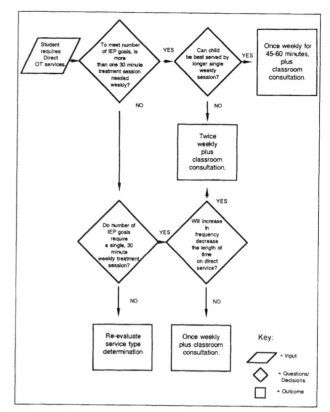

Figure 6. Determination of frequency of direct services. *Note.* OT = occupational therapy, IEP = individualized education program.

Determination of Frequency of Service

The questions used to determine frequency for each service type are presented in Figures 6–8. As with type of service, research on the efficacy of frequency of service is limited. Jenkins et al. (1982) compared two levels of frequency of direct service: once a week versus more than once a week. Results showed a significant difference in outcomes only when the two experimental groups were compared with the control group, which received no direct service. No significant difference was found between the two experimental groups; therefore, the results of this study indicate that the only important factor was whether the child received direct services, not the frequency of the service.

Determination of the frequency of direct service depends partially on the number of IEP goal areas addressed by the occupational therapist (see Figure 6). A large number of goal areas may require more frequent or longer sessions. Traditionally, direct treatment is provided within 30-min sessions. If a child has difficulty making the transition to direct occupational therapy service, a longer treatment session may be more advantageous than an increase in the frequency of sessions. Alternatively, a student may not be able to tolerate longer treatment sessions because of attention deficits and therefore would need two shorter sessions. If the number of IEP goals requires at least one 30-min session, but an increase in

frequency of services to twice weekly will expedite progress toward meeting those goals, then two weekly sessions would be indicated. For example, a student may be in an emotional crisis because he or she cannot keep up with the written demands of the classroom, so the occupational therapist may see the student twice weekly to provide more intensive intervention toward developing a functional means of written communication. Another example would be a child who is on the verge of developing a critical skill and requires a little extra push for the emerging skill to become functional.

Determination of the frequency of monitoring service depends on the student's expected rate of progress in meeting the IEP goals (see Figure 7). Expected rate of progress is related to the difficulty of the skill being taught and the child's ability and motivation to acquire the skill. These elements determine how much and how often the occupational therapist needs to reevaluate the program.

Determination of the frequency of consultation service depends on the particular environmental (human and nonhuman) adaptations needed to meet the IEP goals, the education staff's skill in implementing these adaptations, and the student's ability to use these modifications to be functionally independent (see Figure 8). Adaptations to the human environment may include altering the education staff's expectations of the student or

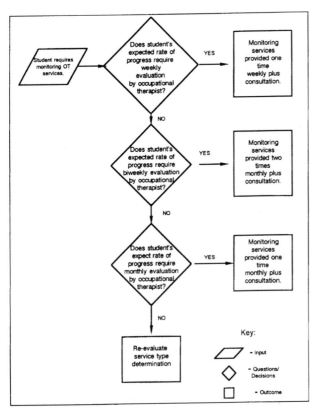

Figure 7. Determination of frequency of monitoring services. *Note.* OT = occupational therapy.

what occupational therapy can realistically do for children in the educational setting (Royeen & Marsh, 1988). The use of specific criteria, such as the 12-month discrepancy between mental age and skills tested by occupational therapists, may not be a sensitive enough guideline for preschoolers, but the clinical reasoning process used for service determination will be the same for preschool and school-age children. The questions will always return to the child's ability to function in the educational environment.

Many practical factors can influence a therapist's decision of whether to place a student on the caseload. However, allowing services to be determined by staffing, schedules, and space can lead to provision of token services, long waiting lists, angry parents, and dissatisfied administrators (King, 1988). Parents who have had to cope with the stress of having a child with special needs and who have had to fight for services may push for more services than needed, because they believe that more services will mean greater progress toward a nondysfunctional child (Huebner, 1990). Dunn (1988) pointed out that "the intent of Public Law 94–142 is that the type and amount of service provision may not be determined by parental wishes or district resource limitations such as space or personnel shortages, but by the student's needs" (p. 718).

working with the education staff on developing and implementing strategies to allow the student to be functionally independent. Adaptations to the nonhuman environment may include providing adaptive equipment including typewriters, laptop computers, and feeding equipment; recommending the use of study carrels, breaks in schedule, or a specific type of paper or writing instrument; or adapting the format of tests and work sheets.

Discussion and Implications

The decision-making process presented reflects an initial attempt by the occupational therapists of the Wake County Public School System to look at how they think about service provision decisions. The process is not a criterion of eligibility for service determination, but an attempt to develop a consistent and justifiable approach to making decisions regarding occupational therapy service provision. As public funding becomes less available, occupational therapists are being further pressed to define and justify occupational therapy services. With the expansion of services to the 3- to 5-year-old population mandated in the Education of the Handicapped Act Amendments of 1986 (Public Law 99–457), occupational therapists must present a clear picture to administrators and parents as to

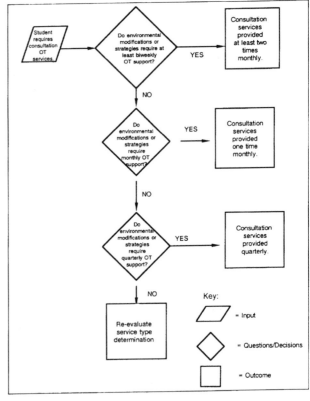

Figure 8. Determination of frequency of case consultation services. *Note.* OT = occupational therapy.

934

Following an articulated clinical reasoning process will increase consistency in decision making among staff therapists and among a particular therapist's cases. Reaching occupational therapy service decisions through a clinical reasoning process enables the therapist to explain these decisions to parents, teachers, area therapists, and outside agencies. Another reason to develop a clearly articulated clinical reasoning process related to school-based services is its value as a training tool for newly graduated therapists and for those entering school-based practice from other practice areas.

The assumptions underlying this clinical reasoning process need further research to determine efficacy and validity. Some assumptions that need further testing include the following: (a) Does the use of an articulated clinical reasoning process increase consistency of decision making among staff? (b) Is use of discrepancy criteria a valid measure for determining the need for occupational therapy services? (c) Is the multiservice provision approach a valid means of providing occupational therapy service in the public schools?

The use of an articulated clinical reasoning process enables occupational therapists working in public schools to define their role as providers of a related service separate from other disciplines. Implementing this process ensures the development of educationally relevant, not clinically based, occupational therapy goals on the IEP. As teachers, parents, and administrators are better able to see a direct link between occupational therapy services and educational progress, the value of all types (direct, monitoring, and consultation) of occupational therapy service provision in the school system will increase. ▲

Acknowledgments

This paper was made possible through the collaborative efforts of the occupational therapists of the Wake County Public School System; the guidance and support of Ai Li Lee, MS, OTR/L, Ruth Humphry, PhD, OTR/L, and Jane Rourk, OTR/L, FAOTA; and the support of Juanita Van Liere.

References

American Occupational Therapy Association (1989a). *Guidelines for occupational therapy services in school systems* (2nd ed.). Rockville, MD: Author.

American Occupational Therapy Association (1989b). Uniform terminology for occupational therapy—second edition. *American Journal of Occupational Therapy, 43*, 808–815.

Ayres, A. J. (1976). *Interpreting the Southern California Sensory Integration Tests.* Los Angeles: Western Psychological Services.

Barrows, H. S., & Feltovich, P. J. (1987). Clinical reasoning process. *Medical Education, 21*, 86–91.

Carr, S. H. (1989). Louisiana's criteria of eligibility for occupational therapy services in the public school system. *American Journal of Occupational Therapy, 43*, 503–506.

Coutinho, M. J., & Hunter, P. L. (1988). Special education

and occupational therapy: Making the relationship work. *American Journal of Occupational Therapy, 42*, 706–712.

Dunn, W. (1988). Models of occupational therapy service provision in the school system. *American Journal of Occupational Therapy, 42*, 718–723.

Dunn, W. (1990). A comparison of service provision models in school based occupational therapy services: A pilot study. *Occupational Therapy Journal of Research, 10*, 300–320.

Dunn, W., & McGourty, L. (1989). Application of uniform terminology to practice. *American Journal of Occupational Therapy, 43*, 817–831.

Education of All Handicapped Children Act (Public Law 94–142). (1975).

Education of the Handicapped Act Amendments of 1986 (Public Law 99–457), 20 U.S.C., § 1400.

Giangreco, M. (1990). More concerns [Letter to the editor]. *American Journal of Occupational Therapy, 44*, 470.

Gilfoyle, E., & Farace, J. (1981). The role of occupational therapy as an education-related service—Official Position Paper. *American Journal of Occupational Therapy, 35*, 811.

Gillette, N., & Mattingly, C. (1987).The Foundation—Clinical reasoning in occupational therapy. *American Journal of Occupational Therapy, 41*, 399–400.

Huebner, R. (1990). Occupational therapy in the schools. *Occupational Therapy Forum, 5*, 1–5.

Individuals With Disabilities Education Act (Public Law 101–476), 20 U.S.C., § 1400. (1990).

Jenkins, J. R., Sells, C. J., Brady, D., Down, J., Moore, B., Carmen, P., & Holms, R. (1982). Effects of developmental therapy on motor impaired children. *Physical & Occupational Therapy in Pediatrics, 2*(4), 19–28.

Kielhofner, G., & Burke, J. P. (1980). A Model of Human Occupation, part 1, conceptual framework and content. *American Journal of Occupational Therapy, 34*, 572–581.

King, L. J. (1988). Can occupational therapy survive in the public schools? *Occupational Therapy Forum, 3*, 1–5.

Mattingly, C. (1991). What is clinical reasoning? *American Journal of Occupational Therapy, 45*, 979–986.

Mattingly, C., & Gillette, N. (1991). Anthropology, occupational therapy, and action research. *American Journal of Occupational Therapy, 45*, 972–976.

Ottenbacher, K. (1982). Occupational therapy and special education: Some issues and concerns related to Public Law 94–142. *American Journal of Occupational Therapy, 36*, 81–84.

Pelland, M. (1987). A conceptual model for the instruction and supervision of treatment planning. *American Journal of Occupational Therapy, 41*, 351–359.

Rainforth, B. (1990). Concerns about Louisiana criteria [Letter to the editor]. *American Journal of Occupational Therapy, 44*, 469-470.

Reilly, M. (1969). The educational process. *American Journal of Occupational Therapy, 23*, 299–307.

Rogers, J. (1982). The spirit of independence: The evolution of a philosophy. *American Journal of Occupational Therapy, 36*, 709–715.

Rogers, J. (1983). Eleanor Clarke Slagle Lectureship—Clinical reasoning: The ethics, science, and art. *American Journal of Occupational Therapy, 37*, 601–616.

Rogers, J., & Holm, M. (1991). Occupational therapy diagnostic reasoning: A component of clinical reasoning. *American Journal of Occupational Therapy, 45*, 1045–1053.

Rogers, J., & Masagatani, G. (1982). Clinical reasoning of occupational therapists during the initial assessment of physically disabled patients. *Occupational Therapy Journal of Research, 2*, 195–219.

Royeen, C., & Marsh, D. (1988). Promoting occupational

therapy in the schools. *American Journal of Occupational Therapy, 42,* 713–717.

Saltz, D. L. (1991, February 7). Study delves into process of clinical reasoning. *OT Week, 5,* pp. 4–7.

Spencer, K. (1990). More concerns [Letter to the editor]. *American Journal of Occupational Therapy, 44,* 471–472.

Stephens, L. (1989). Occupational therapy in the school system. In P. Pratt & A. Allen (Eds.), *Occupational therapy for children* (2nd ed., pp. 593–611). St. Louis: Mosby.

Takata, N. (1980). Introduction to a series: Occupational behavior research for pediatric practice. *American Journal of Occupational Therapy, 34,* 11–12.

and can almost automatically pull together the medical and psychosocial aspects of the patient's condition. They use analytic abilities in an almost automatic way. Achieving this intuitive sense takes time, practice, and experience. DePoy (1990) further identified the mastery of occupational therapy as that which includes personal characteristics (e.g., commitment to practice, creativity, intelligence) combined with well-developed knowledge; extensive and varied experiences; and individuality in behaviors, actions, and reasoning processes.

I recalled these definitions as I observed the group of Level II fieldwork students. In some areas, the students appeared to be moving rapidly back and forth through the beginning levels of this progression, from novice to advanced beginner. The expectations of the supervisors, however, appeared at times to be greater than they should have been for students at an advanced beginner stage.

The following thoughts and questions came to mind. Are the expectations of student clinical supervisors in general greater than the capabilities of students at this level of experience? Are these "great expectations" facilitating or hindering the learning process and development of the students? Can an entry-level student even begin to reach the novice level during a Level II fieldwork experience? Are supervising therapists even aware of the various levels of skill acquisition and this progression of development?

This led me to think about entry-level occupational therapists. Are they expected to become experts too quickly? Do we allow our clinicians the time necessary to attain mastery? Clinicians are allowed to supervise students after 1 year of experience, but clinicians at this stage are little more than novices or advanced beginners themselves. Are they too demanding of the students whom they are supervising?

I believe that heads of occupational therapy departments should encourage their staff members to learn about the levels of skill acquisition and then explore their own levels of skill acquisition. Those who have great levels of skills could possibly be paired with those who are still in the first few levels of skill acquisition and a mentoring process could be initiated. Literature on occupational therapy, nursing, and leadership all support the importance of role models and mentors as a effective strategy for development of staff members (Benner, 1984; Bennis, 1989; Cohn & Czycholl, 1991; Rogers, 1982; Sabari, 1985; Schon, 1983, 1987; Slater & Cohn, 1991). Additionally, once occupational therapists have identified their own skill acquisition levels, perhaps they will then recognize reasonable expectations for students on fieldwork experiences. More experienced therapists could possibly oversee therapists with lower skill levels when these latter therapists are supervising students. This might assist new supervisors to develop ways of facilitating skill acquisition in the students.

Granted, I have presented some reflections and questions, but no answers. It seems to me, however, that all occupational therapists (not just academic educators and clinical supervisors) should think seriously about the issues raised by the research and articles on clinical reasoning in our profession. ■

Questions (But No Answers) About Clinical Reasoning and Student Supervision

■ Paula Kramer, PhD, OTR, FAOTA

I recently had the opportunity to observe some senior students in their Level II fieldwork placements, and I thought about the literature relating to skill development and mastery. Dreyfus and Dreyfus (1986) described a model of skill acquisition that includes the following five stages: novice, advanced beginner, competent, proficient, and expert. Slater and Cohn (1991) clearly articulated these five levels and related them to clinical practice in the following ways.

Stage 1—Novice. "The novice recognizes various facts and features relevant to the acquisition of new skills and learns rules for determining actions based on those facts and features" (Slater & Cohn, 1991, p. 1040). The novice will concentrate first on the condition of the patient. The interaction between therapist and patient is seen as secondary.

Stage 2—Advanced beginner. "Once novices gain more experience with patients, they learn to consider additional cues, which enable them to consider elements that relate to the patient as an individual" (Slater & Cohn, 1991, p. 1040). At this point, the occupational therapist begins to see the patient and the condition within a context. There is still limited ability in sorting out crucial data.

Stage 3—Competent. The competent practitioner can view the situation as a set of facts, but tends to see more facts than the beginner and can distinguish which facts are the most important or crucial at any given time. The experienced occupational therapist can attend to more patient cues than the novice therapist.

Stage 4—Proficient. "Proficient therapists perceive a situation as a whole rather than as isolated parts" (Slater & Cohn, 1991, p. 1041). Because of their experience, proficient occupational therapists can recognize the subtleties of clinical problems and have a sense of direction (i.e., where to go with the patient). The proficient practitioner will also designate some features of a patient's case as important and allow other aspects to fade into the background.

Stage 5—Expert. The expert therapist knows the rules and guidelines of their profession, but lets them stay in the background. Experts have an intuitive judgment about what features of a case are important and what aspects should be given the most attention at any particular time. They can identify the most relevant cues of the patient

References

Benner, P. (1984). *From novice to expert: Excellence and power in clinical nursing practice.* Reading, MA: Addison-Wesley.

Bennis, W. (1989). *On becoming a leader.* Reading, MA: Addison-Wesley.

Cohn, E. S., & Czycholl, C. M. (1991). Facilitating a foundation for clinical reasoning. In E. B. Crepeau & T. LaGarde (Eds.), *Self-paced instruction for clinical education and supervision: An instructional guide* (pp. 159–182). Rockville, MD: American Occupational Therapy Association.

DePoy, E. (1990). Mastery in clinical occupational therapy. *American Journal of Occupational Therapy, 44,* 415–422.

Dreyfus, H., & Dreyfus, S. (1986). *Mind over machine—The power of human intuition & expertise in the era of the computer.* New York: Free Press.

Rogers, J. C. (1982). Sponsorship: Developing leaders for occupational therapy. *American Journal of Occupational Therapy, 36,* 309–313.

Sabari, J. S. (1985). Professional socialization: Implications for occupational therapy education. *American Journal of Occupational Therapy, 39,* 96–102.

Schon, D. (1983). *The reflective practitioner: How professionals think in action.* New York, NY: Basic Books.

Schon, D. (1987). *Educating the reflective practitioner.* San Francisco, CA: Jossey-Bass.

Slater, D. Y., & Cohn, E. S. (1991). Staff development through analysis of practice. *American Journal of Occupational Therapy, 45,* 1038–1044.

Paula Kramer, PhD, OTR, FAOTA, is Professor and Chair, Department of Occupational Therapy, Kean College of New Jersey, 311 Willis, Union, NJ 07083. She serves as Newsletter Editor for the Education Special Interest Section.

Teaching Strategies for the Development of Clinical Reasoning

Maureen E. Neistadt

Key Words: curriculum • education

A primary aim of occupational therapy education is to teach students how to think like practitioners, that is, how to engage in clinical reasoning. Since the early 1980s, occupational therapy clinical reasoning research has elucidated a language that describes the various types of thinking therapists use in clinical practice, a language that has the potential to make previously tacit thought processes accessible to conscious examination and improvement. Occupational therapy educators can use that language to make their teaching of clinical reasoning more explicit to students. This article examines occupational therapy teaching methods using the language of clinical reasoning, categorizing them by the types of clinical reasoning they promote. Current clinical reasoning language is reviewed, and teaching strategies to facilitate the various types of clinical reasoning are described.

Maureen E. Neistadt, ScD, OTR/L, FAOTA, is Assistant Professor, Occupational Therapy Department, University of New Hampshire, Hewitt Hall, 4 Library Way, Durham, New Hampshire 03824-3563.

This article was accepted for publication October 6, 1995.

Clinical reasoning, the thought process occupational therapists use during evaluation and treatment, is central to practice (Dutton, 1995; Mattingly & Fleming, 1994). Teaching clinical reasoning is, therefore, vital to the professional preparation of occupational therapy students (Royeen, 1995). The various types of clinical reasoning that occupational therapists use in practice have been well explained in the literature (e.g., Fleming, 1991a, 1991b; Mattingly 1991a, 1991b; Rogers & Holm, 1991; Schell & Cervero, 1993). Various strategies for teaching some of these types of reasoning have also been described (e.g., Cohn, 1989; Neistadt, 1987, 1992; VanLeit, 1995). However, to date, no one has examined teaching strategies for all types of occupational therapy clinical reasoning in a single article. This article reviews clinical reasoning teaching strategies, using the different types of occupational therapy clinical reasoning as an organizing framework.

Clinical Reasoning

Clinical reasoning is not new to occupational therapy. Therapists have always engaged in clinical reasoning, and educators have always sought to teach students how to think like therapists. Although these thought processes are not new, the language that we now have available to describe those thought processes is relatively new. This naming of our thought processes provides advantages for both therapists and educators. For therapists, the current clinical reasoning terminology can help to (a) improve clinical decision making through giving therapists tools for self-conscious reflection on their decisions; (b) improve abilities to explain the rationales behind therapist decisions to clients, family members, team members, and insurance carriers; and (c) improve job satisfaction by making therapists more aware of the complexity of their work (Hall, Robertson, & Turner, 1992; Parham, 1987; Slater & Cohn, 1991; Terry & Higgs, 1993). For educators, the current clinical reasoning language can (a) allow more explicit mentoring of clinical reasoning, (b) help students develop more precise thought processes sooner, and (c) give students a vocabulary for self-evaluation and improvement of their clinical reasoning skills (Dutton, 1995; Royeen, 1995).

If occupational therapy educators are to derive the potential benefit of current clinical reasoning language, they must use that language to describe their teaching methods. Just as clinical practice may be strengthened when therapists become consciously aware of thought processes that were previously automatic or tacit, so too can education become more effective when educators explicitly tell students what types of reasoning various assignments are meant to foster.

The development of clinical reasoning follows a continuum through the following stages: novice, advanced beginner, competent, proficient, and expert (Benner, 1984; Dreyfus & Dreyfus, 1986; Dutton, 1995; Slater & Cohn, 1991). A novice is "characterized by the rigid application of rules and principles learned in school" (Dutton, 1995, p. 8), regardless of the circumstances of a particular case. A novice therapist or student performs a complete sensory evaluation on all clients in a physical dysfunction setting—even on those who are not suspected of having sensory problems—because he or she learned in school that a thorough physical dysfunction evaluation includes a detailed sensory evaluation.

An advanced beginner can modify rules and principles for specific situations (i.e., "situational thinking" [Dutton, 1995, p. 8]) but still has difficulty prioritizing evaluation information. The advanced beginner therapist will use goniometry to measure only those joints that appear to have less than full range on observation of functional movement but will see decreased range at any joint as an occupational therapy problem, even if the client does not experience any functional limitations from some of those reduced ranges.

The competent therapist is able to adjust procedures to specific situations and perceive the relative importance of different pieces of information about a client but may still have difficulty altering initial treatment plans. The competent therapist will identify as occupational therapy problems only those range of motion deficits that cause functional limitations. However, this therapist may be resistant to changing the treatment activity planned for a given day (i.e., switching from active range of motion exercises to kitchen activities) because he or she has difficulty in seeing quickly how different activities can be modified to accomplish given treatment goals.

The proficient therapist has the flexibility to alter treatment plans as needed in the treatment process and has a clearer sense than therapists in earlier developmental stages of the client's total situation, including the physical and social aspects of the potential discharge situation. The proficient therapist can easily change his or her treatment activity, at the client's request, from teaching active range of motion exercises to making tea because he or she understands the symbolic and practical importance of kitchen activities for the client and can see how to adapt the tea task to elicit maximal active range of motion from the client.

Expert therapists seem to be able to organize their approach to treatment more from client cues than from preconceived plans of therapeutic action. The expert therapist can begin an initial evaluation from any data point and gather information in whatever sequence is dictated by a particular client situation. Experts are able to recognize client problems and potentials quickly on the basis of their recognition of patterns from previous clinical experiences.

It is not reasonable to expect occupational therapy students to graduate as competent, proficient, or expert therapists. Those levels of clinical reasoning require years of clinical practice and continuing education. However, it is possible for students to enter practice as novices or advanced beginners who are capable of progressing to higher levels of clinical reasoning if their academic preparation for Level II fieldwork has given them an awareness of the types of reasoning they will be using in practice (Benner, 1984). This awareness of clinical reasoning concepts can help students learn about their thinking and doing in clinical practice simultaneously, intensifying the learning derived from clinical experience (Pesut & Herman, 1992). Educators can foster that awareness by explicitly naming the types of reasoning different assignments and learning experiences are meant to promote.

The types of clinical reasoning that have been identified in the occupational therapy literature to date include narrative reasoning, interactive reasoning, procedural reasoning, pragmatic reasoning, and conditional reasoning. *Narrative reasoning* deals with the client's occupational story and focuses on the process of change needed to reach an imagined future (Clark, 1993; Mattingly, 1991a). The occupational story answers the following questions:

1. What activities and roles were important to this client before his or her injury or illness?
2. What valued activities and roles can this client perform now?
3. What valued activities and roles are possible in the future, given his or her residual disability?
4. Which valued activities and roles would the client choose as priorities for the future?

Interactive reasoning deals with how the disability or disease affects the client (i.e., the client's illness experience) and focuses on the client as a person (Crepeau, 1991; Fleming, 1991b). Interactive reasoning has also been termed the *community aspect of practice* (Hasselkus & Dickie, 1994) because it deals with the therapeutic relationship the therapist forms with a client and his or her caregivers.

Procedural reasoning involves identifying occupational therapy problems and implementing treatment strategies via systematic gathering and interpreting of client data. This thought process, which has also been called *scientific reasoning* (Rogers, 1983; VanLeit, 1995), typically involves hypothesis generation and testing and focuses on the client's disease or disability (Fleming, 1991b; Mattingly & Fleming, 1994). Hasselkus and Dickie (1994) referred to procedural reasoning as analogous to their craft dimension of practice, which represents the actual doing of clinical practice (i.e., the evaluation and treatment techniques that therapists use day to day). The part of procedural reasoning that deals with evaluation and identification of occupational therapy problems has been termed diagnostic reasoning (Rogers & Holm, 1991).

Pragmatic reasoning considers the treatment environment and therapist values, knowledge, abilities, and experiences and focuses on the treatment possibilities within a given treatment setting. Therapists use this thought process to integrate consideration of practical factors such as clients' insurance coverage and social supports into their decisions about treatment recommendations (Creighton, Dijkers, Bennett, & Brown, 1995; Schell & Cervero, 1993).

Conditional reasoning involves an ongoing revision of treatment to meet the client's needs and focuses on the client's current and possible future social contexts (Fleming, 1991b). Conditional reasoning has also been called the *change dimension of practice* (Hasselkus & Dickie, 1994) and can be viewed as an integration of interactive, procedural, and pragmatic reasoning within the context of the client's narrative.

Ideally, an occupational therapist would use all of these types of reasoning during evaluation and treatment. Narrative reasoning would delineate the client's occupational story. The occupational story, or narrative, is the context for understanding the exact nature of occupational disruptions and the meaning of those disruptions for any given person. The ultimate aim of occupational therapy treatment is for the therapist and client to collaboratively reformulate the client's occupational story, via the other types of reasoning, to project a future that includes continued occupation with adaptations for disability. Teaching strategies to promote student development of all these types of reasoning have been described in the occupational therapy, physical therapy, and nursing literature.

Teaching Strategies

Because all occupational therapy curricula seek to teach clinical reasoning, the teaching strategies reviewed and described in this article can be integrated into existing courses within any curricula. It is not necessary to offer specific courses on clinical reasoning. In fact, integrating

clinical reasoning teaching throughout a curriculum is very effective in helping students connect all their course work with clinical reasoning skills and transfer their reasoning from the classroom to the clinic (Higgs, 1992; Terry & Higgs, 1993). Generally speaking, facilitation of pragmatic and conditional reasoning is most appropriate toward the latter part of a curriculum, after students feel somewhat comfortable with their basic narrative, interactive, and procedural reasoning skills (Cohn, 1989; Dutton, 1995). Table 1 categorizes different teaching strategies according to the type of clinical reasoning those strategies facilitate. These teaching strategies come from the literature and my teaching experiences. The following sections analyze the characteristics of assignments appropriate to facilitating specific types of reasoning and describing selected strategies.

Narrative Reasoning

The first three strategies listed in Table 1 for narrative reasoning aim to help students understand the narrative concept of life stories. These assignments help students appreciate that we all live and create our own life stories every day and that those life stories can be changed and altered unexpectedly by illness and disability. Crepeau (1991), for example, suggests that novels like Miller's (1990) *Family Pictures* and personal accounts of disability like Murphy's (1990) *The Body Silent* can "enhance our understanding of the effects of disability on persons and their families" (p. 1024). A more complete list of suggested readings is provided in Peloquin and Davidson's (1993) article.

Asking students to write narratives, or stories, about persons with disabilities who they have met in Level I fieldwork or in classroom settings is another way to foster narrative clinical reasoning skills. Students can be asked to focus these stories on the possible future of a person with a disability and on how this person's past and present might be reflected in that future. This type of writing shifts students out of the "chart talk" (Mattingly & Fleming, 1994, p. 60) of medical terminology associated with procedural reasoning into a more client-centered storytelling mode.

To apply the general concept of client narratives to clinical practice, students need specific instruction on how to build occupational narratives with clients. Orienting students to interview instruments such as the Canadian Occupational Performance Measure (Pollock, 1993) or the Patient Participation System (Payton, Nelson, & Ozer, 1990), which focus on the activity preferences of clients, is a way to help students translate the concept of occupational narrative—a life story of occupation (Clark,

678

September 1996, Volume 50, Number 8

32 | Cognitive Learning Styles and Clinical Reasoning

Table 1
Teaching Strategies for Different Types of Clinical Reasoning

Narrative Reasoning	Interactive Reasoning	Procedural Reasoning	Pragmatic Reasoning	Conditional Reasoning
Reading and analyzing literature about disability experiences (Crepeau, 1991; Kautzmann, 1993; Peloquin, 1989, 1995; Peloquin & Davidson, 1993)	Reading and analyzing literature about disability experiences (Crepeau, 1991; Peloquin, 1989, 1995; Peloquin & Davidson, 1993)	Case study exams (Schwartz, 1991)	Ethical case scenarios (Neuhaus, 1988)	Systems treatment plans
Writing narratives about clients met (Mattingly & Fleming, 1994)	Writing journals and reflective papers (Crepeau, 1991; Tryssenaar, 1995)	Formal debates (Field, 1992; Higgs, 1992)	Systems treatment plans	Level I fieldwork
Writing autobiographical papers that make students aware of their own narratives	Analyzing own therapeutic style (Peloquin & Davidson, 1993)	Classroom as clinic (Neistadt, 1987, 1992) Guest speakers or actors (VanLeit, 1995) Videotapes	Level I fieldwork (Zimmerman, 1995)	Paradigm case analysis (Farrell & Bramadat, 1990)
Administering Canadian Occupational Performance Measure (Pollock, 1993)	Receiving faculty feedback (Sands, 1995)	Level I fieldwork (Levine & Gitlin, 1990; Neistadt & Cohn, 1990; Zimmerman, 1995)		Stimulated recall (Farrell & Bramadat, 1990)
	Classroom as clinic (Neistadt, 1987, 1992)	Videotaping (Cohn, 1989; Farrell & Bramadat, 1990)		Professional self-talk (Rogers, 1982)
	Level I fieldwork (Rydeen, Kautzmann, Cowan, & Benzing, 1995)	What and why questions (Cohn, 1989)		
	Methods of collaborative goal setting (Payton, Nelson, & Ozer, 1990)	Metacognitive questions (Pesut & Herman, 1992)		

1993)—into concrete clinical procedures for building that narrative.

Interactive Reasoning

The strategies listed in Table 1 for interactive reasoning are meant to either heighten students' awareness of illness experiences, promote insights about their interactional styles and therapeutic qualities, or provide opportunities for them to practice therapeutic interactions with actual clients. Reading literature on disability experiences (Crepeau, 1991; Peloquin, 1989, 1995; Peloquin & Davidson, 1993) can help students understand how different persons experience illness. Additionally, Peloquin (1989) suggested that by reading this type of literature, students can "reflect on and affirm the importance of relationships and caring in practice by comparing and contrasting those various characteristics most conducive to helping" (p. 225).

Students can use journals and reflective papers to become more aware of their feelings, their therapeutic capacities, and the feelings of clients (Crepeau, 1991; Neistadt, 1987; Peloquin & Davidson, 1993; Tryssenaar, 1995). They also can use self-evaluations of their interac-

tive styles, such as the ones suggested by Peloquin and Davidson (1993) and the one presented in Appendix A, to become aware of their therapeutic capacities.

Faculty feedback about clinically related behaviors can augment students' awareness of their behavioral styles. Sands (1995), for example, described the use of a Personal and Academic Performance Summary (PAPS) in Orange County Community College's Certified Occupational Therapy Assistant Program in New York state. Faculty members (two full time, two part time) use the PAPS to reach consensus on each first-year student's clinically related attitudes, interpersonal skills, and behaviors, and each student meets with two faculty members to review the completed PAPS. Sands has used this process for 5 years with more than 100 students and "found that making a connection between students' behaviors and attitudes and their potential performance in a therapeutic environment has given students an incentive to engage in a realistic form of self-evaluation that has produced beneficial results" (p. 151).

Interaction with actual clients, in either classroom or Level I fieldwork settings, has also been found to facilitate students' interactive reasoning skills. For example,

Rydeen, Kautzmann, Cowan, and Benzing (1995) of Eastern Kentucky University found that students involved in a faculty-supervised Level I experience in an Alzheimer's day-care and respite program "developed an awareness of the personal, familial, and social ramifications of Alzheimer's disease [and of] the individuality of each program participant" (p. 117).

Ideally, interactive reasoning in occupational therapy is used to form a partnership with clients (Fleming, 1991b; Peloquin, 1990). Students are helped to implement this collaboration in practice if they are given instruction about exactly how to involve clients and their caregivers in goal setting and treatment planning. Payton et al. (1990) delineated specific guidelines on client interviewing for the purpose of collaborative goal setting. Payton and Nelson have been using this system successfully at the University of Virginia for 5 years to teach physical therapy and occupational therapy students how to collaborate with clients (C. E. Nelson, personal communication, July 17, 1995).

Procedural Reasoning

Much of the occupational therapy curricula is focused on teaching students procedural reasoning (i.e., the evaluation and treatment skills occupational therapists use in practice). The teaching strategies listed in Table 1 for procedural reasoning are meant to increase the effectiveness of that teaching by making it more directly related to clinical practice. A continuum of practice-related experiences is represented in this list, from paper case studies (Field, 1992; Higgs, 1990; Schwartz, 1991), to simulated clinical experiences (Neistadt, 1987, 1992; VanLeit, 1995), to actual clinical experiences (Levine & Gitlin, 1990; Neistadt & Cohn, 1990; Zimmerman, 1995).

Schwartz (1991), for example, has suggested that case study exams are a more effective way to promote clinical thinking than multiple-choice tests aimed at testing students' recall of course content. Case study exams are a way to help students apply procedural information to clinical situations. Appendix B provides an example of a case study exam format that I developed for the Rehabilitation of the Upper Extremity course at the University of New Hampshire. This format combines case studies and multiple-choice questions, a practical format for large lecture courses. Students are given the case studies and study questions before the exam to guide their studying toward clinical problem solving and away from straight memorization.

Higgs (1990) described an interesting use of paper case studies in a physical therapy curriculum at the University of Sydney in Australia. This learning experience requires students to work in groups of three to prepare hypothetical case studies about clients who seek physical therapy services. These case studies are then presented to two groups of three to four students who are responsible for making diagnostic, treatment, and evaluation decisions about the case presented. The creation of these case studies requires students to research the signs and symptoms of particular diagnoses and accurately depict a possible set of physical therapy problems that might be associated with those diagnoses, a more active process than having a typical case presented and explained by an instructor. Higgs found this case study assignment and ensuing discussions to be very effective in promoting students' diagnostic and procedural reasoning skills. Field (1992) has used a similar format in the physical therapy program at the University of Miami where two teams of two students each formally debate treatment options for paper case studies provided by the instructor.

Relative to simulated clinical experiences, I have found a classroom-as-clinic methodology to be effective in promoting students' diagnostic reasoning skills. In these experiences, students are asked to (a) generate tentative occupational therapy problem lists from preliminary diagnostic and social information about guest speakers with disabilities and (b) revise those lists after actually meeting and interviewing the guest speakers. Students are graded on the accuracy of their problem lists relative to those of an experienced therapist. Both lists relate directly to clinical practice—the first represents the mental hypotheses a therapist might generate after an initial chart review, and the second represents the summary problem list from an initial evaluation. This same format could be used with actors posing as clients (VanLeit, 1995) or with videotapes of clients being evaluated by experienced occupational therapists.

Level I fieldwork can provide an opportunity for students to learn hands-on techniques with actual clients. For example, Zimmerman (1995) described a cooperative education model for Level I fieldwork where occupational therapy students mostly function as paid occupational therapy aides.

Cohn (1989) suggested that videotaping students' interactions with actual clients and later discussing their clinical reasoning in those sessions, with reference to the videotapes, is an effective way to improve their procedural reasoning abilities. Cohn also suggested that asking students what and why questions about their clinical decisions can help them develop and articulate their reasoning processes. Similarly, Pesut and Herman (1992) suggested that nursing students can be helped to develop their reasoning by answering metacognitive questions about their clinical behaviors. Metacognitive questions force persons to think about how they are thinking. Appendix C lists adaptations of Pesut and Herman's questions that could be used to help occupational therapy students critique their reasoning during or after Level I experiences.

Pragmatic Reasoning

The teaching strategies listed in Table 1 for pragmatic reasoning seek to sensitize students to some of the practical issues of clinical practice (e.g., reimbursement, documentation, staffing and equipment resources) and their ethical implications (Neuhaus, 1988). The systems treatment plan, for example, is an assignment developed by Ruth Smith at the University of New Hampshire for the senior-level occupational therapy course, Systems of Therapeutic Intervention in Physical Dysfunction. Through a series of field trips and guest lectures, this course orients students to many of the settings in which they might work as physical dysfunction therapists. On their field trips, students meet and interview an actual client for whom they need to write a systems treatment plan. The guidelines for the systems treatment plan are as follows:

1. Describe how the system affects the client and his or her family members or caregivers. Be sure to comment on the appropriateness of the system for this client.
2. Describe the system factors that guide occupational therapy intervention (i.e., regulations, reimbursement, institutional or departmental policies).
3. Describe precautions you consider important for this client in this setting.
4. List the problems you would address with this particular client in this setting.
5. Describe for each problem the types of treatment activities you would use for this client in this particular setting (types = broad categories of activities such as activities of daily living) and the level of client performance you would expect at the time of discharge from this setting.
6. Describe how the system aids and hinders the occupational therapist responsible for this client's program.

This assignment helps students expand their notion of a treatment plan to include consideration of the practical factors that can affect their work with clients.

Conditional Reasoning

The teaching strategies listed in Table 1 for conditional reasoning are meant to give students experience with in-

tegrating narrative, interactive, procedural, and pragmatic reasoning in the planning or implementation of treatment. Level I experiences that allow students to work with some of the same clients for several weeks so that they can develop an appreciation for client change over time are particularly effective for promoting conditional reasoning. Levine and Gitlin (1990), for example, described a teaching model where occupational therapy students work individually with community-based clients with chronic disabilities over the course of a semester (6–10 visits averaging 1 hour or more). The students used a participant–observer approach to data collection to identify the client's world, functional performance, social interactions and networks, and environment. That information was used as the basis for collaborative problem solving with clients about adaptive equipment or activity modifications to meet the client's identified needs. This fieldwork model forces students to use all types of clinical reasoning in a real clinical situation. Faculty members can also help students pull the different aspects of clinical reasoning together by modeling conditional reasoning through "professional self-talk" (Rogers, 1982, p. 29), that is, through explaining their thought processes during videotaped or recalled exemplar clinical incidents (Farrell & Bramadat, 1990).

Conclusion

In the current health care climate, occupational therapists need to be effective and efficient enough in their clinical thinking to deliver quality client services in the context of constantly changing organizational structures. To function well in this environment, entry-level practitioners need to progress quickly to the competent therapist stage of clinical reasoning, be able to alter their procedures as needed for specific situations, and prioritize client problems. Teaching strategies that are explicitly aimed at improving the clinical reasoning skills of occupational therapy students may speed their ultimate progression through the stages of clinical reasoning by helping them learn about their thinking and doing simultaneously during their clinical experience.

Many of the clinical reasoning teaching strategies suggested in this article will sound familiar to faculty members in occupational therapy educational programs. What may not sound familiar is the description of these learning experiences in terms of the types of clinical reasoning they are likely to facilitate. By specifically naming the types of reasoning they are trying to help students develop, occupational therapy educators can help them become aware of their own clinical reasoning skills and lay the foundation for the continued development of occupational therapy graduates' clinical reasoning abilities. ▲

Appendix A
Analysis of Therapeutic Self Assignment

One of the most important tools that you bring to the therapeutic situation is your self. The purpose of this paper is to help you start thinking about that self in a focused way so that you become more aware of the personal resources that you can bring to therapeutic relationships.

In an 8- to 10-page paper:

1. Describe your personal style, referencing the following qualities. In your descriptions, include examples of illustrative behaviors that you have demonstrated in clinical helping relationships. (You may want to reflect on your Level I experiences.) The following qualities are in alphabetical order—you do not have to follow this order in your paper. Rather, we would like you to choose whatever organization works best for you. The comments after each quality are meant simply to give you some ideas or to clarify the concepts.

   a. Affect, emotional tone (enthusiastic, energetic, serious, low key)
   b. Attending and listening (including your ability to reflect back on and add to what the speaker has said)
   c. Cognitive style (detail or gestalt oriented, abstract or concrete, ability to understand diverse points of view)
   d. Confidence (not only what you feel, but also what you think you show to others)
   e. Confrontation (can you do it and with whom?)
   f. Empathy (for what emotions, in what situations?)
   g. Humor (do you use it, and if so, how?)
   h. Leadership style (directive, facilitative, follower)
   i. Nonverbal communication (facial expressiveness, eye contact, voice tone and volume, gestures)
   j. Power sharing (need to control, comfortable with chaos)
   k. Probing (when are you comfortable doing it, with whom, and about what?)
   l. Touch (do you use it automatically or consciously, when, where, and with whom?)
   m. Verbal communication (vocabulary, use of vernacular, ease of speaking)

2. Summarize what you see as your strengths and weaknesses relative to establishing therapeutic relationships.

3. In anticipation of your upcoming Level II fieldwork experience, delineate areas or skills that you would like to improve and suggest strategies for doing so.

You will be graded on your organization, the clarity of your writing (including how well your examples illustrate your descriptions), and your thoroughness in completing the assignment. Content here is personal and, therefore, not gradable.

Note. Developed by Maureen E. Neistadt, ScD, OTR/L, FAOTA, for the Interactive Reasoning Seminar at Tufts University, Medford, Massachusetts, 1989.

Appendix B
Case Study Exam Example

Case Study

M. G. is a 24-year-old woman who is a right-handed, married, computer programmer with no children. For the past few months, she has been working a lot of overtime and has often worked 70 hours per week. She has gone to her physician complaining of intermittent numbness in her wrists and hands and pain in her upper arm. When she first started having problems with her hands about 2 weeks ago, she was experiencing intermittent pins and needles in her wrists and hands and pain in her upper arm. Her hands are now swollen, particularly over their dorsal surfaces. She is experiencing more symptoms in her right hand than in her left. She has been referred to occupational therapy as an outpatient for splinting.

Study Question

What is M. G.'s medical diagnosis? What sensory and motor problems would you expect to find in M. G.'s hand as a result of the diagnosis? What types of grasps would she be likely to have trouble with? List five activities that might be difficult for her and explain why those particular activities would be hard.

   Test Questions
   1. M. G.'s most likely medical diagnosis is:
      a. Reflex Sympathetic Dystrophy
      b. cumulative trauma disorder in her wrists
      c. Thoracic Outlet Syndrome
      d. compression of her cervical nerve roots
   2. M. G.'s pattern of swelling indicates:
      a. damage to the dorsal structures in her hands
      b. inflammation in the dorsum of her hands
      c. poor posture at her workstation
      d. the inflammation at the site of her diagnosis has overtaxed the lymphatic drainage and venous return systems

Appendix C
Metacognitive Questions for Students to Ask Themselves During Evaluation and Reassessment

Data Search
   "What decisions have I made to narrow my data search?"
   "Have I used all available types and sources of data?"
   "Have I collected all the data I need?"
   "Am I clear on the meaning of the data?"

Cue Clustering
   "What are some possibilities for clustering of cues?"
   "What experiences have I had before with these cues and how did I cluster them?"
   "Is there a logic to the cue clusters?"
   "Have I distinguished relevant from irrelevant cues?"
   "What diagnostic hypotheses am I generating based on cues clustered?"
   "Are the diagnostic hypotheses within the domain of [occupational therapy] practice?"

Planning

"How do I plan to turn the problem into an outcome?"

"What [occupational therapy] interventions do I plan to influence the [problem]?"

"Creatively, what [occupational therapy] interventions can I develop to influence the [problem]?"

"Are my plans useful, effective, and efficient?"

Reassessment

"Do the [occupational therapy] interventions need to be revised?"

"Does the patient outcome need to be revised?"

"Does the problem/etiology need to be revised?"

"Do the cue clusters need to be revised?"

"Does the data search field need to be reshaped?"

(Pesut & Herman, 1992, pp. 152–153)

References

Benner, P. (1984). *From novice to expert. Excellence and power in clinical nursing practice.* Reading, MA: Addison-Wesley.

Clark, F. (1993). Occupation embedded in a real life: Interweaving occupational science and occupational therapy, 1993 Eleanor Clarke Slagle Lecture. *American Journal of Occupational Therapy, 47,* 1067–1078.

Creighton, C., Dijkers, M., Bennett, N., & Brown, K. (1995). Reasoning and the art of therapy for spinal cord injury. *American Journal of Occupational Therapy, 49,* 311–317.

Crepeau, E. B. (1991). Achieving intersubjective understanding: Examples from an occupational therapy treatment session. *American Journal of Occupational Therapy, 45,* 1016–1025.

Cohn, E. S. (1989). Fieldwork education: Shaping a foundation for clinical reasoning. *American Journal of Occupational Therapy, 43,* 240–244.

Dreyfus, H. L., & Dreyfus, S. E. (1986). *Mind over machine. The power of human intuition and expertise in the era of the computer.* New York: Free Press.

Dutton, R. (1995). *Clinical reasoning in physical disabilities.* Baltimore: Williams & Wilkins.

Farrell, P., & Bramadat, I. J. (1990). Paradigm case analysis and stimulated recall: Strategies for developing clinical reasoning skills. *Clinical Nurse Specialist, 4,* 153–157.

Field, E. (1992). Use of debate format to facilitate problem-solving skills and critical thinking. *Journal of Physical Therapy Education, 6,* 3–5.

Fleming, M. H. (1991a). Clinical reasoning in medicine compared with clinical reasoning in occupational therapy. *American Journal of Occupational Therapy, 45,* 988–996.

Fleming, M. H. (1991b). The therapist with the three-track mind. *American Journal of Occupational Therapy, 45,* 1007–1014.

Hall, L., Robertson, W., & Turner, M. A. (1992). Clinical reasoning process for service provision in the public school. *American Journal of Occupational Therapy, 46,* 927–936.

Hasselkus, B. R., & Dickie, V. A. (1994). Doing occupational therapy: Dimensions of satisfaction and dissatisfaction. *American Journal of Occupational Therapy, 48,* 145–154.

Higgs, J. (1990). Fostering the acquisition of clinical reasoning skills. *New Zealand Journal of Physiotherapy, 18*(3), 13–17.

Higgs, J. (1992). Developing clinical reasoning competencies. *Physiotherapy, 78,* 575–581.

Kautzmann, L. N. (1993). Linking patient and family stories to caregivers' use of clinical reasoning. *American Journal of Occupational Therapy, 47,* 169–173.

Levine, R. E., & Gitlin, L. N. (1990). Home adaptations for persons with chronic disabilities: An educational model. *American Journal of Occupational Therapy, 44,* 923–929.

Mattingly, C. (1991a). The narrative nature of clinical reasoning. *American Journal of Occupational Therapy, 45,* 998–1005.

Mattingly, C. (1991b). What is clinical reasoning? *American Journal of Occupational Therapy, 45,* 979–986.

Mattingly, C., & Fleming, M. H. (1994). *Clinical reasoning: Forms of inquiry in a therapeutic practice.* Philadelphia: F. A. Davis.

Miller, S. (1990). *Family pictures.* New York: Harper Paperbacks.

Murphy, R. F. (1990). *The body silent.* New York: Norton.

Neistadt, M. E. (1987). Classroom as clinic: A model for teaching clinical reasoning in occupational therapy education. *American Journal of Occupational Therapy, 41,* 631–637.

Neistadt, M. E. (1992). The classroom as clinic: Applications for a method of teaching clinical reasoning. *American Journal of Occupational Therapy, 46,* 814–819.

Neistadt, M. E., & Cohn, E. S. (1990). Evaluating a Level I fieldwork model for independent living skills. *American Journal of Occupational Therapy, 44,* 692–699.

Neuhaus, B. E. (1988). Ethical considerations in clinical reasoning: The impact of technology and cost containment. *American Journal of Occupational Therapy, 42,* 288–294.

Parham, D. (1987). Nationally Speaking—Toward professionalism: The reflective therapist. *American Journal of Occupational Therapy, 41,* 555–561.

Payton, O. D., Nelson, C. E., & Ozer, M. N. (1990). *Patient participation in program planning: A manual for therapists.* Philadelphia: F. A. Davis.

Peloquin, S. M. (1989). Sustaining the art of practice in occupational therapy. *American Journal of Occupational Therapy, 43,* 219–226.

Peloquin, S. M. (1990). The patient–therapist relationship in occupational therapy: Understanding visions and images. *American Journal of Occupational Therapy, 44,* 13–21.

Peloquin, S. M. (1995). The fullness of empathy: Reflections and illustrations. *American Journal of Occupational Therapy, 49,* 24–31.

Peloquin, S. M., & Davidson, D. A. (1993). Brief or New—Interpersonal skills for practice: An elective course. *American Journal of Occupational Therapy, 47,* 260–264[1].

Pesut, D. J., & Herman, J. (1992). Metacognitive skills in diagnostic reasoning: Making the implicit explicit. *Nursing Diagnosis, 3,* 148–154.

Pollock, N. (1993). Client-centered assessment. *American Journal of Occupational Therapy, 47,* 298–301.

Rogers, J. C. (1982). Teaching clinical reasoning for practice in geriatrics. *Physical and Occupational Therapy in Geriatrics, 1,* 29–37.

Rogers, J. C. (1983). Eleanor Clarke Slagle Lectureship—1983; Clinical reasoning: The ethics, science, and art. *American Journal of Occupational Therapy, 37,* 601–616.

Rogers, J. C., & Holm, M. B. (1991). Occupational therapy diagnostic reasoning: A component of clinical reasoning. *American Journal of Occupational Therapy, 45,* 1045–1053.

Royeen, C. B. (1995). A problem-based learning curriculum for

---

[1]See reference list at the end of article for additional reading sources.

occupational therapy education. *American Journal of Occupational Therapy, 49,* 338–346.

Rydeen, K., Kautzmann, L., Cowan, M. K., & Benzing, P. (1995). Three faculty-facilitated, community-based Level I fieldwork programs. *American Journal of Occupational Therapy, 49,* 112–118.

Sands, M. (1995). Brief or New—Readying occupational therapy assistant students for Level II fieldwork: Beyond academics to personal behaviors and attitudes. *American Journal of Occupational Therapy, 49,* 150–152.

Schell, B. A., & Cervero, R. M. (1993). Clinical reasoning in occupational therapy: An integrative review. *American Journal of Occupational Therapy, 47,* 605–610[2].

Schwartz, K. B. (1991). Clinical reasoning and new ideas on intelligence: Implications for teaching and learning. *American Journal of Occupational Therapy, 45,* 1033–1037.

Slater, D. Y., & Cohn, E. S. (1991). Staff development through analysis of practice. *American Journal of Occupational Therapy, 45,* 1038–1044.

Terry, W., & Higgs, J. (1993). Educational programmes to develop clinical reasoning skills. *Australian Journal of Physiotherapy, 39,* 47–51.

Tryssenaar, J. (1995). Interactive journals: An educational strategy to promote reflection. *American Journal of Occupational Therapy, 49,* 695–702.

VanLeit, B. (1995). Using the case method to develop clinical reasoning skills in problem-based learning. *American Journal of Occupational Therapy, 49,* 349–353.

Zimmerman, S. S. (1995). Brief or New—Cooperative education: An alternative Level I fieldwork. *American Journal of Occupational Therapy, 49,* 153–155.

---

[2]See reference list at the end of article for additional reading sources.

38 | Cognitive Learning Styles and Clinical Reasoning

The Classroom as Clinic: Applications for a Method of Teaching Clinical Reasoning

Maureen E. Neistadt

Key Words: education • evaluation studies

This study examined the efficacy of one method for teaching diagnostic reasoning to occupational therapy students. During a clinical reasoning seminar in their first academic year, 80 entry-level occupational therapy master's degree students in three successive classes were given three different levels of exposure to classroom-as-clinic or in-class evaluations of adults with physical or psychosocial disabilities. During the following summer, most students completed their first Level II fieldwork experience. Students' grades for a second-year classroom-as-clinic experience with adults with physial disabilities were then compared across groups to determine the relative effect of the different seminar formats and fieldwork experiences. Students who had experienced in-class evaluations during their first academic year wrote significantly more accurate second-year evaluations than those who had not. Students who had completed psychosocial Level II fieldwork experiences were as accurate on their evaluations as students who had had physical dysfunction fieldwork experiences. The results suggest that in-class evaluations improve students' diagnostic reasoning skills.

Maureen E. Neistadt, ScD, OTR/L, is Assistant Professor, Occupational Therapy Department, University of New Hampshire, Hewitt Hall, Durham, New Hampshire 03824–3563. At the time of this study she was Assistant Professor, Tufts University–Boston School of Occupational Therapy, Medford, Massachusetts.

This article was accepted for publication April 10, 1992.

Skill in clinical reasoning is essential for effective occupational therapy practice (Fleming, 1991; Parham, 1987; Rogers, 1983; Slater & Cohn, 1991). "Clinical reasoning is a dynamic process of inquiry in action that takes place in the context of occupational therapy evaluation and treatment" (Tufts University–Boston School of Occupational Therapy [BSOT], 1990, p. 3). Schwartz (1991) recently highlighted the need for occupational therapy education programs to develop and implement teaching methodologies that encourage the development of students' clinical reasoning abilities.

In 1987, I described a *classroom-as-clinic* method designed to teach occupational therapy students the clinical reasoning process associated with evaluation and treatment planning. A previous study demonstrated that this method improved occupational therapy students' abilities to accurately analyze preassessment data and formulate appropriate treatment plans (Neistadt, 1987). Students in that study engaged in classroom-based evaluations of adults with physical disabilities at the end of an occupational therapy curriculum, after they had taken all of their nonelective course work and before they had begun their Level II fieldwork experiences. One question raised by that study was whether in-class evaluations of adults with physical or psychosocial disabilities would effectively teach clinical reasoning earlier in an occupational therapy curriculum. The present study addressed this question.

Literature Review

Rogers and Masagatani (1982) and Rogers (1983) originally described therapists' thought processes during initial evaluations as involving a sequence of deduction, induction, dialectical reasoning, and ethical reasoning. Therapists, said these authors, begin their evaluations with a review of clients' charts or other preassessment information that might be available or both. From this review, therapists form hypotheses about possible problems of clients through a process of deduction. Therapists evaluate their clients, then modify their preassessment hypotheses by considering the specific details of clients' cases (induction) and deciding between different interpretations for clients' behaviors (dialectical reasoning). Therapists then work with their clients to establish treatment priorities consistent with the clients' value systems (ethical reasoning).

More recently, Rogers and Holm (1991) referred to the thought processes that occupational therapists use during initial evaluation as *diagnostic reasoning*. Diagnostic reasoning "is the sequence of decisions that leads to occupational therapy diagnosis" and "is one component of the clinical reasoning involved in the occupational therapy process" (Rogers & Holm, 1991, p. 1045). The occupational therapy diagnosis "describes the actual or potential effects of disease, trauma, developmental disorders, age-associated changes, environmental deprivation, and other etiologic agents on occupational status" (Rogers & Holm, 1991, p. 1045). This occupational therapy diagnosis becomes the foundation for collaborative treatment planning with the client.

According to Rogers and Holm (1991), the diagnostic reasoning process involves both problem sensing and problem definition. "A therapist senses a problem by framing it, that is, by deciding what will be included in the picture. The picture inside that frame is the clinical image" (Rogers & Holm, 1991, p. 1045). This formation of clinical images begins during the chart review stage of assessment and is influenced by the reason for occupational therapy referral; the practice setting; the experience and frames of reference of the therapist; and the client's condition, age, and sex. The severity of the client's condition will also influence the clinical image (Rogers & Holm, 1991). This clinical image would include mental hypotheses about the client's potential problems—hypotheses formed through deductive reasoning about the information available from the chart review and other preassessment information (Rogers, 1983; Rogers & Masagatani, 1982).

Problem definition is a process in which the therapist concisely and precisely describes and names the client's problems. "As a result of this descriptive process, the therapist's clinical image of a client becomes more like the actual client encountered in the clinic" (Rogers & Holm, 1991, p. 1045). Therapists engage in the problem-definition process during the initial evaluation of a client. Rogers and Holm presented an information-processing perspective on problem definition that sees the therapist as a data processor and the client and the client's living situation as the data field. The therapist "collects, organizes, analyzes, and synthesizes data about a client's occupational status" (Rogers & Holm, 1991, p. 1048). As a data processor, the therapist uses "four basic processes: cue acquisition, hypothesis generation, cue interpretation, and hypothesis evaluation" (Rogers & Holm, 1991, p. 1048). Cues are data to which therapists attend. Therapists interpret the cues gathered during initial evaluation to test their preassessment hypotheses and to form and test new hypotheses. They use dialectic process to weigh the relative merits of alternative hypotheses and ethical reasoning to consider the influence of clients' values and motivations on problem definitions.

As Rogers and Holm (1991) have suggested, diagnostic reasoning is only one component of occupational therapists' clinical reasoning process. Fleming (1991) has suggested that occupational therapists simultaneously use three different ways of thinking: procedural, interactive, and conditional. Therapists use *procedural reasoning* to focus on diagnosis and disability by following a logical medical decision-making process of problem identification, goal setting, and treatment planning that uses their medical, technical, and occupational knowledge.

Fleming's procedural reasoning corresponds to Rogers and Holm's diagnostic reasoning. Therapists use *interactive reasoning* during meetings with clients to try to understand how the client makes sense of the disability or disease and how that disability or disease interferes with the roles and activities that give that person's life meaning. Therapists use *conditional reasoning* to think about the client's future, "given the constraints of the physical condition within the client's personal and social context" (Fleming, 1991, p. 1013).

During chart review, therapists use primarily procedural (diagnostic) reasoning. Experienced clinicians might also use conditional reasoning at this stage to begin forming an image of the client's future, given the diagnosis, prognosis, and social and vocational history. During a client evaluation, therapists combine procedural (diagnostic), interactive, and conditional reasoning to observe, elicit, and interpret cues so they can develop a treatment plan that is meaningful to the client.

Cohn (1991) stated that occupational therapy clinicians and clinical educators frequently complain "that academic programs do not adequately prepare students for the uncertainties inherent in the challenges of practice" (p. 969). Perhaps these complaints arise because the traditional teaching and testing methodologies of higher education cannot foster the complex array of reasoning skills that occupational therapists must use in practice. More experiential teaching modes that use testing methods linked to clinical practice might teach clinical reasoning better (Schwartz, 1991). The primary purpose of the present experimental study was to see whether a modified classroom-as-clinic method in the first year of an entry-level master's degree program would improve the clinical reasoning skills of students by the second year of their program, as measured by performance in a classroom-as-clinic experience at the beginning of the second academic year. A secondary purpose was to assess the effects of Level II fieldwork experiences on these students' second-year classroom-as-clinic performances.

Method

Design

A post hoc experimental design was used to compare the second year classroom-as-clinic performances of three independent groups of students. As a result of ongoing curriculum development, three successive groups of students were given three different levels of exposure to classroom-as-clinic or in-class evaluations of adults with physical or psychosocial disabilities during a clinical reasoning seminar in the second semester of their first academic year.

Subjects

The subjects in this study were 80 entry-level master's degree students at Tufts University–Boston School of Occupational Therapy, Medford, Massachusetts. Subjects were members of three successive groups of students attending the university between the years 1989 and 1992 (for Group 1, $n = 21$; Group 2, $n = 31$; Group 3, $n = 28$). Their ages ranged from 22 years to 40 years. Five subjects were men and 75 were women. The average preadmission grade point average was 3.1 for all three groups of students.

All subjects took their basic science, pathology, and introductory occupational therapy course work in their first academic year. As part of the first academic year's work, all subjects participated in clinical reasoning seminars on observation skills and interactive reasoning during their first and second semesters, respectively. Subjects also took either a psychosocial or physical dysfunction course in the second semester of their first year, to prepare them for a first summer Level II fieldwork corresponding to the dysfunction course they had taken. Some subjects elected not to do a Level II fieldwork that first summer for personal or financial reasons. In the first semester of the second year, all subjects participated in an advanced occupational therapy course that used the classroom-as-clinic teaching method. The second-year course work included clinical reasoning seminars on procedural and conditional reasoning in the first and second semesters, respectively. Additional course work in pediatrics and in the major dysfunction course not taken in the first year was also offered. Most subjects completed their second Level II fieldwork in the summer after the second academic year, with the remaining subjects completing their first and second Level II fieldwork at this time.

For Group 1, the interactive reasoning seminar did not include contact with persons with physical or psychosocial disabilities. The goal in this first seminar was to improve subjects' self-awareness so that they would be able to interact as therapeutic agents with future clients. Lectures and small group exercises about interviewing, empathy, and nonverbal communication were used. Subjects expressed dissatisfaction with the lack of client contact in this seminar. Consequently, the interactive seminar for Group 2 included in-class student group interviews with persons with physical or psychosocial disabilities. Faculty thought that this interview experience helped students develop their interactive reasoning skills, but that it did not force students to use interactive reasoning in conjunction with procedural and conditional reasoning, as would be required in clinical evaluations and treatment. Therefore, the interactive seminar for Group 3 included modified classroom-as-clinic experiences.

Course outlines, testing methods, and Level I fieldwork for all courses but the interactive seminar remained constant during the study period. Group 3 had a different instructor than Groups 1 and 2 for two psychosocial courses and one pathology course. Otherwise, course instructors remained constant throughout the study period.

Procedure

The format of the classroom-as-clinic experience was based on Rogers' model of clinical reasoning during initial evaluation (Rogers, 1983) and has already been described in detail (Neistadt, 1987). During these experiences, the subjects were expected to write a problem-goal-plan list after reviewing limited preassessment information (i.e., diagnosis and social situation) and to revise that list after interviewing a guest participant with a physical or psychosocial disability. In the original classroom-as-clinic method, which was used in the advanced occupational therapy course at the beginning of the subjects' second year, subjects did not receive any information on the diagnosis of the guest participant before the day of the in-class evaluation and were expected to write their first problem-goal-plan list in the 30 to 40 min immediately preceding their meeting with the guest participant. For this first second-year evaluation, the guest participants all had conditions diagnosed as central nervous system dysfunction. In the modified in-class evaluation used in the first-year interactive reasoning seminar for subjects in Group 3, subjects received preassessment information about the guest participants 1 week in advance and were given 1 week to work on their initial problem-goal-plan lists at home, using their books and class notes as references. For all in-class evaluations, subjects met in small groups with one guest participant for 90 min and then wrote revised problem-goal-plan lists which they then handed in at the end of class.

The grades on the problem-goal-plan lists represented the percentage of correct problems that the subjects recorded from a list of expected problems for a given diagnosis or guest participant. The preassessment or chart review *correct problems lists* were derived from the Uniform Occupational Therapy Evaluation Checklist (American Occupational Therapy Association, 1981). Problem areas specific to particular diagnoses were selected from this list according to the occupational therapy literature and the instructor's clinical experience. The postassessment or evaluation correct problems lists were also derived from the uniform checklist and were based on the clinical experience of the instructor and the clinical observations of the faculty coleaders in the guest participants' groups. The grading procedure, course instructor, and guest participants were the same for all three subject groups.

Results

Subjects' grades on the chart review and evaluation problem-goal-plan lists for the first classroom-as-clinic experience in the second year were analyzed with two-way analyses of variance and Tukey pairwise comparisons (Cody & Smith, 1987). Subject group during the first year and Level II fieldwork during the first summer were the independent variables, and grades on the second-year problem-goal-plan lists were the dependent variables in these analyses. A significance level of .05 was used.

Chart Review Lists

For the chart review lists, there was no significant effect for either subject group [F (2, 71) = 2.47, p = .0919] or type of Level II fieldwork [F (2, 71) = 0.60, p = .5495]. Tukey pairwise comparisons showed no significant differences in chart review grades among any of the three subject groups (see Tables 1 and 2).

There was a significant group by Level II fieldwork interaction [F (2, 71) = 3.05, p = .0224] in the chart review analysis of variance. When the sample was sorted by groups, one-way analyses of variance with Level II fieldwork as the independent variable and chart review grades as the dependent variable showed a significant Level II fieldwork effect only for Group 1 [F (2, 18) = 4.36, p = .0286]. Tukey pairwise comparisons for this group showed significant differences in chart review grades between subjects who had had physical dysfunction Level II fieldwork and those who had had psychosocial Level II fieldwork. The former scored an average of 90.7%; the latter, an average of 79.7%.

Evaluation Lists

For the evaluation lists, there were significant effects for both group [F(2, 71) = 11.74, p = .0001] and Level II fieldwork [F(2, 71) = 4.27, p = .0177]. There was no significant group by Level II fieldwork interaction [F(2, 71) = 1.12, p = .3558]. Tukey pairwise comparisons showed significant differences in evaluation list grades among all three groups (see Table 1) and between those subjects who had had physical dysfunction Level II fieldwork and those who had not done any Level II fieldwork in the preceding summer (see Table 2). Paired t-test comparisons showed that only Group 3, with the in-class evaluation experience, improved significantly from the chart review to the evaluation list grades (see Table 2).

Table 1
Tukey Pairwise Comparison of Average Grades for Subject Groups

Group	Chart Review Lists		Evaluation Lists	
	M (%)	SD	M (%)	SD
1 (n = 21)	87.1	9.4	84.5	9.1
2 (n = 31)	90.4	9.9	90.9	9.0
3 (n = 28)	92.8	6.5	97.3	4.9

Note. For Group 1, the interactive reasoning seminar did not include contact with persons with physical or psychosocial disabilities. For Group 2, the interactive seminar included in-class student group interviews with persons with physical or psychosocial disabilities. For Group 3, the interactive seminar included modified classroom-as-clinic experiences.

Table 2
Tukey Pairwise Comparison of Average Grades for Level II Fieldwork Experiences

Level II Fieldwork	Chart Review Lists		Evaluation Lists	
	M (%)	SD	M (%)	SD
Physical dysfunction (n = 32)	90.9	8.2	94.3	8.8
Psychosocial dysfunction (n = 34)	90.5	9.2	90.3	9.1
None (n = 14)	89.1	10.1	87.7	9.3

Note. Preadmission grade point average was comparable for all Level II fieldwork groups.

Discussion

Results suggest that the use of in-class evaluations of adults with physical or psychosocial dysfunction during the first year of an entry-level master's program helps students to develop their clinical reasoning skills. The general consistency of instructors, content, and teaching and testing methods for other courses in the curriculum during the study period strongly suggests that the results are related to the in-class evaluation variable. Subjects who had experienced in-class evaluations during their first academic year were significantly more accurate than those who had not experienced in-class evaluations in writing evaluation problem-goal-plan lists for an in-class evaluation experience in the second academic year. Results for both the chart review and evaluation lists are discussed below.

Chart Review Lists

Subject groups. The lack of significant differences between the three different subject groups on the second-year chart review lists suggests that skill with this part of the evaluation process is not strongly affected by interaction with adults with physical or psychosocial disabilities in the first academic year. Although not statistically significant, a trend emerged showing that subjects with interview experience in the first year did better than those with no interview experience and that those with a modified classroom-as-clinic experience did better than those with only interview experience (see Table 1).

In my previous classroom-as-clinic study, I reported that students had repeatedly said that "meeting adults with disabilities helps them to make sense of and 'picture' the theoretical information they have learned in the classroom" (Neistadt, 1987, p. 634). The interview experiences may have given subjects some beginning clinical images (Rogers & Holm, 1991) of people with particular disabilities, and retrieving these images may have helped them write more accurate chart review lists in the second academic year. Subjects who were forced to contrast their preassessment and postassessment images in the modified classroom-as-clinic experience may have had more vivid and accurate clinical images to draw on in the second year of their program.

Fieldwork experiences. The lack of significant differences among the three different Level II fieldwork experiences (physical dysfunction, psychosocial dysfunction, none) on the second-year chart review lists suggests that skill with this part of the evaluation process is also not strongly affected by interaction with adults with physical or psychosocial disabilities during fieldwork. However, there was a trend for subjects with psychosocial Level II fieldwork to do better than those without Level II fieldwork experience and for those with physical dysfunction Level II fieldwork to do better than those with psychosocial experience (see Table 2).

The preassessment list is primarily an exercise in problem sensing (Rogers & Holm, 1991). Subjects without Level II fieldwork would have missed intensive practice with the problem-sensing process. The psychosocial Level II fieldwork would have given subjects practice with problem sensing for adults with psychosocial dysfunctions, whereas the physical dysfunction Level II fieldwork would have provided practice with problem sensing for adults with physical disabilities. Because the guest participants in the second-year classroom-as-clinic examined here all had physical disabilities, one would expect the physical disability Level II fieldwork problem-sensing experience to be more applicable; however, the differences between the performances of all subjects who had done psychosocial and physical dysfunction Level II fieldwork were not significant. The significant difference in chart review accuracy between subjects with different Level II fieldwork experiences within Group 1 is most likely related to a few weak subjects in the psychosocial group whose grades lowered the entire psychosocial average. Rogers and Holm have said that "diagnostic reasoning is generic to all practice areas" (Rogers & Holm, 1991, p. 1047). These chart review results suggest that the problem-sensing part of diagnostic reasoning, in particular, can be generalized across treatment settings.

Evaluation Lists

Subject groups. The significant differences among the three subject groups on the second-year evaluation lists suggests that students' skill with this part of the evaluation process is strongly affected by interaction with adults with physical or psychosocial disabilities in the first academic year. Subjects with interview experience in the first year did significantly better than those without interview experience, and those with a modified classroom-as-clinic experience did significantly better than those with either no interview or only interview experience (see Table 1).

This result suggests that the classroom-as-clinic experience provided subjects with practice in using the combination of interactive, procedural, and conditional reasoning that Fleming (1991) has said is essential to clinical evaluation. Practice in constantly switching from one type of reasoning to the other during a time-pressured meeting with an adult with a disability may help students to hone their problem-definition skills (Rogers & Holm, 1991). That is, the first year in-class evaluations seemed to make subjects more proficient at observing, eliciting, and interpreting cues during an initial interview. Consequently, in their second year, subjects could describe guest participant problems more accurately than could subjects who had not experienced the classroom-as-clinic method. The finding that only the subjects who had the classroom-as-clinic experience in their first year improved significantly from the chart review to evaluation lists in their second year further supports the notion that this teaching method improves students' reasoning abilities during the client evaluation process.

Fieldwork experiences. The lack of significant differences between the subjects with physical dysfunction Level II fieldwork and psychosocial Level II fieldwork experiences on the second-year evaluation lists suggests that Level II fieldwork in either practice setting provides students with generalizable experience in combining procedural, interactive, and conditional reasoning to yield accurate client-specific problem definitions. The trend for subjects with physical dysfunction Level II fieldwork to do better than those with psychosocial Level II fieldwork (see Table 2) may relate, again, to practice with the population seen in the second-year classroom-as-clinic experience. Rogers & Holm (1991) have suggested that recency, intensity, and frequency of practice with particular populations will influence the accuracy of problem definition, even though the general process of diagnostic reasoning can be applied across practice settings.

The significant difference between subjects with physical dysfunction Level II fieldwork and those without Level II fieldwork on the second-year evaluation lists probably also relates to the Level II fieldwork practice the former had with the population seen in second-year classroom-as-clinic experience. The lack of significant differences in evaluation list scores between subjects with psychosocial dysfunction Level II fieldwork and those without Level II fieldwork may relate to the lack of Level II fieldwork practice for either group in evaluating a physical dysfunction population, but the trend was for the subjects with psychosocial Level II fieldwork to score better than those without Level II fieldwork. This trend probably reflects the former's Level II fieldwork practice with diagnostic and interactive reasoning.

Conclusion

The results of this study suggest that the use of the classroom-as-clinic teaching method in the first year of an entry-level master's program helps to improve students' clinical reasoning during the clinical evaluation process. The use of this method early in an occupational therapy curriculum may also give students an experiential base for

Cognitive Learning Styles and Clinical Reasoning | 43

their concurrent and subsequent didactic and theoretical learning. Belenky, Clinchy, Goldberger, and Tarule (1986) suggested that providing experience as a base for theoretical learning is an important part of what they called *connected teaching*. The small student group interview component of the classroom-as-clinic experience and the processing of the experiences in subsequent classes (Neistadt, 1987) allow for collaboration and evolution of personal knowledge through open discussion, which is another aspect of connected teaching (Schwartz, 1991).

Research on the effect of the classroom-as-clinic method on Level II fieldwork and early practice performance would be helpful in further validating this teaching method. Additional research on the relative effect of different aspects of the method might help refine the method and provide guidelines on modifications needed for different groups of students at different points in occupational therapy curricula.

Provision of training in clinical reasoning may be the best educational strategy for preparing clinicians to meet the complex demands of modern practice. This study has examined the relative efficacy of one method for providing that training. Other methods for teaching clinical reasoning need to be developed, tested, and shared so that occupational therapy can continue to evolve to meet the ongoing challenges of health care provision. ▲

References

American Occupational Therapy Association. (1981). Uniform Occupational Therapy Evaluation Checklist. *American Journal of Occupational Therapy, 35,* 817–818.

Belenky, M. F., Clinchy, B. V., Goldberger, N. R., & Tarule, J. M. (1986). *Women's ways of knowing.* New York: Basic.

Cody, R. P., & Smith, J. K. (1987). *Applied statistics and the SAS programming language* (2nd ed.). New York: North-Holland.

Cohn, E. S. (1991). Nationally Speaking—Clinical reasoning: Explicating complexity. *American Journal of Occupational Therapy, 45,* 969–971.

Fleming, M. H. (1991). The therapist with the three-track mind. *American Journal of Occupational Therapy, 45* 1007–1014.

Neistadt, M. E. (1987). Classroom as clinic: A model for teaching clinical reasoning in occupational therapy education. *American Journal of Occupational Therapy, 41,* 631–637.

Parham, D. (1987). Nationally Speaking—Toward professionalism: The reflective therapist. *American Journal of Occupational Therapy, 41,* 555–561.

Rogers, J. C. (1983). Eleanor Clarke Slagle lectureship–1983—Clinical reasoning: The ethics, science and art. *American Journal of Occupational Therapy, 37,* 601–616.

Rogers, J. C., & Holm, M. B. (1991). Occupational therapy diagnostic reasoning: A component of clinical reasoning. *American Journal of Occupational Therapy, 45,* 1045–1053.

Rogers, J. C., & Masagatani, G. (1982). Clinical reasoning of occupational therapists during the initial assessment of physically disabled patients. *Occupational Therapy Journal of Research, 2,* 195–219.

Schwartz, K. B. (1991). Clinical reasoning and new ideas on intelligence: Implications for teaching and learning. *American Journal of Occupational Therapy, 45,* 1033–1037.

Slater, D. Y., & Cohn, E. S. (1991). Staff development through analysis of practice. *American Journal of Occupational Therapy, 45,* 1038–1044.

Tufts University–Boston School of Occupational Therapy. (1990). *Master's degree programs in occupational therapy.* Medford, MA: Tufts University.

Ethical Considerations in Clinical Reasoning: The Impact of Technology and Cost Containment

Barbara E. Neuhaus

Key Words: ethics, professional • values clarification

This article raises, but does not answer, the kinds of questions that need to be asked by responsible occupational therapists in the 1980s—ethical questions that deal with technological advances on the one hand and limited resources on the other. The article examines moral dilemmas that practitioners and students face when making clinical decisions in a climate where technology and cost containment may overshadow the needs of the individual patient. A review of the literature on clinical reasoning, technology, and cost containment provides the background for a discussion of specific issues of quality of life for the occupational therapist. Implications for education and practice are presented, with suggestions for further consideration.

Barbara E. Neuhaus, EdD, OTR, FAOTA, is Associate Professor and Director of Programs in Occupational Therapy, Columbia University, New York, New York 10032.

The complex nature of clinical reasoning has intrigued and plagued physicians, philosophers, psychologists, and educators since the time of Hippocrates, when doctors first insisted on the importance of observation of patients, refined by reason. Many disciplines have rightfully claimed a stake in the work on clinical reasoning. The debate on whether to label clinical reasoning art or science continues in the growing tension between what Elstein (1976) calls the scientific-actuarial and the artist-intuitionist models of clinical judgment. While the former attempts to use logic or decision theory to transform the process into a respectable science, the latter declares that it is an art, not subject to scientific analysis, and that it can be improved only as one might increase one's skill at painting or music. Rogers (1983) has settled the argument by proposing, "Without science, clinical inquiry is not systematic; without ethics, it is not responsible; without art, it is not convincing" (p. 616). Using her thoughts as a guide, it seems safe to say that clinical reasoning incorporates scientific and artistic elements directed to a specific practical end: a right action for a particular patient, given that person's situation at the time of the decision (Pellegrino & Thomasma, 1981). Since this process calls for judgment and decision making as well, the ethical elements must be equally recognized as significant factors.

Within the last decade, ethical issues have assumed increasing importance in clinical decisions. To date, the fundamental questions about effective clinical reasoning remain unanswered. In fact, they are further complicated by questions that are deeply troubling, often with multiple, conflicting opinions. In the current climate of high technology, cost containment, accountability, and quality assurance, clinicians and students must grapple with strong external pressures that can easily overshadow the needs of the individual who is perilously balancing on the threshold between autonomy, self-determination, and competence on one side and disability, dependence, and possibly death on the other.

In the 1950s the teaching of ethics still dealt mainly with such issues as not accepting gratuities from patients and not sitting on patients' beds. Now students are engaged early in their professional education in discussions of justice surrounding allocation of scarce resources. "Who shall be treated when not all can be treated?" has become a question of immediate relevance to students in their first encounters with extreme staff shortages. The sword of cost containment hangs over the heads of students and their supervisors when a monetary value is placed on human life. Hippocrates' basic, timeless admonition, "above all, do no harm," has an added dimension since technological advances have created an increasing population of survivors of heroic life-saving efforts for whom issues of quality of life are central. As occupational therapists approach the last decade of the 20th century, they are forced to reexamine personal and professional values and goals that have been the keystone of their clinical reasoning as health professionals. Engelhardt (1986) graphically describes the tensions experienced by all highly developed scientific and technological societies. He states:

> We are at present committed to providing the best of care, equally to all, while maintaining provider and receiver choice, though at the same time engaging in cost containment. It should be clear that one cannot pursue all of these four goals at the same time. We confront a conflict of values and goals. (p. 40)

This conflict becomes apparent in the education of students who are faced with baffling clinical problems that call for special reasoning, judgment, and decision making. Observing students on the arduous journey from patient history through the satisfactory resolution of a problem heightens one's awareness of the number of competing variables that vie for attention. It also points up our limited understanding of the intellectual and emotional processes involved in clinical reasoning.

The purpose of this article is to examine moral dilemmas that confront occupational therapy practitioners and students as they approach clinical decisions in a climate where technology and cost containment efforts may overshadow the needs of the individual patient. The discussion seeks to acknowledge the forceful presence of ethical issues that must be addressed in the teaching and application of clinical reasoning.

Literature Review

Clinical Reasoning

A review of the recent health care literature on clinical reasoning reveals the pervasive nature of ethical questions raised by practitioners in several disciplines. Earlier work on clinical reasoning rarely covered these issues. Up to the late 1960s there was a paucity of empirical data on clinical reasoning. In the 1970s the most definitive work was carried out by Elstein, Shulman, and Sprafka (1978), who studied the clinical reasoning of physicians in an environment that approximated medical practice. They hoped to understand the skills, strategies, competencies, or attributes that characterize the performance of skilled clinicians in order to improve or accelerate the manner in which medical students might learn to master those skills. They also explored the differences between medical problem solving and the psychological in-

vestigations of cognitive processes that had characterized all studies of problem solving in the 1950s and 1960s. These earlier studies looked at such artificial tasks for learning and cognition as rats in mazes, cats in problem boxes, and humans with memory drums. The scientists created novel situations that did not allow earlier experiences to influence the subject's performance. Elstein and his associates, along with other medical educators, postulated that clinical problem solving *does* rely heavily on past experience and the particular features of the problem being approached. These features are characterized by ambiguity, uncertainty, and inconsistency and call for development of a limited number of hunches or hypotheses to be tested in selecting the "best fit" solution for the problem at hand. Several other features distinguish clinical reasoning from general reasoning: For the health professional, there is not one right answer but, rather, multiple options, all of which may be resolutions or compromises and not solutions that are correct for all time. Similarly, clinical reasoning generally begins with incomplete information, and the reasoning is adjusted as new information is acquired or retrieved. This has led an anonymous, somewhat cynical thinker to define clinical reasoning as "the process of making adequate decisions with inadequate information" (Elstein, Shulman, & Sprafka, 1978, p. VIII).

In her Eleanor Clarke Slagle lecture, Rogers (1983) deplored the limited attention given to explicating the thinking that guides practice, despite the obvious importance of clinical judgment in the occupational therapy process. She developed an "intellectual device" (p. 602) for viewing the scientific, ethical, and artistic dimensions of clinical reasoning from the questions the therapist seeks to answer through clinical inquiry. Her model was based on a scheme of clinical judgment in medicine presented by Pellegrino and Thomasma (1981). Because of its relevance to the ethical questions presented here, this scheme for analysis of clinical judgment is further developed in this article.

To date, the only descriptive research on occupational therapists' clinical reasoning is the groundbreaking pilot study by Rogers and Masagatani (1982) of 10 therapists engaged in assessment of patients with physical problems in medical settings. The therapists' perspective for assessment focused on musculoskeletal and self-care functions, and they appeared to experience difficulty in giving reasons for their actions and explaining how they proceeded from one step to the next. Most recently, Pelland (1987) described a method of teaching clinical reasoning for treatment planning. Gillette and Mattingly (1987) reported on current clinical reasoning research in which therapists are observed during treatment and later view themselves on videotape while they explain the rationales for their actions. However, among all of these studies only the 1982 Slagle lecture (Rogers, 1983) examined the ethical components.

The model proposed earlier by Pellegrino (1979) is useful for analysis of clinical judgment. He asks three generic questions that must be answered if the process of clinical judgment is to be complete and authentic: What can be *wrong?* What can be *done?* What *should* be done? The first question, What can be wrong? yields a diagnostic answer which, in the case of occupational therapy, is a functional profile: What can this person do? What can't he or she do, and why? The second question, What can be done? is a therapeutic one that allows the occupational therapist to suggest a multitude of potential options that might benefit the patient, given the current problem, the patient's life-style and goals, and the prognosis. The third question, What should be done? moves the process out of the scientific into the value-laden realm. Here many factors must be weighed against each other: quality of life, dignity of death, and expense to society and patient, balanced with the personal values of the patient, the personal and professional values of the therapist and other health professionals, and the expectations of the treatment setting. What should be done also calls for an examination of what should *not* be done, what *might* be done, and what *must* be done.

In making the right decisions for an individual patient, the personal, social, economic, and psychological characteristics of the patient must be simultaneously considered (Pellegrino, 1979). All of this is familiar territory to the occupational therapist. However, to what extent therapists weigh the pros and cons of making judgments about choice of treatment has not been documented.

Technology

The impact of technology on clinical reasoning is receiving increasing attention in lay and professional publications. Clinical technology differs from industrial technology by its proximity to the patient (Thoma, 1986). This may engender fear in the patients, especially if the technology is mismanaged or not understood by them. Thomasma (1984) suggests that "the focus upon life-prolongation by using machines and life-support systems leads to an image of man as increasingly dependent" (p. 38). On the other hand, the use of computerized systems (automated diagnosis and automated treatment) may lead to loss of contact with health care personnel. The danger in both situations is the worship of technology, which may result in the personnel's admiration of the machine and neglect of the patient.

The use of artificial devices to prolong life has been widely debated in lay and professional literature. This use may result in a vision of individuals as technological products. Sidler (1986) states that "almost any aspect of human activity that has been impaired could potentially be aided to some degree through the use of microcomputers as processors, manipulators or controllers" (p. 56).

It must not be construed from the preceding that the beneficial aspects of technology are not clearly recognized. The advent of the computer has dramatically enlarged the scope of occupational therapists' effectiveness; other types of rehabilitation technology have also contributed immeasurably to the quality of life of severely disabled individuals (see *American Journal of Occupational Therapy,* Special Issue, Nov. 1987). However, since the focus of this article is on ethical considerations, interventions that are clearly beneficial are not discussed.

Cost Containment

The literature on cost containment also raises ethical concerns. Richards (1984) proposed that hospitals have become rationing agents who are asked to make moral choices that are actually political and social responsibilities. Availability of care has been restricted by economics and payer decisions and by individual characteristics of the patient, such as age, ethnic origin, or health status. No matter what is done, Richards contended, someone will get hurt. On the same theme, *OT Week* ("HCFA faces . . . ," 1987) reported that, as a result of delegating primary decision-making authority to private fiscal intermediaries without adequate supervision or regulatory mandate, Medicare patients and providers of home health care services are faced with "irrational and unexplained coverage determinations" (p. 12). These fail to take into consideration the needs of the individual patient, the attending physician's opinion, and community medical practice.

The President's Commission for the Study of Ethical Problems in Medicine and Biomedical Research (1983b) was charged by Congress to address the ethical implications of differences in the availability of health services. After 3 years of study, the commission concluded that society has an ethical obligation to ensure equitable access to an adequate level of health care without excessive burdens. However, the definition of these concepts was left to society.

In summary, the impact of regulatory, technological measures has drastically affected the context in which clinical reasoning must take place. *Clinical* reasoning alone is not enough; there must be *moral* reasoning as well in order to focus on the precise nature of the patient's problem and identify the conflicts and their origin.

Occupational Therapy Issues

Quality of Life

The changing nature of practice has brought these issues into the day-to-day reality of the practitioner. For the occupational therapist, clinical reasoning has generally been conceptualized as a model that aims to shift autonomy, control, and responsibility from the professional back to the patient. Occupational therapy students learn to reason in a framework where the "just right" amount of challenge (Rogers, 1982, p. 712) is presented to the patient for eliciting physiological and psychological output toward the highest level of independence possible. This emphasizes the congruence of the clinical decision with the individual's particular position at that time. It is an upbeat, optimistic approach that views the patient and therapist as working together toward a previously set, mutually determined goal. However, the therapist has increasingly less control over whom to treat, when, and how. While life-saving measures have restored life to many people who had already relinquished control and care to others, economic realities have placed time and justification constraints on the health professional in attempting to meet previously agreed on goals. It is difficult to set realistic priorities that have some meaning for the patient when the patient's length of hospital stay has been determined on the basis of a diagnostic category that denies the individuality of patients in general as well as the specific needs of that particular person. Equally, goals for increased quality of life begin to sound hollow when patients' lives are governed by the fear of power failures that could extinguish life or the fear of discharge before survival skills have been attained.

Quality of life has always been a difficult concept to define and measure. It can only be described individually by each person and depends on present lifestyle, past experience, hopes for the future, dreams and ambitions. It must take into account the impact of illness and treatment (Calman, 1984). Policing of regulations regarding informed consent may be limited to merely checking the record for the presence of a signed consent to proceed. Patients are rarely given opportunities to examine the choices or the consequences. By the very fact that they are human beings holding out hope to those in their care, health professionals may guide patients toward a choice in favor of a new technique or treatment without full exploration of the consequences. Thomasma (1986) suggested that the informed consent process does not clearly inform patients or families that the end result might be a state of existence worse than the previous state. "The patient is neither brought to a better quality of life than he had before the operation nor left alone peacefully to die" (p. 1477).

As both a blessing and a curse, technology has removed the inevitability of death from incurable illness or serious injury a step farther and has thereby increased the complexity and the value conflicts that need to be addressed. Schoenberg (1984) raised this point with a probing question:

> Life may be sustained by respirators, cardiac stimulators and other technology, draining the emotional and financial resources of the family, straining overtaxed facilities and scarce personnel of hospitals and creating emotional problems for caretakers. Is it the physician's responsibility to preserve a patient's life, simply because advances make it possible to accomplish? (p. 216)

Although occupational therapists are generally not on the front line of decisions about saving lives, they *are* on the front line in dealing with the consequences of life-saving measures and the technological measures that make survival possible. When an already heavy caseload is further taxed by the addition of a patient who is comatose after a head injury or an 87-year-old patient who has just survived the third cerebrovascular accident through heroic life-saving measures, the occupational therapist comes face to face with some of the most difficult quality-of-life questions. Although answers to scientific questions may be found in accumulating data and testing hypotheses, technical questions are resolved by coming to grips with values and making value judgments (Rogers, 1983). Here, especially, students and practitioners need to examine more closely their own moral, cultural, and religious views about living and dying, dependence and independence, and quality of life in order to design therapeutic programs that preserve their patients' values and represent a mutual understanding between themselves and the patient (Rogers, 1983).

One of the decisions of the President's Commission for the Study of Ethical Problems (1983a) was that "no one has an obligation to provide treatment that would, in his judgment, be countertherapeutic" (p. 44). However, the decision to treat or not to treat must also include an evaluation of the meaning of existence with varying impairments. Great variation exists among these essentially evaluative elements between patients, their families, physicians, and other health professionals and policy makers.

Ethics is not just what one does, but why one does it (Churchill & Cross, 1986). Here, again, the ethical responsibility is to be concerned for the quality of life experienced by the patient, in spite of trends toward an emphasis on technique and objectivism (Yerxa, 1980). It is also the therapist's responsibility to examine questions of dependence caused by using machines and life support systems to prolong life. To what extent are questions about self-determination and autonomy relevant when the patient is dependent on a machine for every heartbeat?

Financial Constraints

The question of health care costs and their ethical implications has received considerable attention from all service providers. A widely shared view has been that if one *can* do something in health care to assist a patient, it *should* be done. Now that principle is being examined. Which treatment should be funded? For whom? At whose expense? (Richards, 1984). Further, who is to decide eligibility, who is to pay for the costs incurred, and what regulatory guidelines are necessary?

A major ethical issue, and one that is all too familiar to occupational therapists, is the denial of treatment to a medically qualified person because of inability to pay or ineligibility for third-party payment. Of equal importance is the concern about federal regulations, such as the 1982 Health Care Financing Administration ruling that requires 3 hours of occupational therapy or physical therapy per day for rehabilitation patients. Such concentrated treatment may not increase the patients' progress but may merely increase the cost of rehabilitation ("Length of Stay," 1987). The moral dilemma here, as Intaglia and Hollander (1987) pointed out, is deciding what to do when a patient does not really need another hour of occupational therapy. In this situation, occupational therapists are faced with the moral dilemma of whether to comply with the regulation when their clinical experience and professional judgment cause them to question the underlying tenet that more has to be better. This becomes a problem particularly when the diagnosis-related group (DRG) determination has discharged the patients "sicker and sooner" from an acute care setting and the patients are therefore less able to be engaged in an intensive 3-hour schedule of therapy.

A further issue is raised in the patient–therapist relationship when the patient must pay for part or all of the care out of pocket. To what extent are patients made aware of alternate delivery systems and plans so that they can decide whether occupational therapy might be of greater value to them than some other service? Each of these issues presents therapists with weighty ethical questions that challenge their reasoning and their integrity.

Implications for Education and Practice

An approach to dealing with moral, ethical dilemmas needs to be incorporated into the repertoire of all practitioners. Early in their education and repeatedly in practice there must be open acknowledgment that it may not always be possible to decide the right thing to do in a clinical situation. In fact, there may not be one best decision, but merely one that is the better of several less desirable options. It is possible, however, to assure that the options have been considered in a systematic way, through open communication, awareness of feelings and values, and clarification of the issues involved.

For the occupational therapist, there are recurring paradoxes and resulting dilemmas that call for a response: having the knowledge, the clinical judgment, and the technical expertise but not the funding to enhance a patient's quality of life; having limited amounts of time or resources and deciding who is entitled to them; having the tools of science and struggling not to be entrapped by them. These realities seem far removed from the idealism that is a normal developmental step for students. They see themselves becoming paragons of intellectual ability, moral integrity, and creative skill, dealing wisely and humanely with every patient's special needs and omnipotently confronting and solving patient problems. At the same time, they are subject to feelings of helplessness that surface during early encounters with patients. These feelings are confirmed by witnessing inconsistency, ambiguity, and instability in moral dilemmas in which there are at least two compelling alternatives (Harron, Burnside, & Beauchamp, 1983). Most disquieting is the patient's tenuous situation. Students yearn for some security and consistency, and they lack the two ingredients that might offer a sense of direction: facts and experience. Feelings of ineffectuality may result in anger toward the patient, followed by feelings of guilt (Schoenberg & Carr, 1984). Faculty and clinicians, recalling their own struggles at a similar stage, must be able to retrace with the student their own developmental steps in gaining a more realistic perspective on the limits of power, as well as the potential for helping to effect change in a cold, uncaring health system.

A useful and timely learning experience that brings ethical questions closer to reality for students also depicts the diversity of personal, ethical, and moral values. This is a class exercise that asks students to rank seven patients who have been referred to occupational therapy for a variety of acute medical and psychosocial problems. The patients are of varying ages and have differing social support systems. Students are told that, because of staff shortages, only two patients can be accepted for immediate treatment. Whom will they select? Why? In the discussion that follows there are as many different choices as there are students. Some will select the child, because she has a lifetime ahead of her; others may select the young mother who must be discharged next week; still others will choose the old man who is near death and whose quality of life needs should be met. Each student builds a strong case for his or her decision—a choice that reflects personal, ethical, and moral values about life.

The most helpful role models for students and practitioners are those who can openly discuss their own feelings about ethical questions and who can help others carefully examine their responsibilities to the patient, their employer, the profession, and, ultimately, to themselves. Over the past several years, students have repeatedly underscored their need to talk about ethical issues in an environment that permits open exploration of questions for which there are no clear answers. Although they initially expressed anxiety about the lack of certainty in planning for patients, they later welcomed the opportunity to have a faculty member challenge them in exploring all sides of an issue.

Every individual has deeply rooted values and beliefs about what is right and wrong and the kinds of decisions with which one can and cannot live. The norms and attitudes of different occupational therapists reflect the pluralism of attitudes and ethical norms in society. For this reason, important decisions based on value judgments should not be made independently, but rather in a group of colleagues. As practitioners move out of the social structure of the institution and have fewer opportunities for obtaining a variety of opinions, they may find themselves isolated and helpless when faced with ethical questions. The importance of finding mentors or a community of colleagues with whom to raise the questions cannot be overemphasized. Increasingly, all health professionals are recognizing the need for further access to the study of ethics and the logical analysis of ethical problems to guide them in making the most moral, humane decisions for their patients. Scientists have found ways to sustain life; now society must assume responsibility for supporting and nurturing that life. Clearly, these questions will not go away; rather, they must be accepted as a sobering legacy for the 21st century.

Conclusion

This article has examined moral, ethical questions facing health professionals in a time of high technology and cost containment efforts. Clinical reasoning in 1988 requires far more extensive preparation of occupational therapists in areas that up to a few years ago were left to other disciplines, such as business, law, and economics. This calls for a close partnership of clinicians and educators. Students and practitioners need opportunities for reasoning about issues and for considering the external pressures and internal value systems that will affect judgment. Occupational ther-apy personnel need to learn to live with questions of conscience as part of their professional responsibility.

References

Calman, K. C. (1984). Quality of life in cancer patients—An hypothesis. *Journal of Medical Ethics, 10,* 124–127.

Churchill, L. R., & Cross, A. W. (1986). Moralist, technician, sophist, teacher/learner: Reflections on the ethicist in the clinical setting. *Theoretical Medicine, 7,* 3–12.

Elstein, A. S. (1976). Clinical judgment: Psychological research and medical practice. *Science, 194,* 696–700.

Elstein, A. S., Shulman, L. S., & Sprafka, S. A. (1978). *Medical problem solving: An analysis of clinical reasoning.* Cambridge, MA: Harvard University Press.

Engelhardt, H. T. (1986). The importance of values in shaping professional direction and behavior. In *Occupational therapy education: Target 2000.* (Proceedings of forum on promoting excellence in education, pp. 39–43). Rockville, MD: American Occupational Therapy Association.

Gillette, N., & Mattingly, C. (1987). The Foundation: Clinical reasoning in occupational therapy. *American Journal of Occupational Therapy, 41,* 399–400.

Harron, F., Burnside, J., & Beauchamp, T. (1983). *Health and human values.* New Haven, CT: Yale University Press.

HCFA faces legal storm over home care denials. (1987, April 16). *OT Week, 1*(13), pp. 12–14.

Intaglia, S., & Hollander, R. (1987). The 3-hour therapy criterion: A challenge for rehabilitation facilities. *American Journal of Occupational Therapy, 41,* 297–304.

Length of stay is stable, but rehab costs increase. (1987, April 9). *OT Week, 1*(12), p. 4.

Pelland, M. J. (1987). A conceptual model for the instruction and supervision of treatment planning. *American Journal of Occupational Therapy, 41,* 351–359.

Pellegrino, E. D. (1979). The anatomy of clinical judgments. In H. T. Engelhardt, S. F. Spicker, & B. Towers (Eds.), *Clinical judgment: A critical appraisal.* Dordrecht, Holland: D. Reidel Publishing Co.

Pellegrino, E. D., & Thomasma, D. C. (1981). *A philosophical basis for medical practice: Toward a philosophy and ethic of the healing profession.* New York: Oxford University Press.

President's Commission for the Study of Ethical Problems in Medicine and Biomedical and Behavioral Research. (1983a). *Deciding to forego life-sustaining treatment.* Washington, DC: U.S. Government Printing Office.

President's Commission for the Study of Ethical Problems in Medicine and Biomedical and Behavioral Research. (1983b). *Securing access to health care.* Washington, DC: U.S. Government Printing Office.

Richards, G. (1984). Technology costs and rationing issues. *Hospitals, 58,* 80–88.

Rogers, J. C. (1982). The spirit of independence: The evolution of a philosophy. *American Journal of Occupational Therapy, 36,* 709–715.

Rogers, J. C. (1983). Clinical reasoning: The ethics, science and art. *American Journal of Occupational Therapy, 37,* 601–616.

Rogers, J. C., & Masagatani, G. (1982). Clinical reasoning of occupational therapists during the initial assessment of physically disabled patients. *Occupational Therapy Journal of Research, 2,* 195–219.

Schoenberg, B. (1984). Management of the dying patient. In A. C. Carr, A. H. Kutscher, & M. Meyer (Eds.), *Bernard Schoenberg: Contributions to psychiatry, education of the health professional, thanatology and ethical values.* New York: Foundation of Thanatology.

Schoenberg, B., & Carr, A. C. (1984). Educating the health professional in the psychosocial care of the terminally ill. In A. C. Carr, A. H. Kutscher, & M. Meyer (Eds.), *Bernard Schoenberg: Contributions to psychiatry, education of the health professional, thanatology and ethical values.* New York: Foundation of Thanatology.

Sidler, M. R. (1986). Impact of technology on rehabilitation—Computer applications in occupational therapy. *Occupational Therapy in Health Care, 3,* 56–78.

Thoma, H. (1986). Some aspects of medical ethics from the perspective of bioengineering. *Theoretical Medicine, 7,* 305–317.

Thomasma, D. C. (1984). The goals of medicine and society. In D. H. Brock, Ed., *The culture of biomedicine: Studies in Science and culture* (Vol. I, pp. 34–54). Newark, DE: University of Delaware Press.

Thomasma, D. (1986). Bioethical issues in organ transplantation. *Southern Medical Journal, 79,* 1471–1484.

Yerxa, E. (1980) Occupational therapy's role in creating a future of caring. *American Journal of Occupational Therapy, 34,* 529–534.

Acknowledgement

I would like to express my sincere appreciation to the many students, colleagues, and patients who inspired the conceptual development of this article.

TEACHING CLINICAL REASONING
FOR PRACTICE IN GERIATRICS

Joan C. Rogers, PhD, OTR

ABSTRACT. Allied health education involves integration of theory and clinical practice. In this paper, gerontological concepts are applied to clinical practice through *professional self-talk*. This is a case study teaching strategy which documents the clinical reasoning process and affective reactions of the therapist as they unfold in interaction with the patient. It aims at conveying content in a real-life context and at providing a model of clinical decision making. *Professional self-talk* is particularly appropriate for teaching geriatrics because of the rudimentary state of knowledge and practice in this area.

Professional education in the health fields aims at imparting the knowledge underlying practice, and the skills and attitudes needed to competently serve clients. The educator is challenged to develop teaching techniques that relate thought to action. Schein (1), for instance, encouraged "a form of education that permits basic science, applied science and clinical modes to be taught simultaneously in an integrated fashion (p. 46)."

Professional self-talk is an instructional strategy which aims at developing a working relationship between subject matter, the problem-solving process, and professional and personal values. Self-talk is defined as the thoughts that we communicate to ourselves about our experiences which in turn control the way we feel and act (2). *Professional self-talk* refers to thoughts that we communicate to ourselves about the client-professional encounter which in turn controls our actions and feelings regarding the treatment process. The following examples illustrate the relationship between experience, self-talk, feeling, and action.

Professional self-talk is a case study teaching approach which documents the clinical reasoning process and affective reactions of the clinician as they unfold in interaction with the client. The prac-

Dr. Rogers is an Assistant Professor, Department of Medical Allied Health Professions, Division of Occupational Therapy (Wing B Medical School 207H) University of North Carolina, Chapel Hill, N. C. 27514. This paper was presented at the Annual Conference of the Association for Gerontology in Higher Education, Denver, Colorado, 1980.

Physical & Occupational Therapy in Geriatrics, Vol. 1(4), Spring 1982

29

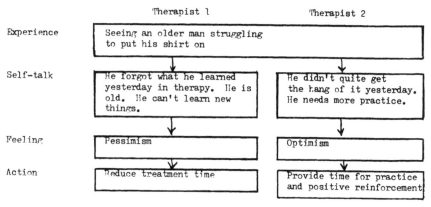

Table 1

titioner shares his decision-making rationales, as he establishes therapeutic goals, priorities, and methods. *Professional self-talk* is appropriate for both the planning and interactive phases of intervention. It provides a record of the factors that are considered in formulating plans. Changes in these plans stemming from a lack of response to treatment and from progress are verbalized. The student enters into the mind and emotion of the experienced practitioner from initial contact through discharge. *Professional self-talk* helps the student to think like a professional by demonstrating how a professional thinks. In this way, the student gains insight into how biopsychosocial data are integrated and used in problem-solving, why theoretical perspectives may change during therapy, why treatment is modified, and how feelings are managed.

Appropriateness for Teaching Gerontological Concepts

Strategies that bridge the theory to practice gap, although useful for teaching any clinical approach are particularly appropriate for gerontological practice. First, the knowledge base in gerontology is only developing and much of what is available is fragmentary. Thus, the connection between theory and parctice is more elusive than it is in more established disciplines. Professional self-talk assists the student in identifying the usefulness of concepts in particular situations.

Second, just as the knowledge base in gerontology is rudimentary, so too is each profession's base for gerontological practice. Each profession selects from gerontology, the concepts and theories most in keeping with its philosophical perspective and professional science. These concepts must then be organized so as to give meaning and direction to treatment. To teach a subject matter, one must organize it in some way. *Professional self-talk* provides a mechanism for identifying significant concepts and for organizing them around the problem-solving process. It requires the educator to be involved in clinical practice. This is particularly important since many instructors who are called on to teach gerontology in professional curricula have had no special training in gerontology or specialized practice with older persons. The involvement in clinical activity required to develop teaching cases from a *professional self-talk* perspective, mitigates against arm chair practice.

Lastly, much of the integration of thought, action, and emotion in professional curricula occurs during field work under the tutelage of a clinical instructor. Traditionally, work with the elderly has been assigned a low priority and negative attitudes toward older persons have been well documented among health care workers (3). Because of the present shortage of gerontologic practitioners, good professional role models may not be available in student training centers. Opportunities for learning by example or modeling may thus be limited. *Professional self-talk* has the capabilities of furnishing a descriptive model of the intervention process.

Case Illustration

The use of *professional self-talk* in teaching will now be illustrated by five excerpts from an actual self-report of an occupational therapist. Afterwards, ways of varying the technique will be pointed out, the advantages of the technique will be discussed, and cautions in using it will be presented.

The case selected for analysis is that of an 80 year old widowed male admitted to the rehabilitation unit of the hospital, secondary to a cerebral vascular accident that resulted in left hemiparesis:

Excerpt 1

Experience:	Mr. B. is lying in bed. Egg yolk and coffee are spilled all over the bed clothes. The room smells of feces. This is our first contact.
Self-talk:	"If our eyes hadn't met, I could leave. I have a weak stomach. He is dirty, smelly and old. Priority for admission should have been given to the young patient with multiple sclerosis. Mr. B. is an uninteresting case."
Feelings:	Repulsion; annoyance
Action:	Introduce myself; explain my function as an occupational therapist.

Experience: Mr. B. says that his working days are over and that he
            doesn't need an occupational therapist.
Self-talk: "He wouldn't understand occupational therapy even if I
            told him."
Feelings: Hopelessness; indifference
Action: No explanation; temporary termination of the encounter

This excerpt emphasizes the awareness and expression of negative affect, particularly the valuing of youth over maturity, the ageism that "you can't teach an old dog new tricks," and the stereotypic attitude that dirty, smelly, and old go together.

Excerpt II

Experience: Planning the initial assessment
Self-talk: The areas of self-care, sensation, perception, general
            physical endurance, voluntary motor control, leisure
            skills, homemaking, and work history are appropriate
            for hemiplegic evaluation. Comparing these evaluation
            procedures with Lawton's (4) hierarchy of behavioral
            areas will help me to check on the completeness of my
            assessment. (See Figure 1.)

            This points out a deficiency in social role. I will need
            this information before developing a treatment plan, so
            that I will know who needs to be included in the patient
            education sessions. I will discuss this with the social
            worker.

            The first thing that I will test is Mr. B.'s ability to feed
            himself. This is a good place to start since our first
            contact indicated problems in feeding. By observing
            feeding, information will also be gained on visual per-
            ception, and if Mr. B. uses his affected arm, on the
            extent of voluntary control. Feeding is also a good place
            to start since the problems experienced secondary to
            stroke are usually remediated with assistive devices.
            Being able to feed oneself again soon after the onset of
            disability, can head off feelings of helplessness and in-
            competence as discussed by Bengtson (5) in regard to
            the social breakdown and reconstruction syndromes.

            I will also assess the sensory status of the right upper
            extremity and general physical endurance at the first
            session.
Feeling: competence; in-control
Action: Schedule first evaluation session

Figure 1

OCCUPATIONAL THERAPY EVALUATIONS
CLASSIFIED ACCORDING TO LAWTON'S HIERARCHY

Lawton's Hierarchy of Behavioral Areas	Occupational Therapy Evaluations
Social Role...................................	
Effectance....................................	Leisure/Inventory
Instrumental Self-maintenance...................	Work history including homemaking
Physical self-maintenance......................	Feeding, Grooming, Dressing
Perception-cognition...........................	Orientation to time and space, Visual perception, Memory, Functional speech, Problem-solving abilities
Functional health	Sensation of the left upper extremity, General physical endurance, Voluntary motor control of the left upper extremity, Functional ambulation

In this excerpt, rationales for decisions concerning the evaluation procedures are made explicit—including the sequence in which the procedures are to be done. Occupational therapy theory concerning the treatment of adult hemiplegia is aligned with the gerontological models of Lawton and Bengtson.

Excerpt III

Experience: Mr. B.'s lunch tray is 45 minutes late. Mr. B. brings his left hand to his mouth. He is unable to use it to feed himself because he can't hold a spoon. He is drooling out of the right side of his mouth. He chokes when swallowing.

Self-talk: "Someone should do something about the late trays. The Dietary Department habitually throws everyone off schedule. Mr. B.'s use of his left arm probably places him at stage 5 or 6 of Brunnstrom's (6) stages of neuromuscular recovery. This is good. Full voluntary usage may be feasible. Drooling and choking suggests that a detailed evaluation of oral-motor status is in order. If

           Mr. B. were a child, I would feel more comfortable about how to proceed. He really cooperated very well with the testing. He does present some interesting problems!"

Feelings: Annoyance; confusion; excitement

Action: Exploration of oral-motor assessment procedures and treatment techniques

In the affective area, this excerpt concentrates on a change of attitude toward Mr. B., who is now perceived as cooperative and as a challenge to the therapist's professional skill. Constraints on the treatment situation arising from inter-department factors are also pointed out. In the cognitive area, the application of oral-motor procedures, to adults, which were developed and used primarily with children, is questioned. Formulation of a hypothesis regarding recovery is illustrated at an early stage in the evaluation process.

Excerpt IV

Experience: Stimulated by a request to discuss his recreational interests, Mr. B. is talking at length about his life.

Self-talk: "I need to assess leisure skills in order to decide on an appropriate activity to improve grasp in the left hand. Preserve me from the occupational therapists, God, she means well but I'm too busy to make baskets. I want to relive a day in July . . . This review is healthy."

Feeling: Patience

Action: Listen

This excerpt illustrates a change in plans initiated by the client and the acquiescence of the therapist to that change. The lines from Elise Maclay's poem, "Occupational Therapy (7)," prompt thoughts of the life review as an adaptive process (8).

Excerpt V

Experience: Discharge planning

Self-talk: "According to Lawton's hierarchy of behavior (4), Mr. B. is at the self-maintenance level of competence. Hence, based on Golant and McCaslin's model (9) which relates service-packages to Lawton's hierarchy, independent living should be feasible, if community support services are available. Mr. B. needs someone to clean his home and to bring groceries. If such services are not available, he will need a sheltered living situation.

Feelings: Concern over pre-mature institutionalization

Action: Instruct the certified occupational therapy assistant to get information on the services available in Mr. B.'s community.

This excerpt illustrates the use of two gerontological models to assist decision making regarding independent living and the delegation of a task by the professional to an assistant.

Variations

The *professional self-talk* technique may be modified in several ways. In the excerpts given above, frames of reference, such as Lawton's hierarchy of behavior, were merely mentioned. This approach assumes that students are already familiar with the subject matter through prior study or from course reading assignments. If this is the case, the primary gain from using *professional self-talk* is to emphasize that these models assist in understanding this particular case. If students have had prior exposure to the material, they can be called on to give a summary of the theorist's ideas. Such repetition provides a review of the subject matter and thus reinforces it. If students have not been exposed to the models, *professional self-talk* may be interspersed with mini-lectures.

It is also advantageous to have the students summarize the cognitive and affective content, and to reflect on changes that occur in these areas as treatment progresses. This may be done by having them identify what is being illustrated, in the same manner as this was done in the summaries provided at the end of each of the excerpts. Underlying assumptions and principles may be made explicit.

As students become involved in field work, they can present their own self-reports and get feedback on their decisions. Similarities and differences in the rationales and feelings; of different students, of the same students at different times, and of skilled versus beginning practitioners, may be analyzed. Comparisons may also be based on age and disease entities.

Advantages and Drawbacks

The professional process—be it in occupational therapy, physical therapy, nursing, or teaching—is essentially a decision-making process. Information is collected, classified, analyzed, and summarized and is used to determine patient's problems, goals, and prescriptions. *Professional self-talk* emphasizes these decision-making processes by making them explicit. All too frequently professional education concentrates on perfecting isolated skills, such as how to assess leisure interests and how to strengthen weak muscles. Putting these bits and pieces together to solve a particular patient's problems is generally left to fieldwork. However, even then, the student is required to assume the clinician's reasoning from the behavior observed. *Professional self-talk* identifies decision-making as the pivotal skill of the intervention process. It seeks to develop this skill by demonstrating "how the mind works that directs the hands." It also fosters the attitude of reflecting on decisions in order to learn from them.

A second advantage of *professional self-talk* is that it provides a model of real rather than ideal thinking. Although the scientific method is generally upheld as the paradigm par excellence for professional thinking, naturalistic studies have indicated that this is modified in various ways in practice. Physicians (10) for instance, systematically deviate from the scientific method by formulting diagnostic hypotheses early in the evaluative process. The decision-making process in many of the allied health fields is less prescribed than it is in medicine. The range of options for treatment is broader and client preferences are taken into account to a greater extent. *Professional self-talk* helps the student appreciate the working methods of the practitioner.

Thirdly, *professional self-talk* is problem-centered as well as process-oriented. Subject matter is introduced as it relates to what is being done or what is being contemplated. Thus, it attempts to make information more relevant to students by permitting them to see it in relation to a practical problem that is to be solved.

A final advantage of using *professional self-talk* as an instructional tool lies in its capacity to integrate the process of value clarification with cognitive learning. The educational process has frequently concentrated solely on instilling the professional, "objective" attitude, in spite of the evidence that personal biases enter into professional decisions. *Professional self-talk* provides a stimulus for analyzing how attitudes influence behavior. The management of positive as well as negative reactions to patients and of patients to treatment may be shared. Such self-disclosure facilitates the development of personal relationships with students. When students are lectured to, they go away informed. When the instructor shares himself or herself, they go away moved.

Like every technique, *professional self-talk* has drawbacks as well as advantages. Although problem-centered, the student is only passively involved in instruction, via lecture, and the exercise is essentially theoretical. There is also the danger that the reasoning presented may be interpreted as the way to think rather than as an example of the thinking process. Furthermore, an instructor may not wish to reveal her thoughts and feelings. Finally, using *professional self-talk* as an educational device assumes that it is theory-based. If this is not the case, the technique loses its value.

In spite of the drawbacks, *professional self-talk* holds potential for demonstrating the theory to practice connection and for facilitating the development of professional thinking in treating the older patient.

REFERENCES

1. Schein EH: *Professional Education*. New York: McGraw-Hill Book Co., 1972.

2. Lembo J: *Help Yourself*. Niles, Ill.: Argus Communications, 1974.

3. Wolk RL, Wolk RB: Professional workers' attitudes toward the aged. *J Am Geriatrics Soc* 19: 624-639, 1971.

4. Lawton MP: Assessing the competence of older people. In: *Research Planning and Action for the Elderly* edited by D. P. Kent, R. Kastenbaum, and S. Sherwood. New York: Behavioral Publications, Inc., 1972, 122-143.

5. Bengtson VL: *The Social Psychology of Aging*. Indianapolis: The Bobbs-Merrill Co., Inc., 1973.

6. Brunnstrom S: *Movement Therapy in Hemiplegia*. New York: Harper and Row, 1970.

7. Maclay E: Green Winter: *Celebrations of Old Age*. New York: Reader's Digest Press, 1977.

8. Butler R: The life review: An interpretation of reminiscence in the aged. *Psychiatry* 26: 65-76, 1963.

9. Golant SM, McCaslin R: A functional classification of services for older people. *Journal of Gerontological Social Work* 1: 187-209, 1979.

10. Elstein AS, Shulman LS, Sprafka SA. *Medical Problem Solving: An Analysis of Clinical Reasoning*. Cambridge, Mass.: Harvard University Press, 1978.

Clinical Reasoning and New Ideas on Intelligence: Implications for Teaching and Learning

Kathleen Barker Schwartz

Key Words: curriculum • education, occupational therapy

Some recent research efforts have been focused on the attainment of a better understanding of intelligence and reasoning. One such study is the Clinical Reasoning Study funded by the American Occupational Therapy Association and the American Occupational Therapy Foundation. Other studies have been conducted by theorists of human development. The findings of both groups reveal three common themes: the multiple aspects of intelligence, the importance of understanding the patient's story, and the use of the caring perspective. This article examines these shared themes and discusses their implications for new directions in occupational therapy curricula.

Kathleen Barker Schwartz, EdD, OTR, FAOTA, is Associate Professor, San Jose State University, One Washington Square, San Jose, California 95192–0059.

This article was accepted for publication June 26, 1991.

The Clinical Reasoning Study, funded by the American Occupational Therapy Association and the American Occupational Therapy Foundation, has defined several themes that elucidate central aspects of clinical reasoning. *Clinical reasoning* is described as a complex intellectual process that surpasses logical thought (Fleming, in press). It is depicted as a process that involves the therapist in a phenomenological approach to making sense of the patient's condition (Mattingly, 1991b) and evokes the therapist's use of a caring perspective in establishing a collaborative relationship with the patient (Fleming, 1991; Mattingly, 1991a). These three themes—the multiple aspects of intelligence, the importance of understanding the patient's story, and the use of a caring perspective—are echoed in the research of several prominent theorists in human development who are concerned with new ways of viewing intellectual and moral development. That similar concepts are being discussed in both the human development literature and the Clinical Reasoning Study reflects a movement toward a new view of intelligence. In the present article, I have examined common themes underlying this movement in the hope of providing a better understanding of possible implications for occupational therapy. These ideas are further applied to the classroom, and teaching strategies are proposed that center on this view of reasoning.

Multiple Aspects of Intelligence

Fleming (1991) postulated that therapists use different types of reasoning in their clinical practice. A logical mode is used when thinking about the patient's performance problems, an interactive mode when trying to understand the patient as a person, and a projective mode when thinking about the patient's future functioning. This description of reasoning differs greatly from that found in the medical literature, in which clinical reasoning is defined solely in terms of logical problem solving (Fleming, in press). Until recently, the psychology profession has emphasized logical, or rational, thought as the critical intellectual capacity.

The model posed by Piaget (Gruber & Voneche, 1977) of a unified center of operation (i.e., intelligence) that leads to the desired reasoning (i.e., logical and abstract) was challenged by Gardner (1985), who proposed instead a theory of multiple intelligences. Gardner posited that several kinds of intelligence exist and that different results are achieved depending on the type of intelligence used. The intelligences he defined were linguistic, musical, logical-mathematical, spatial, kinesthetic, and personal. He argued that people use these intelligences in varying proportions, according to need and ability. Expressing a viewpoint similar to Gardner's, Fleming (1991) proposed that therapists use more than one intelligence during a therapy session. Indeed, Fleming found that therapists use their movement and sensory capabilities (what Gardner would call *spatial* and *kinesthetic intelligence*) as well as their problem-solving mode (what Gardner called *logical-mathematical intelligence*). In addition, Fleming said that the therapeutic process depends on the therapist's ability to engage the patient in a meaningful relationship (what Gardner called *personal intelligence*).

Gardner's (1985) ideas have fueled a debate within human development circles, with those opposing him arguing that what he defined as an intelligence is really more of an ability than a cognitive process. Those sharing Gardner's view argue that intelligence is not monolithic and that the study of all possible modes of intelligence can lead to a better understanding of how we reason. Supporters of Gardner's view of multiple intelligences include Sternberg (1988) and John-Steiner (1985). Sternberg proposed a model of multiple intelligence drawn from case studies and an analysis of the history of intelligence theory. John-Steiner, who studied male and female artists, scientists, and writers, proposed that there are several kinds, or languages, of thought. Together, the works of Gardner, Sternberg, and John-Steiner represent a movement in human development to replace the traditional view of a unified intellect with a view of multiple intelligences. The premise of the therapist with the three-track mind posited by Fleming (1991) echoes this movement to define multiple modes of reasoning.

Understanding the Patient's Story

Luria (1976) has added to our understanding of intelligence through his writings on cognitive development. Perhaps more importantly, he has played a key role in the movement to emphasize the clinician's responsibility to acquire a full understanding of the patient. He has published what experts consider to be two of the most illuminating clinical studies done in this century (Luria, 1972, 1987). These studies offer a vivid portrayal of cognitive dysfunction that goes far beyond the traditional discussion of diagnosis. Luria enables the reader to understand the disability by portraying the patient's life as that person experiences it and tries to make sense of it.

Sharing Luria's (1972, 1987) view, Bruner (1986) posited that we must "understand the ways human beings construct their worlds" (p. 46). He asserted that these constructs are not arbitrary, but rather, reflect intellectual and psychological processes founded on individual's beliefs and values. He saw the clinician's role as one of "interpreting a person," and he argued that this can only be done when one understands the narrative of the person's life story (p. 39). Sacks (1985) illustrated Bruner's point by using his "clinical tales" to portray the patient's "essential being," which he said was relevant to neurology in that the patient's personhood and disease "cannot be disjoined" (p. xiv). Similarly, Coles (1989) described how

his knowledge of narrative enables him to enter another patient's life and to understand that person through listening to his or her story.

Mattingly (1989, 1991b) described how the occupational therapist uses a narrative mode of reasoning to develop an understanding of the meaning of disability from the patient's perspective. In the narrative mode of reasoning, training in daily living activities means more than simply skill building. It symbolizes the patient's experience of loss of former capacities as well as his or her attempt to acquire new ways of behaving and understanding. The patient, in effect, has to write a new chapter in his or her life story, and the therapeutic experience in part shapes how that chapter is written. Contrary to studies of clinical problem solving that presume a focus on diagnosis, Fleming (1991) found that therapists spend a considerable amount of their reasoning time trying to understand the patient's current functioning and predicting future performance capabilities. By discovering the patient's underlying values and beliefs, the occupational therapist is able to incorporate this knowledge into the therapeutic process. Knowledge of the patient's story enables treatment dedicated to the patient's reclamation of self and creation of a new image (Mattingly, 1991a).

Taylor (1989) shared this view when she argued that health professionals need to understand the self-images that their patients create and, if possible, to nurture optimism within the therapeutic process. Like Bruner (1986), Sacks (1985), Coles (1989), and Luria (1987), she underscored the importance of eliciting the patient's life story and urged that an understanding of this life story is as important a part of the therapeutic process as the establishment of the diagnosis. The idea that knowledge of both the diagnosis and the patient's life story constitutes the best treatment approach is borne out in the Clinical Reasoning Study.

A Caring Perspective

Gilligan's (1982) *In A Different Voice* marked the beginning of a new vantage point from which to view moral and intellectual development. Until that time, Kohlberg's (1981) theory of moral development had offered the predominant view. Gilligan's research was prompted in part by curiosity as to why women generally scored lower than men on Kohlberg's stages of moral development. Her findings suggested that Kohlberg's schema presumed a particular kind of thinking, one that relied on abstract principles such as truth, justice, and equality to resolve moral dilemmas. Gilligan called this the *justice perspective*. In contrast, Gilligan found that the perspective most prevalent among women was what she called the *caring perspective*. Those holding a caring perspective used concerns about relationships and persons to decide their moral dilemmas. This initial theorizing has been substantiated in recent research (Gilligan, Ward, & Taylor, 1988). The studies confirm that both the justice and the caring perspectives exist and that men tend to hold the former perspective while women tend to hold the latter. Gilligan cautioned, however, against making this finding the basis for simplistic views about male and female behavior. Studies indicate that children of both sexes are capable of using the caring and justice perspectives. The research suggests that environmental influences play a major role in the adoption of a particular perspective in adulthood and that adults may change their perspective as they grow older and redefine their values.

A characteristic of the caring perspective is the desire to strengthen relationships. According to Gilligan et al. (1988), "from the perspective of someone seeking or valuing care, relationship connotes responsiveness or engagement . . . a connection" (p. xviii). In a study of medical students, those holding a caring perspective noted the powerful therapeutic potential of a strong relationship between patient and caregiver (Gilligan & Pollak, 1988). Similarly, Mattingly (1991a) argued that a strong therapeutic relationship underlies successful therapy. She explained that only a patient strongly committed to the therapeutic process gains from it and that commitment necessitates that the patient and therapist share a similar view of treatment. Such sharing evolves through a relationship founded on trust and caring.

The difficulty in using the caring perspective within a medical context is evidenced in Fleming's (1991) discussion of the interactive mode of reasoning. She defined this reasoning as dominated by concern for the person and for his or her reaction to the therapist and the treatment. Although Fleming found that therapists in the Clinical Reasoning Study engaged in this mode of reasoning, they were generally silent about it. Therapists were concerned that administrators, physicians, and third-party payers would not deem these interactions to be a legitimate part of medical treatment. The failure of the medical model to value this aspect of treatment, however, did not cause therapists to abandon it, but rather, to "go underground" (i.e., they continued to address this aspect of treatment but did not discuss it openly) (Fleming, 1991). A similar phenomenon was noted by Gilligan, Lyons, and Hanmer (1989) in their study of adolescent girls. They found that when the girls' valuing of relationships was not reaffirmed by school administrators and teachers, they would retain their beliefs but speak about them only among themselves. These examples illustrate the difficulty that groups have when they hold a perspective that is not recognized by those in the environment, whether it be a school or hospital. The studies done by Gilligan and colleagues have alerted us to the existence of the caring perspective and its importance in adolescent and adult development, whereas the Clinical Reasoning Study documents the importance of the caring perspective in the therapeutic process.

Implications for Teaching and Learning

The knowledge from the research on intelligence and clinical reasoning suggests the following direction for occupational therapy education.

Teach to all modes of reasoning. This involves recognition of the different ways of knowing and of designing learning experiences that emphasize the various facets of intelligence. It means a shift from teaching facts toward guiding the development of reasoning capability through experiential and cooperative learning (Slavin, 1985). The experiential model of teaching affects curriculum content decisions in that emphasis is placed on the learning of critical concepts rather than of facts or techniques. The different modes of reasoning should be given equal time in the curriculum. Thus, although we must teach the logic of problem solving, we must also teach students interactive reasoning. Moreover, a focus on the teaching of reasoning requires a shift in the method of evaluation from a quantitative to a qualitative mode of measurement. For example, a videotape of a student working with a patient at the beginning and end of the semester provides a more reliable measure of interactive reasoning ability than does a multiple-choice exam. Similarly, a case study that requires students to apply their knowledge is a more valid measure of reasoning ability than is a test that measures factual retention.

Teach a narrative approach to patient evaluation. Because clinical reasoning requires the therapist to use a phenomenological approach in making sense of the patient's condition, students need to learn how to use a narrative reasoning mode when evaluating patients. For students to understand all of the aspects of the patient, they must learn about the patient's beliefs and values and develop an understanding of what disability means to that particular person's life. One way to elicit such information is through interviews that encourage patients to discuss their feelings about illness and disability. Another is to use evaluations that assess interests, values, and roles. Although students are generally well grounded in such evaluations as range of motion and muscle testing, ways of evaluating that can yield data about the meaning of disability are rarely emphasized. By encouraging students to use qualitative as well as quantitative assessments and by familiarizing them with the phenomenological approach to understanding patients, we can promote the development of narrative reasoning. It could be argued that in doing so, we are educating students to use an approach that is not supported by third-party payers. In response, however, we can pose the question, "Who should be shaping occupational therapy education?" The Clinical Reasoning Study offers evidence that narrative reasoning is an integral part of the therapeutic process. Occupational therapy curricula can help to give this underground activity more credibility by teaching students narrative reasoning and ways to justify its use within the medical model.

Use a connected teaching approach. Belenky, Clinchy, Goldberger, and Tarule (1986) described *connected knowing* as an educational orientation that includes the sharing of common experiences and discussion of the feelings that inform ideas. They contrasted connected knowing with what they called *separate knowing,* which is an orientation to learning characterized by impersonal and objective reasoning. Separate knowing dominates higher education in that the professor demands that the students acquire a facility for logic and problem solving based solely on abstract reasoning. This approach is commonly referred to as *critical thinking* in higher education curricula (Paul, 1990). However, Fleming (in press) found that occupational therapists use methods other than logic-based reasoning to make decisions. Similarly, Belenky et al. suggested that although women were capable of mastering a logical approach, they remained uncomfortable using this approach exclusively. The women preferred a more collaborative approach to knowing. Rather than beginning with theory and logic, they found it more fruitful to begin with a discussion of experience and use that as a basis for problem solving. Thus, Belenky et al. recommended a connected teaching approach, wherein experience precedes theoretical abstraction. This approach has the benefit of demystifying theory by making it accessible through illustration in practice. Using the connected teaching approach, the teacher demonstrates the process of sharing concepts and examining them for their aptness. This enables students to see their teacher as someone who, like themselves, forms ideas and tests them out. Thus, the ownership of knowledge shifts from teacher to student, and the classroom becomes the center for the learning and testing of ideas. Classroom activity that involves discussion of experiences and case studies that illustrate theory in practice are two examples of methods that can stimulate connected learning. Fieldwork provides a wonderful opportunity to engage in connected learning. The cases are no longer simulated, but real, and the testing of ideas becomes the basis for treatment. Indeed, the success of clinical education may in part be due to its ability to engage the student in connected learning.

Conclusion

Recent research in intelligence and clinical reasoning suggests that education should be redirected from the teaching of facts and techniques to the teaching of methods that stimulate higher-level reasoning capabilities. Whereas multiple modes of reasoning seem to be inherent in clinical practice, these several modes of knowing need to be addressed in the curriculum. The research confirms what occupational therapists have intuitively known: Caring is an important aspect of patient care, and knowing our patients means more than simply learning about their diagnosis. It reinforces the holistic view of patient treatment proposed by our profession's founders (Schwartz, in press).

In a broader context, the ideas discussed in this paper coincide with the accountability movement in higher education (Wolff, 1990), a movement that originated with the legislature and also with the public to express their growing dissatisfaction with the products of higher education. The movement calls for a change in the traditional methods of teaching and measurement, that is, lecture and multiple-choice exam, on the grounds that they are ineffective in stimulating higher-level problem solving. Although many innovative ideas, such as those proposed in this paper, have been tried in various forms (McKeachie, 1990), there has been no sustained, systematic movement in higher education toward the use of these more effective teaching methods. In addition to a call for change in teaching methods, there is a growing demand for outcomes assessment with which to measure teaching effectiveness (Committee on College and University Teaching, Research, and Publication, 1990). The measurement of students' performance depends on our ability to define intelligence and reasoning.

The ideas expressed in this article are pertinent and suggest a valuable approach to guide occupational therapy educators as they develop the best methods by which to assess and teach the kind of reasoning that will lead to better-prepared practitioners. ▲

References

Belenky, M. F., Clinchy, B. M., Goldberger, N. R., & Tarule, J. M. (1986). *Women's ways of knowing.* New York: Basic.

Bruner, J. (1986). *Actual minds, possible worlds.* Cambridge, MA: Harvard University Press.

Coles, R. (1989). *The call of stories.* Boston: Houghton Mifflin.

Committee on College and University Teaching, Research, and Publication. (1990). Mandated assessment of educational outcomes. *Academe, 76,* 34–40.

Fleming, M. H. (1991). The therapist with the three-track mind. *American Journal of Occupational Therapy, 45,* 1007–1014.

Fleming, M. H. (in press). Difference between assumptions about thinking and observations of the clinical reasoning strategies of occupational therapists. *American Journal of Occupational Therapy.*

Gardner, H. (1985). *Frames of mind: The theory of multiple intelligences.* New York: Basic.

Gilligan, C. (1982). *In a different voice.* Cambridge, MA: Harvard University Press.

Gilligan, C., Lyons, N. P., & Hanmer, T. J. (1989). *Making connections.* Troy, NY: Emma Willard School.

Gilligan, C., & Pollak, S. (1988). The vulnerable and invulnerable physician. In C. Gilligan, J. V. Ward, & J. M. Taylor (Eds.), *Mapping the moral domain* (pp. 245–262). Cambridge, MA: Harvard University Press.

Gilligan, C., Ward, J. V., & Taylor, J. M. (Eds.). (1988). *Mapping the moral domain.* Cambridge, MA: Harvard University Press.

1036

Gruber, H., & Voneche, J. (Eds.). (1977). *The essential Piaget.* New York: Basic.

John-Steiner, V. (1985). *Notebooks of the mind: Explorations of thinking.* Albuquerque: University of New Mexico Press.

Kohlberg, L. (1981). *The philosophy of moral development.* San Francisco: Harper & Row.

Luria, A. R. (1972). *The man with a shattered world: The history of a brain wound.* Cambridge, MA: Harvard University Press.

Luria, A. R. (1976). *Cognitive development.* Cambridge, MA: Harvard University Press.

Luria, A. R. (1987). *The mind of a mnemonist: A little book about a vast memory.* Cambridge, MA: Harvard University Press.

Mattingly, C. (1989). *Thinking with stories: Story and experience in clinical practice.* Unpublished doctoral dissertation, Massachusetts Institute of Technology, Cambridge, MA.

Mattingly, C. (1991a). The narrative nature of clinical reasoning. *American Journal of Occupational Therapy, 45,* 998–1005.

Mattingly, C. (1991b). What is clinical reasoning? *American Journal of Occupational Therapy, 45,* 979–986.

McKeachie, W. J. (1990). Research on college teaching: The historical background. *Journal of Educational Psychology, 82,* 189–200.

Paul, R. (1990). *Critical thinking.* Rohnert Park, CA: Center for Critical Thinking and Moral Critique.

Sacks, O. (1985). *The man who mistook his wife for a hat.* New York: Summit.

Schwartz, K. B. (in press). Education and occupational therapy: A shared vision. *American Journal of Occupational Therapy.*

Slavin, R. E. (1985). *Learning to cooperate: Cooperating to learn.* New York: Plenum.

Sternberg, R. J. (1988). *The triarchic mind: A new theory of human intelligence.* New York: Penguin.

Taylor, S. E. (1989). *Positive illusions: Creative self-deception and the healthy mind.* New York: Basic.

Wolff, R. A. (1990, June). *Assessment and accreditation: A shotgun marriage?* Paper presented at the Fifth American Association for Higher Education Conference on Assessment, Washington, DC.

Relationship Between Occupational Therapy Student Learning Styles and Clinic Performance

(education, occupational therapy; fieldwork; learning)

Elaine M. Stafford

Scores from the Learning Style Inventory (LSI), Your Style of Learning and Thinking (SOLAT), and Fieldwork Performance Reports (FWPRs) were used to assess the relationship between learning styles and clinic performance of 33 occupational therapy students who graduated from the University of Puget Sound in May 1983. The LSI was administered during the first semester of professional studies. The SOLAT was administered during the second fieldwork experience. There were significant correlations between scores from both learning style instruments and components of the Physical Disabilities Fieldwork Performance Report (PDFWPR) and Mental Health Fieldwork Performance Report (MHFWPR) scores. Results indicate that a logical, sequential cognitive style enhanced PDFWPR scores, but negatively affected some MHFWPR scores. A preference for active experimentation contributed to both PDFWPR and MHFWPR scores. Regression analysis identified the LSI Active-Reflective score as the best predictor of the PDFWPR total. Results suggest further research to assess learning styles as predictors of clinic performance and guides for curriculum design.

Effective clinic performance is the ultimate goal of occupational therapy education. The value of fieldwork experience in achieving that goal has been recognized and affirmed by practitioners and educators throughout the history of the profession (1, 2). Occupational therapy is among the 20 fastest growing occupations, according to recent US Bureau of Labor Statistics, and the bureau predicts continued growth for allied health professions through 1995 (3). Despite dimensions of change that are affecting professional education (1, 4), the role of fieldwork as a vital complement to academic preparation can be projected through the next decade.

Katz and Mosey (5) stated that the number of applicants for graduate and undergraduate programs in occupational therapy is greater than the number of available openings. Programs, therefore, must attempt to accept those students who are most qualified upon entry and

most likely to function effectively as practitioners and professional leaders. In addition, Katz and Mosey suggested that research to identify factors contributing to fieldwork performance may help clarify curriculum design. Presseller (1) showed that facilitating the application of theory to practice is the most difficult task in the educational process.

Numerous studies have correlated students' performance in fieldwork settings with scores from a variety of instruments, including the Florida Placement Examination (6, 7), the Minnesota Multiphasic Personality Inventory (7), the Strong Vocational Interest Blank (7, 8), the Allport-Vernon-Lindzey Study of Values (8), the Edwards Personal Preference Schedule (8), and grade point averages (5, 6, 8, 9). Some correlations have been found to be significant at the level of $p \le .05$ (5–7), but most have had little value in

Elaine M. Stafford MOT, OTR, is a therapist for Bethel School District No. 403, Spanaway, WA 98387.

predicting performance in a clinical setting. Anderson and Jantzen (6) concluded "... It appears that the predictors and criteria are merely unrelated" (p 77). They noted the importance of predicting success as early as possible, preferably before the student makes a commitment to the professional program. Bailey, Jantzen, and Dunteman (7) indicated that the Strong Vocational Interest Blank may have more predictive value than other measures, but their results were inconclusive.

All of the references cited concluded that there is a need for more research to determine predictors for clinic performance in occupational therapy. Ford (9) noted that clinical experience usually occurs near the end of the educational process and that performance in the clinic may be the student's first indicator of success or failure as a clinician. Accurate predictors would serve not only as preselection criteria but also as guides for student advisement and for planning effective instruction (10–12).

A recent study by Teske and Spelbring (4) pointed out that a pattern of declining college enrollment is forecast for the next 20 years. This pattern will be accompanied by changes in the characteristics of higher education students, including an increase in the number of nontraditional students (e.g., older women, minorities, and high school dropouts). Teske and Spelbring suggested that educational strategies in response to change include the modification of occupational therapy curriculum designs and fieldwork patterns and the promotion of "development in the areas of student learning styles, teaching methodology, and student evaluation" (4, p 672). In view of the changing applicant pool,

Holm (2) stressed the need for educational programs to use selection criteria that represent occupational therapy professional practice.

Numerous studies reflected interest in the personality types and affective behaviors of occupational therapy students (2, 13–15). In addition to traditional achievement measures, personality characteristics are commonly considered in admissions procedures (16–18). However, Dietrich (19) contended that many affective constructs are poorly defined and that "the development of allied health personality profiles is still in its infancy" (p 230). She pointed out that personality may change with maturation and experience and that the nontraditional student may present a different profile from the "college-age" applicant on standardized tests developed from a particular framework of psychology. Lacefield (20) also emphasized the varied changes that may occur during the time committed to professional studies. He stated that the curriculum should be designed to reinforce and augment the characteristics for which students were originally selected.

Rezler and French (12) compared personality types and learning styles of undergraduate occupational therapy students with those of students in five other allied health professions. Results indicated the need for longitudinal studies of learning styles to test the hypothesis that students will exhibit higher motivation and achievement levels if they are allowed to learn according to their preferences. Rezler and French also asserted that teaching styles would need to be compatible with learning preferences.

Llorens and Adams (10) surveyed 77 occupational therapy students over a three-year period us-

ing the Canfield-Lafferty Learning Styles Inventory, which focuses on affective components of teaching-learning situations. Based on the results, some changes in the presentation of course material were made at the group level in response to learning style preferences. In addition, scores from the Canfield-Lafferty inventory were used in advising some individual students. Although the authors concluded that accurate, highly individualized programming was not possible with data from the instrument, the results of the study were used effectively to increase faculty and student awareness of learning style preferences.

Using a pretest-posttest design, Rogers and Hill (11) studied the learning style preferences of two groups of occupational therapy students. Learning style preference was defined as "the preferred mode of obtaining knowledge" (p 78). They administered the Learning Preferences Inventory developed by Rezler and French (12) before and after a period of basic professional course work. Results were not consistent between samples, but they suggested that an educational program may influence learning style preference through teaching strategies that foster attitudes and reinforce behaviors congruent with a particular mode of learning.

Cunningham and Trickey (21) used Kolb's Learning Style Inventory in a preliminary study to determine the correlation between learning styles and performance in academic and clinical course work. No significant correlation was found between any of the learning styles and fieldwork performance. However, results led to the conclusion that further investigation is warranted.

The purpose of this study is to

examine the relationship between learning styles and clinic performance.

Methods

Subjects

Subjects were selected from occupational therapy students who graduated from the University of Puget Sound in May 1983. Those individuals included in the study met the following criteria:

1. Both required Fieldwork II experiences were completed by April 1, 1984.

2. Fieldwork Performance Reports were returned by April 15, 1984.

3. Written permission was granted for all scores to be used in this study.

Eighty-nine percent of the graduating class, 29 women and 4 men, met the criteria for the inclusion. Twenty-six of the subjects were undergraduates; the remaining seven were graduate students.

Instruments

Two instruments were used to assess learning styles. *Your Style of Learning and Thinking—Form C* (SOLAT) (22) seeks to classify subjects according to style of processing information. The self-administered test is based on extensive analysis of research concerning cerebral hemispheric functions. Each of 40 items presents the subject with three choices that represent a cognitive style characterized by right or left hemisphere domination or by integration. The instrument evaluates an individual's tendency toward processing information in a logical, sequential, systematic fashion described as being typical of the left hemisphere (SOLAT-L); in a more intuitive, synthetic, appositional manner char-

acteristic of the right hemisphere (SOLAT-R); or in a style that uses a logical, an intuitive, or an integrated approach as needed (SOLAT-I).

The second instrument used, Learning Style Inventory (LSI), was designed to assess strengths and weaknesses in learning styles and is based on Kolb's experiential learning theory (23, 24). Kolb's theoretical model describes a cycle in which experiences are used to develop concepts, which then guide the selection of new experiences. The learning process as reflected by the model involves two primary dimensions. The first is represented by an axis with Abstract Conceptualization at one end and Concrete Experience at the other. The second is represented with Active Experimentation at one end and Reflective Observation at the other.

A nine-item, self-description questionnaire asks respondents to order by rank four words in a way that best describes their learning styles. One word in each item represents one of the four steps in the experiential learning cycle. By adding the scored items in each column, respondents obtain four scores that indicate their relative preference for each learning mode. Two composite scores are computed from column totals—the Abstract Conceptualization total minus the Concrete Experience total (Abstract-Concrete) and the Active Experimentation total minus the Reflective Observation total (Active-Reflective). A positive Abstract-Concrete score indicates that the subject prefers abstract conceptualization to concrete experience; a negative Abstract-Concrete score indicates the opposite. The magnitude of the score reflects the strength of the preference. The

Active-Reflective score is interpreted in the same manner.

Only the composite scores were used in the present study. However, the Abstract-Concrete and Active-Reflective scores can be plotted in quadrants formed by the axes of the two dimensions. Dominant learning styles identified by the quadrants are described in the manual (23).

Clinical performance was assessed using the Level II Fieldwork Performance Report (FWPR). The FWPR is divided into five components: Data Gathering, Treatment Planning, Treatment Implementation, Communication Skills, and Professional Characteristics. The FWPRs were scored according to the AOTA Scorer's Guide (25), and there were 212 possible points. Scores for each subject were obtained for fieldwork in mental health dysfunction by using the MHFWPR and physical disabilities by using the PDFWPR.

Procedure

All subjects completed the LSI in the fall of 1981 during their first semester. Scores for the SOLAT and written permission to use all scores for this study were obtained during the second Fieldwork II experience. FWPR scores were computed when the clinical experiences were completed in mental health dysfunction and physical disabilities settings.

Pearson product-moment correlation coefficients were computed to determine the relationship between FWPR component scores and the learning style variables. To determine whether a combination of variables could predict outcomes on the FWPR, the researcher used a stepwise multiple regression that selected a combination of variables producing the maximum R^2 (the

Table 1

percentage of one variable explained by another variable) improvement on each step. Multiple regressions were also performed on the combination of variables to determine the relative contribution of each learning style variable to the FWPR score variance. A significance level of $p \le .05$ was established.

Results

Table 1 gives information that describes the sample. Table 2 presents the Pearson product-moment correlation coefficients of the various learning style indicators and the FWPRs. A significant correlation was found between the SOLAT-L and PDFWPR Professional Characteristics scores. There were significant positive correlations between the LSI Active-Reflective score and all of the PDFWPR component scores. Significant negative correlations were found between the SOLAT-L and MHFWPR Treatment Planning, Treatment Implementation, and total scores. There was a significant positive correlation between the LSI Active-Reflective score and the MHFWPR Communication Skills score.

A multiple regression revealed that the five learning style indicators accounted for 39.4% of FWPR score variance in physical disabilities. An analysis of variance yielded an F-ratio (variance between scores divided by variance within scores) significant at the $p \le .05$ level. The learning styles accounted for 17% of the FWPR score variance in mental health dysfunction, but this result was not significant.

The stepwise regression (which selects in descending value order the independent variables that contribute most to changes in the dependent variable) showed that each of the five learning style scores significantly affected variance in the physical disabilities FWPR total. Results are summarized in Table 3. Stepwise regression did not indicate that any of the learning style scores contributed significantly to changes in the mental health dysfunction FWPR total. However, it was noted that the LSI Active-Reflective and SOLAT-L scores, which contributed most to changes in the physical disabilities FWPR total, also contributed most to changes in the mental health dysfunction FWPR total. For mental health dysfunction, the SOLAT-L score entered the regression first, and both scores affected variance in the MHFWPR total at a level of $p \le .10$.

Discussion

The findings suggest that a learning style characterized by logical, systematic processing of infor-

Table 1
Statistics Showing Subjects' Learning Style and Fieldwork Performance Variables (N = 33)

Scores	Mean	SD	Range
SOLAT-R	11.970	5.382	4–26
SOLAT-L	11.061	4.697	2–21
SOLAT-I	16.910	5.960	5–34
LSI Abstract-Concrete	−.242	5.391	−11–12
LSI Active-Reflective	3.727	5.479	−9–12
PDFWPR	194.394	15.332	139–212
MHFWPR	197.394	11.546	170–212

SD, standard deviation. SOLAT-R, Your Style of Learning and Thinking—Right. SOLAT-L, Your Style of Learning and Thinking—Left. SOLAT-I, Your Style of Learning and Thinking—Integrated. LSI, Learning Style Inventory. PDFWPR, Physical Disabilities Fieldwork Performance Report. MHFWPR, Mental Health Fieldwork Performance Report.

Table 2
Correlation Coefficients for Learning Styles and FWPR Components

Learning Style	Data Gathering	Treatment Planning	Treatment Implementation	Communication Skills	Professional Characteristics	Total
Physical Disabilities Fieldwork						
SOLAT-R	.045	.149	.395	−.063	−.262	−.045
SOLAT-L	.245	.115	.178	.264	.307‡	.249
SOLAT-I	−.237	−.234	−.183	−.159	−.018	−.164
LSI Abstract-Concrete	−.048	−.128	−.078	.004	−.070	−.072
LSI Active-Reflective	.675*	.567*	.535*	.461†	.397†	.558*
Mental Health Dysfunction Fieldwork						
SOLAT-R	−.092	.151	.279	.104	.065	.158
SOLAT-L	−.161	−.380‡	−.362‡	−.219	−.062	−.304‡
SOLAT-I	.205	.161	.030	.071	−.009	.094
LSI Abstract-Concrete	−.127	−.108	.161	.046	−.063	.008
LSI Active-Reflective	−.090	.214	.228	.345‡	.264	.255

*$p \le .001$.   †$p \le .01$.   ‡$p \le .05$.
FWPR, Fieldwork Performance Report. SOLAT-R, Your Style of Learning and Thinking-Right. SOLAT-L, Your Style of Learning and Thinking—Left. SOLAT-I, Your Style of Learning and Thinking—Integrated. LSI, Learning Styles Inventory.

Table 3
Contribution of Learning Style Variables to FWPR Total in Physical Disabilities

Learning Style	R^2	R^2 change*	F-ratio	$p \leq$
LSI Active-Reflective	.3116	.3116	14.035	.001
SOLAT-L	.3595	.0479	8.421	.01
LSI Abstract-Concrete	.3713	.0118	5.709	.01
SOLAT-I	.3716	.0002	4.139	.05
SOLAT-R	.3940	.0225	3.512	.05

*R^2 change × 100 = percent of variance of PDFWPR total accounted for by each learning style variable.

FWPR, Fieldwork Performance Report. LSI, Learning Style Inventory. SOLAT–L, Your Style of Learning and Thinking—Left. SOLAT–I, Your Style of Learning and Thinking—Integrated. SOLAT–R, Your Style of Learning and Thinking—Right. PDFWPR, Physical Disabilities Fieldwork Performance Report.

mation (SOLAT-L) may be more relevant in physical disabilities settings than in mental health dysfunction settings. In contrast, clinic performance in mental health dysfunction may be enhanced by a more intuitive, appositional style of processing information (SOLAT-R) or by the ability to employ a systematic, holistic or integrated approach as needed (SOLAT-I).

The results indicate that a preference for active experimentation, that is, for "doing," for "testing implications of concepts in new situations" (23, pp 1–2), is an important factor in fieldwork performance. The mean LSI Active-Reflective score reflected this preference among the sample (see Table 1). These findings are congruent with previous studies that indicated the preference of occupational therapy students for direct experience (10) and learning practical skills (11, 12).

Multiple regression analysis indicated that simultaneous consideration of the learning style variables contributed significantly to the predictive power of these variables for the PDFWPR total but not for the MHFWPR total. Katz and Mosey (5) suggested that criteria used to assess student performance in occupational therapy physical disabilities courses may be more objec-

tive and discriminate more finely than criteria used in mental health dysfunction courses. Cunningham and Trickey (21) found the relationship between academic course work and physical disabilities fieldwork to be stronger than that between academic course work and fieldwork in mental health dysfunction. If it is true that physical disabilities courses afford a more objective evaluation of students, it may be because the criteria for evaluating clinic performance in physical disabilities are more objective and provide finer discrimination among students. The findings of this study suggest that further research is necessary to assess possible differences among the criteria used to evaluate students in physical disabilities practice and in mental health dysfunction settings.

The five learning style variables accounted for 39.4% of the variance in the PDFWPR total. Stepwise regression analysis determined that the LSI Active-Reflective score contributed 31.16% of the variance, isolating this learning style variable as the single best predictor in the study. The SOLAT-L score was the next highest contributor at 4.79%. Although the other three learning styles contributed only a small percentage to PDFWPR total variance, the con-

tribution of each was also statistically significant (see Table 3). These findings suggest that the evaluation of students' learning styles may identify a profile of predictors of clinical performance outcomes in physical disabilities.

Gay (26) stated that correlation coefficients below 0.50 are inadequate for purposes of group or individual prediction, "although a combination of several variables in this range may yield a reasonably satisfactory prediction" (p 188). Coefficients for significant correlations between learning style and FWPR variables in this study ranged from .304 to .675 (see Table 2). The statistical analysis indicated that LSI and SOLAT scores, considered in combination, may serve as substantial predictors of clinical performance scores (see Table 3).

Intercorrelations between SOLAT and LSI scores were below .150, and none was significant. The low level of intercorrelation indicated that instruments were independent measures of learning style and that therefore each may contribute meaningfully to formulating a professional profile.

Recommendations for Future Research

The findings of this study suggest several directions for further research on learning styles and clinic performance. Further research may determine the influence of learning styles on clinic performance in mental health dysfunction settings and establish the predictive power of the learning style variables. Also, when considered with findings from similar examinations of learning styles and clinic performance in physical disabilities, such research may contribute to the development of student selection criteria that more accurately reflect the practice of occupational therapy (2).

Others have suggested research to study the effects of time and curriculum on learning styles (11). In the present study, SOLAT scores may have been affected by the educational process. However, the low correlations between most SOLAT scores and fieldwork performance scores did not indicate a major effect.

Additional recommendations for further research include the exploration of using knowledge of occupational therapy student learning styles in the design and presentation of professional course content (10). Student advisement is another area in which the use of learning styles evaluation results may be examined for value in minimizing potential problems in clinic performance. Wong (27) noted, "Improvement in teaching strategies alone will not guarantee transfer of knowledge to the clinical practice. Since learning is a self-active process, the student must assume an active role in order to promote transfer of learning" (p 166). Understanding learning style strengths and weaknesses may facilitate the educational process for students and educators and guide both toward achieving the goal of effective clinic performance.

Summary

Scores from the LSI and SO-LAT were correlated with FWPR component scores for 33 occupational therapy students in physical disabilities and mental health dysfunction fieldwork. Results indicate that a logical, sequential cognitive style enhanced clinic performance in physical disabilities, but negatively affected some components of performance in mental health dysfunction settings. A preference for active experimentation correlated significantly with all components of the PDFWPR and with MHFWPR Communication Skills. The LSI Active-Reflective score emerged as the single best predictor in the study. The SO-LAT-L and LSI Active-Reflective scores contributed most to variance in both PDFWPR and MHFWPR totals.

ACKNOWLEDGMENTS

This research was completed in partial fulfillment of the requirements for the master's degree in occupational therapy at the University of Puget Sound, Tacoma, Washington.

REFERENCES

1. Presseller S: Fieldwork education: The proving ground of the profession. *Am J Occup Ther* 37:163–165, 1983
2. Holm MB: *Occupational Therapy Selection Criteria and Educational Processes: An Integrated Model*, doctoral dissertation. Lincoln, NE: University of Nebraska, 1980
3. Dataline: OT among twenty fastest growing occupations. *Occup Ther News* 38:6, March 1984
4. Teske YR, Spelbring LM: Future impact on occupational therapy from current changes in higher education. *Am J Occup Ther* 37:667–672, 1983
5. Katz GM, Mosey AC: Fieldwork performance, academic grades, and preselection criteria of occupational therapy students. *Am J Occup Ther* 34:794–800, 1980
6. Anderson HE, Jantzen AC: A prediction of clinical performance. *Am J Occup Ther* 19:76–78, 1965
7. Bailey JP, Jantzen AC, Dunteman GH: Relative effectiveness of personality, achievement and interest measures in the prediction of a performance criterion. *Am J Occup Ther* 23:27–29, 1969
8. Lind AI: An exploratory study of predictive factors for success in the clinical affiliation experience. *Am J Occup Ther* 24:222–226, 1970
9. Ford AL: A prediction of internship performance. *Am J Occup Ther* 33:230–234, 1979
10. Llorens LA, Adams SP: Learning style preferences of occupational therapy students. *Am J Occup Ther* 32:161–164, 1978
11. Rogers JC, Hill DJ: Learning style preferences of bachelor's and master's students in occupational therapy. *Am J Occup Ther* 34:789–793, 1980
12. Rezler AG, French RM: Personality types and learning preferences of students in six allied health professions. *J Allied Health* 4:20–26, 1975
13. Delworth UM: Interpersonal skill development for occupational therapy students. *Am J Occup Ther* 26:27–29, 1972
14. Wise BL, Page MS: Empathy levels of occupational therapy students. *Am J Occup Ther* 34:676–679, 1980
15. Greenstein LR: Student anxiety toward level II fieldwork. *Am J Occup Ther* 37:89–95, 1983
16. Blaisdell EA Jr, Gordon D: Selection of occupational therapy students. *Am J Occup Ther* 33:223–229, 1979
17. Johnson RW, Arbes BH, Thompson CG: Selection of occupational therapy students. *Am J Occup Ther* 28:597–601, 1974
18. Mann WC: Interviewer scoring differences in student selection interviews. *Am J Occup Ther* 33:235–239, 1979
19. Dietrich MC: Putting objectivity in the allied health student selection process. *J Allied Health* 10:226–229, 1981
20. Lacefield WE: Skill domains for allied health professions. *J Allied Health* 10:188–197, 1981
21. Cunningham MJ, Trickey BA: The correlation of learning styles with student performance in academic and clinical course work. *Occup Ther J Res* 3:54–55, 1983
22. Torrance EP, Reynolds C: *Norms-Technical Manual for Your Style of Learning and Thinking—Form C*. Athens, GA: University of Georgia, Department of Educational Psychology, 1980
23. Kolb DA: *Learning Style Inventory Technical Manual*. Boston: McBer, 1976, pp 1–2
24. Kolb DA, Rubin IM, McIntyre JM: *Organizational Psychology: An Experiential Approach*. Englewood Cliffs, NJ: Prentice-Hall, 1971, pp 23–29
25. *Field Work Experience Manual for Academic Field Work Coordinators, Field Work Supervisors, and Students*, interim document. Rockville, MD: American Occupational Therapy Association, 1977
26. Gay LR: *Educational Research*, 2nd edition. Columbus, OH: Charles E. Merrill, 1981
27. Wong J: The inability to transfer classroom learning to clinical nursing practice: A learning problem and its remedial plan. *J Adv Nurs* 4:161–168, 1979

The American Journal of Occupational Therapy **39**

The *Guide to the Preparation of Fieldwork Objectives for Occupational Therapy Students* developed by a committee of the University of Kansas Occupational Therapy Council on Education in response to Charge 13 from the Commission on Education of the American Occupational Therapy Association. The *Guide* was adopted by the Commission in April of 1977. In October of 1977, the *Guide* was accepted by the Representative Assembly with a mandate that it be published in *The American Journal of Occupational Therapy*.

I.   *General Introduction*

This document was developed by a committee chaired by members of the Commission on Education of the American Occupational Therapy Association and represents the educational (academic and fieldwork) programs at the University of Kansas. A working committee was selected by the chairs of the committee, and the Local Council of the University of Kansas was enlisted to provide input, feedback, and general assistance with this project.

The original task of this committee was to write a set of national fieldwork objectives. As work progressed on this task, writing specific behavioral objectives for all fieldwork experiences was seen as an overwhelming and unrealistic undertaking. The approach would seem to impose unnecessary constraints upon individual fieldwork centers, and inhibit, rather than encourage, flexibility. Instead, it was decided to produce a document that could be seen as a guide to the preparation of fieldwork objectives, rather than as the objectives themselves; it was hoped that this would be a more useful approach.

II.   *Purposes/General Objectives for Fieldwork*

The purposes and general objectives for fieldwork experience are as follows:

1. To provide students with the opportunity to practice with actual patients/clients/consumers the skills learned in the academic program.
2. To provide verification of the knowledge acquired in the academic program.
3. To provide the opportunity for students to expand the knowledge acquired in the academic program.
4. To provide students with the opportunity to refine the interpersonal skills and attitudes necessary for effective interaction with persons having physical, psychosocial, and/or developmental deficits; people with different values and backgrounds; and with other members of the health care team.
5. To provide students with feedback on their on-the-job performance, and to provide guidance for modifying that performance to improve effectiveness.
6. Subsequently, to promote the development of self-evaluation and problem-solving skills.
7. To provide the student with role models in direct service to patients/clients/consumers.
8. To ease the transition from the role of student to the role of occupational therapy practitioner.

The objective for the student's performance is: the student will meet the general objectives stated for the curriculum as they apply to the particular fieldwork facility to which the student is assigned.

III.   *Instructions for Using the Guide*

This *Guide* is divided into two major sections—direct and indirect services. Within each section there is a suggested task inventory based upon the material found in several documents listed in the reference section of the *Guide*. For selected items, examples of possible enabling activities are listed. In addition, some have samples of specific behavioral objectives that might apply to a given setting. All examples of enabling activities and specific behavioral objectives are enclosed in boxes so that they may be differentiated from the items in the task inventory.

Functions of the therapist and assistant are noted. It is assumed that the occupational therapist can perform all the tasks identified as appropriate for the assistant, when the situation demands.

Terms used in this project may be defined as follows:

Enabling Activity—activity that allows or assists the student to develop and/or demonstrate requisite skill in one or more subtask items.

Specific Behavioral Objective—statement of expectation for student behavior, including specific behavior, condition(s) under which the behavior is to occur, and criterion or criteria to be met.

The following is a recommended procedure for developing and using fieldwork objectives:

1. Identify appropriate entry-level tasks and sub-tasks, using this inventory or one developed by a given curriculum and taking into consideration any national, state, and local requirements that apply.
2. Identify enabling activities that can be offered in a given setting for as many subtasks as feasible (to be done by the fieldwork facility).
3. Write specific behavioral objectives that apply to enabling activities (to be done by fieldwork facility; may be done in collaboration with student).
4. Select and modify objectives to be met in keeping with the particular and unique characteristics of the curriculum(a) from which students are accepted by the facility and the needs and interests of the individual student, in the form of a learning contract between student and center.
5. Modify this contract by mutual consent of student and facility as the student's progress may indicate during the fieldwork experience.

Fieldwork Objectives

IV. *Direct Services*

A. **Screening**
Determine which patients/clients would benefit from occupational therapy services based on precise statements of criteria.

	COTA	OTR
1. Identify type of information needed.		x
2. Obtain information through—		
(a) Written sources.	x	x
(b) Interview with patient/client.	x	x
(c) Observation of patient/client.	x	x
(d) Discussion with others who may be involved in patient/client treatment program.	x	x
3. Identify needs for further evaluation.		x
4. Record data.	x	x
5. Summarize and interpret data.		x

Enabling Activities
A. 1. Have students observe a screening interview, then interpret the results orally or in writing.
2. Have students read a medical chart, then summarize and interpret data which are pertinent to potential need for occupational therapy services.

	COTA	OTR
6. Recommend general need for occupational therapy services.		x
7. Report findings verbally and/or in writing to appropriate persons.	x	x

B. **Evaluation**

Evaluate patients/clients with a wide range of physical, psychosocial, and developmental dysfunction, focusing on strengths and weaknesses.

	COTA	OTR
1. Select evaluation instruments/plan methodology for data collection.		x
2. Administer evaluation/collect data on occupational performance through—		
(a) Interview.	x	x
(b) Observation.	x	x
(c) Testing.	x	x
3. Record results/scores.	x	x

Enabling Activities
B. 1. Have student observe client performing an activity, then record observations pertinent to a specific performance skill.
2. Have a student record results of a standardized performance test as therapist administers the test.

	COTA	OTR
4. Compare results/scores to norms.	x	x
5. Interpret and synthesize findings to identify strenghts and weaknesses.	x	x
6. Report findings verbally and/or in writing to appropriate persons.	x	x
7. Administer evaluation/collect data on performance components through—		
(a) Interview.		x
(b) Observation.		x
(c) Testing.		x

Enabling Activities
B. 3. Have student observe client performance of an activity to identify a specific performance skill.
4. Have student administer a standardized test designed to identify skills and deficits in specific performance components.
Specific Objective
(a) The student shall administer to a client selected by the supervising therapist at least one Southern California Sensory Integrative Test and score and interpret it to at least 85% accuracy.

8. Record results/scores.

	COTA	OTR
8.		X

9. Compare results/scores to norms.
10. Interpret and synthesize findings to identify strengths and weaknesses.
11. Report findings verbally and/or in writing to appropriate persons.

	COTA	OTR
10.		X
11.		X

C. Program Planning

Utilize all available data to establish in collaboration with patient/client and significant others, realistic short- and long-term objectives and methods for implementation of occupatinal therapy.

1. Occupational therapy service programs designed to prevent deterioration in occupational performance.*
   (a) Set goals and priorities.
   (b) Select and plan use of occupational therapy techniques, media, and activities.
   (c) Discuss plans with client, family, and significant others.

	COTA	OTR
(a)	X	X
(b)	X	X
(c)	X	X

Enabling Activities
C. 1. Give student health maintenance case samples with established occupational therapy goals and have student select activities to meet these goals.
   2. Have student discuss an approved self-care plan with client family.

2. Occupational therapy service programs designed to restore/develop occupational performance skills.*
   (a) Set goals and priorities.
   (b) Select and plan use of occupational therapy techniques, media, and other activities.
3. Occupational therapy service programs designed to restore, develop, or prevent deterioration of performance component functioning.
   (a) Set goals and priorities.
   (b) Select and plan use of occupational therapy techniques, media, and activities.

	COTA	OTR
2(a)		X
2(b)		X
3(a)		X
3(b)		X

> *Review the theoretical basis and rationale from which treatment is derived. Consider limitations, barriers, contraindications, and precautions for treatment.

D. Program Implementation

Implement occupational therapy and document appropriately.

1. Discuss overall goals with client/ family.
2. Guide client selection of various appropriate activities/techniques.
3. Prepare, structure/adapt materials and environment necessary for selected activities/techniques.

	COTA	OTR
1.		X
2.	X	X
3.	X	X

Enabling Activities
D. 1. Have student construct an assistive device as part of client's occupational therapy program.
   2. Have student prepare work area before client comes to occupational therapy.

4. Instruct/supervise other staff in selected activities/techniques.
5. Instruct client/family in selected activities/techniques.
6. Engage client/family in selected activities/techniques.
7. Direct client performance.
8. Establish relationship that enhances optimal client performance.

	COTA	OTR
4.	X	X
5.	X	X
6.	X	X
7.	X	X
8.	X	X

Enabling Activities
D. 1. Have student practice role-playing an initial encounter with client.
   2. Videotape student's interaction with client, then have student review the tape and discuss with supervisor ways to improve the interaction.
Specific Objective
   (a) Using a videotape of an interaction between the student and client, the student and supervising therapist shall review the tape together and identify at least three ways in which the student could have facilitated the interaction.

9. Observe/measure client performance.
10. Elicit client/family (subjective) response regarding performance.
11. Report/record #7, 8, and 9.
12. Analyze/summarize client performance.

	COTA	OTR
9.	X	X
10.	X	X
11.	X	X
12.		X

	COTA	OTR
13. Collaborate with other disciplines to integrate client program.	X	X
14. Implement discontinuance/ transfer of treatment, considering need for and method of treatment continuity.		X

E. **Re-Evaluation**
Periodically evaluate effectiveness of occupational therapy and communicate appropriate objective and subjective information regarding evaluation, treatment planning implementation, and re-evaluation with patient/client, other involved health professionals, and significant others.

	COTA	OTR
1. Determine need for and scope of re-evaluation.		X
2. Repeat specific evaluation.	X	X
3. Compare results to previous data.	X	X

	COTA	OTR
4. Describe change on basis of findings.	X	X
5. Compare change to stated goals of the treatment program.	X	X
6. Evaluate effectiveness of program.		X
7. Recommend changes as indicated.	X	X

V.   *Introduction to the Indirect Services Section of This Guide*

With the increasing demand for expansion of health care services, including occupational therapy, there is a need for occupational therapy practitioners—even at the entry level—to have skills not only in providing direct client services but also in providing indirect services (sometimes referred to as support functions). Both direct and indirect services need to be accomplished in order to ensure that potential consumers of occupational therapy services will have access to those services appropriate to their needs and of high quality, and that these services may be provided by appropriately credentialed and competent personnel. Such indirect services include, but are not limited to, establishment of new occupational therapy programs and activities designed to ensure continued competency and encourage excellence in occupational therapy practitioners.

It is a rare individual who is prepared to perform the indirect service functions independently at the entry level. A wide variation in degree of expertise in these functions may be expected. However, the authors of this *Guide* believe that all students in occupational therapy should be encouraged to develop skills to provide indirect services whenever and to whatever extent possible. In many cases, these skills may be seen as variations of skills required to perform direct services.

Keeping in mind the need for varying degrees of supervision, consultation, and collaboration, the authors present the indirect services section of this *Guide* as an overview of possible functions, suggestions for a variety of enabling activities that might be provided in various fieldwork settings, and a sampling of specific behavioral objectives such as might be written where various learning activities in the area of indirect services are to be provided.

VI.   *Indirect Services*

Note: All items *A-E* are applicable to both levels of students. Primary application for COTAs is in the areas of health maintenance and self-care. Primary application for OTRs is in the areas of remediation and developmental facilitation.

A. **Consultation/Collaboration**
Determine need for and use consultation/collaboration.
   1. Identify when consultation/collaboration is needed.
   2. Identify type of consultation/collaboration needed.
   3. Identify available consultative/collaborative resources.
   4. Request and use consultation/collaboration as needed.

B. **Screening**
Determine the needs for occupational therapy services in various communities as well as in particular clinical settings.
   1. Identify type of information needed.
   2. Identify sources of information needed.

3. Identify methods of obtaining information needed.
4. Obtain information about community/clinical setting.
5. Evaluate information obtained in order to identify potential patient/client/consumers of occupational therapy services.
6. Describe potential patient/client/consumers/of occupational therapy services.
7. Define patient/client/consumer's general needs for such services.
8. Identify potential sources of support for occupational therapy services.
9. Describe potential support for occupational therapy sources.
10. Define strategies for securing such support.
11. Formulate recommendations regarding types of occupational therapy services that could meet the general needs of clients in a given community or clinical setting.
12. Formulate recommendations regarding ways in which occupational therapy services could be supported in a given community or clinical setting.

Enabling Activities
B. 3. Have student write a report recommending ways in which a new occupational therapy program could be supported in a given community or facility.
   4. Have student formulate recommendations for securing additional support for an existing occupational therapy program.

C. **Evaluation**
Describe specific problems that can be completely or partially resolved through provision of occupational therapy services in a given setting.
   1. Select and plan methodology for collection of data to identify specific needs of persons who could benefit from occupational therapy services, including preventive services, treatment, rehabilitation, and health maintenance.
   2. Select and plan methodology for collection of data to identify:
      a. Facilities required to meet identified needs.
      b. Personnel required to meet identified needs.
   3. Select and plan methodology for collection of data to identify specific sources of support for the various occupational therapy services identified as needed.
   4. Collect data to identify: nonoccupational therapy services available to meet some identified needs, quality of existing services, services needed, facilities and personnel needed, and specific sources of support for these.
   5. Interpret data: Identify, describe and summarize.

(a) Needs of persons in community/clinical setting for occupational therapy services.
(b) Willingness of community to accept and use such services.

Enabling Activities
C. 1. Have student survey a local nursing home, then report on specific occupational therapy approaches/techniques needed in that nursing home.
   2. Have student interview administrator and key staff members in nursing home, then describe to supervisor impressions of their willingness to accept a new occupational therapy program, using supporting evidence.
Specific Objective
(a) The student shall interview the administrator and key staff members in a local nursing home and, using supporting evidence and data collected during the interviews, describe to the supervising therapist the student's impression of the feasibility of a new occupational therapy program.

6. Interpret data: Identify, describe, and summarize facilities and personnel required to provide needed occupational therapy services.
7. Interpret data: Identify, describe, and summarize specific sources of support for needed occupational therapy services.
8. Summarize evaluative data and interpretation of findings in a written report.

D. **Planning and Implementation**
Demonstrate an ability to plan and implement programs to meet the needs for occupational therapy service.
   1. Draw accurate conclusions from evaluative data.
   2. Identify overall goals that apply to the setting.

Enabling Activities
D. 1. Have student search through official documents of facility to identify statements that relate to the goals of the setting.
   2. Have student interview key personnel to elicit information on overall goals.

3. Identify appropriate expectations/hopes of sponsoring agent.
4. Develop program objectives within limitations of available resources.
5. Identify priorities in establishing long-term and short-term goals.
6. Identify steps in achieving overall goals.
7. In collaboration with consumers and sponsoring agents, mutually agree on steps and a plan of action to be taken.

8. Incorporate into plan support of:
   (a) maintenance of professional standards.
   (b) continued professional development, i.e., workshops, conferences, etc.
9. Select and plan specific programs, considering the media, techniques, and skills necessary to meet the needs of the sponsoring agency and its patients/clients.
10. Select and plan specific occupational therapy programs in keeping with current and established practice.
11. Plan budget to implement program.
12. Formulate additional occupational therapy recommendations(s), as needed, to coordinate with and support other health services and programs.

13. Interpret occupational therapy services to other disciplines and to all those persons who will be affected by the planned program.
14. Obtain staff and use as necessary:
   (a) recruit.
   (b) hire.
   (c) orient.
   (d) supervise.
15. Order supplies and equipment as necessary.
16. Develop fee system as necessary.
17. Develop a system of client referral.

18. Develop a record-keeping system.
19. Interpret occupational therapy services to the public.
20. Obtain volunteer assistance as needed:
   (a) recruit.
   (b) screen.
   (c) train.
   (d) supervise.
21. Coordinate program with other disciplines and collaborate as appropriate.
22. Change and adapt program as needed.

E. **Re-evaluation**
Engage in continuing review of professional effectiveness.
1. Re-describe results of screening, evaluation, planning, and implementation.
2. Identify new problems/needs.
3. Discuss findings with consultant(s).
4. Seek additional information.
5. Establish new priorities, new focus.

6. Consider new options and consequences, select new strategies.
7. Implement new strategies in orderly manner.
8. Seek and use opportunities for professional growth and development.

F. **Research**
Use research as a means for continuing education and adaptation of skills according to professional level.

	COTA	OTR
1. Formulate hypotheses.		X
2. Develop research design.		X

Enabling Activities

F. 1. Have student develop a research design to cover a longitudinal case-study approach with a single client over the duration of the fieldwork assignment.

2. Have student develop a design for survey research

	COTA	OTR
3. Use a monitoring/evaluation system that will consider intervening variables.		X
4. Plan methodology for collection of data.		X
5. Implement plan for data collection.	X	X
6. Evaluate results of collected data:		
(a) Apply methods of observation and measurement.		X
(b) Employ concepts of reliability and validity.		X
7. Report results and discuss implications.		X

Enabling Activities

F. 3. Have student write up case study research project.

4. Have student write a report on a survey to submit for publication.

	COTA	OTR
8. Critically evaluate studies done by others.		X
9. Review current research for new information to improve services.	X	X

VII. *References and Recommended Readings*

Bloom, Benjamin, Editor: *Taxonomy of Educational Objectives*, New York: Longmans, Green, 1956.

Entry Level Functions of the Registered Occupational Therapist, Certified Occupational Therapy Assistant and Occupational Therapy Aide, American Occupational Therapy Association, 1973.

Essentials of an Accredited Educational Program for the Occupational Therapist, American Occupational Therapy Association, 1973.

Essentials of an Approved Educational Program for the Occupational Therapy Assistant, American Occupational Therapy Association, 1975.

Mager, Robert F, Beach, Kenneth M: *Developing Vocational Instruction*, Palo Alto: Fearon Publishers, 1967.

Mager, Robert F: *Goal Analysis*, Belmont, CA: Fearon Publishers, 1972.

Mager, Robert F: *Preparing Instructional Objectives*, Palo Alto: Fearon Publishers, 1962.

Roles and Functions of Occupational Therapy Personnel (particularly *Appendix A*), American Occupational Therapy Association, N01-AH-24172.

****

Members of the Committee to Develop National Fieldwork Objectives:

Dorothy Anne Penner, Editor, and Co-Chair

Nancy Mashak, Co-Chair

Working Committee:

Kay Heather	Barbara Kleinman
Karin Chapman	Sue Meredith
Betty Bulkley	Jane Underwood
Ellen Roose	Joane Wyrick

Consulting and Feedback Committee:

Members of the Council on Education of the University of Kansas, Occupational Therapy Department.

Nedra Gillette and various fieldwork supervisors for the occupational therapy program at Columbia University.

Naomi Greenberg and various fieldwork supervisors for the occupational therapy assistant program at LaGuardia Community College.

Kathlyn Reed, University of Oklahoma.

Various students in the occupational therapy curriculum at the University of Kansas.

Adopted by the Commission on Education, April 1977.

SECTION TWO

Research on Educational Outcomes Related to Fieldwork

Fieldwork is a broad subject that represents both practice and education, and the debate continues whether practice precedes education or vice-versa. This suggests that more outcomes studies and research studies on the efficacy of fieldwork are needed to provide the specialty practice of fieldwork a knowledge and "number" base.

This section contains articles that discuss general research methodologies and results in the larger scheme of fieldwork. The articles cover the spectrum from fieldwork cost-effectiveness to the proper use of the fieldwork evaluation form for occupational therapy students. The articles are replete with references to the need for further research and qualitative studies to support the development of fieldwork as we approach the 21st century.

How important is fieldwork? Important enough that every one of us credentialed as an OTR or COTA has had to complete fieldwork successfully. Each of us has most likely experienced Maslow's hierarchy of needs to stay afloat financially and emotionally on fieldwork. There is strict adherence to state and certification boards for requirements. Additionally, the fieldwork process entrusts students to represent occupational therapy to consumers in an intellectual, professional, and ethical manner. Clinical education research will always change as the healthcare market changes and new clinical competencies emerge. In occupational therapy, our fieldwork scholars are the clinical supervisors, students, and faculty. We need more solid information on the value of fieldwork in various settings, on the fieldwork process, on the estimation of fiscal benefit, on the effect of fieldwork on choice of employment, and on the reliability and validity of standard fieldwork evaluations.

Whether you believe that fieldwork drives practice or practice drives fieldwork, clinical education is still a driving force in our profession.

The Value of Psychosocial Level II Fieldwork

Anne W. Atwater, Christine G. Davis

Key Words: education, occupational therapy • holistic health • mental health occupational therapy

The shortage of occupational therapists choosing to practice in mental health and the increase of therapists electing to specialize in other areas led to a pilot study designed to gather information regarding the value of psychosocial Level II fieldwork. A survey was mailed to 152 practicing occupational therapists who had graduated from Colorado State University in Fort Collins between 1983 and 1988; of the surveys returned, 116 were used in this study. The results indicate that the psychosocial Level II fieldwork experience provides therapists with valuable training and experience regardless of their current area of practice or specialization. The results also suggest that to preserve the holistic approach that occupational therapists offer their clients, psychosocial Level II fieldwork must remain a requirement of occupational therapy programs.

Anne W. Atwater, OTS, is an Occupational Therapist at the Kalispell Regional Rehabilitation Center, Kalispell, Montana. At the time of this study she was a graduate student at Colorado State University, Fort Collins, Colorado, and was completing her Level II fieldwork at St. Patrick Hospital, Missoula, Montana.

Christine G. Davis, MOT, OTR, is an Occupational Therapist at the WorkAbility Program, North Colorado Medical Center, Greeley, Colorado, and at the Brain Injury Recovery Program, Fort Collins, Colorado. At the time of this study, she was Assistant Professor, Department of Occupational Therapy, Colorado State University, Fort Collins, Colorado. (Mailing address: 1164 East Fourth Street, Loveland, Colorado 80537)

This article was accepted for publication January 25, 1990.

A decline in the number of occupational therapists working in mental health settings is a current trend in the field of occupational therapy. Fewer occupational therapists are now working in long- or short-term psychiatric settings and more are employed in private practice, public schools, or home health care agencies (Gibson, 1984). Between 1973 and 1986, the percentage of registered occupational therapists practicing in psychiatric hospitals and community mental health centers declined from 18% to 8.5%; for certified occupational therapy assistants, it declined from 26.6% to 12.2% (American Occupational Therapy Association [AOTA], 1987). A review of the literature indicates that this trend is shared by other medical disciplines (Arnswald, 1987; Fagin, 1981; Mitsunaga, 1982; Nielsen, 1979). Arnswald stated that fewer nurses are choosing psychiatric nursing for both employment and graduate study, and between 1971 and 1976, there was a 27% decrease in the number of first-year residents practicing in psychiatry (Nielsen, 1979).

The small number of practitioners in mental health greatly concerns our profession and is exacerbated by a general shortage of therapists (Bonder, 1988). Psychosocial educators in occupational therapy have also identified the paucity of students going into psychiatric practice as a problem facing occupational therapy in mental health today (Barris & Kielhofner, 1986).

Trends in health care provision that cause a shift in focus are not new to occupational therapy. These trends can be directly related to factors that affect society as a whole (Tiffany, 1983). With roots firmly planted in the foundation of mental health since the early 1900s, occupational therapy has undergone many changes and has emerged as a profession that is involved in the treatment of many physical and psychological disorders. Although many therapists tend to categorize occupational therapy as dealing with either physical dysfunction or psychosocial issues, the two must be considered together in the treatment of an individual. This holistic treatment approach is a major component of our philosophical base and has been a unique characteristic of occupational therapy throughout the years (Tiffany, 1983).

As the focus of occupational therapy has shifted over the years to meet the needs of society and the challenges of the ever-changing health care system, educational programs for students have had to respond. In light of the current trend, that is, the decline in the number of occupational therapists working in mental health settings and the increase of therapists specializing in other areas, educational programs face two challenges. The first is to decide whether to continue to require psychosocial Level II fieldwork, because so few students are electing to specialize in this area. Research concerning the career choices of occupational therapists indicates that fieldwork experience has the greatest effect on the development of a therapist's preference for a specific area of clinical practice (Christie, Joyce, & Moeller, 1985) and that a positive fieldwork experience is one of the most influential factors determining specialty choice (Ezersky, Havazelet, Scott, & Zettler, 1989). We may assume, therefore, that the decline of therapists choosing to practice in mental health would be further affected if occupational therapy students were not required to participate in a psychosocial Level II fieldwork experience.

The second challenge of educational programs is to determine whether knowledge and experience with mental health disorders is essential to the holistic practice of occupational therapy. How would the holistic, philosophical base of future occupational therapists be influenced if participation in psychosocial Level II fieldwork were no longer mandatory?

Although psychosocial Level II fieldwork has been a part of our educational programs for many years, no research has been conducted to determine the value of such fieldwork. The present pilot study was designed to gather information from practicing occupational therapists, regardless of their area of clinical practice or specialization, concerning the value of their psychosocial Level II fieldwork experience.

Method

Psychosocial Level II fieldwork is a 12-week internship or affiliation in a mental health setting that is undertaken by occupational therapy students after completion of their academic course work. Throughout this paper, the terms *psychosocial* and *mental health* will be used interchangeably, and the terms *Level II fieldwork experience, internship,* and *affiliation* will be used synonymously.

We designed a three-part questionnaire to use in this study. In the first part, the respondents were asked to identify the focus of their current practice as primarily psychosocial, physical dysfunction, both, or other. They were also asked to indicate their work setting, age, and years in practice, and the percentage of their practice that involves psychosocial issues.

In the second part of the questionnaire, the respondents were asked to rate their interest in, contact with, and fear of working with mental health clients prior to their Level II fieldwork. They were also asked to rate their psychosocial academic course work in terms of preparation for their Level II internship experience and to indicate if they had participated in a Level I psychosocial practicum experience.

The third part of the questionnaire dealt with the

respondents' perceptions of the relationship between their psychosocial fieldwork experience and their current practice as an occupational therapist. Did their psychosocial affiliation have an impact on the area they chose for clinical practice, and if so, was the impact positive or negative? Did the psychosocial internship provide experiences and training of value to them in their current practice? If the respondents indicated that the fieldwork was valuable, they were asked what aspects of the experience were particularly valuable. They were also asked if there was a specific aspect or experience provided by their psychosocial fieldwork that they believed could not have been gained from their physical dysfunction placement. The final question asked respondents if they felt psychosocial fieldwork should be required for all occupational therapy students, and space was left for additional comments concerning this issue. The questionnaire was mailed to 152 registered occupational therapists who had graduated from Colorado State University between 1983 and 1988. The sample was randomly selected by AOTA, drawing from a population of current AOTA members who met the above criteria. A postcard reminder was sent to all those who had not responded within 2 weeks. Raw data were analyzed with the Biomedical Data Processing Statistical Software (Regents of University of California, 1985).

Results

Of the 152 surveys mailed, 127 (83.5%) were returned. Of those returned, 11 were eliminated from the data analysis because of incomplete data, thus yielding a sample size of 116 (76.3%).

The mean age of the respondents was 28.8 years (range = 22 to 49 years). The mean number of years in practice was 3½ (range = 0 years [for a respondent who had never practiced] to 10 years [for a respondent who had had experience as a certified occupational therapy assistant]). A total of 54.3% of the respondents indicated that the focus of their current practice was primarily physical dysfunction; 8.6%, psychosocial; 7.8%, both areas; and 29.3%, other (e.g., pediatrics).

The largest percentage of respondents (56.8%) indicated that they worked in a hospital, a rehabilitation center, or a school system. When the respondents were asked what percentage of their current practice involved psychosocial issues, 97.4% indicated that they dealt with psychological issues as part of their clinical practice.

The respondents were evenly divided concerning Level I (practicum) participation in a mental health setting: 50% had participated in a 40-hr practicum in a psychosocial setting, and 50% had not. When asked to rate the adequacy of their psychosocial academic course work in preparation for their mental health Level II fieldwork, 15.5% indicated that their course work was less than adequate; 57%, adequate; 24.1%, more than adequate; and 3.4%, excellent.

The respondents were asked to rate their interest in mental health issues, experience or contact with mental health patients, and fear of working with mental health patients before their psychosocial internship. The surveys showed that, before their Level II fieldwork experience, 55.2% of the respondents had a moderate or high interest in mental health issues, more than 80% had either minimal or no experience with mental health patients, and 67.2% believed they had either minimal or no fear of such patients.

More than half (57.8%) of the respondents indicated that they had done their mental health fieldwork in a psychiatric hospital; 26.7%, in a general hospital. Only 4.3% had done their fieldwork at a community mental health center, and 11.2% of the respondents chose other, with 6 of those specifying a Veterans Administration setting.

More than half (55.2%) of the respondents indicated that the psychosocial Level II fieldwork had influenced their career choice, whereas 44.8% indicated that it had not. Of those who indicated that it had an impact, 53.1% said the impact was positive, and 46.9% said it was negative. When asked if the psychosocial Level II fieldwork experience provided training and experiences that were valuable in current practice, 85.3% of the respondents viewed it as valuable. The one-way chi-square (goodness-of-fit test) indicated that this was significant ($\chi^2 = 56.56$, $df = 1$, $p < .001$). Of the respondents who indicated that such experience was of no value to their current practice, 35% attributed this to poor site selection and believed that a more positive setting may have been valuable. Forty-seven percent of the respondents indicated that although their particular experience was not valuable, psychosocial internships should still be required.

To gather more specific information about the value of the internship experience, we asked the respondents to indicate what aspects of their psychosocial fieldwork they considered valuable. They were to indicate *yes* or *no* for three listed aspects: leading small groups, psychosocial theory application, and dealing with feelings and emotions. The fourth category, other, allowed the respondents to list other aspects that they found to be of specific value. Most of the respondents (75.9%) indicated that learning to deal with their own and others' feelings and emotions was a valuable aspect of their experience, and 57.8% indicated that leading small groups (group dynamics) was another valuable aspect of their experience. Forty-four percent valued applying psychosocial theory, and 32.8% indicated other valuable aspects of their psychosocial fieldwork experience. An open-ended question asked if there was a particular aspect

of the psychosocial fieldwork experience that gave the respondents what they could not have gotten from their physical dysfunction internship; 75.9% of the respondents cited specific examples.

The final survey question asked if psychosocial Level II fieldwork should be required of occupational therapy students; 84.5% answered yes. The one-way chi-square test indicates that this is significant ($\chi^2 = 53.80$, $df = 1$, $p < .001$). Of the 18 respondents who indicated that psychosocial fieldwork should not be required, 10 (55.5%) believed that students should be able to choose between a psychosocial internship and a pediatric, hand therapy, or other specialized area for their second fieldwork experience. Space left for additional comments elicited concern from most respondents about this issue. These comments are summarized below.

Discussion

This pilot study indicates that the psychosocial fieldwork experience is valuable to occupational therapists, regardless of their area of clinical practice or specialization, and that such fieldwork should be included in the educational program.

A major concern expressed by the respondents was that the holistic approach traditional to occupational therapy would be greatly threatened if the psychosocial internship were no longer required. Many respondents believed that through their psychosocial internship they learned how to deal with the mental health issues (e.g., anger, depression, grief) that they encounter daily in their work with clients and families. Many respondents indicated that their psychosocial internship allowed them to get to know themselves better and to deal more assertively with clients, a skill they found beneficial in their current practices.

The respondents who indicated that the Level II experience was not valuable or that it should not be required generally fit into two categories: (a) those who had had a negative psychosocial fieldwork experience (attributed to poor supervision or what they believed to be an inadequate site selection) and (b) those who had already selected their area of practice and thought their time would have been better spent in their area of specialization. The respondents who had had a negative experience indicated that educational programs should more carefully screen fieldwork sites and supervisors to ensure that students have an adequate experience. The respondents who indicated that students should have a choice recognized the trend toward specialization in occupational therapy and identified the need to address specialization in fieldwork.

Although this study has a number of limitations, it does raise several questions that warrant further ex-

Research on Educational Outcomes Related to Fieldwork | 83

amination. Additional research is needed to determine if the survey results would hold true for graduates of other educational facilities and for therapists who have been practicing for more than 5 years. Research is also needed to determine if the holistic approach of occupational therapy would be affected if the psychosocial Level II fieldwork were no longer required. The prompt and substantial return rate (83.5%) of this survey, along with the wealth of additional comments submitted, indicate that this is a topic of interest and concern to practicing occupational therapists and one that needs to be more fully addressed.

An additional area for future research would be to determine the sequence in which students should complete their fieldwork placements. Several respondents indicated that they found it beneficial to complete their psychosocial Level II fieldwork first because of the insight it gave them during their physical dysfunction internship.

Study Limitations

The subjects for this study were limited to those who had graduated from Colorado State University between 1983 and 1988. We chose to perform this study in a location in which the psychosocial academic course work as well as the Level I (practicum) and Level II fieldwork requirements were known to be relatively consistent over time. Because the population was limited in years of practice and to one educational facility, the results may not be consistent with a random selection of all occupational therapists.

A second limitation of this study was the small number of subjects who indicated that the focus of their practice was primarily psychosocial. Because the response in this area was so small, we could not use chi-square tests to determine relationships between a therapist's current focus of practice and other selected variables without violating the assumption of expected frequencies.

A third limitation of this study was that the average length of practice for occupational therapists responding to the survey was 3.5 years. Perhaps many of the positive values attributed to psychosocial Level II fieldwork (e.g., assertiveness, dealing with one's own and others' feelings) were in fact maturational and increased with experience and time in practice, regardless of the psychosocial fieldwork experience. We hope that a future, controlled study will prove or disprove this point.

Conclusion

The concerns over the declining number of occupational therapists practicing in mental health and how educational programs will meet this challenge prompted this pilot study. The results indicate that therapists perceive that psychosocial Level II fieldwork (a) provides valuable training and experience to occupational therapists regardless of the focus of their current practice or specialization and (b) is a vital part of our educational program and should continue to be included in the training of future occupational therapists. ▲

Acknowledgment

We wish to thank Susan M. Thornton, MS, for her editorial assistance.

References

American Occupational Therapy Association. (1987). *1986 Member data survey: Interim report no. 1.* Rockville, MD: Author.

Arnswald, L. (1987). Not fade away. *Journal of Psychosocial Nursing, 25,* 31–33.

Barris, R., & Kielhofner, G. (1986). Beliefs, perspectives, and activities of psychosocial occupational therapy educators. *American Journal of Occupational Therapy, 40,* 535–541.

Bonder, B. R. (1988, December). Occupational therapy: Issues in mental health. *Mental Health Special Interest Section Newsletter,* pp. 1–3.

Christie, B. A., Joyce, P. C., & Moeller, P. L. (1985). Fieldwork experience, part I: Impact on practice preference. *American Journal of Occupational Therapy, 39,* 671–674.

Ezersky, S., Havazelet, L., Scott, A. H., & Zettler, C. L. B. (1989). Specialty choice in occupational therapy. *American Journal of Occupational Therapy, 43,* 227–233.

Fagin, C. M. (1981). Psychiatric nursing at the crossroads: Quo vadis. *Perspectives in Psychiatric Care, 19.* 99–106.

Gibson, D. (1984). Guest Editorial: The dearth of mental health research in occupational therapy. *Occupational Therapy Journal of Research, 4,* 131–149.

Mitsunaga, B. K. (1982). Designing psychiatric/mental health nursing for the future: Problems and prospects. *Journal of Psychosocial Nursing and Mental Health Service, 20,* 15–21.

Nielsen, A. C. (1979). The magnitude of declining psychiatric career choice. *Journal of Medical Education, 54.* 632–637.

Regents of University of California. (1985). *Biomedical Data Processing Statistical Software.* Los Angeles: Author.

Tiffany, E. G. (1983). Psychiatry and mental health. In H. L. Hopkins & H. D. Smith (Eds.), *Willard and Spackman's occupational therapy* (6th ed., pp. 267–285). Philadelphia: Lippincott.

84 | Research on Educational Outcomes Related to Fieldwork

Perceptions of the Purpose of Level I Fieldwork

Lisette N. Kautzmann

Key Words: education, occupational
therapy • educational objectives • fieldwork

The purpose of this study was to examine perceptions of the purpose of Level I fieldwork. Academic faculty members, fieldwork supervisors, and students were asked to rank their 10 most valued choices from a list of proposed objectives. Responses were tabulated by frequency, summed, and analyzed.

The results show that objectives from the category of student involvement in the occupational therapy treatment process were ranked most frequently and that objectives associated with understanding the clinical program and facility were ranked the least often. Statistically significant differences between academic and fieldwork educators were identified on two items: (a) "Receive feedback on beginning strengths and weaknesses in professional behavior" and (b) "Opportunity to develop a treatment plan." Both academic and fieldwork educators differed significantly with students on six items: (a) "Develop an awareness of the patient as a whole person," (b) "Develop a beginning awareness of patterns of practice in occupational therapy delivery systems." (c) "Participate in supervisor/supervisee relationship and experience working out communication and personality differences," (d) "Introduction to evaluation and treatment techniques," and (e) "Opportunity to develop a treatment plan." By clarifying the perceptions of the academic faculty, the fieldwork supervisors, and the students, Level I fieldwork will be strengthened and improved.

Lisette N. Kautzmann, EdD, OTR, FAOTA, is an Assistant Professor in the Department of Occupational Therapy at Eastern Kentucky University, Richmond, Kentucky 40475.

Clinicians and academicians agree that fieldwork links theory with practice. The importance of the fieldwork experience is also evidenced by its continuous inclusion in the American Occupational Therapy Association (AOTA) *Essentials for an Approved Educational Program for Occupational Therapists* from 1923 to the present (AOTA, 1983). While the Association has developed a structure and guidelines for Level II fieldwork, the Level I experience has received less attention from the national level. Level I fieldwork, which is broadly defined, is intended to be responsive to the needs and resources of each academic program. The 1983 AOTA *Essentials* describe Level I fieldwork as experiences designed to be an integral part of the didactic courses for the purpose of directed observation and participation in selected fieldwork settings (AOTA, 1984). Personnel qualified to supervise Level I students includes occupational therapy staff, teachers, social workers, public health nurses, ministers, probation officers, and physical therapists. Fieldwork objectives are to be developed collaboratively by academic and fieldwork educators.

Major variables that occur in the delivery of Level I fieldwork are in the academic curriculum and in fieldwork supervision. The variations that occur in individual academic programs' institutional mission, organization, resources, and philosophical base influence curriculum design and the delivery pattern of all courses, including Level I fieldwork. The availability of personnel to supervise students is also a primary factor in determining the character of the Level I experience.

This diversity in academic programs makes it difficult to generalize about the educational management of Level I fieldwork beyond limited geographical regions. The issue of educational management is complicated further when several schools share fieldwork sites. Thus it has become increasingly difficult to negotiate the delivery of Level I fieldwork in a manner that will meet the needs of academic programs, fieldwork programs, and students. Leonardelli and Caruso (1986) indicated that if academic and fieldwork educators became aware of and understood each other's objectives, they would be closer to making Level I fieldwork a more satisfying experience. The purpose of this investigation was to contribute to the clarification of the purpose of Level I fieldwork by identifying and statistically analyzing the valued choices of academic faculty members, fieldwork supervisors, and students within one geographic area.

Literature Review

The literature on Level I fieldwork, model programs, and fieldwork supervision is not extensive. One of the studies that contributed to the understanding of Level

I fieldwork was conducted by Leonardelli and Caruso (1986). In this study, academic and fieldwork educators were surveyed to identify their preferences in fieldwork objectives, responsibility for management of the fieldwork experience, and scheduling patterns. Also included were questions on cost-effectiveness and the potential usefulness of uniform objectives and evaluations. The ranking of objectives reflected differences in opinion between academic and fieldwork educators: Academic educators focused on students' needs, and fieldwork educators were more responsive to patients' needs. Respondents did not identify a preferred scheduling pattern. The level of concern about cost–benefit and provision of quality supervision rose in direct proportion to the number of schools using the center as a Level I fieldwork site. The availability of continuing education, access to school resources, in-services, and clinical and research consultation was identified as compensation that could help offset cost–benefit concerns. The development of uniform objectives and an evaluation instrument received both support and criticism. Although it was thought that uniform objectives would provide more consistency in determining expectations for students' performances and have the potential to serve as guidelines, they were also considered to be too general or too restrictive for some fieldwork sites. Fieldwork educators who supervised students from several schools supported the development of a uniform evaluation. However, they expressed concern that a uniform evaluation might be too general, not objective, and not able to measure performance accurately.

Alternative models of fieldwork have been described by several authors. The development of a Level I placement in a federal correctional institution was discussed by Platt, Martell, and Clements (1977). The placement was developed by occupational therapy faculty members, and the program was staffed by students working under faculty supervision. Students showed gains in the areas of personal resourcefulness, group leadership skills, and ability to identify clients' needs. They also learned to identify the role of occupational therapy within the context of the institution and experienced the satisfaction and challenges of clinical practice.

Several models of Level I fieldwork that used students as program staff working under the direction of occupational therapy faculty supervisors have also been reported (Kramer, 1985; Cole, 1985; and Kimball, 1983). The program presented by Kramer was located in college-based demonstration classes on communication for handicapped children. Students developed competency in the following areas: beginning skills in evaluation, data analysis, treatment planning and intervention, writing behavioral goals,

and interacting with other professionals. Cole's program was located in a Veterans Administration hospital. This program provided students with an exposure to a disabled population and the opportunity to practice evaluation and treatment techniques and documentation skills. In Kimball's model, the rationale and procedure for developing a community occupational therapy clinic was discussed. Level I experiences were offered in the areas of pediatrics, physical disabilities, psychosocial dysfunction, and blindness.

Nontraditional, community-based fieldwork programs have been described in two articles. In the first study, Cromwell and Kielhofner (1976) presented a model of training that prepares students for community practice. Students were assigned to human services programs that did not provide occupational therapy services. They gathered data about the agency and used the information to design an activity-focused program that met health needs. Supervision was shared by members of the academic faculty and agency personnel. In the second study, a practicum experience in a camp for diabetic children was described (Gill, Clark, Hendrickson, & Mason, 1974). Students were able to apply their knowledge of growth and development, define the role of occupational therapy in a nontraditional setting, and learn about childhood diabetes.

Three sequentially oriented fieldwork experiences were designed by the occupational therapy faculty at the University of Texas Medical Branch at Galveston (1981). Faculty members structured learning experiences to move from simple to complex taxonomic levels and thus provide a sequential orientation to clinical practice.

Studies by Christie, Joyce, and Moeller (1985a, 1985b) confirmed the importance of the fieldwork supervisor as a role model in the development of professional behavior at both levels of fieldwork. Beginning and experienced fieldwork supervisors differed in supervisory style. New supervisors felt the need to control all aspects of clinical learning and preferred a rigidly structured fieldwork program that was applied to all students regardless of individual need. In contrast, experienced fieldwork supervisors recognized that students share some responsibility for the success or failure of the clinical learning experience. They also realized the importance of assessing the needs of the individual student and adjusting the structure of the fieldwork experience to meet these needs. Christie et al. also found that fieldwork supervisors' flexibility seemed to increase with experience and appeared to be directly related to their increased confidence in their abilities as student supervisors. Another finding was that student growth was facilitated by open communication, good interpersonal skills, and a supportive, caring environment.

Methods

A questionnaire was used to collect information on perceptions of the purpose of Level I fieldwork. Questionnaire items were developed by a group of 50 occupational therapy academic and fieldwork educators during a brainstorming exercise designed to produce a number of Level I fieldwork objectives. The educators, working in small groups, generated individual, written lists of objectives that were shared verbally and pooled to form a master list. When the master lists from each group were combined, 24 objectives were identified. These proposed objectives clustered around the following categories: (a) objectives related to student involvement in the occupational therapy treatment process, (b) items concerning students' understanding of the clinical program and the facility, (c) objectives focusing on the role of the occupational therapist, and (d) items associated with students' growth as emerging health professionals.

Questionnaire respondents were instructed to rank, in descending order, their 10 most valued choices from the list of 24 proposed objectives. After field testing, the questionnaire was mailed to all 27 academic faculty members in Wisconsin and all 136 occupational therapy fieldwork supervisors that provide a Level I fieldwork experience to Wisconsin occupational therapy students. The questionnaire was then distributed to 49 University of Wisconsin–Milwaukee senior occupational therapy students. Their responses to each item were tabulated by frequency, summed, and analyzed. The mean scores for each item were computed and compared between groups using a two-tailed independent t test at the .05 level of significance.

Results

Nineteen of the 27 academic faculty members (70%), 71 of the 136 fieldwork supervisors (52%), and 46 of the 49 students (93%) completed and returned the questionnaire. Two academic faculty members and 10 fieldwork supervisors returned unranked question-

Table 1
Rank Order of Responses, Including 10 Most Valued Items

Item Number	Description	Rank		
		AF	FWS	S
Student Involvement in the Treatment Process				
1.	Develop an awareness of the patient as a whole person.	10	9	
2.	Provide initial clinical exposure to occupational therapy through observation of clinical application of theory.	3	1	3
3.	Provide hands-on experience with patients.	1	5	1
4.	Provide opportunities for student–patient interaction.	2	2	6
5.	Introduction to evaluation and treatment techniques.	8	4	2
6.	Opportunity to practice writing skills.			7
7.	Opportunity to develop a treatment plan.			9
Student's Understanding of the Program and Facility				
8.	Orientation to the treatment philosophy of the facility.			
9.	Opportunity to observe continuity of care.			
10.	Develop a beginning awareness of patterns of practice in occupational therapy delivery systems.	7	6	
11.	Observe interdisciplinary cooperation.			
12.	Exposure to a disabled population.		8	
13.	Exposure to the scope of the facility.			
Role of the Occupational Therapist				
14.	Observe role model of OTR–COTA interaction.			
15.	Observe role model of therapist–client interaction.	5	3	8
16.	Observation of a role model of lifelong learning and recognition that occupational therapy practice is a dynamic process.			
17.	Opportunity for observation of professionalism.			
Student's Growth as Emerging Health Professionals				
18.	Provide opportunities for the student to observe problem solving in practice situations and to begin to develop his/her own style and flexibility.	9		5
19.	Receive feedback on beginning strengths and weaknesses in professional behavior.	6	10	4
20.	Participate in supervisor/supervisee relationship and experience working out communication and personality differences.			
21.	Provide a screening/counseling process for students regarding Level II fieldwork and career choices.			
22.	Opportunity for the student to identify specific interests and skills.			
23.	Provide opportunities for students to explore their feelings about their interactions with patients and their reaction to the observed practice of occupational therapy.	4	7	10
24.	Opportunity for the student to start focusing on others, with less concern for how others are affecting him- or herself and more concern for his or her own impact on others.			

Note. AF = Academic faculty; *n* = 19. FWS = Fieldwork supervisors; *n* = 71. S = Students; *n* = 46.

naires; their comments indicated that they felt all the objectives were valuable. The results of the questionnaire are summarized in Table 1.

Of the top ten objectives chosen by each group, the top five for both faculty members and fieldwork supervisors as well as the top six for students were in the category of student involvement in the occupational therapy treatment process. Students did not include any objectives in the category of understanding the clinical program and the facility in their rankings.

In order to determine whether or not there was a significant difference in the perceptions of the purpose of Level I fieldwork between faculty members, fieldwork supervisors, and students, the mean scores of each rank-ordered item on the 24-item list were computed for each group and compared between groups using a two-tailed independent t test at the .05 level of significance. At this level, the critical value of t was 1.960. Items with fewer than five responses from any group were not compared. The results of the comparison are presented in Table 2.

Academic and fieldwork faculty respondents differed significantly in their perceptions of the purpose of Level I fieldwork in only two areas. The former group placed a higher value than the latter group on Item 19, "Receive feedback on beginning strengths and weaknesses in professional behavior." Although neither group ranked Item 7, "Opportunity to develop a treatment plan," statistically fieldwork supervisor respondents valued this item more than academic faculty respondents.

There were significant differences between academic faculty and student perceptions on six items.

Academic respondents valued the following items more than student respondents: Item 1, "Develop an awareness of the patient as a whole person," Item 10, "Develop a beginning awareness of patterns of practice in occupational therapy delivery systems," Item 20, "Participate in supervisor/supervisee relationship and experience working out communication and personality differences," and Item 23, "Provide opportunities for students to explore their feelings about their interactions with patients and their reaction to the observed practice of occupational therapy. Student respondents valued Item 5, "Introduction to evaluation and treatment techniques," significantly more than did academic faculty respondents. Again, even though academic faculty respondents did not rank Item 7, "Opportunity to develop a treatment plan," as a preferred choice, statistically students valued this item more than did faculty members.

Fieldwork supervisor respondents also differed from student respondents on six items. The former group valued the following items more than the latter group: Item 1, "Develop an awareness of the patient as a whole person," Item 10, "Develop a beginning awareness of patterns of practice in occupational therapy delivery systems," Item 20, "Participate in supervisor/supervisee relationship and experience working out communication and personality differences," and Item 24, "Opportunity for the student to start focusing on others, with less concern for how others are affecting him- or herself and more concern for his or her own impact on others." There was a statistically significant difference between groups on Item 24, even though it was not ranked by either group. Two items, Item 3, "Provide hands-on experience with patients," and Item 19, "Receive feedback on beginning strengths and weaknesses in professional behavior," were valued more by student respondents than by fieldwork supervisor respondents.

Discussion

Since this study was limited to Wisconsin, the results cannot be generalized to other geographical areas. However, the high rate of response from all groups surveyed provides a strong indication of perceptions and values associated with Level I fieldwork in this region. Use of the methodology and findings from this study can serve as a basis for studies in other geographical regions. Additional limitations included the small number of students represented in this study and the possibility that a response bias may have been created by surveying students from only one academic program. The students' emphasis on ranking clinical skills as priority items may have been due to anxiety about their impending Level II affiliations. The use of multiple t tests increases the experimental

Table 2
Intergroup Comparisons ($p \leq .05$)

	Calculated Value of t^a		
Item	Academic Faculty/Fieldwork Supervisors	Academic Faculty/ Students	Fieldwork Supervisors/ Students
1	0.600	2.340*	3,769*
2	0.520	0.859	1.413
3	0.774	0.731	2.278*
4	0.176	0.615	0.299
5	1.872	3.769*	1.805
6	0.253	0.492	0.159
7	2.297*	2.508*	0.429
10	0.500	2.172*	2.317*
11	1.794	0.709	1.817
12	1.598	0.206	1.866
15	1.474	0.337	1.392
17	0.659	0.468	1.474
18	0.595	1.601	1.177
19	2.170*	0.532	2.268*
20	0.017	3.270*	4.079*
23	1.299	2.134*	1.064
24	0.071	1.570	3.633*

Note.[a] Critical value of t = 1.960.
*$p \leq .05$, two-tailed.

error rate and the probability of error in the interpretation of the significance of the results (Ottenbacher, 1983). Therefore, it is suggested that statistical findings under the adjusted rate of 2.576, using the formula $1 - [(1 - \alpha)^c]$, should be viewed cautiously (Ottenbacher, 1983).

The major conclusion of this investigation was that there is strong agreement, particularly between academic faculty members and fieldwork supervisors, on the purpose of Level I fieldwork. All three groups gave highest value to objectives associated with students' involvement in the occupational therapy treatment process. This involvement includes opportunities for observation and active participation in the treatment of patients. Findings indicate that academic faculty members need to consider ways to integrate treatment planning into the design of Level I fieldwork, and fieldwork supervisors should explore alternatives for providing feedback to students on professional behavior. Orientation to the treatment philosophy of the facility and exposure to the scope of the facility were perceived as having low value and priority by all three groups. This would indicate that time spent in orienting students could be reduced and that this could perhaps be accomplished through the use of videotapes and readings.

There is evidence to indicate that students' perceptions of the purpose of Level I fieldwork differ from the perceptions of academic and fieldwork educators. Students are concerned with learning the skills of clinical practice. They want and expect hands-on experience, not just observation. Fieldwork supervisors should be aware that students' primary objectives are to practice and receive feedback on clinical skills and to observe clinicians in action. Additionally, modeling and coaching should be used to help students learn to focus on the needs of patients.

Developmentally, Level I students are looking for professional growth and prefer receiving feedback on their performance over participating in all aspects of the supervisory relationship. The high value placed on feedback echoes the findings of Christie et al. (1985b) regarding the importance of communication in the supervision of fieldwork education and the need to provide regular, timely, and constructive feedback. Students are eager to acquire psychomotor skills and strengthen their identities as health professionals; they are not as interested in the overall aspects of the fieldwork experience, including the need to treat the whole person, to understand the treatment philosophy of the facility, and to learn the patterns of occupational therapy practice. Academic and fieldwork educators can help students bridge this gap by reinforcing these concepts both in the classroom and during fieldwork supervision.

In this study, gathering data from three distinct sources was an important factor in clarifying the purpose of Level I fieldwork. Students' values may not always be considered in decisions on fieldwork. In fieldwork councils, students and academic faculty members are in the minority, and their voices and values may be lost in the majority vote. In other situations, fieldwork educators may not be equally represented in discussions with academic faculty members. By analyzing the responses from these three separate groups, the opinions of each group are clarified and pathways for working together are identified. Decisions regarding Level I fieldwork are frequently made by small groups of people who represent larger constituencies. In these situations verbal skills, assertiveness, persuasiveness, and the power and status of individual group members may affect other group members' objectivity and influence group decision making. By surveying the perceptions and values of the groups involved in Level I fieldwork, the variables and constraints of the group decision making process are eliminated. In addition, the process brings objectivity and breadth to the examination of the purpose of the fieldwork experience.

Summary

Despite the difficulties in the delivery of Level I fieldwork, it is of critical importance to this segment of occupational therapy education that academic faculty members, fieldwork supervisors, and students look beyond their differences, perceive each others' needs, and work together toward strengthening the Level I experience. Identifying and understanding the values and concerns of all groups associated with this level of fieldwork is the first step. Replications of this study in other geographical areas are recommended as follow-up. Mutual understanding can be achieved if findings of this and similar studies are used by fieldwork councils, in negotiations between schools and fieldwork centers, and in the preparation of students for fieldwork. Cooperative effort by all groups associated with Level I fieldwork will improve and strengthen this experience.

Acknowledgment

This paper is based on a presentation made at the 1984 American Occupational Therapy Association Annual Conference in Kansas City.

References

American Occupational Therapy Association. (1983). *Essentials for an approved educational program for occupational therapists.* (Available from AOTA, 1383 Piccard Drive, Rockville, MD 20850.)

American Occupational Therapy Association. (1984). *Guide to fieldwork education.* Rockville, MD: Author.

Christie, B. A., Joyce, P. C., & Moeller, P. L. (1985a).

Fieldwork experience, Part I: Impact on practice preference. *American Journal of Occupational Therapy, 39,* 671–674.

Christie, B. A., Joyce, P. C., & Moeller, P. L. (1985b). Fieldwork experience, Part II: The supervisor's dilemma. *American Journal of Occupational Therapy, 39,* 675–681.

Cole, M. B. (1985). Starting a Level I fieldwork program. *American Journal of Occupational Therapy, 39,* 584–588.

Cromwell, F. S., & Kielhofner, G. W. (1976). An educational strategy for occupational therapy community service. *American Journal of Occupational Therapy, 30,* 629–633.

Gill, A. A., Clark, J. A., Hendrickson, F. R., & Mason, C. L. (1974). A student practicum experience. *American Journal of Occupational Therapy, 28,* 284–287.

Kimball, J. G. (1983, spring). The community occupational therapy clinic: One answer to providing fieldwork I experiences at a rural college. *OT Education Bulletin,* pp. 13–16.

Kramer, P. (1985, fall). A unique Level I fieldwork experience: The student as therapist. *OT Education Bulletin,* pp. 11–12.

Leonardelli, C. A., & Caruso, L. A. (1986). Level I fieldwork: Issues and needs. *American Journal of Occupational Therapy, 40,* 258–264.

Ottenbacher, K. (1983). The issue is: A "tempest" over *t*-tests. *American Journal of Occupational Therapy, 37,* 700–702.

Platt, N. P., Martell, D. L., & Clements, P. A. (1977). Level I field placement at a federal correctional institution. *American Journal of Occupational Therapy, 31,* 385–387.

University of Texas–Galveston, Department of Occupational Therapy. (1981). *Level I preceptorship preceptor manual.* Galveston: Author.

Exploring the Costs and Benefits Drivers of Clinical Education

Susan K. Meyers

Key Words: education • fieldwork, occupational therapy, level II • qualitative method

Objective. *This study was designed to identify monetary and nonmonetary costs and benefits, as well as their drivers, to assist persons in clinical sites who are implementing clinical education to minimize costs and maximize benefits.*

Method. *Qualitative research methodology involved students, student supervisors, administrators, and patients in a hermeneutic dialectic process of identifying costs and benefits of Level II fieldwork in three clinical sites.*

Results. *Different costs and benefits were identified by the different groups of respondents. Drivers, or causes, of these costs and benefits reflected unique environmental factors in each site of data collection as well as common factors across the sites.*

Conclusion. *Clinical education may be enhanced and stress reduced for all persons involved in clinical education through improved communication, structure, education, and support.*

Susan K. Meyers, EdD, MBA, OTR, is Associate Professor and Chair, Department of Occupational Therapy, College of Health and Human Services, Western Michigan University, Kalamazoo, Michigan 49008.

This article was accepted for publication January 4, 1994.

Occupational therapy students are dependent on practitioners in clinical environments to provide them with experiences necessary to integrate and apply theory to practice. The monetary costs and benefits associated with clinical education have been identified in the literature (Chung & Spelbring, 1983; Page & MacKinnon, 1987; Porter & Kincaid, 1977; Schauble, Murphy, Cover-Patterson, & Archer, 1989; Shalik, 1987). The net monetary cost benefits to facilities that provide clinical education to students are (a) revenue generated by students who provide treatment to patients and (b) increased revenue generated by therapists who are freed by students from performing clerical and administrative tasks. However, changes in health care environments, including increases in the number of students seeking clinical education and in the demands for productivity in patient treatment, have created new demands for practitioners responsible for the clinical education of occupational therapy students.

In previous cost-benefit analyses, the use of an a priori theory limited costs and benefits to those that could be monetarily quantified. The rigor required for generalization of conventional research has negated the relevance of factors that may be contextually meaningful, such as nonmonetary costs and benefits of therapists, students, patients, and administrators who have a stake in clinical education. This study was designed to identify monetary and nonmonetary costs and benefits, as well as the drivers of these costs and benefits. Identifying the drivers of costs and benefits may assist persons in clinical sites who are implementing or planning to implement clinical education to minimize costs and maximize benefits to all of the stakeholders in the clinical site.

Methodology

This study used the qualitative research methodology of naturalistic inquiry to collect and analyze data from three clinical education sites over a 6-month period. Study participants included 19 administrators and student supervisors; 14 occupational therapy students who were completing first, second, or third rotations of clinical education; and 6 patients who were being treated by the students.

The major methods of data collection were observation, individual and focus group interviews, and documents review. Data collection and analysis were done simultaneously with a constant comparative method (Glaser & Strauss, 1967; Lincoln & Guba, 1985; Strauss & Corbin, 1990). Each piece of data was grouped with similar pieces of data until clear categories that were salient to the research concern emerged. These categories provided the skeletal shape of the information needed to understand the costs and benefits drivers of clinical education. The data led to additional questions and responses that gave flesh to the skeletal shape by providing a collaborative understanding of costs and benefits drivers of clinical education.

Trustworthiness techniques used to establish rigor for the qualitative research were prolonged engagement, persistent observation, peer debriefing, negative case analysis, progressive subjectivity, and member checks (Guba & Lincoln, 1989). Prolonged engagement was achieved by spending 6 months, or two rotations of clinical education, at each site in order to build a rapport with respondents and gain an understanding of the culture of the setting. Persistent observation, which gave depth to the study, was achieved by multiple observations and interviews with each respondent. This technique led to improved understanding of costs and benefits drivers affecting stakeholders of the clinical education process.

Two peer debriefers, disinterested parties with knowledge of the methodology and understanding of the research questions, were used throughout this study. By posing questions and suggestions, the debriefers helped focus the inquiry and kept my work consistent with the methods of naturalistic inquiry.

Negative case analysis involved looking for alternative constructions, or views, to those most often stated by respondents. As respondents generated these alternative views and discussed them with me and each other, respondents either modified their views as a result of new knowledge, or continued to hold their different views; in either case, they acknowledged that other views were also valuable in understanding the costs and benefits associated with clinical education.

Progressive subjectivity occurred when my own construction changed as a result of being better informed by respondents. Member checks provided the mechanism to ensure that a construction was in fact that of the respondent as he or she reported it. At the end of each observation or interview, data that I recorded were reviewed with the contributing respondent. Respondents either verified the accuracy or elaborated on their concerns and clarified their viewpoints. At the conclusion of the study, drafts of the final constructions of costs and benefits drivers of clinical education were distributed to all respondents for their agreement regarding data accuracy. This procedure led to additional clarification, which continued until all respondents agreed that the final construction was accurate, regardless of whether they agreed with the views of others. An audit trail referenced each piece of data reported by respondents to its source. The sources of all data have been kept anonymous.

Results

The results of the analysis indicated that students, student supervisors, administrators, and patients constructed costs and benefits drivers differently. Summaries and comparisons of costs and benefits drivers appear in Table 1.

The costs and benefits drivers were considerably dif-

Table 1
Level II Fieldwork Costs and Benefits Identified by Respondent Groups

Costs and Benefits	Students	Student Supervisors	Administrators	Patients
Monetary costs				
Cost of treatment			•	•
Travel to site	•			•
Space for students		•	•	
Supplies used by students		•	•	
Loss of income from work	•			•
Loss of revenue		•	•	
Potential liability			•	
Clothing	•			
Housing	•			
Tuition	•	•		
Failure	•	•		
Nonmonetary costs				
Stress	•	•		•
Frustration	•	•		•
Loss of esteem	•	•		•
Responsibility		•		
Annoyance to staff members	•			
Illness from stress	•			
Failure	•			
Monetary benefits				
Revenue		•	•	
Recruitment		•	•	
Cost savings	•		•	•
Nonmonetary benefits				
Learning	•	•	•	•
Relationship formation	•	•	•	•
Stay current in practice		•	•	•
Satisfaction		•	•	
Self-esteem	•	•		
Excitement	•	•		
Peer support	•		•	
Attention				•
Professional commitment		•	•	
Prestige	•			
Decreased patient load		•		

ferent among student supervisors both across the three clinical sites and within each site. Stress was a nonmonetary cost for all student supervisors, but this stress was driven by different situations indigenous to each site. In some sites, student supervisors identified external pressures to lower standards for student performance so that students who performed poorly would pass the clinical education experience. In two sites, student supervisors reported feeling stressed by organizational structure over which they believed they had little control. In two sites, there were conflicting constructions of nonmonetary cost drivers among student supervisors and their administrators in the organization, which created additional stress for therapists, students, and patients in the sites. When these types of conflicts existed, students identified them as contributors to a stressful clinical education experience.

There were some similarities among student supervisors' constructions of nonmonetary cost drivers. Students' egocentrism and dependence on their supervisors drove costs in all three clinical sites. Some students' behaviors, such as delayed response to treatment team members (especially when this was mentioned by other health care providers), contributed to the student supervisors' negative image of the profession. Student supervisors had to take their own work home in the evenings as a result of the time they spent supervising their students during the day. Although student supervisors from all sites agreed on these drivers of nonmonetary costs, administrators did not identify these drivers. However, administrators agreed that students might be a cause of frustration to student supervisors.

All student supervisors identified the same monetary costs. Student supervisors and administrators agreed that there was minimal cost associated with providing students materials such as manuals and supplies in the clinics. Greater costs were associated with space needed for students in the sites, especially when space was scarce. Another cost was lost revenue driven by the need for student supervisors to spend time educating students instead of treating patients. When students were assigned the task of preparing patients' charges, they missed some of the charges due to inexperience with the billing process.

Student supervisors and administrators agreed that monetary benefits were gained from students treating patients, especially after students completed the first half of a clinical education rotation. Cost savings resulted from hiring students to become staff therapists in the sites studied.

Identification of nonmonetary benefits of clinical education was similar across sites. Student supervisors said they experienced satisfaction and increased knowledge because of their work with students. Students gave their supervisors positive feedback, and supervisors believed that they were doing a service to the profession by educating future clinicians. Student supervisors kept current in treatment techniques and research related to patient care so that they would be better able to teach their students. Students brought new ideas with them to the clinics and completed projects and assignments that were beneficial to their supervisors. When students were performing well, their supervisors had additional time to spend with patients or in other related activities. Students were credited with bringing a freshness and new enthusiasm for clinical practice, which some of the student supervisors identified as a benefit. Administrators in the three sites also tended to be in agreement with these benefits of clinical education.

Students at the three sites identified similar monetary costs drivers, including housing, utilities, and food. All had to pay tuition to their academic institutions for credit hours they received for clinical education. These costs were driven by the requirement to complete assigned clinical education as part of their academic programs. Transportation was another monetary cost, because most students lived a distance from the clinical sites and incurred local transportation expenses. Some students traveled from another city or state for clinical education. Some students needed to purchase clothing to wear in the clinics because the clothes they owned were not suitable for the clinic. A few students lost revenue from jobs they either gave up or reduced hours for in order to devote their time and energy to their clinical education experience.

Students across the three sites also identified similar nonmonetary costs. Students experienced considerable stress as a result of their clinical education. This stress resulted in symptoms of illness and some absences from the clinic. As some students became more stressed, their performance worsened. This set in motion a vicious cycle in which the students' stress led to poor performance, which in turn resulted in negative feedback from their supervisors. The negative feedback exacerbated the students' stress and, in at least one case, was identified as the cause of student failure. Some of the drivers of stress identified by the students included being watched by supervisors; having trouble with critical thinking, time management, and communication; lacking skills in specific treatment techniques; fearing failure; having heard negative comments about the clinical education site or the supervisors in the site; dealing with the reality of very sick patients; and adjusting to the role of worker. Adapting from a student role to a worker role was especially difficult for students during a first clinical education experience. Just getting to work through morning traffic and working an 8-hr day were identified as being highly stressful. In addition, most of the students said they took large amounts of work home in the evenings.

Some students were more satisfied than others with their clinical education sites, and this satisfaction mitigated the stress they experienced. Students who were in a site that they had requested as their first choice for clinical education were more satisfied than students who were not placed in their first choice sites. Students who were in a site in which they were fairly certain they wanted to continue working after completing their clinical education were the most satisfied and the least stressed.

All of the student respondents agreed that they experienced no monetary benefits from being in the clinical sites studied. They did not identify future monetary benefits that would result from this education process. They did identify cost savings because they did not have to buy textbooks for clinical education. Several students said that their parents were supporting them through clinical education—another form of cost savings.

Nonmonetary benefits were similar for all students who participated in this study. Students learned skills necessary for clinical practice; they also learned more about themselves. Learning in the clinics was driven by exposure to patients and supervisors. Application of theories and techniques learned in school were integrated and given relevance in the clinic settings. Students increased their confidence in their abilities when they were successful in treating patients and received positive feedback from supervisors. Students identified contact with supervisors as helpful in shaping both a professional image and a sense of belonging to a professional group. Some of the drivers decreasing stress identified by the students were receiving a good orientation to the site; having other students with whom to share the clinical education experience; and receiving manuals and handouts that specified expected performance in the sites. Almost anything that increased the structure of the clinical education experience was considered a stress reducer by students.

Costs and benefits identified by the patients were different from those of the other groups of respondents. Patients discussed major monetary costs due to illness and treatment that were not specifically related to treatment in a clinical education environment. They identified nonmonetary costs associated with separation from families and loss of functional abilities due to their illnesses. However, patients identified benefits resulting specifically from the services they received in a clinical education environment. They learned about their illnesses or injuries from supervisors' explanations to students about the treatment process. Patients said that if a supervisor trusted a student, the student must be capable of doing a good job and that the treatment he or she received from that student was of good quality. Patients saw little difference in skill levels between students and student supervisors. Some patients identified differences in attitudes between students and student supervisors. In the sites where student supervisors were more stressed by their working conditions, patients identified students as more enthusiastic than student supervisors about work.

Students and student supervisors identified different reasons for student failures. Student supervisors said that students were not adequately prepared for the work in clinic sites; that students had difficulty because of poor technical, problem-solving, and communication skills; and that students demonstrated inadequate self-awareness. Students said that failures were a result of inadequate supervision, poor communication, inadequate feedback, lack of structure, and personality clashes with supervisors. Students accepted responsibility for contributing to their own failures. Some of the student supervisors shared responsibility for student failures, saying that they could have intervened sooner to prevent failures.

Conclusion

Although the results of this study are not generalizable, information about costs and benefits drivers of clinical education may be useful to other clinical education sites.

Bureaucratic organizational structures of the three sites contributed to nonmonetary costs of clinical education for students and student supervisors. Decisions made at high levels of the organization were transmitted to persons at lower levels for implementation; however, persons providing direct services to patients believed that high-level decision makers were not adequately informed to make those decisions. The discrepancy between student supervisors and administrators regarding the drivers of costs and benefits appeared to be a result of inadequate communication across hierarchical lines.

When student supervisors were not satisfied with administrators of their work units, there was a direct effect on the clinical education of students; students who heard their supervisors talking about their dissatisfaction became stressed. Student supervisors who were the most stressed seemed to be the least satisfied with the responsibility of educating students. When student supervisors were cohesive with other supervisors in their work units, clinical education was a positive experience for students. Student supervisors' report of satisfaction with autonomy in their work and with their relationships with each other and with their administrators seemed to result in the best environment for providing clinical education to students.

As data collection for this study progressed, respondents began to make changes in their environments. Communication improved among respondents, and more structure was provided for students in some sites. Administrators' concerns with what was occurring in clinical education sites appeared to increase. Some of the changes that were made to improve clinical education appeared to be the result of the interactive nature of the research methodology used in this study. Naturalistic inquiry seemed to be the catalyst for turning ideas expressed by respondents into actions that would maximize benefits and minimize costs of clinical education.

Recommendations

The goals of cost-benefit analysis are to maximize benefits and minimize costs. On the basis of this study, the following six guidelines are recommended to facilities that want to establish or improve existing clinical education programs and reduce stress to all persons involved.

1. Establish effective communication between administrators and student supervisors related to worker satisfaction. Informal and consistent communication between administrators and subordinates lessens stress in the work environment and enhances clinical education.
2. Decentralize decision making related to task performance within the clinic sites, including decisions related to clinical education. Persons with direct contact with students in the work environment have the greatest information with which to make decisions about scheduling, supervising, and terminating students. Decentralized decision making allows decisions to be made quickly and

to be made in response to changes in the environment. If decentralized decision making is not possible, the administrator responsible for making decisions should spend time in the clinic site and be willing to discuss and negotiate decisions with those subordinates responsible for carrying out the tasks of clinical education.

3. Offer education and support to supervisors. Student supervisors in clinics that have well-established, successful education programs, in which student supervisors and students have satisfying experiences, should share their methods with student supervisors in other sites who have less satisfying experiences. This sharing of information may be accomplished through supervisor support groups or individual mentoring of a new supervisor by a more experienced supervisor who enjoys working with students.

4. Provide students with a structured learning experience. A clearly defined structure for clinical education assists students in adapting to a work environment and maximizes their performance. Such a structure includes frequent formal evaluation of students so that the students know how they are performing. Students should also be accountable for tasks in the site; a checklist of performance expectations would be helpful to both students and their supervisors.

5. Establish criteria for student performance. Academicians who send students into clinical education sites should be aware of the requirements for student performance in each site. Students should be prepared to adequately perform tasks required in the clinic sites. Additional course content, including training in assertive behavior, criti-cal thinking, and time management, may need to be added to improve student success. (In this study, students had more difficulty with general behaviors than with specific treatment techniques.)

6. Limit some clinical education sites to students who are in a second or third rotation of clinical education. (In this study, when a clinical site required specialized skills, students on a first rotation had great difficulty performing while adjusting to the new role of worker.) ▲

References

Chung, Y. I., & Spelbring, L. M. (1983). An analysis of weekly instructional input hours and student work hours in occupational therapy fieldwork. *American Journal of Occupational Therapy, 37*, 681–687.

Glaser, B., & Strauss, A. (1967). *The discovery of grounded theory: Strategies for qualitative research.* Chicago: Aldine.

Guba, E. G., & Lincoln, Y. S. (1989). *Fourth generation evaluation.* Newbury Park, CA: Sage.

Lincoln, Y., & Guba, E. (1985). *Naturalistic inquiry.* Beverly Hills, CA: Sage.

Page, S. S., & MacKinnon, J. R. (1987). Cost of clinical instructors' time in clinical education: Physical therapy students. *Physical Therapy, 67*, 238–243.

Porter, R. E., & Kincaid, C. B. (1977). Financial aspects of clinical education to facilities. *Physical Therapy, 57*, 905–908.

Schauble, P. G., Murphy, M. C., Cover-Paterson, C. E., & Archer, J. (1989). Cost effectiveness of internship training programs: Clinical service delivery through training. *Professional Psychology: Research and Practice, 40*(2), 17–22.

Shalik, L. D. (1987). Cost-benefit analysis of level II fieldwork in occupational therapy. *American Journal of Occupational Therapy, 41*, 638–645.

Strauss, A., & Corbin, J. (1990). *Basics of qualitative research: Grounded theory procedures and techniques.* Newbury Park, CA: Sage.

Field Work Experience Ratings

and

Certification Examination Scores
as Predictors of Job Performance and Satisfaction
in Occupational Therapy

J.E. Muthard
J.D. Morris
L.M. Crocker
J.E. Slaymaker

The American Occupational Therapy Association's certification instruments, the Certification Examination for Occupational Therapists Registered and the Field Work Performance Report, were examined in terms of their ability to predict future job performance and satisfaction of occupational therapists. A job satisfaction questionnaire was administered to 208 occupational therapists, and their supervisors rated them on a job performance instrument. The resulting correlations between these work adjustment variables and the previously administered certification instruments failed to reveal any predictive ability. Some plausible reasons for these negative results and possible directions for further research into this professional screening process were explored.

Within the past ten years health and rehabilitation professions have intensified their study of the nature and quality of their training programs, the knowledge, skills, and competencies of their members, the use and training of supportive personnel, and the quality of patient care. In 1972 the American Occupational Therapy Association (AOTA) developed a new, standardized instrument for assessing

J.E. Muthard, Ph.D., Head, Rehabilitation Research Institute, College of Health Related Professions, University of Florida, Gainesville.

*J.D. Morris, Ph.D., Assistant Professor, College of Education, Georgia Southern College, Statesboro, Georgia.

* L.M. Crocker, Ph.D., Assistant Professor, College of Education, University of Florida.

J. Slaymaker, M.A., O.T.R., Associate Professor, Department of Occupational Therapy, College of Health Related Professions, University of Florida.

*Former staff members of the Rehabilitation Research Institute.

Note: The phrase currently in use for "clinical affiliation" is "Field Work Experience."

the performance of occupational therapy students in their field work experiences. On the Field Work Performance Report (FWPR), supervisors rate the extent to which students display desirable professional skills and behavior in their field work. The development of the FWPR and its subsequent field testing and validation are described in the AOTA Manual for the FWPR (1) and in a subsequent paper (2). The development of the FWPR provided an exceptional opportunity to study the relationships between FWPR ratings and measures of professional knowledge as well as indices of job satisfaction and job performance on the first job following graduation. This follow-up study describes the extent to which two measures designed to assess the occupational therapy student's readiness to enter full professional status—the FWPR and the Certification Examination for Occupational Therapists (CEOT)—relate to supervisors' ratings of the occupational therapists' initial job performance and feelings of job satisfaction. The purpose of including job satisfaction was to explore the predictability of a worker-oriented criterion.

Despite the long use of clinical affiliation ratings and the CEOT, studies of the relationship between these pre-professional measures and either undergraduate academic performance or postgraduate employment success have been sparse and limited. Two studies (3, 4) of occupational therapists showed no significant correlations between lower-division undergraduate grades and clinical affiliation Report of Performance in Student Affiliations (RPSA) ratings. As part of a larger study, Lind (5) investigated the relationship between selected grades and RPSA ratings and found no significant correlations. In that same study Lind used multiple regression analysis to determine whether or not the subtests of three personality and interest inventories predicted success in clinical affiliation. Although she obtained statistically multiple correlations, the results are of questionable practical value since the two groups studied were small (25 and 50), and the correlations between any test variable and the RPSA scores were quite low. In a somewhat similar study, Bailey, Jantzen,

FIELD WORK EXPERIENCE

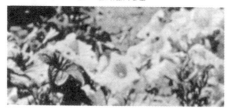

and Dunteman (6) found that the scales of the Strong Vocational Interest Blank, Minnesota Multiphasic Personality Inventory, or the Florida Placement Examination did not correlate with ratings on the RPSA; only 1 scale of the 44 represented by these 3 inventories was found to be significantly predictive of clinical affiliation success.

Although the prediction and assessment of clinical or job performance has concerned educators and researchers in many professional disciplines during the past decade, efforts have thus far led to refined measures and methodologies rather than results useful for supporting or modifying existing professional curricula. In a thorough examination of the performance evaluation problem in medicine, Barro (7) reports that "no system of measurement now available allows us to determine objectively who are the high and low performing physicians. Lack of validation in terms of patient outcomes is the primary shortcoming of many of the approaches currently being used or developed, and efforts to establish such validity should be the focus of future endeavors in this field." A large-scale study of California nurses (8) showed that State Board and National League for Nursing achievement scores were not related to ratings of clinical performance but that they were somewhat related to overall GPA, nursing theory grades, and Otis IQ scores. A recent review of the validity studies of the National Teacher Examinations (9) showed much the same result among educators. The two studies that examined the relationship between supervisor ratings for practice teaching and Weighted Common Examinations Total scores, which equate year-to-year teaching achievement performance, were not encouraging. Six such correlations examined ranged from -.03 to .18, with a median value of .11, which indicates little relationship between field work performance and test scores.

Methodology

Sample. Participants in this study were 208 occupational therapy graduates from among 1,012 therapists who had participated in an earlier national validation study of the Field Work Performance Report (FWPR) administered during their field work experiences. The therapists included had: (1) successfully completed their field work and graduated from an accredited program; (2) been working for at least one year; (3) signed a

consent form permitting researchers to contact his or her employer (only 165 of the original 1,012 therapists were excluded from the sample because of a refusal to sign); (4) completed the job performance and satisfaction questionnaires.

Instruments. The predictive measures used in this study were the CEOT, the FWPR, and the Hiring Rating Form (HRF).

Since 1972 the CEOT has been administered by the Psychological Corporation in cooperation with the AOTA. The total score of this comprehensive 250-item multiple-choice examination is used to make pass/fail decisions. Although designed as a comprehensive test, part scores for ten topical areas are available to examinees and to occupational therapy teaching programs. The first two parts cover basic knowledge in the biological and behavioral sciences. Four parts relate to clinical areas (CEOT-CL) including medical and surgery, neurology, orthopedics, and psychiatry. The final four parts relate to occupational therapy principles (CEOT-OTP) for the same clinical areas. There is no published data on the reliability and predictive validity of recent versions of the CEOT. Staff of the AOTA, however, report that the total scores of the forms of the CEOT used in testing this sample were internally consistent (Kuder-Richardson 21 coefficients of .82, .85, and .87). Reliability information was not available for the individual topic areas. Content validity for the CEOT is claimed on the basis of the methods used for item development and selection. Scores on the CEOT were transformed to standard scores for the minor differences in the number of items in each content area on the parallel forms administered in 1972-1973.

The FWPR was developed by the AOTA to serve as the official standardized instrument (1) for certification of clinical competence. Each of the items on this scale is a behavioral statement depicting a single element of good practice in occupational therapy (for example, "Selects evaluation methods or tools which are appropriate for a change in treatment or program."). The test items sample performance areas on data gathering, treatment planning, treatment implementation, communication skills, and professional characteristics. Clinical supervisors rated student performance on each item on a four-point scale that indicated the relative performance on each item on a four-point scale that indicated the relative frequency or proportion of times the student displayed the desired behavior. A complete description of the developmental procedures was reported in the Manual (1) prepared for its users. Evidence of concurrent validity with the HRF (.62 - .76), inter-rater reliability (.76), and internal consistency (.97) for the FWPR has been reported earlier (2).

The Hiring Rating Form (HRF) was also completed by two of the student's supervisors during clinical internship. This rating, which reflected the supervisor's willingness to employ the student if a vacancy existed, was considered an immediate criterion of overall performance. In an earlier study (2) the product moment correlations between FWPR and HRF ratings by independent judges assessing the same performance were .64 and .62.

The criterion measure for job performance was the therapist's rating by his/her immediate occupational therapy supervisor on a modified form of the Minnesota Satisfactoriness Scale (MSS) (10). The MSS is a published standardized questionnaire that employers have used to assess the job satisfactoriness of individual employees in a wide range of blue collar, technical, and professional occupations. Three response alternatives of "not as well," "about the same," and "better" indicate the employer's perception of the employees' relative performance in many areas. With the publisher's permission the instrument was modified so as to be more applicable to occupational therapists by substituting "facility" for "company" in all items where it appeared, by adding six items related directly to performance in occupational therapy, and by deleting two items. To distinguish between this version of the MSS and the original, it is hereafter called the Job Satisfactoriness Inventory (JSI). Factor analysis of the modified instrument's 31 items suggested subscore dimensions of general satisfactoriness, conformance (CON), personal adjustment (PA), and clinical performance (CL). The general satisfactoriness score was derived from a sum of the choices on all 31 items with a resultant coefficient alpha reliability of .95. Similarly, the reliability of the conformance subscale of eight items was .90, the seven item personal adjustment scale was .86, and the six item clinical and performance scale was .86. These empirically derived subscales and reliabilities were consonant with results from earlier studies on the original instrument (11).

The criterion measure for employee job satisfaction was the short-form Minnesota Satisfaction Questionnaire (MSQ) (12). Each item of the MSQ refers to a reinforcer in the work environment (for example, Advancement, Compensation, Working Conditions, and others), and the respondent indicates the degree of satisfaction with that reinforcer in his/her present job. The five response alternatives range from Very Satisfied to Very Dissatisfied. The subscores yielded by this instrument are internal and external satisfaction composed of 12 and 6 items with coefficient alpha reliabilities of .83 and .77, respectively, for the group of occupational therapists in this study. Validity and reliability data for the MSQ have been reported by Weiss and others (12) for a broad range of occupational groups.

Analysis. The scores of the criterion instruments, the FWPR, the total CEOT score, and the clinical and the occupational therapy prin-

Table 1

Correlations* of Pre-Employment Measures of Occupational Therapist's Ability with Measures of Job Performance and Satisfaction
(N = 208)

Pre-Employment Measures	Supervisor Job Ratings				Job Satisfaction	
	Total	PA	CL	CON	Intrinsic	Extrinsic
FWPR	.08	−.11	.09	.04	.18†	.13
NCETOTAL	.07	−.03	.07	.06	.00	.06
NCECL	.04	−.01	.03	.05	−.03	.04
NCEOTP	.08	−.05	.10	.06	.06	.10
Hiring Rating	.14	.19†	.07	.10	.25†	.15

* Pearson product-moment correlation coefficients.
† Statistically significant at the .05 alpha level.

ciples part scores for the CEOT and the HRF, were cross-correlated (Table 1). In addition, the CEOT part scores were intercorrelated.

Results

It is clear from Table 1 that performance on pre-employment measures did not predict subsequent supervisor ratings of job success or occupational therapist self-ratings of job satisfaction. Even though three correlations were "statistically significant," their small size suggests that their "practical significance" is negligible. This means that neither FWPR or CEOT scores are predictive of how well an occupational therapist will be rated on an initial job nor how satisfied the occupational therapist will be on that job. In a more rigorous test of their independence (13) the total scores of the CEOT, FWPR, and the JSI were found to be mutually independent.

Perhaps the most surprising finding was the lack of a relationship between the FWPR and subsequent supervisor ratings of job satisfactoriness. One possible reason for this lack of relationship between two "on the job" rating scales may be that the instruments sample different performance domains. In order to partially test this proposition, the FWPR and JSI were examined to identify parallel questions. In general, most of the six questions added to the MSS overlapped in content with the FWPR. However, the individual correlations among three almost verbatim "matches" related to performance in "gathering necessary information for planning treatment," "modifying treatment plans to meet patient needs," and "communication with patients,"

The American Journal of Occupational Therapy **153**

FIELD WORK EXPERIENCE

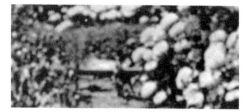

as well as the correlation between the sum of these parallel items were all below .10. In addition, only 8 of the resulting 1643 cross-correlations between FWPR and MSQ items were above .20, and none was above .25. A difference in the perception of "good" occupational therapy performance between field work supervisors and employers in the field may therefore be suggested.

As the data in Table 1 show, the job satisfaction of the recently graduated occupational therapists had little or no relationship with earlier FWPR and HRF ratings and scores on the CEOT examination. The slight positive

relationship between the ratings received by the occupational therapists in clinical affiliation and later satisfaction with the intrinsic elements of the job (the work activities and responsibilities) does not have practical value for career planning.

When ten parts of the CEOT were correlated with job performance and job satisfaction scores, no significant relationships were found. (Correlations ranged from -.13 to .17, with a median r of .02.) The intercorrelations of the part scores, section scores, and totals are shown in Table 2. As Table 2 shows, the clinical areas and occupational therapy principles part scores do have stronger relationships with the scores for their respective section than with the other section. The correlation of part scores with their respective section scores is spuriously high because each part score is a component of its section score. Furthermore, the CEOT scores for clinical areas and occupational therapy principles sections correlate to a moderately high degree and are as predictive of the total CEOT score

Table 2

Intercorrelations of NCE Subtests, Part, and Total Scores Among Occupational Therapists

	02	03	04	05	06	07	08	09	10	TOTAL	CL	OTP
NCE01	.37	.40	.37	.40	.42	.23	.33	.27	.23	.68	.56	.41
NCE02		.33	.32	.25	.49	.21	.34	.24	.48	.70	.50	.50
NCE03			.29	.30	.39	.16	.24	.32	.26	.58	.70	.38
NCE04				.28	.41	.21	.32	.38	.16	.61	.70	.42
NCE05					.30	.18	.34	.28	.16	.55	.67	.38
NCE06						.32	.32	.39	.35	.74	.74	.54
NCE07							.19	.27	.11	.44	.31	.62
NCE08								.28	.23	.57	.43	.66
NCE09									.19	.58	.48	.68
NCE10										.58	.33	.60
NCETOTAL											.88	.85
NCECL												.65
NCEOTP												

01 Biological Science
02 Behavioral Science
03 Medical and Surgical Conditions
   (Clinical)
04 Neurology (Clinical)
05 Orthopedics (Clinical)
06 Psychiatry (Clinical)

07 Medical and Surgical Conditions
   (OT Principles)
08 Neurology (OT Principles)
09 Orthopedics (OT Principles)
10 Psychiatry (OT Principles)
CL Clinical subscore
OTP OT Principles subscore

Correlations > .18 are significant at the .01 level of confidence.

as they can be within the limits of their reliability.

Discussion

Although it is somewhat discouraging that two primary measures of the occupational therapy students' readiness for admission to full professional status are not predictive of early job success, this finding is consistent with experiences in other professions. Studies of the value of student teacher grades and the National Teacher Examination scores as predictors of later job success have shown little or no relationship with later job ratings (9). Parallel studies in the fields of nursing (8) and medicine (14, 15) have yielded equivocal results between pre-professional ratings and tests and subsequent measures of job success. Clearly, the general failure to find pre-professional measures predictive of later success in the profession is not unique to the occupational therapy profession. The question of why two primary screening measures prerequisite to admission to professional status were found to have no relation to later job success is still present.

One possible explanation may involve the nature of the work and the supervisor's expectations of students in field work that may differ from the expectations for practicing therapists. In field work settings student supervisors usually see themselves primarily as teachers and advisors to the students rather than as colleagues who would give only general direction to a peer who is relatively autonomous. These relationships may not only differ, but there may also be differences in the tasks assigned to occupational therapy students and those assigned to a new staff member. Differences in task assignments might also lead to different expectations for competency.

Another aspect is that the supervisors on the job typically have had responsibility for selecting the new occupational therapists who join their staff, whereas field work supervisors do not have such a personal investment in the individuals who come to their facilities. Thus, many supervisors might be expected to assess the staff they selected as being relatively successful in their overall job performance, and hold to different standards for students in field work.

Another possible explanation for the lack of relationship between the FWPR and the job ratings may have arisen from differences in the preparation of the raters for doing their assessment job. In the case of the FWPR, the field work supervisors had copies of the newly developed FWPR available prior to or early in the student's field experiences and may have had an opportunity to rate several students on it. That is, they knew what was to be observed systematically beforehand. In the case of the supervisors who responded to the JSI, the supervisors had no such preparation and therefore had to recollect past observations in order to evaluate the staff member. Consequently, interrater reliability could be expected to be lower in the use of the JSI than in the field work assessment.

One hypothesis that can probably be eliminated is the view that the type-of-setting strongly affects individual student ratings on the FWPR and as a consequence reduces its predictive validity. Since the data from the two major types of settings, physical dysfunction and psychosocial dysfunction, were available for a substantial portion of the students participating in this study, this question was examined by determining the correlation between the ratings for the same students in the two settings. The correlation between these scores (.88) makes clear that differences in types of affiliation did not lead to different FWPR assessments.

Why the CEOT scores do not predict job success criteria is somewhat disconcerting, but there may be a simple explanation, since the general finding that student grades do not predict later job success is closely parallel. The post hoc explanation of some professional leaders in occupational therapy is that CEOT scores alone cannot be expected to predict the professional performance skills and competencies needed to function effectively in the complex milieu of health and rehabilitation settings. Primarily, they do not tap the interpersonal skills and attitudes therapists need for effective occupational therapy practice. In short, possessing occupational therapy knowledge does not in itself lead to job success in occupational therapy.

The simplest explanation for the lack of association between the CEOT and ratings of early job success is that its primary purpose was to identify individuals who lacked the minimum knowledge deemed necessary to render effective occupational therapy services. Thus, the designers of the CEOT did not intend to differentiate the acceptable from the most knowledgeable therapist. Within that stated purpose, the CEOT should not be expected to correlate significantly with job performance. It follows that educators and others using the CEOT findings should regard them as indicative of the level of basic knowledge mastered and not necessarily predictive of future professional performance. Thus, one clearly needs to give more weight to facets of competency and personality in estimating professional potential.

An alternative explanation for the lack of relationship between job success and the FWPR and the CEOT may be that the JSI is not an appropriate measure of job success. This explanation would hinge on the judgment of occupational therapy professionals of the adequacy of the variables covered in the JSI. The validity and reliability of the parent form of the JSI for assessing workers in a wide range of occupations, including other professional jobs, would seem to support its probable utility

FIELD WORK EXPERIENCE

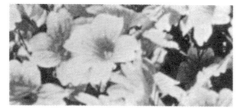

for making a general judgment of occupational therapy performance. This criticism is further weakened by the lack of relationship between parts of the JSI drawn from the FWPR and parallel parts of the FWPR.

The initial concern with the lack of predictive value of critical standards in a student's progress toward professional status may not be warranted. Ebel (16) suggests that if a test has high content validity, then it may not be necessary for it to have high predictive validity. That is, the validity of the FWPR and the CEOT may rest on the extent to which they reliably assess those elements of the student's preparation that occupational therapy practitioners and educators judge necessary for entering the profession. This may not be as self-serving as it sounds in that requiring all entrants into the profession to pass the FWPR and the CEOT assures basic entry level knowledge but not the totality of personal and professional skills necessary to function effectively as an occupational therapist. Such an interpretation would suggest that the effective occupational therapist displays traits on the job that are critical to effective job performance, but which are not assessed by either the FWPR or the CEOT. Some traits that come to mind include interpersonal skills such as tact, judgment, warmth, and likeability.

Since the ultimate criterion of an occupational therapist's performance is effectiveness in helping a client or patient move toward more effective physical and/or social functioning, it would seem reasonable to consider the possibility of undertaking a sampling study that would look more intensively at the extent to which therapists contribute to such goals. Using the opinions of patients would, of course, be one way to do this, but an approach developed in the mental health field, Goal Attainment Scaling (17), would appear to be a sounder and more direct method for asessing a therapist's effectiveness. This method systematically individualizes not only a statement of the problems, but also the level of outcomes that, in light of the total factors in the patient's background, are likely to be highly favorable, very unfavorable, or something in between. From such individualized assessments of the therapist the summary findings for a small sample of specific patients would then represent the therapist's overall functional capacity. The use of such fairly intensive and basic measures of occupational

therapy success, together with such instruments as the FWPR, the CEOT, or a proficiency examination, might well lead to different conclusions about the strengths and limitations of each of these measures as well as the limitations or viability of supervisors' ratings on the job.

Although this study failed to show that the CEOT or the FWPR had predictive validity for specific indices of later job success or jobssatisfaction, it does not justify a recommendation to discard these instruments or even to claim they are invalid. The findings do suggest, however, the need for further systematic examination of the relationship between these measures and job success criteria acceptable to the profession. If further studies also find that the FWPR and the CEOT scores are nonpredictive of job success, it may be appropriate to question their use as intermediate criteria for all types of measures and inventories designed to guide students who are considering occupational therapy as a program or faculty charged with selecting students.

●

REFERENCES

1. Slaymaker JE, Crocker LM, Muthard JE: Field Work Performance Report Manual. Rockville, MD, American Occupational Therapy Association, 1974
2. Crocker LM, Muthard JE, Slaymaker JE, Samson L: A performance rating scale for evaluating clinical competence of occupational therapy students. *Am J Occup Ther* 29: 81-86, 1975
3. Anderson HE, Jantzen AC: A prediction of clinical performance. *Am J Occup Ther* 19:76-78, 1965
4. Englehart HV: An investigation of the relationship between college grads and on-the-job performance during clinical training of occupational therapy students. *Am J Occup Ther* 11: 97-107, 1957
5. Lind AL: An exploratory study of predictive factors of success in the clinical affiliation experience. *Am J Occup Ther* 24: 222-226, 1970
6. Bailey, Jr, JP, Jantzen AC, Dunteman GH: Relative effectiveness of personality, achievement and interest measures in the prediction of a performance criterion. *Am J Occup Ther* 23: 27-29, 1969
7. Barro AR: Physician performance measurement. *J Med Educ* 48: 1051-1092, 1973
8. Taylor CW, Nahm H, Quinn M, et al: Report of measurement and prediction of nursing performance, Part I. (US Public Health Service Grant No. NU00062 report), University of Utah, 1965
9. Quirk TJ, Witten B, Weinberg SF: Review of studies of the concurrent and predictive validity of the national teacher examinations. *Rev Educ Res* 43: 89-113, 1973
10. Gibson KL, Weiss DJ, Dawis RV, Lofquist LH: Manual for the Minnesota satisfactoriness scales. University of Minnesota: Bulletin 53: 1970
11. Carlson RE, Dawis RV, England GW, et al: The measurement of employment satisfactoriness. University of Minnesota: Bulletin 37, 1963
12. Weiss DJ, Dawis RV, England GW, Lofquist LH: Manual for the Minnesota satisfaction questionnaire. University of Minnesota: Bulletin 45, 1967
13. Bartlett MS: A note on the multiplying factors for various Chi-squared approximations. *J Royal Stat Soc*, Ser B, 16: 296-298, 1954
14. Gough HG, Hall WB, Harris RE: Evaluation of performance in medical training. *J Med Educ* 39: 679-692, 1964
15. Wingard JR, Williamson JW: Grades as predictors of physicians' career performance: An evaluative literature review. *J Med Educ* 48: 311-322, April 1973
16. Ebel, RL: Must all tests be valid? *Am Psychol* 16: 640-647. 1961
17. Kiresuk TJ: Goal attainment scaling at a county mental health service. *Eval Monogr*, 1 (special issue): 12-18, 1973

R30302

Cost–Benefit Analysis of Level II Fieldwork in Occupational Therapy

Linda Dean Shalik

Key Words: costs and cost analysis • education, occupational therapy • fieldwork

This cost–benefit study of Level II (professional-level) fieldwork included 180 student-supervisor pairs from 12 occupational therapy educational programs. Costs and benefits were measured in time (valued at market rates) spent by students in patient treatment and by supervisors in fieldwork-related duties. Various factors were also evaluated to determine their relationship to overall cost or benefit.

Results indicated a mean benefit of $4,700 for 12-week placements. Costs generated in the first few weeks of placement were generally recovered by the 6th week, with benefits gradually increasing, then declining slightly through the end of the fieldwork. Greater economic benefits resulted from physical dysfunction and psychiatric placements than from pediatric placements, and with second and third student experiences as compared with first experiences.

Linda Dean Shalik, PhD, OTR/L, is Assistant Professor in Occupational Therapy at the University of Florida. (Mailing address: J-164 JHMHC, University of Florida, Gainesville, Florida 32610.)

The rising cost of health care has been a major national concern in recent years. The increase in health care expenditures, up from 4.6% of the gross national product (GNP) in 1950 to approximately 10.5% of the GNP in 1985 (Arnett, Cowell, Davidoff, & Freeland, 1985), has been the impetus for the initiation of cost containment measures such as prospective payment systems (Curtin & Zurlage, 1984; Dowling, 1979). To adjust to the constraints imposed by these new payment systems, hospital administrators have begun to study all aspects of hospital expenditures to determine where costs can be reduced. One area scrutinized has been the costs attributed to clinical education for both medical and allied health students. This has become necessary because reimbursement agencies have shown resistance to continuing the payment of these costs (Chung, Spelbring, & Boisonneau, 1980; Frum, 1986).

The accuracy of the assumption made previously that clinical education programs constitute an overall cost to health care institutions (Busby, Leming, & Olson, 1972; Pratt & Hill, 1960) is now being called into question. In this paper the results of a national study of the costs and benefits of Level II fieldwork in occupational therapy are presented. In addition to the overall findings of costs and benefits, variables that contribute to the net cost or benefit are also identified.

Review of the Literature

Cost–benefit analysis is a branch of normative or welfare economics in which the value or goodness of a project is evaluated by economic criteria. It is defined as "an attempt to ascertain the net benefit (total benefit less total cost) of a policy or project" (Sassone & Schaffer, 1978, p. 11). The process of a cost–benefit analysis involves the identification, valuation, and discounting of all costs and benefits across the lifetime of a project (including direct, indirect, and external effects) and the comparison of these costs and benefits. Once this comparison has been made, the economical desirability of the project can be evaluated (Prest & Turvey, 1965). The application of cost–benefit analysis has rapidly expanded in the health care sector (Warner & Hutton, 1980), where the lack of normal market incentives has permitted the skyrocketing of prices (Dittman & Smith, 1979; Klarman, 1974).

A few studies of the costs and benefits of clinical education programs have been conducted in both allied health and medical education, with emphasis on either time investments by students and supervisors (since the major costs have been defined in terms of personnel time rather than in terms of other factors) or on actual monetary costs and benefits. These studies were generally limited to single educational institutions or small geographic areas.

In their research at the Hartford Hospital, Freymann and Springer (1973) reported that the costs of medical, nursing, and allied health educational programs were more than recovered through the addition of "hospital-essential" services provided by students in these programs. In their study of time investments in allied health clinical placements, Keim and Carney (1975) found that supervisors perceived neither an overall benefit nor an overall cost as a result of placement of occupational therapy students in their fieldwork sites. Similarly, Chung et al. (1980) reported that fieldwork sites were breaking even with the placement of Level II occupational therapy fieldwork students. Burkhardt (1985) also reported roughly equal time investments on the part of supervisors and students in the Level II fieldwork placements at the University of Michigan Hospitals.

Through an analysis of the effect that student placements had on productivity, Leiken, Stern, and Baines (1983) found that the presence of occupational therapy, physical therapy, and radiology technology fieldwork students had a positive impact on productivity (number of treatment outputs) in clinical settings. Lapopolo (1984) found that physical therapy students on fieldwork assignment in the San Francisco area generated an average daily benefit of $89 per student, while Pobojewski (1978) determined that radiology technology students generated a yearly benefit of more than $45,000 in the hospital he studied. Only Hammersberg (1982) reported an overall cost of fieldwork placement to the clinical facility as reported by the fieldwork supervisors in various technical-level allied health fields.

Little is known about the variables that influence the costs or benefits of clinical placements. In their study of the effect of the presence of medical students on physicians' productivity, Pawlson, Watkins, and Donaldson (1980) found a greater loss in productivity associated with the more advanced students than with 1st-year students. In other words, loss in productivity was minimal when the student role was purely an observational one. However, Leiken et al. (1983) reported that Level II fieldwork students had a positive impact on productivity (treatment output) in the occupational therapy clinics studied whereas the presence of Level I students had no effect on productivity. Similarly, Porter and Kincaid (1977) reported differences in the degree of benefit derived from the placement of junior- and senior-level physical therapy students: Benefits were greater with seniors than with juniors.

Chung et al. (1980) compared the effects on costs and benefits of students in first versus second fieldwork assignments and found no difference between the two groups. Chung et al. concluded that expanded studies were needed to compare the costs and benefits of "undergraduate and graduate entry-level education; agencies that treat physical dysfunction, psychosocial dysfunction, and other categories of disability; . . . and first, second, and third placements" (Chung & Spelbring, 1983, p. 687). These suggestions for further research, as well as certain portions of the methodology used in the study by Chung et al. (1980) formed the basis of the questions asked and the structure of the research reported here.

Purpose of the Study

The purpose of this study was to determine if there is an overall cost or benefit to the clinical sites as a result of Level II occupational therapy fieldwork placements. Additionally, the study was to determine whether selected variables are significantly related to the overall benefit or cost of the fieldwork placement.

Method

Identification of Costs and Benefits

Costs and benefits of Level II fieldwork were identified and valued strictly from the institutional (or fieldwork site) point of view. Direct costs included the time spent by the supervisor and other professional staff in preparation and supervision during the student placement. This included time spent in one-to-one supervision of the student, meetings, preparation and administration of the fieldwork experience, and in formal teaching or instructional sessions.

Other sources of possible cost were identified as the provision of room and board for students and the payment of stipends. Although data regarding these factors were gathered, they were not included in the overall cost–benefit equation because of the inconsistency in their occurrence from site to site and because of concerns about the ability to maintain confidentiality in the data collection phase. Finally, indirect costs, such as those associated with space and overhead, were considered marginal and were therefore not included.

Benefits were identified as arising from time spent by the student treating patients independently (in individual or group sessions), doing administrative work (including treatment planning and documentation), attending meetings, and performing clerical duties or the duties of an aide. Indirect benefits, such as recruiting advantages were viewed as marginal and were therefore not included in the cost–benefit equation.

Valuation of Costs and Benefits

Time spent by supervisors (cost) was valued according to the average charge per 15-minute treatment unit in the sites participating in the study. This was justified by the assumption that time not spent supervising students would be available to the institution for income generation in the form of treatment revenue. Similarly, time spent by students in the independent treatment of patients was also valued according to the 15-minute treatment charge, since institutions commonly charge the same amount for patient treatment regardless of who performs the treatment. However, time spent by students in group treatment was valued only at the rate of one treatment per 15-minute period; thus the students' inexperience in coordinating the simultaneous treatment of several patients was taken into consideration.

Time spent by the students in other professional duties, such as attendance at meetings and treatment planning (administrative work) was valued according to the average salary of therapists at the participating institutions. Finally, students' contributions in the form of clerical duties or the duties of an aide were valued at the current minimum hourly wage. These values were determined on the basis of what it would cost to replace the students by appropriate personnel in these functions and by taking into account that the students' performance in Level II fieldwork is assumed to approach that of the entry level therapist (AOTA, 1985).

The following equations represent the calculations of costs and benefits in the study.

For costs, the equation is $C = T(G + M + P + I)$.

(C = cost; T = treatment charge, prorated to hourly rate; G = general one-to-one supervision [time]; M = meetings [time]; P = preparation and administration [time]; I = formal instructional sessions [time].)

For benefits, the equation is $B = T(PI + PJ) + S(A + M) + W(D)$.

(B = benefit; T = hourly treatment charge; PI = individual patient treatment [time]; PJ = joint or group patient treatment [time]; S = average hourly salary for an occupational therapist; A = administrative work [time]; M = meetings [time]; W = minimum wage; D = clerical or aide duties [time].)

By subtracting the costs from the benefits, a single number, called the net present value (NPV) became the dependent variable. Ordinarily in a cost–

Table 1
Weekly Mean NPV (Expressed in Dollars)
With All Variables Combined

N	Mean	SD	Min. Value	Max. Value	SEM
180	397.02	639.56	−1413.00	2069.00	47.66

Note. NPV = net present value.

Table 2
Weekly Mean NPV (Expressed in Dollars)
by Academic Degree

Degree	Mean	SD	Min. Value	Max. Value	SEM
Bachelor's $n = 129$	389.07	648.42	−1413.00	2069.00	57.09
Master's $n = 51$	417.12	622.41	−694.00	1679.00	87.15

Note. NPV = net present value.

benefit analysis, the net present value would be discounted over the lifetime of the project, but this step was eliminated because of the short lifetime (less than 1 year) of the fieldwork placement (Klarman, 1974). A positive NPV indicated an overall benefit, whereas a negative NPV indicated a cost to the fieldwork site. The equation to determine NPV was simply NPV = B − C.

The Independent Variables

Of particular concern in the study were those factors that would contribute to the resulting NPV of the fieldwork placement. The degree level of the student (bachelor's or basic master's level), the age of the student, the number of fieldwork experiences, the type of fieldwork, and the week of fieldwork were identified as factors that could influence the overall cost or benefit.

It was believed that greater experience in life, academic studies, and fieldwork (the variables of age, degree level, and number of fieldwork experiences) might cause a student to perform more independently and thus bring about greater benefits while decreasing costs to the fieldwork sites. It was also speculated that different types of fieldwork settings might be structured to either foster or inhibit independence on the part of students and thus would affect the costs or benefits of placement. Finally, the variable of week of fieldwork was included, since it was found to affect the overall benefits in previous research (Chung et al., 1980). It could also be argued that as students gain skill and expertise in a particular fieldwork site, their value to the site increases.

Recruitment of Subjects and Data Collection

Directors of 12 occupational therapy educational programs agreed to participate in the study, and they provided the information, such as students' and supervisors' names and addresses, that was needed for implementing the study. Included were seven bachelor's level programs and five basic master's level programs, with a total of 384 students assigned to Level II fieldwork during the 1985 summer fieldwork period.

All students and their fieldwork supervisors in this group were contacted. Each student–supervisor

Table 3
Overall Weekly Mean NPV (Expressed in Dollars) by Week of Fieldwork

Week	Mean	SD	Minimum Value	Maximum Value	SEM
Week 1 ($n = 12$)	−462.75	388.12	−986.00	340.00	112.00
Week 2 ($n = 13$)	−175.31	559.17	−976.00	712.00	155.00
Week 3 ($n = 17$)	156.35	507.35	−637.00	1099.00	123.00
Week 4 ($n = 17$)	107.59	680.04	−1413.00	1494.00	164.90
Week 5 ($n = 12$)	595.75	536.38	−379.00	1265.00	154.80
Week 6 ($n = 16$)	212.68	598.84	−694.00	1647.00	147.70
Week 7 ($n = 15$)	664.93	562.06	−56.00	2069.00	145.10
Week 8 ($n = 18$)	686.00	406.70	5.00	1432.00	95.85
Week 9 ($n = 16$)	858.06	492.48	160.00	1679.00	123.10
Week 10 ($n = 18$)	617.11	414.67	25.00	1375.00	97.73
Week 11 ($n = 15$)	720.87	650.62	−475.00	1934.00	167.90
Week 12 ($n = 8$)	731.25	484.06	156.00	1668.00	171.10
Week 13 ($n = 3$)	144.67	399.13	−305.00	457.00	230.40

Note. NPV = net present value.

pair was asked to complete three, 1-week time logs indicating how much time the student spent treating patients and how much time the supervisor spent supervising students. The student's log included items for recording time investment in the activities specified in the benefit equation, and the supervisor's time log included items for time spent in the activities outlined in the cost equation.

Additionally, a questionnaire, sent to all participating fieldwork sites and completed anonymously, was used to determine therapists' average annual salary, per-unit treatment charges, and the overall incidence of stipends, room and board subsidies, or other perquisites given to students on Level II assignments.

Analysis of the Data and Results

Responses from a total of 230 (60%) student–supervisor pairs were received. By using a method of sequential sampling of responses from the student–supervisor pairs, a final data set of 180 pairs was obtained. These pairs represented 156 clinical sites in 32 states.

Site questionnaires were returned from 167 fieldwork sites, but not all items had been completed on all questionnaires. With responses from 149 sites, it was found that the average salary for supervising therapists was $11.38/h. The average hourly treatment charge was $61.35, with 95 sites responding to this item.

The statistical analysis included the calculation of descriptive data and the use of a multiple regression analysis to determine the significance of each independent variable in predicting NPV while controlling for the covariates (Agresti & Agresti, 1979; Kerlinger & Pedhazur, 1973). Because previous research (Chung et al., 1980) and a preliminary review of the descriptive data indicated the possibility of a curvilinear relationship between week of fieldwork and NPV, a quadratic variable was added to the analysis to test

for curvilinearity. In addition, because the variable of type of fieldwork is qualitative, with four types (or levels), it was evaluated separately using an F test to evaluate the increase in prediction it brought to the regression model.

Descriptive Analysis

Tables 1 to 5 show the descriptive results. In Table 1 the weekly mean NPV across all variables is given. This is followed by tables that demonstrate the mean weekly NPV for the following independent variables: degree level, week of fieldwork, number of fieldwork experiences, and type of fieldwork. These tables clearly indicate that the clinical sites in the study derived a financial benefit from the Level II fieldwork placement of occupational therapy students, with a mean weekly benefit of nearly $400, and a mean benefit from the 12-week and 13-week placements of $4,700 and $4,850, respectively. This benefit appeared to exist regardless of degree level, number of fieldwork experiences, or type of fieldwork, although some differences appeared to exist among these groups.

Results from the site questionnaire regarding payments or perquisites given to students in return for their work in Level II fieldwork indicated that 40% of

Table 4
Weekly Mean NPV (Expressed in Dollars) by Number of Fieldwork Experiences

Experience	Mean	SD	Min. Value	Max. Value	SEM
First ($n = 116$)	381.85	629.24	−986.00	2069.00	58.42
Second ($n = 57$)	440.23	651.27	−1413.00	1934.00	86.26
Third ($n = 3$)	88.00	196.85	−138.00	222.00	113.60

Note. There were four responses with no designation for number of fieldwork experiences.
NPV = net present value.

Table 5
Mean NPV (Expressed in Dollars) by Type of Fieldwork

Type of Fieldwork	Mean	SD	Minimum Value	Maximum Value	SEM
Physical Dysfunction ($n = 77$)	520.47	734.50	−1413.00	2069.00	83.70
Pediatric ($n = 8$)	63.63	388.99	−694.00	659.00	137.50
Psychiatric ($n = 91$)	315.57	547.60	−986.00	1347.00	57.40
Geriatric ($n = 4$)	540.25	688.14	−475.00	1014.00	344.00

Note. NPV = net present value.

the sites provided either room or board benefits for students, with the mean value of these benefits estimated at $36 per week. Only six sites (10%) reported providing stipends, which averaged $75 per week. An additional 10% indicated that room-and-board benefits plus some financial remuneration were provided; the average value of these benefits was $58 per week.

Inferential Analysis

The results of the regression analysis are given in Tables 6 and 7. Of the independent variables built into the model, the variables of number of fieldwork experiences and week of fieldwork and the quadratic variable indicating curvilinearity between week of fieldwork and NPV were found to be significantly related to the NPV. Conversely, no relationship was found between degree level and NPV and between students' age and NPV.

Significance was also found in adding the variable of type of fieldwork to the model ($p < .05$). Differences found between the specific types of fieldwork are shown in Table 7. A significant difference occurred between NPVs in physical dysfunction fieldwork and pediatric fieldwork. Geriatric and psychiatric placements were found to generate benefits similar to the benefits generated by physical dysfunction placements.

Figure 1 illustrates the relationship between NPV and the variables of week, type of fieldwork, and number of fieldwork experiences. The incidence of first fieldwork assignments in pediatric settings was nil; therefore, this particular combination was not graphed. Curves for psychiatric and geriatric fieldwork placements would be similar to those for physical dysfunction. The figure also shows the break-even point, that is, the point at which the fieldwork sites would be expected to recover the initial costs of the fieldwork placement and to begin receiving a financial benefit.

Discussion

From the descriptive and statistical analysis, it is apparent that, with the possible exception of pediatric placements, a 12- or 13-week Level II fieldwork place-

Table 6
Results of the Multiple Regression Analysis: Source

Source	df	Sum of Squares	Mean Square	R-Square
Regression	8	23150884	2893861	.335
Error	164	45949790	280182	
Total	172	69100674		

ment brings about an overall benefit to the fieldwork site. As a result of the time invested in orienting and teaching the student, a cost is incurred during the first few weeks of the placement. This cost is subsequently recovered between the 3rd and 5th weeks (see Figure 1). From this point on, the placement becomes an overall benefit to the fieldwork site, generating increasingly greater weekly benefits until the last few weeks. As the end of the fieldwork approaches, the degree of benefit levels off, then declines somewhat in magnitude. This is possibly the result of activities associated with the end of fieldwork: the reassignment of patients to regular clinical staff and the evaluation of students' fieldwork performance.

In considering the effects of the number of fieldwork experiences on NPV, it is clear that as a student gains in experience, the fieldwork site benefits. With the more experienced student, the supervisor has to invest less time in the early weeks of the fieldwork placement; thus, an earlier break-even point occurs. For example, the student on a second fieldwork placement in a physical dysfunction setting would be expected to generate an overall financial benefit for

Table 7
Results of Multiple Regression Analysis: Parameter

Parameter	Estimate	SE	p
Intercept	−859.11	333.70	.0109
Age	2.78	8.92	.7553
Degree	−74.42	101.62	.4650
Fieldwork experience	194.64	87.61	.0277*
Week	290.89	52.61	.0001*
Week 2 (quadratic)	−15.20	3.90	.0001*
X5 (Ped-PD)	−605.91	219.79	.0065*
X6 (Psy-PD)	−166.07	84.34	.0506
X7 (Ger-PD)	−144.40	277.02	.6029

Note. PD = physical dysfunction fieldwork. Ped = pediatric fieldwork. Psy = psychiatric fieldwork. Ger = geriatric fieldwork.
* $p < .05$.

Figure 1
Relationship of Week to NPV for Specific Types of Fieldwork and Number of Fieldwork Experiences

NPV
(in dollars)

NPV	Week 1	Week 2	Week 3	Week 4	Week 5	Week 6	Week 7	Week 8	Week 9	Week 10	Week 11	Week 12	Week 13
1200													
1100								3	3	3	3		
1000							3					3	
900						3		2	2	2	2		3
800					3		2					2	
700						2		1	1	1	1		2
600				3		1						1	
500					2			B	B	B			1
400			3	2		(1)		(B)				B	
300						B		A	A	A	A		B
200		3	(2)	1	B		A					A	
100						A							(A)
0		2	1	B									
0	(3)			A									
−100			1	B	A								
−200	2												
−300		B	A										
−400	1												
−500		A											
−600	B												
−700													
−800	A												
−900													
WEEK	1	2	3	4	5	6	7	8	9	10	11	12	13

Note. NPV = net present value. 1 = physical dysfunction, 1st experience; 2 = physical dysfunction, 2nd experience; 3 = physical dysfunction, 3rd experience. A = pediatrics, 2nd experience; B = pediatrics, 3rd experience. Value marked ( ) indicates week when benefits overcame costs.

the fieldwork site by the 3rd week of placement, as opposed to a student on a first fieldwork placement who would be expected to generate an overall financial benefit by the 5th week of placement.

While differences are found in NPV between types of fieldwork settings, it is suggested that these results be viewed cautiously. In this study, the pediatric sites were not able to break even until the conclusion of a 13-week placement even with students in

their second fieldwork assignments. A more acceptable benefit was generated by students in their third fieldwork placements. While highly significant differences between NPVs for physical dysfunction and pediatric settings were revealed ($p < .0065$, mean difference of $605.91), it must be noted that only eight observations were obtained from pediatric settings, as opposed to 77 observations from physical dysfunction settings. Although the results give a strong indication that a real difference exists between pediatric placements and other types of placements, additional research, with a greater number of participants, is needed to more carefully evaluate this difference.

The benefits of greater academic experience (basic master's degree as compared with bachelor's degree) had no relationship to the overall financial effect of fieldwork to the clinical sites. However, this study compared only one quantitative aspect of performance between bachelor's and basic master's level students. There are possibly other differences, perhaps in the areas of quality of care and knowledge base, between these two educational levels that could influence the delivery of patient care services but were beyond the scope of this study.

The variable of age was not predictive of the overall cost or benefit of fieldwork placement. It seems that the greater life experience of older students was of no particular advantage in facilitating more independent functioning or in lessening costs to fieldwork sites.

Finally, the relatively small costs (average of $36 to $75 per week) of stipends or other perquisites as payment for students' work in Level II fieldwork had little impact on the overall financial benefit to the clinical sites, with the possible exception of pediatric placements. The major impact of perquisites would be to delay the break-even point of the fieldwork placement by a maximum of 1 week.

This research supports the conclusions of previous research on the cost and benefits of fieldwork education and largely refutes the argument that Level II fieldwork constitutes a cost to the clinical sites. This study carries greater weight than previous studies because a more representative sample of the population was used, encompassing a greater number of study participants and 20% of the accredited occupational therapy educational programs.

Educators should be cognizant of the importance of length of fieldwork and number of fieldwork experiences as factors in planning fieldwork experiences. Fieldwork placements of 6 weeks or less would likely bring about a cost to the clinical site and should be avoided, particularly when they are first fieldwork assignments. Some flexibility exists in establishing placements that are longer than 6 weeks, since most placements (other than pediatric) will at least break even beyond this point. Fieldwork sites that are known to require a great amount of student instruction during the first few weeks would probably be more appropriate for longer assignments so that a benefit to the clinical site could be assured.

The research results give preliminary indication that the special case of pediatric fieldwork would require a full 12-week assignment for the clinical site to break even from a cost–benefit point of view. If pediatric sites would accept only third fieldwork placements, these sites would be able to gain some benefit from their time investment. More importantly, however, it appears that further research is warranted (a) to determine the specific aspects of pediatric assignments that make them more costly and (b) to determine what adjustments can be made in the educational process to decrease these costs to the clinical sites.

Summary

Variables in this study that were identified as possibly relating to cost or benefit of fieldwork were age of student, degree level (bachelor's or basic master's), type of fieldwork, week of fieldwork, and number of fieldwork experiences. A total of 384 student–supervisor pairs were contacted from 12 participating occupational therapy educational programs, 180 of which were included in the data analysis.

Results supported previous research in refuting the assumption that Level II fieldwork brings a fiscal burden to fieldwork sites. In fact, an overall mean benefit to the fieldwork sites of approximately $400 per week, or $4,700 to $4,850 for 12- or 13-week assignments was discovered. A curvilinear relationship was found between week of fieldwork and NPV, with early weeks of the fieldwork generating a cost to the clinical sites and later weeks bringing increasing benefits. These benefits were found to level off and decline slightly during the final weeks of the placement. The type of fieldwork placement and the number of fieldwork experiences were found to be significant in predicting the cost–benefit relationship, with specific differences found between physical dysfunction and pediatric placements and greater benefits found for longer fieldwork experiences.

The results suggest that educators should consider length of fieldwork assignments in light of factors such as type of fieldwork and number of fieldwork experiences to assure that fieldwork sites recover their initial investments in student training. Assignments of a minimum of 6 weeks are recommended for first fieldwork placements, with longer assignments suggested for pediatric or other placements known to be difficult.

Acknowledgments

I thank the education program directors, fieldwork coordinators, students, and fieldwork supervisors who assisted and participated in this research. Special thanks go to Lyla Spelbring, PhD, OTR, for her input in the early phase of the research.

References

Agresti, A., & Agresti, B. F. (1979). *Statistical methods for the social sciences.* San Francisco: Dellen.

American Occupational Therapy Association. (1985). *Guide to fieldwork education.* Rockville, MD: Author.

Arnett, R. H., Cowell, C. S., Davidoff, L. M., & Freeland, M. S. (1985). Health spending trends in the 1980's: Adjusting to financial incentives. *Health Care Financing Review, 6*(3), 1–26.

Burkhardt, B. F. (1985). A time study of staff and student activities on a Level II fieldwork program. *American Journal of Occupational Therapy, 39,* 35–40.

Busby, D. D., Leming, J. C., & Olson, M. J. (1972). Unidentified educational costs in a university teaching hospital: An initial study. *Journal of Medical Education, 47,* 243–251.

Chung, Y. I., & Spelbring, L. M. (1983). An analysis of weekly instructional input hours and student work hours in occupational therapy fieldwork. *American Journal of Occupational Therapy, 37,* 681–687.

Chung, Y. I., Spelbring, L. M., & Boisonneau, R. (1980). A cost-benefit analysis of fieldwork education in occupational therapy. *Inquiry, 17,* 216–229.

Curtin, L. L., & Zurlage, C. (1984). *DRGs: The reorganization of health.* Chicago: S-N Publications.

Dittman, D. A., & Smith, K. R. (1979). Consideration of benefits and costs: A conceptual framework for the health planner. *Health Care Management Review, 4*(4), 45–64.

Dowling, W. L. (1979). Prospective reimbursement of hospitals. In L. E. Weeks, H. J. Berman, & G. E. Bisbee, Jr. (Eds.), *Financing of health care* (pp. 249–265). Ann Arbor, MI: Health Administration Press.

Freymann, J. G., & Springer, J. K. (1973). Education and the hospital: Cost of hospital-based education. *Hospitals, 47*(5), 65–67, passim.

Frum, D. (1986). Fieldwork education: Can we afford it? *Occupational Therapy News, 40*(4), 13.

Hammersberg, S. S. (1982). A cost/benefit study of clinical education in selected allied health programs. *Journal of Allied Health, 8,* 35–41.

Keim, S. T., & Carney, M. K. (1975). *A cost-benefit study of selected clinical education programs for professional and allied health personnel.* Arlington, TX: University of Texas at Arlington, Bureau of Business and Economic Research.

Kerlinger, F. N., & Pedhazur, E. J. (1973). *Multiple regression in behavioral research.* New York: Holt, Rinehart, & Winston.

Klarman, H. E. (1974). Application of cost-benefit analysis to the health services and the special case of technologic innovation. *International Journal of Health Services, 4,* 325–352.

Lapopolo, R. B. (1984). Financial model to determine the effect of clinical education programs on physical therapy departments. *Physical Therapy, 64,* 1396–1402.

Leiken, A. M., Stern, E., & Baines, R. E. (1983). The effect of clinical education programs on hospital production. *Inquiry, 20,* 88–92.

Pawlson, L. G., Watkins, R., & Donaldson, M. (1980). The costs of medical student instruction in the practice setting. *The Journal of Family Practice, 10,* 847–852.

Pobojewski, T. R. (1978). Case study: Cost/benefit analysis of clinical education. *Journal of Allied Health, 7,* 192–198.

Porter, R. E., & Kincaid, C. B. (1977). Financial aspects of clinical education to facilities. *Physical Therapy, 57,* 905–908.

Pratt, O. G., & Hill, L. A. (1960). The price of medical education: A dissection of one hospital's expenditures. *Hospitals, 34*(15), 44–47, 104.

Prest, A. R., & Turvey, R. (1965). Cost-benefit analysis: A survey. *The Economics Journal, 75,* 683–735.

Sassone, P. G., & Schaffer, W. A. (1978). *Cost-benefit analysis: A handbook.* New York: Academic Press.

Warner, K. E., & Hutton, R. C. (1980). Cost-benefit and cost-effectiveness analysis in health care. *Medical Care, 18,* 1069–1084.

The Occupational Therapy Level II Fieldwork Experience: Estimation of the Fiscal Benefit

Harold Shalik, Linda D. Shalik

Key Words: costs and cost analysis • education, occupational therapy • services, occupational therapy

A nationwide study, from which the data in this article were taken, suggests that most physical dysfunction and psychosocial Level II fieldwork placements for occupational therapy students represent a financial benefit to the sponsoring institution. This article provides the occupational therapy educator or fieldwork site supervisor with a method for estimating the amount of financial benefit one may anticipate from the assignment of a student to a physical dysfunction or psychosocial Level II fieldwork placement. Time-consuming data collection and interpretation are not necessary to perform this analysis. A formula to predict the fiscal outcome is described. Step-by-step instructions guide the user in applying the formula to a given physical dysfunction or psychosocial Level II fieldwork situation.

Harold Shalik, PhD, OTR/L, is in private practice working as a clinical consultant in occupational therapy. (Mailing address: 1355 NE Archer Road, Archer, Florida 32618)

Linda D. Shalik, PhD, OTR/L, is Assistant Professor of Occupational Therapy, Occupational Therapy Curriculum, University of Florida, Gainesville, Florida.

Various observers have speculated that the costs of Level II fieldwork for the preparation of professional occupational therapists have been borne by the sponsoring facility supervising the fieldwork student; others have suggested that agencies benefit greatly from the additional workforce provided by students. Busby, Leming, and Olson (1972) indicated that hospital administrators viewed student educational programs in hospitals as incurring an overall cost to the institution, with these costs budgeted to the estimated costs for fieldwork education. Frum (1986) reasoned that, as a result of the prospective payment system, institutions and third-party payers did not permit payment for educational purposes. She stated, "Data which demonstrates the positive nature of the student to the total program's productivity during affiliation periods is needed" (p. 13). This article examines such data. The nationwide study from which these data were taken suggests that most physical dysfunction and psychosocial Fieldwork II placements represented a financial benefit to the institution (Shalik, 1986). The statistical analysis of the data by means of a multiple regression procedure has resulted in a formula that may be used by occupational therapists to compare their specific fiscal experience with similar experiences in other fieldwork placements.

Review of the Literature

Time logs have consistently been used to determine how students' time was spent in the fieldwork experience (Arthurson, Mander-Jones, & Rocca, 1976; Gillanders & Heiman, 1971; Payson, Gaenslen, & Stargardter, 1961). Freymann and Springer (1973), by computing direct and indirect expenditures in fieldwork education for medicine, nursing, and allied health, concluded that students provided manpower at a level that exceeded the costs of their education programs. Partially through the use of faculty logs, Pawlson, Watkins, and Donaldson (1980) found that faculty salaries constituted the primary expense to an institution for fieldwork education, with costs of space and overhead found to be marginal. Chung, Spelbring, and Boissoneau (1980) conducted a cost–benefit analysis of occupational therapy fieldwork involving Eastern Michigan University students and found that the major fiscal cost to the institution resulted from the reduction in the production of agency services, or the use of personnel time in the training of the student. The institution received financial benefits in the revenue produced by students treating patients and in inexpensive labor by students for miscellaneous duties. Shalik (1986) followed up on the methodology and design of the Eastern Michigan University study using 180 supervisor/student responses for a cost–benefit analysis study and concluded that there was an *average* benefit to the agency of $4700 per student for a 12-week placement.

The Data Base

The data base used to predict fiscal cost or benefit for a Level II fieldwork placement was generated from Shalik's survey, which was completed during 1985 (Shalik, 1986). Table 1 shows that there were 156 occupational therapy fieldwork sites involved in the data collected. The sites were located in 32 states. Twelve occupational therapy professional schools located in different areas of the United States cooperated in the study, with 180 students from these schools supplying the log sheets for the data (in conjunction with paired log sheets from their fieldwork supervisors). A detailed discussion of the methodology used to collect these data appears elsewhere (Shalik, 1986).

Data Analysis

Net Present Value (NPV) represents the difference between benefit and cost, with allowance made for the discount rate over the period of the project. Because a fieldwork experience never exceeds 1 year,

Table 1
Clinics, Schools, and Students by States

State	Number of Clinics ($N = 156$)	Number of Schools ($N = 12$)	Number of Students ($N = 180$)
Alabama	2	1	8
Arizona	2	0	0
Arkansas	2	0	0
California	27	2	26
Colorado	2	0	0
Connecticut	1	0	0
Delaware	1	0	0
Florida	13	1	19
Georgia	2	0	0
Illinois	5	0	0
Indiana	5	0	0
Iowa	2	0	0
Kansas	1	0	0
Maryland	4	0	0
Massachusetts	2	0	0
Michigan	13	2	33
Minnesota	1	0	0
Mississippi	1	0	0
Montana	1	0	0
Nevada	1	0	0
New York	1	0	0
North Carolina	5	1	4
North Dakota	2	0	0
Ohio	15	1	28
Oklahoma	2	0	0
Pennsylvania	4	0	0
South Carolina	2	1	9
Tennessee	3	0	0
Texas	12	1	20
Virginia	8	1	10
West Virginia	5	0	0
Wisconsin	9	1	23

Table 2
***R* Square Change: Summary of Stepwise Regression Procedure for Dependent Variable NPV at .05 Significance Level for Entry**

Step	Variable Entered	Number In	Partial *R* Square	Total *R* Square
1	Week	1	.2271	.2271
2	Week^2	2	.0616	.2887
3	Pediatric Fieldwork	3	.0114	.3001
4	Fieldwork Sequence	4	.0160	.3161

Note. NPV = Net Present Value.

the discount rate is not a factor in the NPV for this particular fieldwork experience analysis (Sassone & Schaffer, 1978). If one subtracts the *cost* of a fieldwork experience (supervisor's input) from its *benefit* (student's input), the result is the NPV. Thus, NPV equals benefit minus cost. If the NPV is positive, the result is a fiscal benefit; if it is negative, the result is a fiscal cost. Thus the single outcome of NPV expresses either cost or benefit, based on the difference between these two variables.

Using the single-outcome variable NPV, we performed a stepwise regression, using covariates to predict the NPV outcome. The covariates deemed best suited for the prediction were (a) the types of fieldwork, (b) the week of the fieldwork, and (c) the fieldwork sequence (i.e., first, second, or third fieldwork experience). A curvilinear relationship existed between week and NPV; that is, the NPV increases with time, reaches a maximum point, and then starts a gradual decline beyond that point as time progresses. To account for this relationship a quadratic variable for the week (e.g., Week^2) was added to the prediction equation.

Results

The original equation for the prediction of NPV, for any specified week, was as follows:

$$\text{NPV}(n) = -824.65 + 294.45 \,(\text{Week})$$
$$- 15.57 \,(\text{Week}^2) + 166.97 \,(\text{Fieldwork Sequence})$$
$$- 537.33 \,(\text{PedsFW})$$

The multiple *R* for this equation was .562, which accounted for about 31.6% of the variance in the NPV criterion variable.

Table 2 shows the percent of variance each predictor variable contributes to the NPV. Table 3 shows the distribution of the sequence of the fieldwork experience (i.e., first, second, or third experience). The third experience has only three paired responses. Table 4 shows the type of fieldwork experiences: pediatric fieldwork experiences have eight paired responses, and geriatric fieldwork experiences have four.

Table 3
Total Number of Fieldwork Experiences by Sequence ($N = 176$)

Fieldwork Experience Number	Total
1	116
2	57
3	3

How to Use the Prediction Equation

The prediction equation for a complete affiliation is as follows:

$$\text{NPV TOTAL} = \text{NPV}(1) + \text{NPV}(2) + \text{NPV}(3)$$
$$\ldots + \text{NPV}(X), \text{ where}$$

X	= total weeks of affiliation (e.g., 6, 12, or 13 weeks)
n	= 1, 2, 3, . . . , to X (n is the subset designation for each NPV. It is read "NPV for Week 1, or Week 2, etc." n and "week" are always the same number.)
Week	= 1, or 2, or 3, . . . , or X
Week²	= (Week) × (Week)
Fieldwork Sequence	= 1 or 2 (designate 3 or more as 2)

Example. To understand how to use the prediction equation, consider the following case:

Type of Fieldwork: Psychosocial or Physical Dysfunction
Length of Fieldwork Experience: 4 weeks
Fieldwork Sequence: Second Fieldwork Experience

Therefore:

$$X = 4$$
$$n = 1, 2, 3, \text{ and } 4$$
$$\text{Week} = 1, 2, 3, \text{ and } 4$$
$$\text{Fieldwork Sequence} = 2$$

$$\text{NPV TOTAL} = \text{NPV}(1) + \text{NPV}(2) + \text{NPV}(3) + \text{NPV}(4)$$

The formula for predicting a single week is

$$\text{NPV}(n) = -824.65 + 294.45 \, (\text{Week})$$
$$- 15.55 \, (\text{Week}^2) + 166.97 \, (\text{Fieldwork Sequence})$$

Substitute for (n), (Week), (Week²), (Fieldwork Sequence):

$$\text{NPV}(1) = -824.65 + 294.45 \times (1) - 15.55$$
$$\times (1 \times 1) + 166.97 \times (2) = -212$$

$$\text{NPV}(2) = -824.65 + 294.45 \times (2) - 15.55$$
$$\times (2 \times 2) + 166.97 \times (2) = 36$$

$$\text{NPV}(3) = -824.65 + 294.45 \times (3) - 15.55$$
$$\times (3 \times 3) + 166.97 \times (2) = 253$$

$$\text{NPV}(4) = -824.65 + 294.45 \times (4) - 15.55$$
$$\times (4 \times 4) + 166.97 \times (2) = 438$$

Thus,

$$\text{NPV TOTAL} = (-212) + (36)$$
$$+ (253) + (438) = +515$$

Interpretation of the Example. Given the example of a psychosocial or physical dysfunction fieldwork placement, which is the student's second fieldwork placement, with a duration of 4 weeks, there is a net benefit to the sponsoring institution of approximately $515.00 per student. This example demonstrates that it costs the institution $212 for the student's first week of fieldwork, a net cost of $212. There is a $36 benefit the second week, but this is still a net cost of $176 for the 2-week period. However, by the third week the benefit increases to $253 for Week 3, resulting in a net benefit for the 3-week period of $77. Thus, it is not until the third week that there is an overall benefit to the institution. It is obvious that the longer the fieldwork experience, the greater the net benefit to the institution for Week 3 and beyond.

Limitations

Table 3 shows that the third fieldwork sequence experience is based on only three student/supervisor pairs. The reader should not rely on a separate projection for the third fieldwork experience because of the small number of observations, but should treat the second and third fieldwork experiences exactly the same.

Table 4 shows that the original prediction equation was based in part on eight pediatric student/supervisor pairs. The analysis shows that this group of eight observations is significantly different from the psychosocial and physical dysfunction groups. The prediction formula used in this article is not recommended for a pediatric affiliation because of the small number of pediatric observations. More data will be required to predict the cost or benefit for a pediatric affiliation.

The prediction equation developed here has the probability of being accurate in 95 out of every 100

Table 4
Total Number of Fieldwork Experiences by Type ($N = 180$)

Type of Fieldwork	Total
Psychosocial	91
Physical Dysfunction	77
Pediatric	8
Geriatric	4

fieldwork experiences (or, stated in another way, inaccurate in 5 out of every 100 experiences). Thus, it may be used either for estimating the benefit one may anticipate in any given physical dysfunction or psychosocial fieldwork experience, or it may be used to confirm data that are created for any given fieldwork experience by means of a specific cost–benefit analysis for that case. The user is cautioned not to place sole reliance on this prediction equation in institutional negotiations without having other substantiating data.

Cross-Validation

The prediction equation developed in this article is based on a single sample from the total population. It is reasonable to assume that each time such a sample is taken a somewhat different equation will be developed. To determine the proposed equation's ability to give a good estimate of the NPV TOTAL when applied to a new and similar group, a cross-validation technique was used.

Huck, Cormier, and Bounds (1974) advocated the following:

> The technique of cross-validation involves four simple steps. (1) The original group of people (for whom both predictor and criterion scores are available) is randomly divided into two subgroups. (2) Just one of the subgroups is used to develop the prediction equation. (3) This equation is used to predict a criterion score for each person in the second subgroup (i.e., the subgroup that was not used to develop the prediction equation). (4) The predicted criterion scores for people in the second subgroup are correlated with their actual criterion scores. A high correlation (that is, significantly different from zero) means that the prediction equation works for people other than those who were used to develop the equation. If the individuals in future studies are not too much different from those in the cross-validation procedure, the researcher is justified in using the prediction equation for groups other than the original. (pp. 159–160)

Using this technique, the prediction equation for any given week was as follows:

$$NPV1 = -713.3 + 294.1 \ (\text{Week}) - 15.65 \ (\text{Week}^2).$$

With the new prediction equation, a criterion score for NPV1 was created for the second subgroup, $n = 90$. Using SAS PROC CORR (SAS terminology for *Procedure Correlation, SAS,* 1985), variables NPV (from original data set) and NPV1 (predicted NPV from NPV1 equation), a 2×2 correlation matrix was developed. A correlation between NPV and NPV1 of 0.49843 was found, which was significant at the .0001

level. It can be concluded that the prediction equation can be used for groups other than the original.

The Prediction Formula

A prediction formula has been developed for educators and fieldwork site supervisors to estimate the fiscal benefit for a Level II fieldwork experience for psychosocial or physical dysfunction settings. The prediction equation takes the form:

$$NPV = -824.65 + 294.45 \ (\text{Week}) - 15.55 \ (\text{Week}^2)$$
$$+ 166.97 \ (\text{Fieldwork Sequence})$$

If the NPV is positive, it represents a benefit; if it is negative, it represents a cost. The above prediction formula is for any given week from 1 to 13. Therefore, in a 12-week fieldwork experience, the NPVs for Weeks 1 through 12 are summed, with the total representing the cost or benefit for the total fieldwork experience. Table 5, developed from the above prediction formula, shows that students in their first experience represent (after a 12-week fieldwork experience) a $4967 benefit and that students in their second or third experience represent a $6971 benefit. A cross-validation study used to correlate the *known* NPV with the *predicted* NPV proved significant at the .0001 level and suggested that the prediction equation created in this article can be used for similar groups other than the original. The data for the physical dysfunction ($n = 77$) and psychosocial experiences ($n = 91$) are sufficiently large to justify generalization to the total population.

Discussion and Conclusion

The ability to predict a cost or benefit for a Level II fieldwork experience offers the occupational therapy educator, the fieldwork site supervisor, and the administrator the opportunity to control the cost of a Level II fieldwork placement. Short affiliations, which are subject to high start-up costs in the early weeks and a downturn of fiscal benefits in the final weeks, should be discouraged if financial cost is a factor to the department or institution. The longer the affiliation, up to 13 weeks, the more fiscal benefits the sponsoring organization may expect to realize.

Educators, when organizing their placement

Table 5
Net Present Value by Week Number and Fieldwork Sequence Number for Physical Dysfunction or Psychosocial Fieldwork Placement

Fieldwork Sequence	Week Number												
	1	2	3	4	5	6	7	8	9	10	11	12	13
1	−379	−510	−424	−153	273	822	1464	2167	2899	3631	4331	4967	5510
2	−212	−716	77	515	1108	1824	2633	3502	4402	5301	6168	6971	7680
3	Suggest using Fieldwork Sequence 2												

Research on Educational Outcomes Related to Fieldwork | **113** schedules, may take into consideration that students in their second or third affiliation bring more fiscal benefits to a placement than do students in their first fieldwork experience. Rotation among students in their first and those in their second or third experience, for a given fieldwork site, may balance the fiscal benefit realized for the placement. A curriculum designed for students to be placed in their first fieldwork experience between their junior and senior years automatically provides a lesser benefit to a given fieldwork site than does a curriculum that permits a rotation of placement (i.e., with students beginning their fieldwork experience after their senior year).

References

Arthurson, J., Mander-Jones, T., & Rocca, J. (1976). What does the intern do? *Medical Journal of Australia, 1,* 63–65.

Busby, D. D., Leming, J. C., & Olson, M. J. (1972). Unidentified educational costs in a university teaching hospital: An initial study. *Journal of Medical Education, 47,* 243–251.

Chung, Y., Spelbring, L., & Boissoneau, R. (1980). A cost-benefit analysis of fieldwork education in occupational therapy. *Inquiry, 17,* 216–229.

Freymann, J. G., & Springer, J. K. (1973). Cost of hospital-based education. *Hospitals, 47,* 65–67.

Frum, D. C. (1986, April). Fieldwork education: Can we afford it? *Occupational Therapy News,* p. 13.

Gillanders, W., & Heiman, M. (1971). Time study comparisons of three intern programs. *Journal of Medical Education, 46,* 142–149.

Huck, S. W., Cormier, W. H., & Bounds, W. G. (1974). *Reading statistics and research.* New York: Harper & Row.

Pawlson, L. G., Watkins, R., & Donaldson, M. (1980). The costs of medical student instruction in the practice setting. *Journal of Family Practice, 10,* 847–852.

Payson, H. E., Gaenslen, E. C., & Stargardter, F. L. (1961). Time study of an internship on a university medical service. *New England Journal of Medicine, 254,* 439–443.

SAS user's guide: Statistics (version 5 ed.). (1985). Cary, NC: SAS Institute.

Sassone, P. G., & Schaffer, W. A. (1978). *Cost-benefit analysis: A handbook.* New York: Academic Press.

Shalik, L. D. (1986). *Cost-benefit analysis of Level II fieldwork for bachelor's-level and basic master's-level students in occupational therapy.* Unpublished doctoral dissertation, University of Florida, Gainesville.

Level I Fieldwork: Creating a Positive Experience

Susan Swinehart, Susan K. Meyers

Key Words: fieldwork, occupational therapy, level I • program evaluation • qualitative method

Qualitative research methodology was used to explore the purpose of level I fieldwork among occupational therapy students, clinical educators, and faculty respondents at one academic program. Differences in purposes among the three groups of respondents created different fieldwork expectations and outcomes. These differences underlined the importance of communication among students, clinical supervisors, and faculty in planning fieldwork to meet the needs of all three groups. Interpersonal skills, rather than academic skills, emerged as most important to student success in clinical education. Other factors that promote optimal level I fieldwork experience are understanding the purpose, level of commitment, clarity of expectations, timing, structure, and evaluation of the experience.

Susan Swinehart, MS, OTR, is Assistant Professor and Coordinator of Admissions, Indiana University School of Medicine, School of Allied Health Sciences, Department of Occupational Therapy, 1140 West Michigan Street, CF 311, Indianapolis, Indiana 46202–5119.

Susan K. Meyers, EdD, OTR, is Associate Professor and Director, Occupational Therapy Program, College of Allied Health Sciences, University of Tennessee–Memphis, Memphis, Tennessee.

This article was accepted for publication August 8, 1992.

Level I fieldwork is an important educational component for occupational therapy students. Although the American Occupational Therapy Association (AOTA) provides a purpose statement, purposes expressed by those engaged in level I fieldwork seem ambiguous (AOTA, 1983). Changes in health care provision, such as reduction in fiscal resources and personnel shortages, have challenged those clinicians responsible for providing level I fieldwork (AOTA, 1985; Masagatani & Bishop, 1991; Teske & Spelbring, 1983). Level I fieldwork is the first clinical experience for occupational therapy students, setting the tone for current and future collaborative relationships among students and academic and clinical educators.

Literature Review

Level I fieldwork was described as providing an important opportunity for the student to develop clinical role models (Christie, Joyce, & Moeller, 1985a, 1985b). Wittman, Swinehart, St. Michael, and Cahill (1989) reported that occupational therapy graduates identified supervision and patient contact as the most valuable experiential aspects of level I fieldwork but generally viewed the experience as negative.

Two studies examined level I fieldwork objectives. Leonardelli and Caruso (1986) compared the rank ordering of level I fieldwork objectives by academic and clinical educators. Hands-on experiences and uniform fieldwork objectives were ranked more important by academic educators than by clinical educators. Clinicians cited cost effectiveness as a major concern and requested "more structure from the schools so less time is spent planning" (p. 262).

Kautzmann (1987) compared ranking of level I fieldwork objectives among students, academic educators, and clinical educators. The results led to recommendations that academic educators improve integration of theory with treatment planning and that clinical educators develop better methods of providing feedback to students regarding their professional behavior. Students requested more patient contact, observations of clinicians, and feedback regarding their skills.

Brown, Caruso Streeter, Stoffel, and McPherson (1989) built on the work of Leonardelli and Caruso (1986) and Kautzmann (1987) to develop the Wisconcil level I fieldwork evaluation form. The evaluation categorized behaviors into 5 groups: interpersonal interactions, professional behavior, data gathering and observation, program planning and implementation, and verbal and written communication. The evaluation form is currently used in Wisconsin and has had some national distribution. There are no reported data on the validity or reliability of the Wisconcil evaluation instrument.

Crist (1986) discussed the collaborative nature of fieldwork, whereas Bell (1986) said that for effective collaboration to take place, all participants must understand each others' perspectives of the level I fieldwork experience. Masagatani and Bishop (1991) indicated that students, clinical educators, and academic educators can have "very different viewpoints and behavior patterns" (p. 10).

The literature describes important elements, processes, and recommendations for level I fieldwork. The purpose of this study was to better understand the effect of level I fieldwork on students, clinical educators, and academic educators by evaluating the process in one academic program to maximize its positive effects on students and clinicians.

Method

This study was conducted through naturalistic inquiry (Lincoln & Guba, 1985; Guba & Lincoln, 1989; Meyers, 1989). Focus was on a single baccalaureate academic program. Level I fieldwork in this institution was begun in the second semester of the occupational therapy program and continued for two semesters. In this institution, students were offered options of a 1-week clinical experience when classes were not in session or ½ day a week for 7 weeks concomitant with classwork. The 1-week fieldwork experiences were available during the summer between the students' junior and senior years. Level I fieldwork was randomly assigned, except for students who requested nontraditional placements (community programs without occupational therapist on site).

Data were collected in clinical environments where level I fieldwork was occurring and during seminar discussions with students. Focus groups of students, faculty, and clinical educators brought respondents together to elaborate on data collected and to respond to data collected from other respondent groups. Approximately 70 students, 30 clinical educators, and 10 faculty, including two classes of students followed from first to last level I fieldwork experiences, contributed to this study over a 2-year period.

Level I fieldwork sites were selected to represent the spectrum of occupational therapy practice, including mental health, acute physical disabilities, rehabilitation, pediatrics, geriatrics, inpatient and outpatient programs, and nontraditional sites. Data were collected through observations, in-depth interviews, and a review of documents. Respondents engaged in successive interviews, learning from, enhancing and rebutting other respondents' ideas over a 2-year period of data collection and analysis. Similar bits of data were grouped together to form themes that defined and critiqued level I fieldwork.

Trustworthiness of the results was assumed through the following activities. At the conclusion of each interview, collected data were reviewed with the respondents for verification of accuracy. Negotiated understanding be- tween respondents and investigators occurred during this process of member checking (Lincoln & Guba, 1985). The investigators debriefed each other to raise additional questions for inquiry and to assure adherence to the inquiry methodology. Throughout the process of data collection, an audit trail was created that referenced each bit of data to its original source (Guba & Lincoln, 1989; Schwandt & Halpern, 1988).

Results

What emerged from the study was a description of level I fieldwork that represented the views of all respondents. The issues that emerged were purpose or purposes of the experience, commitment, expectations, timing, structure, and evaluation methods and process.

Purposes

Nine purposes of level I fieldwork were identified. Agreement of purposes among respondent groups is shown in Table 1. All respondents agreed that one purpose of level I fieldwork was to integrate theory with practice. Students and clinicians agreed that fieldwork should help separate the reality of practice from its ideal and assist students to develop confidence. Students and academicians shared similar perceptions regarding practice choice and role models. Clinical educators and faculty shared the fewest areas of agreement on purposes of level I fieldwork.

Table 1
Comparison of Purpose of Level I Fieldwork

Clinicians Provide Opportunities for Students to	Students Expect Opportunities That Enable Them to	Faculty Expect Clinicians to Provide Students With Opportunities to
Integrate theory and practice		
Apply "hands-on" treatment ↔	Apply theory to practice	↔ Learn while doing
Increase confidence ↔	Develop confidence	
Define occupational therapy ↔	Separate reality from idealism	
	Identify practice choice	↔ Expand exposure to practice settings
	Identify role models ↔	Observe professional role models
Establish patient rapport	⟷	Develop technical and interpersonal skills
Observe patients and therapists during treatment		
		Receive feedback regarding behavior Faculty members expect to validate the curriculum through Level I fieldwork

Note. ↔ Connotes agreement.

When students discussed application of theory and practice, they identified the importance of developing observation skills through clinical observation and feedback from clinicians. Students said that observation skills contributed to the development of critical thinking. One student said, "teachers will be up there talking about this, then you go out and actually see it. It makes you feel good; you are actually getting something out of your classes." Clinical and academic educators agreed that technical and interpersonal therapeutic skills should be developed during level I fieldwork.

Students and clinicians agreed that level I fieldwork increased students' confidence in communication, patient interactions, and knowledge base. They described moving on a continuum from a position of insecurity on the first fieldwork experience to a sense of greater security in later clinical experiences. A student said, "I was always worried about things I would say around the patients. I learned to be comfortable coming up with treatment goals, notewriting, and talking with patients." Clinical educators said that a desired outcome of level I fieldwork was a decrease in students' fears and development of professional confidence. Students distinguished between the textbook picture of clinical conditions and clinical reality. This distinction applied to presenting symptoms and probable diagnoses, clinical treatment schedules, productivity expectations, and reimbursement issues.

Practice choice interests were affected in a variety of ways through level I fieldwork. Students were exposed to a variety of practice environments. Factors that influenced students' practice preferences included perceived success with treatment regimens, types of patients seen in the clinic, attitudes and moods of the clinicians, level of practice autonomy, collegial relationships, and communication. Faculty said that level I fieldwork should expose students to multiple populations and settings.

The role of the clinical educator was viewed as pivotal by students and faculty. Clinicians appeared to underestimate their significance as role models; they did not mention being role models as a purpose of level I fieldwork. Students attributed their success or lack of success within the clinical setting to their relationships and communication with clinicians. The responses of clinicians to students appeared to carry greater weight in practice choice decisions than did actual patient populations or treatment techniques. Faculty described the development of professionalism and interpersonal techniques using clinical role models as central educational elements of level I fieldwork.

Faculty said that level I fieldwork should provide students with feedback regarding their behavior and its potential effect on patients and staff. Feedback was particularly important for students with behavior problems that the academic program had difficulty addressing due to organizational constraints. Faculty also validated the curriculum through students' experiences during level I fieldwork.

Commitment

The perceived commitment of clinical educators influenced the experience of level I fieldwork for students. Commitment was first experienced in students' initial phone calls to the clinic to arrange visits. Students described their clinical educators in terms of being friendly, nice, available, and sensitive to students' situations. Students commented on the frequency and nature of feedback from clinicians, personalities and ages of clinicians (age proximity to students), and organization and preparedness of clinicians. A student said with obvious positive meaning, "she was ready for me." Another student said, "I showed up and the clinician said, 'Oh, I forgot you were scheduled today.'" Students noticed the enjoyment and pleasure that clinicians seemed to receive from their educator role and attributed this to clinicians' sense of commitment. Students were very interested in how clinicians obtained students and whether they had a choice about having students.

A few clinical educators indicated that they had no control over their level I fieldwork involvement; however, the majority indicated that they had sought involvement. Clinicians discussed the positive benefits of level I fieldwork related to students' enthusiasm and interest in clinical practice. Level I fieldwork was described as a recruitment vehicle because it gave students an opportunity to see a clinical site and provided clinicians with a brief opportunity to assess a student's future job potential within their clinic. Clinicians identified their commitment to the continuation of the profession through education. Issues that adversely affected clinicians' motivation included staff shortages, cancellations of level I fieldwork students, and various requirements imposed by the academic program. One clinician said that as pressures for productivity increased, her perceptions of level I fieldwork as a priority decreased. Faculty recognized that clinicians were stressed regarding quality assurance, productivity, and therapist shortages. These issues were seen as having direct, powerful, and adverse effects on clinicians' commitments to clinical education. However, it was believed that clinicians would continue to take level I fieldwork students as part of their responsibility to reciprocate for what they gained during their education process. Faculty recognized that geography played a part in clinicians' willingness to take on level I fieldwork responsibilities; clinicians located in areas more distant from the academic program seemed to be more willing to take students than those in close proximity to the program. This situation may have occurred because these clinicians were less involved in additional academic program projects (e.g. research, guest lectures, committees). Faculty respondents were aware that some level II fieldwork students were supervising level I fieldwork students.

Expectations

Expectations were not consistent across the groups of respondents. Clinicians expected students to take initiative, to be responsible for asking questions in the clinic, and to see that their needs were met. It was the students' responsibility to arrange visits to the clinics to coincide with treatment activities. This responsibility required students to be flexible enough to come early, stay late, or occasionally change the day of a visit. Some clinicians expected students to be willing to try evaluation or treatment techniques, even if the students had not been previously exposed to the evaluation and treatment modalities. Students were expected to exhibit appropriate behavior and dress for the clinic and to appreciate the efforts of clinicians in arranging the education experience. Students were considered egocentric, demanding, and frustrating by clinicians. Clinicians said they wanted to receive feedback from students about the positive and negative aspects of the clinical education experience and they realized that meeting these expectations was difficult for shy students.

Students expected to take some initiative for their education in the clinic by asking questions of therapists. Many students reported expectations for specific sites related to what they heard from peers who had previous experiences in the level I fieldwork sites. One student said that peers "told horror stories" about their experiences. Students in nontraditional sites described difficulty relating what they were doing to occupational therapy practice because there were no occupational therapists in these sites. Students in nontraditional sites often chose to avoid consultation with the faculty member assigned to assist them.

Both student and clinicians had expectations of the faculty. Students wanted explanations of fieldwork assignments because they were not allowed to select level I fieldwork sites. Clinicians expected the faculty to better prepare students in technical and interpersonal skills required in their sites. Clinicians encountered students who had personal problems that the clinicians were uncomfortable addressing and consequently chose to ignore. However, these clinicians were concerned that students with problems can "fall through the cracks" and enter level II fieldwork or practice without having their problems addressed.

Faculty respondents were committed to making level I fieldwork available to students. One academician indicated that she expected students to report a variety of experiences, some "wonderful" and some "horror stories." Faculty stated that it was the school's responsibility to help students apply the wonderful stories to curriculum content or life experiences and turn the horror stories into positive learning experiences by assisting the students in examining their roles in the situation, the effect of those roles, and the clinical conditions present. Faculty expected clinicians to supervise students, meaning that clinicians would deal with behavioral problems by giving students feedback based on observations and expertise. Students were expected to actively engage in the level I fieldwork process. Students were responsible for discussing their concerns with academic or clinical educators. Faculty said that students frequently find themselves in a no-win situation when they are asked to be responsible for evaluation and treatment tools that they have not been prepared to administer. Although faculty said it was the students' responsibility to communicate their situation and concern to clinicians, frequently students' attempts at communicating limit setting had no effect or were perceived negatively by clinicians. There was also the recognition that students' reports were not always accurate given their performance anxiety.

Timing

There were two issues related to timing of fieldwork: sequence of the level I fieldwork experience in relation to courses taken, and the advantages of a 1-week experience versus ½ day a week for 7 consecutive weeks in the same site. Students and clinicians discussed the lack of preparedness of students for the initial fieldwork experience. However, all the respondents agreed that the second semester in the program was the optimal time to initiate fieldwork.

Student respondents were enthusiastic about spending an entire week in the clinic. One week experiences allowed them to develop better rapport with clinicians to ask questions and eliminates school as a distraction thus enhancing their ability to concentrate on clinical activities. When they were in the clinic for ½ day each week, they tended to see the same things repeatedly and not get the gestalt of occupational therapy practice.

Clinicians expressed mixed opinions about the 1-week fieldwork experiences. One said it was too intense for students, making completion of academic and clinical assignments difficult. Another was concerned that students might not have time in 1 week to develop rapport with patients. Conversely, clinicians responding said that students saw more variety of patient treatment in a single week experience and got a better overall view of clinical practice.

Structure

Structure of level I fieldwork was described by students in terms of initial welcome to the clinic, assignments, and supervision. Clinicians who were enthusiastic and took time to stop and establish eye contact with students while explaining expectations made students feel welcome. Students were pleased when they had assigned locations to sit and review charts or write notes while in the clinic.

Written schedules were appreciated by students. All students were required by their school to write progress notes, complete one case study, and participate in weekly practicum seminars. However, there was no consistency in clinic requirements. Some students had observational experiences, whereas other students provided patient treatment. Most clinicians planned carefully for students. They gave students clinic notebooks and access to available educational resources. Some students were asked to keep journals that were discussed with clinicians.

Several fieldwork sites provided students with a different clinical educator each week. Students found this less desirable than having a single supervisor throughout the fieldwork experience. Students said each supervisor had different expectations and it was hard to form relationships and ask questions when they did not know the clinician.

In multidisciplinary departments, some students had difficulty with role blurring. They found it difficult to differentiate occupational therapy from physical therapy or recreational therapy. In nontraditional sites, students said they had no one to talk to about occupational therapy and they missed this opportunity.

Faculty provided course syllabi to fieldwork level I sites to clarify educational content and to facilitate students' fieldwork experiences. However, they were not certain whether these had any meaning to clinicians.

Evaluation Methods and Process

At the conclusion of fieldwork, students and clinicians exchanged evaluations. Initially, students were surprised that an evaluation process occurs. Most students reported being pleased with evaluation results. However, students and clinicians expressed concerns that the evaluation forms did not address areas considered important to professional development. Evaluation forms designed by the education program to resemble AOTA's Fieldwork Level II evaluation forms primarily quantified performance for a grade rather than giving students information about how to modify professional skills and behaviors. One student said, "there were pages of numbers. I went through looking for 3 or below, that's what I was concerned about!"

Students often hesitated to give feedback to clinicians about fieldwork experiences. A student said, "I can't imagine writing anything negative about the place, even if I did find something there." Another student said, "I think if you have negative things you should write them so the next student won't have to go through that." When students were supervised by multiple clinicians, they were frightened by the thought of those clinicians meeting to discuss their performance to assign a score. Students said they performed better for some clinicians than for others and they were concerned about who would have the most influence on the final score.

Some students who had not received feedback throughout fieldwork had no idea how their final scores would look. A student said, "I haven't a clue, because she doesn't say anything." Some clinicians were uncomfortable receiving feedback from students. One student reported that her clinical educator did not allow any discussion about the facility during the evaluation session. Faculty respondents expressed concern about the format of the evaluation. The current format tended to reinforce students' focus on numerical scores (e.g., did I meet the minimum competency standards?) rather than the overall content of the evaluation feedback. One faculty member hypothesized that the two major reasons students failed a fieldwork experience were inadequate time management skills and behavior problems. Faculty respondents speculated that perhaps the evaluation format needed examination and alteration to improve quality of feedback.

Discussion

Transference of the data gleaned from this study of one academic program will have to be assessed by the reader to determine its application to other programs that use a similar format. Data from this study would need to be shared with students and clinical educations within individual settings to see whether similar problems or concerns are evident.

Students, clinical educators, and faculty respondents identified numerous factors that enhanced or detracted from level I fieldwork. Many of these factors centered on the need for improved communication. Clinical educators and faculty identified the need to increase their dialogue regarding student behavioral problems; specifically, to clarify the roles of clinical educators and faculty in addressing student interpersonal skill development, to identify the behavioral expectations of students within the clinic, and to anticipate potential intervention strategies.

Respondent feedback in this study supported the findings of Leonardelli and Caruso (1986), which indicated that level I fieldwork participants have different objectives for the experience, along with differing perspectives on the importance of the objectives. The lowest level of agreement was found between the clinical educators and faculty, again reinforcing the premise of Masagatani and Bishop (1991) that clinical educators and faculty have varied perspectives.

Clinical educators in this study cited the development of student confidence through clinic exposure as a major element of level I fieldwork; however, they tend to minimize their role in this process. Faculty and student respondents both indicated that they see the clinical educator's role as critical. Student respondents attributed their success or lack of success in the clinic to their clinical supervisor. Student response in this study is consistent with the results of Christie et al. (1985a, 1985b). Faculty attribute a student's integration of professionalism and interpersonal techniques to the role modeling of clinical educators.

Student and faculty respondents indicated that level I fieldwork provided a hands-on introduction to practice areas within occupational therapy that students had not previously been exposed to. This exposure to new areas expanded some students' practice choice consideration. Clinical educators described level I fieldwork as an opportunity for students to learn about a given practice area and as an opportunity for the clinical facility to engage in recruitment activities. When level I fieldwork is viewed as a vehicle to expand practice preference consideration as well as an opportunity for recruitment, it becomes a potentially powerful tool in addressing labor shortages that exist within the program.

Recommendations

Specific behavioral and learning objectives might be developed by each fieldwork site in conjunction with referring academic programs so that students would have a clearer understanding of what is expected of them and what they could expect in return from the clinical educator. Given differences in the perspectives of clinicians and faculty, collaborative development of a baseline of clinical expectations is necessary to ensure that specific clinical activities and curricula content are compatible.

Increased awareness by clinicians regarding the significance of their role modeling and its effect on the student is indicated. This issue could be addressed during AOTA's Annual Council on Education (COE) meeting. Local COEs could be encouraged to follow up with workshops involving students, clinicians, and faculty.

The implementation of a level I fieldwork evaluation has real meaning to clinicians and students. Ideally the evaluation would be short and concise with a relevant behavioral focus that allows application in a wide variety of settings. As evaluations are developed and put into use, data should be gathered to allow analysis of reliability and validity. Concurrently, clinicians, students, and faculty need to be involved in discussions regarding their perceptions about the value of an evaluation's ability to provide relevant and helpful information.

The discomfort associated with communication of problem behaviors with students by clinical educators and faculty could be anticipated, acknowledged, and routinely addressed through national and local COE meetings that focus on communication issues and possible intervention strategies. As issues and intervention plans are identified, these ideas could be incorporated into the level I fieldwork objectives.

Conclusion

The results from this research project conducted at one university support the results of previously cited level I fieldwork investigations. Issues involving clarification of expectations, performance evaluation, and communication are critical. The most influential factor identified in this study was the clinical educator's role as professional guide, teacher, and potential mentor. Level I fieldwork was also described as a vehicle for early recruitment. In future research it would be interesting to have more information about what practice areas are made available to students for level I experiences. If level I fieldwork is viewed as an opportunity to recruit, what effect does that focus have on the design and implementation of level I programs, and what, if any, relationship exists between level I and level II fieldwork experiences? ▲

References

American Occupational Therapy Association. (1983). *Essentials for an approved educational program for occupational therapists.* Rockville, MD: Author.

American Occupational Therapy Association. (1985). *Occupational therapy manpower: A plan for progress.* Rockville, MD: Author.

Bell, J. (1986). *The purpose of fieldwork education, proceedings of occupational therapy education: Target 2000* (pp. 85–89). Rockville, MD: American Occupational Therapy Association.

Brown, S., Caruso Streeter, L. A., Stoffel, F., & McPherson, J. J. (1989). Development of a level I fieldwork evaluation. *American Journal of Occupational Therapy, 43,* 677–682.

Christie, B. A., Joyce, P. C., & Moeller, P. L. (1985a). Fieldwork experience. Part I: Impact on practice preference. *American Journal of Occupational Therapy, 39,* 671–674.

Christie, B. A., Joyce, P. C., & Moeller, P. L. (1985b). Fieldwork experience. Part II: The supervisor's dilemma. *American Journal of Occupational Therapy, 39,* 675–681.

Crist, P. A. (1986). Contemporary issues in clinical education. *Monograph of current practice series in occupational therapy I* (3). Thorofare, NJ: Slack.

Guba, E. G., & Lincoln, Y. S. (1989). *Fourth generation evaluation.* Newbury Park, CA: Sage.

Kautzmann, L. N. (1987). Perceptions of the purpose of level I fieldwork. *American Journal of Occupational Therapy, 41,* 595–600.

Leonardelli, C. A., & Caruso, L. A. (1986). Level I fieldwork: Issues and needs. *American Journal of Occupational Therapy, 40,* 258–264.

Lincoln, Y., & Guba, E. (1985). *Naturalistic inquiry.* Beverly Hills, CA: Sage.

Masagatani, G. N., & Bishop, K. F. (1991, March 7). Fieldwork and academic education. *OT Week,* pp. 10–11.

Meyers, S. K. (1989). Program evaluation of occupational therapy level II fieldwork environments: A naturalistic inquiry. *Occupational Therapy Journal of Research, 9,* 347–361.

Schwandt, T. A., & Halpern, E. S. (1988). *Linking auditing and metaevaluation: Enhancing quality in applied research.* Newbury Park, CA: Sage.

Teske, Y. R., & Spelbring, L. M. (1983). Future impact on occupational therapy from current changes in higher education. *American Journal of Occupational Therapy, 37,* 667–672.

Wittman, P., Swinehart, S. A., St. Michael, G., & Cahill, R. (1989). Factors influencing practice choice. *American Journal of Occupational Therapy, 43,* 602–606.

REPORT OF THE COMMITTEE ON TEACHING
METHODS[1]

The committee was assigned the study of practice training, its methods, organization and supervision. Realizing that practice training is a subject in which both the schools and those training the students in the hospitals are equally interested, the committee was divided into two groups; Group A, representing the training schools, and Group B, representing those in the field. Both groups have a distinct contribution to make to the subject, and while they approach it from opposite angles, they agree so well on the main points that it has been relatively easy to make a report with conclusions and recommendations.

Six training schools, The Boston School of Occupational Therapy, Milwaukee-Downer College, Minnesota University, Philadelphia School of Occupational Therapy, St. Louis School of Occupational Therapy, and Toronto University, as well as the following hospitals, representing various services and in widely scattered localities have been used as the basis for this study: Allentown State Hospital, Pennsylvania;[2] Ann Arbor University Hospital, Michigan; James Whitcomb Riley Hospital, Indianapolis, Indiana; Manhattan State Hospital, New York; Norristown State Hospital, Pennsylvania;[2] Robert B. Brigham Hospital, Boston, Massachusetts; Walter Reed General Hospital, Washington, D. C.; and Worcester State Hospital, Massachusetts. In order that the study might not be limited by the practice in these schools and hospitals, but be more comprehensive, the individual members of the committee have expressed themselves on matters of policy and future development; based on a wider experience

[1] Read in part at eleventh annual meeting of the American Occupational Therapy Association held at Minneapolis, Minn., October 10 to 12, 1927.

[2] Material was sent directly from Norristown and Allentown due to the absence from this country of the member of the committee representing Pennsylvania institutions.

287

with the training of students and the hospital situation than these institutions afford.

There were two outstanding questions which confronted the committee at the outset of the study. First, what preparation should be expected of the practice student by the hospital? Second, what educational opportunities should the hospital give the student? These two questions have been studied in detail, because the largest part of the practice training problem is comprehended in their answers.

PART I. PREPARATION OF THE STUDENT FOR PRACTICE TRAINING

1. SCHOOLS OF OCCUPATIONAL THERAPY

The first step of the study was an inquiry into the training of the students in the schools, not with the idea of analyzing the training in detail, but to know the general length and scope of the student's preparation on entering the hospital. The length of training in the schools varies from eight months to four years, and the requirements for practice training range from three to nine months. They are distributed as follows:

	SCHOOL TIME	HOSPITAL PRACTICE TRAINING
Boston School of Occupational Therapy..	9 months	9 months
Milwaukee-Downer College..............	2 and 4 years	9 months
Minnesota University..................	4 years	3 months
Philadelphia School of Occupational Therapy.........................	8 months	6 months
St. Louis School of Occupational Therapy.........................	2 years	6 months
Toronto University..................	2 years	4 months
Present minimum standard............	75 lecture hours 1080 practical hours or 8 or 9 months	3 months

2. COMMENTS OF FIELD WORKERS ON SCHOOL PREPARATION

Group B, or the members of the committee concerned directly with the training of students in hospitals, were asked if they found students sufficiently prepared in design, crafts, theory, recreation and physical education, and hospital conduct and ethics. They were also asked whether they had to give supplementary training in any or all these subjects, and what recommendations they would make to the schools for better preparation.

Design

Two members of the committee felt the students were sufficiently prepared in design, others were non-committal. Miss Montgomery, Director of Occupational Therapy at the Walter Reed General Hospital, who takes students from all the schools in her post-graduate course, says: "Most of the girls need more knowledge of design. Students taking our course are graduates of schools claiming to meet minimum standards."

Miss Clark, Director of the Occupational Therapy Department at the Michigan University Hospital, shows the unique and interesting scheme at Ann Arbor of training the student in design for the particular problems she meets in practice training. She says: "Since our practice work students for the most part are those trained in this hospital, we give them training needed for the practice work they are assigned to at the time."

While those training the students in the hospitals left the impression that lack of training in design is not a serious defect in the school's preparation, nevertheless, half the group admitted they had to supplement the school's training in design, and the following recommendations are made to the schools for better preparation in design:

Dr. Bryan, Superintendent of Worcester State Hospital, Massachusetts: "More applied design."

Miss Clark: "Have students make analysis of project from teaching point of view, also administrative point of view, teaching methods, materials, costs, time needed for preparation of projects, etc."

Miss Montgomery: "More knowledge and application of principles of design; practice in enlarging and adapting good designs to various purposes. Free-hand drawing is necessary in order that a student may design well."

Miss Taylor: "Enlarging and adapting designs to projects."

Mrs. Tompkins: "Appreciation and application."

Norristown: "A working drawing to be made of all articles made in the school."

Crafts

The preparation of the student in crafts was answered by Group B in a way fairly favorable to the present training given in the schools. However, the comment of Mrs. Tompkins, Director of the Occupational Therapy Department at Manhattan State Hospital is particularly well expressed and is appreciated by all those who have practice students under their direction "They seem to lack knowledge of the type of craft to present to patients, also lack knowledge of ways to observe reactions to craft steps." This comment suggests the desirability that all the students should not only know the craft, but the craft analysis and application which are most important in presenting work to sick and disabled persons. A student who had been months in one of the schools expressed amazement when she discovered that she would not be able to teach crafts as she had been taught, with care for design and technique. This is quite often the student point of view and is inevitable when the school is compelled to give the student the greatest knowledge of the processes and tools in the crafts in the shortest possible time. Greater stress, however, must be laid upon crafts being only the means toward a curative end.

All of the members of Group B said they supplemented the training in the crafts. Their comments are as follows:

Dr. Bryan: "Most of their crafts show the need of more practice."

Miss Clark: "My experience leads me to believe the basketry taught in schools should receive more attention."

Miss Conrick, Director of Occupational Therapy at the James Whitcomb Riley Hospital, Indianapolis: "Weaving."

Miss Montgomery: "Weaving, jewelry, metal, woodworking, wood carving, basketry in several cases, pottery, leather work and miscellaneous crafts."

Norristown: "Basketry and weaving."

Miss Taylor, Director Occupational Therapy, Robert B. Brigham Hospital, Boston, Massachusetts: "Basketry and weaving which need a tremendous amount of experience. Craft adaptations to specific disabilities."

Mrs. Tompkins: "Yes. Most of them."

Of the recommendations made to the schools, Miss Montgomery urged: "More attention to knowledge of and use of equipment, for instance learning weaving so that the student is able not only to weave but to care for loom in its details, making warps, threading the loom, mending threads that break, etc. Knowing how to make warps is not learned through the making of one warp. This process should be repeated several times for different looms." Miss Taylor says, "A wider range of crafts, more original problems, more experience in correcting mistakes in crafts, especially weaving and basketry." Mrs. Tompkins, "Classification, varied, mechanical, etc. Methods of linking up with special interests of patients."

Recreation and Physical Exercise

The lack of training in recreation, physical exercise, games, and music was the outstanding defect for practice training in the preparation of the students, indicated in this study by the response of Group B. This is not surprising as it is only recently that the full value of the socializing influence and therapeutic possibilities of recreation and exercise have been appreciated. Dr. Bryan expressed the hope that as much study and stress would be placed upon this phase of occupational therapy in the future as at present is being laid upon the crafts.

Dr. Bryan recommends to the training schools: "A course of 10 lectures similar to the one given by the New York University."

Miss Taylor: "Simple exercises to meet need not met by crafts. Game therapy."

Mrs. Tompkins: "Variety of games, including counterpane games, all kinds of special celebrations, dramatics, musical entertainments possible with home talent. Folk dances."

Theory

There seemed little or no criticism of the student's preparation in the theory of occupational therapy.   Miss Clark outlined the same method of teaching the theory along with the practice in the University Hospital that she used in synchronizing design and craft with practical application.   Dr. Bryan states: "Students come here for training in both theory and practice with mental patients.   They have not had much of this before coming here."

Miss Montgomery says: "Students become so interested in the end product that they lose sight of the effect of the processes upon the patient.   They do not remember why certain processes are followed to produce certain results.   Emphasis should be laid upon the value of the theory of occupational therapy for patients. The real aim of occupational therapy should constantly be uppermost in the mind of the therapist."   Miss Taylor put it very clearly that theory is the function of the practice period as well as of the school.   She said, "Splendid foundation can only be absorbed through experience.   Further theory given during training." As a recommendation to the schools, she suggests, "More medical training, craft analysis and adaptation."   Mrs. Tompkins says: "Students are deficient in psychological principles as to class and group management" and adds, "the students cannot have too broad an understanding of the needs of patients, physical, mental, social, environmental, and the ways to meet them."

Ethics and Hospital Conduct

Again the comments of Group B were very favorable to the schools in their preparation in ethics and hospital conduct. However, this subject can, at best, only be touched and theorized upon in the school, and the fact that there is no real adverse criticism of students' immaturity and inexperience in this regard, reflects well upon the careful vigilance of those responsible for the students in the hospital.

Miss Taylor has expressed the sentiment of almost every member of Group B who said that the answers were sent in reluctantly for fear they might be construed as casting reflection upon the schools, which was farthest from the intention, but that honest answers must be sent to make this study accomplish its purpose. She said: "I feel that training as we are carrying it on is a service to the school and the progress of the profession, not a service to the hospital. Treatment as it is given our patients is of such importance that the responsibility on the therapists is very great. It is not possible to shift that responsibility to young inexperienced students so they must always work under the guidance of the therapist. I do not feel that the questionnaires should be read in the light of criticisms of the schools. I rather hesitate to answer the questions for fear of such an interpretation, but know the desire of the schools and training hospitals is to contribute all in their power to train their students to the highest standards. I hope that frank suggestions will be made to the training hospitals which will raise the quality of our work, and I shall be only too grateful for such suggestions myself."

As criticism has not been withheld, the schools are to be congratulated that the students' preparation has met with so little criticism and so much commendation from those who must adjust students to the hospitals. The recommendations to the schools are constructive, and indicate the constantly increasing standards of work and training which measure growth and progress. These recommendations for more design, more crafts, and craft adaptations, fall in line with the thought of the training schools themselves, who are aware of the shortcomings, but who face the impossibility of giving more in the allotted time. It has been the appreciation of the necessity for giving more training that has prompted the older schools: Boston School of Occupational therapy, Milwaukee-Downer College, Philadelphia School of Occupational Therapy, and the St. Louis School of Occupational Therapy, to lengthen their courses. The development of the teaching of occupational therapy has evolved from the first course of the first school—The Henry Favill School of Occupations—from a six weeks course to the present lengths of college, university, and professional schools.

It is unreasonable to expect the student to be an accomplished designer, proficient in all the crafts, and a competent physical education director at the same time, no matter how long or thorough her training in the school. But it is just as unreasonable to expect the directors of a hospital occupational therapy department to teach elementary design, correct simple craft mistakes, sharpen tools, warp looms, and perform the thousand and one tasks which are the duties of the students. The apparent discrepancy between criticism of the school's preparation of students and the acknowledgment of the need or supplementary training given by Group B, indicates that those responsible for the students in the hospital do not expect them to come fully prepared; but feel their duty is to continue the student's education. They assume the major part of the training in theory, hospital ethics and conduct, hospital processes, record making and application of knowledge to patient disabilities. This appreciation of the teaching function of the director of occupational therapy in hospitals taking practice students, and the willing acceptance of this responsibility, is one of the interesting revelations of this study. It is the greatest asset which the schools can have, for it insures for the students the practical training which it is impossible for the schools to give. The quality and standard of the school will be judged by the type of practice training it can command for its students.

3. PRELIMINARY PRACTICE TRAINING

The step from the school to the hospital is a sudden one. The atmosphere and routine of the two are totally unlike. The student has been the center of interest in the school. The school with its faculty, curriculum, and equipment is organized to serve her. The hospital, on the other hand, is equipped and staffed to serve the patients. The patients have many needs of which occupational therapy is only one. The student from being considered, must now consider. The transition from school to hospital is attended with such real dangers to the student's powers of adjustment that both the schools and hospitals have appreciated the value of giving the students some early contact with patients and some practical experience in dealing with the sick to prepare them for the hospital situation.

Moreover, actual experience with patients and shop problems give the student the right valuation of the essentials in her training course. The student's attitude is apt to be indifferent to tools and equipment, expecting the instructor to keep them in order. The student is primarily interested in the project she is making and resentful of time and effort expended in repair of her inaccuracies. Once, however, she has taught a patient, had to repair his mistakes, mend a warp in the shop loom, her interest shifts from the project to the patient. She notices methods of repairing, is more watchful to prevent mistakes and more ready to do her part in the upkeep of the school looms and equipment.

"Personal lack of ability to adjust themselves to the patients and the hospital," Mrs. Tompkins believes "is one of the outstanding difficulties with students." Miss Clark adds "I think this is always the greatest difficulty with inexperienced workers."

The schools have met this need for practice training preliminary to the hospital in a variety of ways. The combination of training in the University of Michigan and practice in the Ann Arbor hospital has many ideal features.

The Boston School of Occupational Therapy

The Boston School of Occupational Therapy has met the situation for the need of early patient contact in a very interesting and satisfactory way. The school established its own curative workshop or clinic with this end in view. An average of thirty-five patients a month are treated in this clinic. The director of the clinic is a member of the school faculty and a graduate occupational therapist. As the clinic is in the school building, the students have opportunity for daily contact with the patients. They are assigned definite time to observe and mingle with the patients. As the clinic includes mental and orthopedic cases, tuberculosis and children's work, the students see a wide range of disabilities and learn the application of occupational therapy in each. Beside this clinic experience the students are also sent on a number of supervised trips to various types of institutions during their first nine months in training.

Milwaukee-Downer College

Milwaukee-Downer College appreciated the early value of patient contact. The students have had the opportunity for observation and visits to hospitals and social agencies. Through the close affiliation between the college and the Junior League Curative Workshop, the students have had the opportunity to work in the Junior League shop under their director. Commencing in 1928, it is planned that each student will have the experience of caring for a homebound patient, and the students will be detailed to work in the Junior League Curative Workshop and Children's Hospital. The work with the home bound is the logical result of the theoretical courses in economics and sociology, and social service visits. Each student must make her own social contact with the patient, fit her plan into the home environment, outline and carry out a course of occupational therapy under the supervision of the homebound service. The student will study the social, economic, mental, and physical factors in the case, as well as the selection of the occupation, the materials, costs, records, and measurement tests, to know the actual improvement and condition of the patient. This intensive study of the patient is the preparation for considering the patient point of view in the group handling of the cases which the students then learn in the Junior League Curative Workshop and Children's Hospital.

The University of Minnesota

The University of Minnesota has recognized the need for early contact with patients and met it through assignment of students to some occupational therapy department as early as their junior year, for a few hours weekly under supervision of that department. The assignments may be in junior and senior years and in the summer sessions intervening. Work has been with general, tuberculosis, homebound, or mental, and the number of hours has varied.

The new plan which is now being worked out will probably require at least three hundred hours preliminary practice training approximating 30 hours each in general and homebound which will precede approximately 60 hours each in tuberculosis and workshop and concluding with about 80 hours each in orthopedic (children) and mental.

The work is done in the special hospitals of the various types listed with the exception of the work with the homebound which is done with the visiting nurse association.

The work has also included in the past and will continue to include a practical course in medical social service which is a natural part of the sociological courses and gives the student contact and observation in a clinic or ward even before she is assigned to departments for preliminary practice training.

This course in medical social service and the assignment to the supervisor of occupational therapy for the homebound gives the student a very comprehensive view of the patient and an awareness of the multitude of problems she must recognize and respect in working out her plans for the patient, and aligning herself intelligently and harmoniously with others working for and with the patient.

Philadelphia School of Occupational Therapy

In order to bridge the step between the theory of the school and practice of the hospital period and to help students to properly value and understand the theoretical training given in the school, the Philadelphia School of Occupational Therapy plans trips to special classes in the public schools, tuberculosis sanatoria, general hospitals and mental hospitals.   These trips are taken in connection with lectures on mental conditions and under supervision of the doctor in charge and the head aide of the department visited.

The school also makes use of the Curative Workshop, which is on the first floor of the school building and is run as a laboratory for the students.   Each student is scheduled for work in the shop during the second semester of her course and is given individual instruction by the head aide and free access to patients' records.

The St. Louis School of Occupational Therapy

The St. Louis School of Occupational Therapy has a unique and successful way of meeting the problem of early patient contact for the students. In the month of December when the hospital occupational therapy departments are usually pushed with preparations and sales, the students are assigned to various directors with the instructions that they are to do whatever is asked of them, say nothing and bring their questions to the school for later discussion. The students spend one hundred and twenty-five hours in this way within three months after they have started their course. This gives them an insight into the running of a department, and the upkeep of supplies and equipment, as well as the preparation of projects in which the students can assist. They return to the school with a new appreciation of the many phases of occupational therapy and, through discussion of their questions, they assimilate the theory of occupational therapy. The director of the training school is also director of the home service work and the occupational therapy department at Barnes Hospital. As the students may be assigned to home service or Barnes Hospital at any time in their training, the close coördination between the school and practical experience is maintained.

Toronto University

The University of Toronto gives the opportunity for contact with patients after the first year. Two hours are spent in preparation and five hours with mental patients. The same time is given to tuberculous patients and seven hours of contact is spent with patients in a general hospital. Students are also in a curative workshop and institute for the blind. They are under the directors of the respective hospital occupational therapy departments.

Miss Greene, Director of the Boston school, speaks for both the training school group as well as for the field directors when she says: "The concensus of opinion is obviously in favor of considerable hospital and patient contact during the theoretical training period.

"At present the actual amount of time thus spent by the students varies in the individual schools but it is agreed that it is very important that the students have some practical insight into patients' problems prior to entering their hospital training period.

"A clinic workshop under the school roof is recommended as a splendid means by which to allow the student almost constant observation and daily contact, while at the same time not having to interrupt the theoretical study schedule.

"Some time devoted to straight social service visiting is also recommended as a fine means by which to develop the student's ability in approaching patients, meeting situations, and the scheme for work of students during the holiday season as developed by the St. Louis School has many advantages."

4. CONCLUSIONS

Group B were asked if they had any suggestions for reducing the added responsibility and work of training practice students. The replies touching upon the training schools are as follows:

Miss Clark: "Only the indirect one of raising the professional standards and salaries so that only the women of the highest caliber and with fine basic training will be attracted to the training schools."

Miss Montgomery: "Only through better preparatory work before entering upon period of practice training."

Mrs. Tompkins: "Give students more training along the line of hospital ethics and procedure," which strengthens one of the purposes of the preliminary hospital practice training.

The first question—"What preparation should be expected of the practice student by the hospital?" may be answered briefly from the foregoing as:

First: An adequate knowledge of anatomy, kinesiology, psychology, psychiatry, neurology, etc.

Second: An understanding of social service, training in patient contact so that the student has assimilated the theory of occupational therapy and to be sufficiently familiar with hospital ethics and procedure to adjust herself in the hospital with the minimum burden upon the director and with the maximum measure of success for herself.

Third: An elementary knowledge of design; experience in a wide range of crafts, knowledge of tools, materials, equipment, their care and upkeep, processes and their analysis and adaption to the special disabilities; preparation in recreation, games, and physical exercises, and their therapeutic possibilities.

REPORT OF THE COMMITTEE ON TEACHING METHODS

PART III. LENGTH AND DISTRIBUTION OF TIME IN HOSPITAL TRAINING

While the committee were at work on this report a suggestion was received from Mr. Kidner, President, American Occupational Therapy Association, that the committee consider the raising of minimum standards.

The length and distribution of time in practice training falls into three main divisions: first, the length of the student's day and how it is spent; second, time spent in the particular hospital to which the student is assigned, and the variety of experience and services covered in it; and third, the total time spent in practice training and the different types of institutions to which the aide is sent.

1. THE DAY

The number of working hours the student spends in the hospital varies from six and one-half to eight and three-fourths hours a day and are reported as follows:

	HOURS PER DAY	HOURS PER WEEK
Dr. Bryan....................................	8¾	48
Miss Clark................................-	8	44
Miss Conrick................................	7–8	43
Miss Montgomery............................	7½	41
Miss Taylor................................-	6½	35½
Mrs. Tompkins.............................	8	44

The day is spent in routine work in the shop or on the wards. To this is added some theoretical training. This theoretical work (lectures and study) may develop into the ideal day outlined by Dr. Bryan as follows: four hours with patients, three

423

hours preparation, and one hour of class lecture. This arrangement is not only a splendid distribution of time in the day to secure the greatest knowledge and efficiency for the aide, but it is a very definite recognition of the teaching function of the hospital and the necessity for a systematic curriculum that will not leave instruction haphazard to the convenience of the director and staff.

2. TIME AND DISTRIBUTION IN THE HOSPITAL

Each hospital makes a sincere effort to give the student as broad an experience as possible. There are many services to cover in the general and mental hospitals. In the special hospitals, the work must be between bedside, ward, shop, and out-patient service; and with each division there should be lectures and study.

Group B were asked: How long does a student, taking practice training, remain under your supervision, and approximately how is her time distributed between your various services; e.g., bedside, ward, shop, acute, convalescent, recreation, deteriorated, out-patients, etc.? Their answers are as follows:

Dr. Bryan: Students are here 6 months. They work 8 hours per day.

	hours
With patient	4
Preparation	3
Class lecture	1
Total	8

During the six months there are:

	hours
For work with patients	576
For preparation	432
For lectures and class work	144
Total	1,152

Their time is distributed:

	months
Admission service	1
Deteriorated service	1
Chronic service	1

Disturbed service.. 1
Special case work—medical service—bedside........................ 1
Physical exercise and recreation..................................... 1

Miss Clark: Six months one-half day each day or 22 hours per week—children's wards, and shop work under supervision.

Five months about two-thirds day or 28 hours per week—convalescent wards, and small groups of bone and joint cases on acute wards.

Eleven months about three-fourths day or 33 hours per week—neurological and special cases, surgical supply workshop, acute wards, muscle training and recreation.

Miss Conrick: Two months (8 to 9 weeks), and as students are sent to us specifically for children's work, their whole time is spent in the Children's Hospital (ward or bedside work in the a.m. and shop work in the p.m.).

Miss Montgomery: Six months. The distribution of time depends to an extent upon previous training, and an attempt is made to give experience in the fields most needed to round out their training. Very little is done with acute cases.

Miss Taylor: One month, about evenly distributed between bedside, ward, and shop.

Mrs. Tompkins: During entire time of practice. Time is distributed as seems best in order to give student a wide experience.

3. TIME IN VARIOUS TYPES OF INSTITUTIONS

The schools were asked to give the distribution of their practice training time. They answer as follows:

Boston School of Occupational Therapy:

	months
Mental...	6
Workshop and Clinic...	1
Tuberculosis..	1
Orthopedic..	1
	—
Total...	9

All students take same amount of time in each hospital.

Milwaukee-Downer College: Milwaukee-Downer College has

increased the period of practice training to nine months and expects to follow this plan:

	months
Mental	3
Tuberculosis	1
General	1
Children's	1
Curative Workshop	1
Elective	2
Total	9

Minnesota University: The University of Minnesota is increasing the period of time and expects to follow this plan.

	months
General	1
Tuberculosis	1
Workshop	1
Orthopedics (children's)	1
Mental	2
Total	6

(Schedule elastic as to distribution depending on students' needs and plans.)

Philadelphia School of Occupational Therapy:

	months
Mental	3
General	2
Visiting Nurse or Workshop	1
Total	6

(This is general division but elastic to meet individual needs.)

St. Louis School of Occupational Therapy:

	weeks
Mental	6
Tuberculosis	6
General	6
Children	6
Workshop	6
Total	30 (or 6 months)

(Schedule is elastic giving opportunity to individual students.)
Toronto University:

	months
Mental	2
Tuberculosis, General, Workshop, Shop institutes for blind	2
Total	4

The Boston school requires the same amount of time to be spent in each institution regardless of students interests. The other schools strongly recommend the distribution of time listed above but while requiring experience in the various lines, consider the student's choice in allotment of time. While the latter plan has some advantages for the student of special bent, it is deemed best to require each student to have as broad an experience in her practice time as possible, reserving specialization for later or postgraduate training. The opinion of Group B confirms the policy of the schools in limiting the choice of students and insisting on experience in all possible branches.

Dr. Bryan: "The best occupational therapist has experience in all fields. In whatever institution she is in, she may get one of any of these types of patients and if she has specialized, she will not be able to care for anything outside of her specialty."

Miss Clark: "I think if she wished to specialize, that should come after her required training in the other hospitals."

Miss Conrick: "I think if she wishes to specialize that should come after her required training in the hospitals."

Miss Montgomery: "It seems to me that all students should have specializing. They need a general background upon which to build. Is a student equipped to choose her field for specializing before she has had a general knowledge of the various fields or departments, such as mental, tuberculous, orthopedic, etc.?"

Miss Taylor: "I believe she should have experience in each branch as each contributes to her efficiency in another type. A general foundation is the only basis for specializing. A student does not really know which field she is adaptable to without experience in all. I believe a general practice training is necessary for good placement after graduation."

Group B, stressed the need for the emphasis in practice training to be in the mental field.   Dr. Bryan's distribution of time in Worcester State Hospital page—suggests that any time less than six months fails to realize all the possibilities in it for student training.   The training in a mental hospital should be the longest, not only because it takes time to cover the variety of services and types of patients in the mental hospital, but also because a mental factor exists in all types of illness and it is the student's foundation for dealing with this phase of medical, surgical, orthopedic, tuberculosis, cardiac and children's work.   In no other way can the student have the appreciation of mental hygiene, and know so well how to prevent the mental suffering which makes illness tragic.   The late Dr. Thomas W. Salmon said of the mental factor in illness which occupational therapy alleviates: "Occupational therapy will some day rank with anesthetics in taking the suffering out of sickness and with anti-toxins in shortening its duration.   The greater part of distress in chronic diseases is mental and occupational therapy is, thus far, our only means of dealing with this factor."

The schools realize the importance of the students working in various institutions, both general and specialized, so that the students may acquire knowledge of the hospital problem, an intensive knowledge of the specialities, and understand the particular service of occupational therapy in each.

After the mental field, time may be somewhat evenly distributed between work in a general hospital, including medical and surgical cases, and the various specialities such as children's work, home-bound, tuberculosis, orthopedics, cardiac, and curative workshop.   Each has its own technicalities, and some experiences in all must be secured by the training school for its students.

Recommendation

With the idea of lengthening the period of practice training, both groups were asked to recommend an ideal length and distribution of practice training time.   The replies are summarized below.

Dr. Bryan:

	months
Mental	6
Tuberculosis	1
Orthopedic	1
Clinical—children's	1
Total	9

Boston School:

	months
Mental	6
Tuberculosis	2
General, Orthopedic Children's	2
Curative workshop, Home bound, Other services	2
Total	12

Miss Clark:

	hours
Children and shop work	528
Convalescent wards, bone and joint, diseases acute, wards	560
Neurological and special cases, Muscle training, recreation, etc.	1,452
Total	2,540 (or 12 months)

Milwaukee Downer College:

	months
Mental	3
Tuberculosis	1
General	1
Children's	1
Curative workshop	1
Elective	2
Total	9

Philadelphia School:

	months
Mental	2
Orthopedic	2
General	1
Elective (tubercular, cardiac, Visiting Nurse, children)	1

St. Louis School:

	weeks
Mental	(minimum) 6
Tuberculosis	(minimum) 6
General	(minimum) 6
Children's	(minimum) 6
Curative workshop	(minimum) 4
Total	28 (or 7½ months)

Miss Montgomery: 1 year.

Miss Taylor:

	months
Mental	4
Tuberculosis	1
Orthopedic	3
Children's	1
Homebound	1
Total	10

Mrs. Tompkins:

	months
Mental	6
Otherwise	3
Total	9

Miss Tebbets:

	months
General	1
Tuberculosis	2
Workshop	1
Orthopedics (Children)	1
Mental	2
Total	6

or if possible

	months
General	1
Tuberculosis	1
Workshop	1
Homebound	1
Orthopedics (Children)	2
Mental	3
Total	9

From the preceding indication of the desirability of practice training ranging from six months to a year, it is not surprising that almost all the members of both committee groups reporting, agreed that the present minimum standard of three months should be increased. Their answers are:

Dr. Bryan: "Yes, increase to nine months."

Miss Greene: "Yes, increase to nine months."

Miss Clark: "It would seem long enough if the standard is now 6 to 9 months. (Present standard is 3 months)."

Miss Conrick: "Yes, increase to at least six months."

Mr. Dunlap: No answer.

Miss Fulton: "Yes, increase to six months."

Miss Lermit: "Yes, not less than six months."

Miss Montgomery: "Yes, increase to one year."

Miss Taylor: "Yes, increase to 6 months."

Miss Tebbets: Yes, increase to 6 months."

Mrs. Tompkins: "Yes, increase to 9 months."

Norristown: "At least six months, 2 months in each hospital.

Allentown: "Yes."

Miss Fulton sums up the feeling of the training schools regarding the lengthening of the period of practice training when she says: "The consensus of opinion is practically in favor of lengthening the period of practice training. Boston has done so and is planning for further training. Milwaukee-Downer College is also materially lengthening its course and the University of Minnesota feels that it is essential to do so. Philadelphia has just increased its training period, and St. Louis seems to have done so."

The recommendations for the new minimum standard requirements vary from six months to one year. The committee on Teaching Methods is of the opinion that it is desirable to proceed in a conservative manner and therefore recommends that the present minimum standard of three months for practice training be raised to six months.

> (Signed) ELIZABETH UPHAM DAVIS, *Chairman,*
> WILLIAM A. BRYAN, M.D.,
> MARJORIE B. GREENE,
> MARION CLARK,
> WINIFRED CONRICK,
> W. J. DUNLAP,
> FLORENCE FULTON (succeeded by
>   Mrs. Samuel H. Paul),
> GERALDINE LERMIT,
> ALBERTA MONTGOMERY,
> MARJORIE TAYLOR,
> MARION TEBBETS,
> ANNA TOMPKINS.

DISCUSSION

In introducing this report President Kidner said,

This morning's session is, I think, one of the most important because upon the proper training of workers depends the success of our work.

As you know, our association studied the question of minimum standards of training and those standards were promulgated several years ago and have had an extremely good effect on the training of the workers. As I remarked in my address, we are not quite out of the woods yet. There are still so-called schools which are not in any way meeting the standards, but they are becoming fewer as the proper schools become better known.

The preparation of this report has meant an enormous amount of work on the part of the chairman and the members of the committee, and we are indebted to Mrs. Davis and the other members. The papers of Dr. Bryan and Miss Lermit are a discussion of this report and will be read before discussion. Dr. Bryan's paper was then read.

Mrs. Carey (Chicago): I am very enthusiastic over these papers that have been read and am going back to Chicago with the assurance that even though my problems are still heavy I feel more than ever that the national organization is back of me, working at my problems for me.

But I realize very clearly that occupational therapy is making the greatest strides in the mental hospitals and it must necessarily be so because in them are the largest occupational therapy departments. In Chicago the only mental hospitals of any size are Dunning and the Cook County Hospital, so when occupational therapy grows in Chicago it must grow in the general hospitals, and I would like to suggest that Mrs. Davis' committee put a little more thought on the training of students for general hospital work.

I had a student come to me from a school, and though she was a fine craftswoman I found she had had no training in applying her crafts to the patients in a general hospital nor the right approach for this kind of work. I might add that Michael Reese Hospital is a little different from some other hospitals in that we have only acute medical and surgical cases. We have very few chronic patients, so the approach is quite different than it would be in a mental hospital.

Last year, I remember, before I made my talk, I asked Miss Greene about the work in general hospitals and she told me they had no training for pupils in general hospitals.

Also, I think the occupational therapist should be trained in those special crafts that will be of use to tuberculous patients. I would be very grateful if the students in different schools were given a broader experience in hospital work.

Miss Greene: I think Mrs. Carey misunderstood my remark a year ago. My statement was that at that time we were not using any general hospital for our training. Mind you, we were only giving three months total and our general training was taken care of in our own clinic first, and in the Robert Breck Brigham Hospital, which, though mostly orthopedic, has some cardiac and some general work. We also gave several demonstrations and staff clinic meetings at the individual general hospitals around the city.

Now we are in a different position. We are using a splended department at the Massachusetts Eye and Ear Infirmary, which is a branch of the Massachusetts General Hospital. We are also using our own clinic and we have also been able this year to give a month with full maintenance in a tuberculosis hospital in our state. We have not been able to do that before.

I would like to ask Mrs. Carey about the student to whom she refers— was she given a well rounded course, even though emphasis was laid on mental cases?

Mrs. Carey: Yes, as far as crafts were concerned. I was all alone then, my assistant had left, and I was rushed and I possibly couldn't give her as much supervision as necessary.

I had a hyperthyroid patient and of course they have to do "coarse work" as we call it. I persuaded his wife to buy an article of basketry, the making of which I though would not cause him strain. I told my student to take charge. I went down a day and a half later and found she had started him on an Indian weave basket of fine reed and rather intricate pattern. I said: "In your school didn't they tell you what type of craft to give certain types of patients?" and she said: "No— they didn't."

Miss Lermit: The student in question who went to Michael Reese was taken from her practical work in a general hospital before she had completed even a month's work. She was taken without any inquiries being made, when records were available at the school, and I was extremely glad that the lesson was learned, at least in one hospital, when I have said repeatedly: "Leave the students alone until they are ready and let them have their six months' practice work, and when they they are through you will be glad you waited even though you have a hard time getting along." In other words, when superintendents or chief aides are hard-up for assisiants they have no right to go out and persuade students who are in need of financial help to go into their departments.

As soon as that student took the job she wrote, apologizing for doing so, but explained that she did so because she was "dead broke." It is one thing we would all like to have thoroughly understood, that if you give the school a chance to complete training you will not regret it. That student has entered a general hospital of the Veteran's Bureau and reports indicate she has adjusted herself extremely well.

Miss Greene: I am sure that is an excellent point and I agree heartily with Miss Lermit. There is just one other point I would like to make. That is, that it is encouraging to me to hear that in such a center as Chicago there is apparently considerable need for the general worker. Of the positions coming in to us, four out of five are mental and we do feel that the foundation training in which we are now giving emphasis— the mental training—is of the greatest advantage from the standpoint of the whole field. If the student can succeed with the mental training she is a much better worker in the general hospital.

Miss Ross (representing Miss Tebbetts): The University of Minnesota offers a four year course with a B.S. degree in occupational therapy. This includes the arts and crafts, the academic and medical subjects, and and actual time spent on the hospital wards.

This department was organized by Dr. R. O. Beard and is one of the many which make up the College of Education.

I helped Dr. Beard organize this course, and I remember that I insisted on two things: first that the occupational therapy department should belong to the College of Education; and, second, that the chief advisor of this department should always be a medical man. I believe he should be a man who not only sympathizes with the work but also understands it.

We want the very best students that can be found, the most alert, the most intelligent, the best workers. We want these students to have the work at their fingertips—to know their stuff, as the students say. At the same time I agree with Mr. Kidner when he says, "It is the spirit back of the work that counts." And this is where you medical people come in.

During the World War the occupational therapy department of Columbia University, realizing the value of this attitude of mind, insisted that the best possible medical men be obtained to lecture to the army hospital workers. The workers at Minnesota have profited by the experience of the workers at Columbia.

I have heard Dr. Mariette of Glen Lake instructing students in the difficult art of remaking and rebuilding the broken spirit of men; I have seen Dr. Beard create a spirit of coöperation among the doctors, nurses and aides in a hospital by demonstrating the intimate connection and interdependence which exists between their respective lines of endeavor. The rehabilitation and replacement into society of former patients that is being accomplished at the Phalem Park Hospital under the direction of Dr. Gillette and Miss McGregor stands out as an example of what science, good sense and coöperation can accomplish. Such instruction and associations cannot but result in the development of a more scientific, social and practical viewpoint in each individual student.

Mrs. Cox: We have the students from the University of Minnesota come to our hospital for training three times a week, two hours a day and for three months. Miss Tebbetts was going to give me a full-time student but I couldn't take her this year.

The President: I think now the most useful thing we can do is to call on Miss Lermit to give her paper after her long years of training and experience on both sides.

Miss Lermit: Before reading my paper I want to thank Mrs. Davis for this splendid report. I also want to say that both the students and I greatly appreciate the opportunities given for their practice work, through the generous coöperation of Miss Robeson and Mrs. Slagle, in the Kings Park State Hospital, and for Miss Taylor's arranging to accept them at the Robert Breck Brigham Hospital, and Mrs. Keister's and Dr. Stoker's long continued interest and coöperation at Kankakee.

Miss Lermit here read her paper.

Miss Greene: Miss Lermit has certainly given us a very interesting paper. I think many of her points confront us all. I am not going to stand here and try to give you my opinion because, frankly, we agree so generally on all of our principles. We do have many individual problems.

One thing I am interested in is St. Louis being able to send their students to other parts of the country for part of their training. Our students come from all over the United States, and many because they want the advantages of Boston as well as the school. Such an arrangement has not seemed possible for us.

Another problem has been that we haven't had an opportunity of making close, intimate contact with hospitals far removed from our community and we feel that the closest coöperation between the hospital and school is absolutely vital. Miss Lermit has of course brought this out.

Miss Tompkins: In answering the questionnaire, which I understand is to be published, I feel that the various special subjects under discussion were covered quite thoroughly. However, I should like to add one subject which training schools should stress; it is "Ethics."

I am thoroughly in accord with the statement made by Miss Lermit who remarked that it is difficult for the pupil occupational therapist, as she goes out to work in a large hospital, to realize what a small cog either the pupil or her work is in the big hospital machine.

We have had many pupils and few of them have realized what is meant by "Ethics." Therefore, I recommend that more attention be given the subject in training schools.

Miss Sands: I am from the Philadelphia General Hospital, Chief Aide, and we get our students from the Philadelphia school. My suggestions are so radical that I think they will be recognized not as criticisms but as suggestions.

The one thing that has been stressed in the papers and remarks has been the difficulty of adjustment to hospital regime. I think it is perfectly possible to make that adjustment more gradual and also for the student to gain more from her course of instruction if the contacts could be made all through her course. For instance, if she could go to a hospital one day a week or one afternoon a week, and assist in the work she would gradually become used to the hospital before she takes her hospital practice.

I know in some hospitals this isn't considered an advisable plan and one school dean said it wouldn't be advisable from their standpoint because the student wouldn't know enough to be of any use, but I always feel there would be a lot of routine work the student could help in and she would at the same time become used to hospital practice.

If students gave a little time to hospital work all through their course they could get much more out of the course because while taking a craft they would be practicing it. I think that change would be especially valuable to the students. The hospital would gain practically nothing but it wouldn't be inconvenienced.

Another suggestion—I feel I am presuming—is that I think, from my experience, that it would be a good thing for students to major in one or two particular crafts and get what they could out of the others. My reasons for thinking this are that the students come from the school having acquired a slight knowledge of all crafts and they don't have a true craftsman feeling; they don't love their tools.

Of course we all know it takes several years to master a major craft, and why should we expect these girls to get a craftsman feeling by taking three or four majors and a lot of minor crafts in one year? If they could major on one or two major crafts, possibly they couldn't master it as a true craftsman but they would get much more out of it and they would have a better standard.

Also I think a very important thing is a course in ward work, which everybody should take; I mean the real application of minor crafts to ward work, at the same time indicating what type of patients would use it. Then when they come to the hospital they would be able to give these simple crafts to patients on the ward with more facility than they do now.

I don't know whether these are at all possible to carry out but I do think they would make better craftsmen and better occupational therapists.

Miss Ross: We were wondering if we could, if the hospitals would permit it, have the students take one day a week out of their first year. Has that been tried anywhere and do you know of any hospital where it has been tried?

Miss Lermit: In the teachers' college course it was done.

Mrs. Davis: There are five or six pages in the report which answer that question but I have a complete record of the Boston school's practice training. They seem to have solved it most ideally in the clinic. One may say the Boston plan is ideal. You will find in the report how each school is solving the practice training problem, not only to breach *that chasm between the school and hospital, but also how much more* the student gets out of her school work from the practice she gets in the hospital.   Let a girl, for instance, repair a few patients' baskets.   If she has to take out patients' mistakes and repair them she will appreciate accuracy, prevention of mistakes, and want to know how to meet emergencies when she comes back to her school.

The President: During the course of my professional training I am proud to say that I took a course at one of the best arts and crafts schools I know and I speak feelingly when I say I listened the other day to a physician who has been using occupational therapy for many years.   He was one of the first men with whom I came in contact in the hospital field in this country.   He said: "Of course you want good training in arts and crafts, but as I see it, in the hospitals the success of an occupational therapist depends from ten to twenty per cent on arts and crafts and the rest on her knowledge of human people."

Side by side with the craft as it is taught in the best of training schools there must be a well experienced occupational therapist who can interpret daily to the student the things they are doing in relation to the sick patient.

Craft work is one of the tools we put in the hands of the occupational therapist.

Miss Robeson: I agree with Mr. Kidner but he hasn't been a chief aide in a hospital.   When these girls come to you, you ask what they think they can do best and you put them accordingly into a certain unit.   As Dr. Prosser says, if they don't know their craft they cannot teach it, and this is too often true.

I thought Miss Sands made an excellent suggestion.   I would like them to have all their general crafts and then specialize a month or so in some craft to perfect it further.

I was also interested in what Miss Lermit said about these students. They are so willing to be helpful.   I find they are always wanting to help the other aides do their work; often instead of developing their own unit. I believe this is from lack of self-confidence.

Mrs. Tompkins spoke about more emphasis on ethics, and I feel that strongly too.   I was glad Dr. Bryan spoke about loyalty.   I think that should be brought out in the hospital training; loyalty to the hospital; loyalty to your department, and loyalty to the individual in your department.   I find the students are very prone to take sides in petty disputes and I can quite frankly say that with any unit I have had to work with

—the so-called untrained worker is the most loyal supporter of the department; more so than the trained worker.

Miss Lermit was very kind to say that her students derived much good from Kings Park Hospital. I would suggest, Miss Lermit, that you print out what you desire for your students. I have enjoyed very much having them but it would have been quite impossible had not Mrs. Slagle obtained permission from the commissioner.

Miss Taylor: I find the students very much like reflections in mirrors. We expect much of them and if we do not find them to be angels we forget that it is perhaps our reflection we are seeing, not the students.

Every student presents an individual problem which must be solved as such.

In my experience the program of training which Miss Lermit suggests is absolutely necessary. We can have a general outline of training, but I find that I must adapt my program to each separate group in order to do the most for that particular group.

I believe that formal conferences are necessary as well as informal ones. When I chat with the students in the shop during preparation time, I get and give much that is not possible in the more formal atmosphere of staff conference.

The staff workers need to have their interest in training stimulated, not only at the beginning of the students' training, but every day during the time the students are with us. Only this way is the extra burden of training of enough interest to them to make them give the most to it.

Miss Lermit: I am glad I did not send that list; I would not have dared ask for as much as was given.

If I may speak for all of us from the standpoint of the school—the school has had a very different job the last five years from what it had previously. In our training school our first thing is to keep before our minds that our work is "occupation, mental or physical," and we are to prepare people to go into that field. It is very difficult many times to prepare a group of students to do something which could be called "mental" exercise. We take the attitude that we are preparing a group of students to understand the human machine which is composed of three parts, physical, intellectual and mental, and more and more we are stressing the general education of the student rather than the specific.

We are teaching *process* rather than *project*. The process goes on whether you find the medium of its translation through metals, textiles or wood. There is no difference in the *process* of procedure.

When we train the student in regard to understanding the machinery of the human being it is simple enough, though hard to give the understanding of the physical machinery; it is a good deal harder to give the understanding of the nerve and mental machinery as it tends toward an understanding of the head, not the body. We carry psychology through two years, it is taken as a university course, and if students don't get their credit they don't get their diplomas.

All the way through the endeavor of the schools today is to give a general training; we don't prepare for mental hospitals alone, for general, for tuberculosis or for home service, but for *all* of them and it has to be a general view of the situation; to train people to go out and fill in all these situations.

More, I think, than anything, I want to get over for the schools the fact that they have a broad problem to meet, not a highly specialized one.

The whole problem of the training school today is so much more a problem of general education so that one and all of us are struggling to pack into the time we can have the best general education with a specific bent.

Miss Shaffer: We have heard from the teachers and schools and hospitals and I would like to speak from the viewpoint of a student. I think one of the most important things was Mrs. Tompkins' remark on ethics.

Some of us may have a natural gift for getting along with people. A lot do not. And unless you have this conventional training you will not fit in with people; you will always step on somebody.

Miss Lermit spoke of specializing. I don't see how we can specialize very much in the first years of our training. It seems to me if I had specialized the first years in school it would have been absolutely useless to me in the three years at Kings Park but now that I have been able to apply all the arts I have been trained in I can specialize now in a "P. G." course. You have to have your general knowledge first.

I liked the remarks about repairing and undoing bad articles. A mental hospital occupational therapist is trained most in taking out and putting back in again.

Speaking of end problems—when a girl comes out of school without any more training than her hospital part you can't very well have all the end problems in view. Yes, a six months' course will help a lot but I don't think you will get all the end problems until we have been thrown on our own for a year or so.

Miss Clark: We have a very small training course for students who have had some three years university work. We take them only after very carefully considering their personal as well as scholastic qualifications. I really think a combination of theoretical training with practical training is very good. The students have fully four hours a day of theoretical work and the additional four hours per student in practical work—one hour in preparation, one hour in finishing and reports, and the other two with a trained occupational therapist on the wards. It seems to work out very well the first six months; then we give them additional responsibility.

Miss Conrick: One thing that I believe helps us is that the students live in the hospital, receiving full maintenance. They live as students and are expected to follow student rules. Then they go on the ward under the supervision of a graduate aide and they get their adjustment before they are really assigned to special duty.

The President: There is before us the report of the standing committee on teaching methods which has the recommendation that the minimum time spent be six months for hospital training, for hospital practice.

Miss Speed: Mr. President, I move that the report with its recommendation be accepted. The motion was duly seconded by Miss Schaffer and on being put to a vote was carried unanimously.

The President: May I add our sincere thanks to the chairman and members of the committee for the tremendous amount of work they have done, the value being shown by the interest and the discussion? That completing our program for this morning we will now adjourn.

Research on Fieldwork Supervisor Learning and Training

The statement, "just because he (she) makes a good occupational therapist does not mean he (she) makes a good student supervisor," is one of the most critical, yet elemental points to consider about the supervisor-student relationship in fieldwork. Yet, it is also one of the least-referenced topics in fieldwork.

As occupational therapists, we each come to the clinic with different educational and fieldwork experiences, communication styles, and life experiences. These experiences make up the supervisor-supervisee relationship and are responsible for the student's final outcome on fieldwork. A prospective occupational therapy clinical supervisor must make a commitment to student mentoring, not just teaching.

The American Occupational Therapy Association's (AOTA) fieldwork campaign is *Just Say Yes to Fieldwork.* The focus of the campaign is the training of occupational therapists and occupational therapy assistants as supervisors. This training entails not only the clinical competencies that are needed to make a supervisor, but the analysis of individual learning styles, communication styles, adult developmental learning, and professional and ethical behavior. An example of a prime resource on this topic is the *Self-Paced Instruction of Clinical Education and Supervision (SPICES)* (Crepeau & LaGarde, 1991). The potential fieldwork supervisor explores in textbook and workbook activities their individual style, the dominant learning characteristics of others, an analysis of their own teaching experience, and an analysis of their own supervising experience. The participant in *SPICES* describes their

own occupational therapy practice in terms of clinic tools, evaluations, and staff support. *SPICES* activities may also involve the supervisor writing down his or her own philosophy and beliefs on fieldwork and studying professionalism in terms of conflict management, continuing education, and outside professional commitments. *SPICES* is one resource for clinical supervisor training but is by no means the definitive source on clinical education. In fact, this is where the need for occupational therapy research, discussed in Section 2, is linked to the need for more fieldwork supervisor training materials.

This section of the anthology should provide you with a quick start on learning how to be a supervisor, how to develop materials for supervisor training, and ideas for future fieldwork projects. Christie and Joyce (1985) reported that there is a strong correlation between the setting in which occupational therapists choose to work as new graduates and the fieldwork experience.

According to Kathleen A. Curtis (1988), there are nine elements that supervisors should strive for before and during the fieldwork experience:

1. Gain personal understanding of learning styles
2. Team with others
3. Observe student through a learning lens
4. Build on your student's strength
5. Ask your student to think about their own thinking
6. Help your students vary their own styles of learning
7. Ask your student's opinion through open-minded questions

8. Offer choices
9. Examine your "curriculum."

As a supervisor, you must always examine your guiding principles of fieldwork. Do you agree, disagree, regulate, mandate, recommend, suggest, to your student? Does your particular placement need to be traditional? Are you absorbed in the myths of fieldwork? Are you expecting entry-level skills on the first day of fieldwork?

It is important to share with your students any doubts and concerns about fieldwork actions or the program. The idea is to communicate and evaluate with the student how you would change the process the next time so that even the most difficult situations will lead to positive outcomes.

THE AMERICAN JOURNAL

of

OCCUPATIONAL THERAPY

Official Publication of the American Occupational Therapy Association

Buyer's Guide

March-April	1957	Vol. XI, No. 2, Part II

A STUDY OF THE RELATIONSHIP BETWEEN CERTAIN PERSONALITY FACTORS AND SUCCESS IN CLINICAL TRAINING OF OCCUPATIONAL THERAPY STUDENTS*

MARY D. BOOTH, O.T.R.

PROBLEM AND BACKGROUND

Occupational therapists are interested in finding instruments for predicting success of students in the field. In spite of the increasing demand for therapists, there has been little willingness to accept a poor substitute. Grade point average, or the ability to pass the course requirements, are not completely satisfactory predictors of success in a field where personal-social relations are extremely important.[2,6] There is always the exceptionally good academic student who does poorly in clinical training and the student who barely passes the college courses but does well in the hospital situation. Loss of time, money and morale make changes in objectives difficult if not impossible. Therefore, from the point of view of the prospective therapist himself, it is advisable to be able to predict whether he may succeed or not before entering upon a five year educational program.

This study is an attempt to determine whether Guilford's Inventory of Factors STDCR and the Kuder Preference Record can be used as predictors of success of occupational therapists.

DESIGN OF STUDY

Problem. In previous studies of nursing and education students it was found that beyond a minimum level, intelligence is not an important factor in on-the-job success in these fields.[9,10,11,14] Grades which do predict such success are

usually in professional courses which are not available to students making a choice between two vocational objectives. However personality tests, as shown by Beaver, Spaney, Shaw, Schmid, and Seagoe, appear to be of great value in counseling.[1,3,2,10,11]

It would seem that some desirable traits may be measured by the Guilford's STDCR Inventory. The traits measured are social introversion-extroversion, thinking introversion-extroversion, depression, cycloid disposition and rhathymia. Interests as measured by the Kuder Preference Record may also measure relevant interests as inferred above. The nine interests measured are mechanical, computational, scientific, persuasive, artistic, literary, musical, social service and clerical.

The study is an attempt to determine whether or not there is any relationship between the personality traits, as measured by these tests, and success in clinical training and on the registration examination for occupational therapists. This information would be useful in selection of students for occupational therapy schools and in vocational advisement.

Subjects. The study was based on 91 occupational therapy graduates of San Jose State Col-

*An abstract of a thesis presented to the faculty of the department of psychology at San Jose State College, California, in partial fulfillment of the requirements for the degree of Master of Arts.

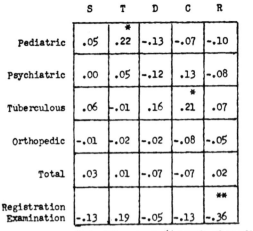

	S	T	D	C	R
Pediatric	.05	.22*	-.13	-.07	-.10
Psychiatric	.00	.05	-.12	.13	-.08
Tuberculous	.06	-.01	.16	.21*	.07
Orthopedic	-.01	-.02	-.02	-.08	-.05
Total	.03	.01	-.07	-.07	.02
Registration Examination	-.13	.19	-.05	-.13	-.36**

*Significant at 5% level of Confidence
**Significant at 1% level of Confidence

Table I. Coefficients of correlation of scores on Guilford's inventory of factors S,T,D,C,R and grades in clinical training and on registration examination (N = 91).

lege. They completed their clinical training and took the registration examination between 1951 and 1954. There were five men and eighty-six women; their ages ranged from twenty-one to forty-one years. The median age was twenty-one. Their mean score on the registration examination was 5.03 and the standard deviation was 7.63. (Grades on the examination are reported in deciles only.) Means of grades on the occupational therapy student clinical training report ranged from 72.5 to 77.9 with standard deviations varying from 7.7 to 10.04.

Tests and Criteria. Guilford's STDCR Inventory and Kuder's Preference Record which are currently administered to all occupational therapy majors at San Jose College were used. Guilford[5] in his manual of directions and norms for the Inventory of Factors STDCR reports that, "A combination of alternate sixths of the items into two pools of approximately equal lists and use of the Spearman-Brown formula gave estimated reliabilities of .92, .89, .91, and .89 for factors S. T, D, C, and R, respectively in a population of 200 (100 men and 100 women) selected at random from the criterion groups." Kuder[8] reported the results of eight studies of the reliability of the subscores of the Preference Record. The coefficients of correlation ranged from .83 to .98 with a mean of .90. The tests were repeated after three days to two months. Herzberg, Bouton and Steiner[7] in a study on the stability of the Kuder Preference Record found reliability coefficients which ranged from .63 for social service and .77 for artistic. The study was based on test and retest 15 to 49 months apart.

There were two criterion measures of success used in this study; one was grades on the occupational therapy student clinical training report, the

other was grades on the registration examination given by the American Occupational Therapy Association.

In order to estimate the reliability of the student training report a Pearsonian coefficient of correlation was computed. An r of +.86 was found. When this was corrected by the Spearman-Brown prophesy formula, the r was equal to +.92. Because the rating scale has only eleven items, it is rather short for such a high reliability coefficient. The range used on the scale is also limited thus theoretically decreasing the reliability. However, it would appear that the rating scale is acceptably reliable.

	Mechanical	Computational	Scientific	Persuasive	Artistic	Literary	Musical	Social Service	Clerical
Pediatric	.12	.00	-.03	-.03	-.08	-.23*	-.08	.09	-.05
Psychiatric	.05	-.02	-.00	-.05	.07	.17	-.15	.11	-.05
Tuberculous	.01	-.20	.02	-.20	.10	.03	-.18	-.19	.04
Orthopedic	-.03	-.02	-.13	.18	.05	.06	.04	.11	.07
Total	-.01	-.03	-.08	-.22*	-.11	-.11	-.13	-.06	-.01
Registration Examination	.03	-.09	.07	-.12	-.09	-.30**	.04	.09	-.14

*Significant at 5% level of Confidence
**Significant at 1% level of Confidence

Table II. Coefficients of correlation of scores on Kuder preference record and grades in clinical training and on registration examination (N = 91).

The registration examination given by the American Occupational Therapy Association consists of 300 multiple choice items. Part I of the examination and Part II have been correlated against each other at every examination. The correlations have ranged from +.75 to +.85. In general, it would seem that the examination is fairly reliable.[4]

Procedure. Pearson's product-moment coefficient of correlation was computed for each factor of the STDCR Inventory and each of the nine interests tested on the Kuder Preference Record with grades in each area of clinical training, with a total score (sum of all clinical training scores) for clinical training, and with the registration examination. The coefficients of correlation were calculated on the basis of raw scores.

Means and standard deviations of scores on Kuder Preference Record were computed for San Jose State College occupational therapy students. These scores were compared with the norms for occupational therapists as given by Kuder and with University of Wisconsin freshmen women.[8] Of the norms reported by Kuder, the latter group of subjects most nearly resembled the general population from which the occupational therapy majors were drawn. Similarly, means and standard deviations of scores on Guilford's STDCR Inventory were computed for occupational therapy students at San Jose State College and compared with students in general at San Jose State College. In order to determine whether the difference between the mean scores of San Jose State College occupational therapy students differed significantly from the mean scores of University of Wisconsin freshman women on the Kuder Preference Record, a *t* ratio was computed. For the mean scores on Guilford's Inventory of Factors STDCR for occupational therapy majors and college students in general at San Jose State College, *t* ratios were also calculated. No *t's* reached the 5% level of confidence for either test.

RESULTS

STDCR Inventory Correlations. The coefficients of correlation for the Guilford STDCR Inventory and grades in clinical training and on the registration examination are shown in Table I. The T score at the 5% level of confidence for 89 degrees of freedom is .206; at the 1% level of confidence it is .269. Only two scores are significant at the 5% level of confidence. They are the coefficient of correlation of the T score (thinking introversion-extroversion) and grade in pediatric clinical training and of the C score (cycloid disposition) and grade in tuberculosis clinical training.

In addition there is a correlation of —.36 between the R factor (rhathymia) and grades on the registration examination. This coefficient of correlation is significant at the 1% level of confidence.

Preference Record Correlations. The coefficient of correlation of scores on the Kuder Preference Record and grades in clinical training and on the registration examination are small (see Table II). However, there is a positive relationship of the order of .30 between "literary interest" as measured on the Kuder Preference Record and grades on the registration examination. This coefficient of correlation is the only one significant at the 1% level of confidence. At the 5% level of confidence there is a negative coefficient of correlation between grades in pediatric clinical training and literary interest. Also at the 5% level of confidence is the coefficient of correlation between the total grade in clinical training and "persuasive interest." The coefficients of correlation between interest in persuasion and grades in tuberculosis and orthopedic clinical training approach the 5% level of confidence.

On the STDCR Inventory the *t* ratios did

not show a significant difference between the mean scores of occupational therapy majors and students in general at San Jose State College.

The T scores did not show a significant difference between the mean scores of San Jose

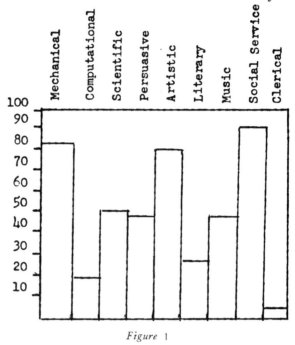

Figure 1

State College occupational therapy majors and University of Wisconsin women on the Kuder Preference Record.

However, on the Kuder Preference Record there seems to be a characteristic profile with scores above the 80% for interests in "mechanical", "artistic," and "social service" and scores below 20% for "clerical" and "computational interests" (see Figure I).

DISCUSSION

Reliability and validity of occupational therapy student clinical training report. It is possible to question the reliability and validity of the occupational therapy student clinical training report since it shares all the problems associated with scales in general.

The reliability of the report may be questioned on several counts, the most important being the number of raters. Since the students were assigned to four medical specialties and to different institutions for similar affiliations, the grading was done by twenty to thirty different raters.

Clinical experience of raters ranged from one to fifteen years. The *Rater's Guide* provided help in standardizing the rating of students. Since San Jose State College occupational therapy students took their training almost exclusively within the State of California, the raters received some uniform instruction through local meetings and individual conference. Additional uniformity of rating was gained since the supervisor was able to observe the student for a period of one to three months. If there was more than one supervising therapist within the hospital, a combined rating was usually given. Students' rating scores were forwarded to the school and not the next affiliation. Bias because of past ratings was thus avoided.

The number and types of patients varies from one hospital to another and also within a hospital from time to time. Consequently, the students were not faced with problems of equal difficulty. Change of personnel both within and without the occupational therapy department may have presented uncontrolled variations.

A student's performance may have been influenced by illness or personal problems and consequently the rating did not represent his real abilities. These errors were partially offset by the long period of training and the supervisor's ability to evaluate the circumstances.

In spite of the above difficulties there is some evidence that the ratings are reliable. A Pearsonian coefficient of correlation, corrected by the Spearman-Brown formula, was found to be .92. Engelhart[3] found ratings in orthopedic clinical training had a reliability coefficient of .81.

Reliability and validity of the registration examination. Engelhart[3] found a correlation of +.34 significant at the 1% level of confidence between the grades on the registration examination and grades in psychiatric clinical training. Correlations of +.23, significant at the 5% level of confidence were found between grades on the registration examination and orthopedic clinical training and a composite score for clinical training. The correlations were probably due to the fact that one-half to two-thirds of the items on the registration examination were based on orthopedics, psychiatry and related basic sciences. She found no relationship between tuberculosis and pediatric clinical training and the registration examination. This is not surprising because of the limited number of items covering these fields. While the r's were low, it would seem that the examination may be valid not only for the course work which it covers but for orthopedic and psychiatric clinical training and for the total grade for clinical training.

Significance of the Correlations. In the present study only six of the eighty-four coefficients of correlation which were computed were significant, four at the 5% level and two at the 1% level of confidence. On the basis of chance alone 4.2 correlations significant at the 5% level would be expected. Hence the significance of the six correlations seem doubtful.

Significant Correlations. One of the largest correlations (see Table II) was found between "literary interest" as measured by Kuder's Preference Record and grades on the registration examination. Phillips,[9] in a study comparing the relationship of the Kuder Preference Record Scales to college marks, notes that the "only reliable r is between 'literary interest' and the Ohio State Psychological Test." The r was +.38. On logical grounds, it would appear that r of +.30 between "literary interest" and grades on the registration examination for occupational therapy majors at San Jose State College may represent a real relationship. Because of this corroborating evidence, it is of some interest to speculate as to the possibility of other correlations which may have real significance.

The registration examination is negatively correlated at the 1% level of confidence with the R score or rhathymic factor (see Table I). It seems likely that the happy-go-lucky person is less apt to spend time studying than the more conscientious student.

The following r's are significant at the 5% level of confidence only and may have occurred by chance alone. An r of —.23 was found between "literary interest" and success in pediatric clinical training. It may be that a high academic interest is disadvantageous in handling children who have a short span of attention and who can grasp only superficial facts about a variety of activities. It is more probable that this correlation appeared by chance.

An r of +.22 was found between the "persuasive interest" and the total score for clinical training. Certainly the motivation of patients, selling his job to the members of a hospital staff and arousing enthusiasm in volunteer workers require the abilities which are indicated by an interest in persuasion. While the coefficient of correlation between "persuasive interest" and success in pediatric and psychiatric clinical training are insignificant, interest in persuasion is close to the 5% level of confidence for both tuberculosis and orthopedic clinical training. The r's are +.20 and +.18 which are very close to the .206 which is significant at the 5% level for 89 degrees of freedom.

It is interesting to note that the coefficient of correlation between tuberculosis clinical training rating and the C factor (cycloid disposition) is +.21, an r significant at the 5% level of confidence. Since rest is the keynote to the treatment of tuberculosis, individuals with an even disposition would be expected to be more successful in a tuberculosis sanatorium than those with a fluctuating disposition. In other fields of occupational therapy the patients need change and stimulation in order to arouse interest in new efforts and enjoyment of new experiences.

(Continued on page 126)

remaining digit needs a mate for purposes of prehension. (2) A normal skin flap may be used to cover the tactile part of the new digit, resulting in essential stereognosis. (3) A normal digit, can be transferred from the same or opposite hand, with nerves and tendons joined to give sensation and motion, but this procedure may be mutilating and nutrition in the new digit will be poor. (4) Most practical is restoration of a new digit by the pedicle method so as to transfer sensation, vascularity and motion. This method applies to furnishing a thumb from a part of the index finger, for example.

It is concluded that a digit fashioned purely for cosmetic reasons has little to recommend it.

D. R. Street, Lt. AMSC (OT)

TREATMENT OF CHECKREIN SHOULDER BY USE OF MANIPULATION AND CORTISONE, Thomas B. Quigley, M.D., *Journal of the American Medical Association*, Vol. 161, No. 9, June 30, 1956.

The treatment of "checkrein shoulder" is discussed by the author following a differential definition of the syndrone, its etiology and pathology. Manipulation techniques are presented. Case studies are reported to illustrate results of the prescribed treatment.

"Checkrein shoulder" is differentiated from "frozen shoulders" by various criteria. There is a history, in a middle aged person, of several weeks of disuse imposed by pain frequently following a minor injury or an episode of inflammation. A gradual return of the lower ranges of shoulder motion is reported but a painful check to the upper ranges of motion is present. Resistance to ordinary treatment measures is usual. Findings include limited passive abduction of the humerus on the scapula at 45° and a limitation of internal and external rotation to about 50% of normal range. Varying degrees of atrophy of shoulder girdle musculature are evident; x-ray findings of demineralization and some calcific deposits may exist. A palpable and audible release of resistance (through an arc of 20° of abduction) during manipulation under anesthesia occurs. This arc is that occupied by the checkrein contracture of the subscapularis muscle in anterior-inferior joint capsule. A resulting free, near normal range of abduction and external rotation is to be expected.

Patients receiving such shoulder manipulations were given corticotropin (ACTH), cortisone, and/or locally injected hydrocortisone acetate to suppress postmanipulation pain.

Of 44 checkrein shoulders so treated over a five year period, the author reports that 33 promptly regained and maintained a normal painless range of motion; 11 improved to some extent, with some degree of pain, of limitation of motion, or both. Duration of symptoms in the latter group was 8.8 months as compared to six months in the former "cured" group. Mention is also made of six "frozen shoulders," not meeting the checkrein criteria, which did not benefit from manipulation procedures. Caution must be exercised, the author warns, lest fracture of the anatomic neck of the humerus result.

—D. R. Street, Lt., AMSC (OT)

APPARATUS AIDS: ADAPTED FLOOR LOOM FOR UPPER EXTREMITY INVOLVEMENT, Cornelius A. Kooiman, O.T.R., M.A., Frederic J. Kottke, M.D., *Archives of Physical Medicine and Rehabilitation*, Vol. 37, No. 6, June, 1956.

It would be impractical to try to describe to the readers of this journal the construction of the apparatus described in the above mentioned *Archives of Physical Medicine and Rehabilitation*. Rather the reviewer suggests that those who are interested in such a piece of equipment refer to this article. A photograph, description of construction, and a list of materials required for construction accompany the article.

The adaptation is "useful for increasing range of motion of the shoulders and especially for providing resistance exercise to the shoulder girdle adductors, depressors and arm extensors to build up endurance for crutch walking."

—Elizabeth M. Nachod, Capt., AMSC (OT)

PROGNOSTIC STUDIES IN CHILDREN WITH CEREBRAL PALSY, Eric Denhoff, M.D., Raymond Holden, M.A., Maurice Silver, M.D., *Journal of the American Medical Association*, Vol. 161, No. 9, June 30, 1956.

This study attempts to evaluate the validity of pneumoencephalography and psychological examinations in the prediction of the future adjustment of cerebral palsied children. The study was performed at the Meeting Street School in Providence, Rhode Island, with a sample group of 50 children with cerebral palsy over a two year period.

Seven diagnostic groupings were established on the basis of pneumoencephalographic findings and clinical diagnosis. From this classification, correlations were run between initial psychological predictions and actual clinical progress with an agreement of 81%, and between pneumoencephalographic predictions and actual clinical progress, with a 72% agreement.

The most reliable prognostic tool was found to be psychological tests. Pneumoencephalography, it was felt, should be reserved for difficult cases, not for routine use. The electroencephalogram was of value only in the diagnosis of seizures in the cases studied.

From the results of this study, it would appear that among the children with cerebral palsy, those most apt to make adequate life adjustments are the ones with spastic hemiplegia, with unilateral brain damage and with intelligence low-average or better, or those of any diagnostic classification who are mildly handicapped and with good intelligence and a relatively normal pneumoencephalogram. Children with spastic quadriplegia, with bilateral brain damage and mental deficiency, have the poorest prognosis for the future.

—D. R. Street, Lt. AMSC (OT)

Personality·Factors . . .

(Continued from page 96)

One other significant coefficient of correlation was found between the T factor and pediatric clinical training. The r was $+.22$, significant at the 5% level of confidence. It is possible that the thinking introvertive type of individual is more sensitive to the moods of interest of children, or this may be a relationship which occurred by chance.

SUMMARY

Occupational therapy students at San Jose College were given the Kuder Preference Record and Guilford's STDCR Inventory. These scores were compared with grades in each field of clinical

---

training, a total grade, and the registration examination in order to see whether the tests could be used to predict on-the-job success. The criteria used were grades on the occupational therapy student clinical training report and the registration examination given by the American Occupational Therapy association.

Pearson's product-moment of correlation was used. At the 1% level of confidence, correlations were found for "literary interest," as measured on the Kuder Preference Record, and for the R factor, as measured on the Guilford STDCR Inventory, with grades on the registration examination.

BIBLIOGRAPHY

1. Beaver, Alma Perry, "Personality Factors in Choice of Nursing," *Journal of Applied Psychology*, 37: 374-379, October, 1953.

2. Crider, Blake, "A School of Nursing Selection Program," *Journal of Applied Psychology*, 27:452-457, October, 1943.

3. Engelhart, Helen, "An Investigation of the Relationship Between College Grades and On-The-Job Performance During Clinical Training of Occupational Therapy Students," Unpublished Master's thesis, San Jose State College, San Jose, 1954, 40 pp. (Abstract carried in this issue.)

4. Fish, Marjorie, O.T.R., Personal communication with the writer, April, 1953.

5. Guilford, J. P., "An Inventory of Factors STDCR," *Manual of Directions and Norms*, revised edition.

6. Healy, Irene and Borg, Walter R., "Personality and Vocational Interests of Successful and Unsuccessful Nursing School Freshmen," *Educational and Psychological Measurement*, 12:767-775, Winter, 1952.

7. Herzberg, Frederich; Bouton, Arthur, and Steiner, Betty Jo, "Studies of the Stability of the Kuder Preference Record, "*Educational and Psychological Measurement*, 41:90-100, Spring, 1954.

8. Kuder, G. F., Revised Manual for the Preference Record, Chicago: Science Research Associates, revised 1946.

9. Phillips, W. S. and Osborne, R. T., "A Note on the Relationship of the Kuder Preference Record Scales to College Marks, Scholastic Aptitude and Other Variables," *Educational and Psychological Measurement*, 9:331-337, Autumn, 1949.

10. Schmidt, John, Jr., "Factor Analysis of Prospective Teachers' Differences, "*Journal of Experimental Education*, 18:287-319, June, 1950.

11. Seagoe, May V., "Prognostic Tests and Teaching Success," *The Journal of Educational Research*, 39: 685-690, May, 1945.

12. Shaw, Jack, "The Function of the Interview in Determining Fitness for Teacher-Training," *Journal of Educational Research*, 45:667-681, May, 1952.

13. Spaney, Emma, "Personality Tests and the Selection of Nurses," *Nursing Research*, 1:4-26, February,3 1953.

14. Thompson, Carolyn Goss, "Some Preliminary Notes on Selecting Students for Training in Occupational Therapy." *The American Journal of Occupational Therapy*, 5:191-192, Sept.-Oct., 1951.

THE AMERICAN JOURNAL OF

Occupational Therapy

OFFICIAL PUBLICATION OF THE AMERICAN OCCUPATIONAL THERAPY ASSOCIATION

THE STUDENT IN PRE-CLINICAL EDUCATION

● **Impressions of a Clinically Oriented Therapist**

RUTH W. BRUNYATE, O.T.R.

For years the Council on Education of the American Occupational Therapy Association has expressed the wish that an exchange of personnel could occur on some regular and predictable basis between the members of the faculty of each occupational therapy curriculum and the therapists who supervise the student's clinical affiliations. The need for a sensitivity to the other's role on the part of both faculty and clinical directors has also been expressed by the registration committee in its effort to keep test material abreast of current academic teaching and in line with field practice.

Such efforts fail because sheer mechanics abort most attempts to implement the philosophy. Faculty members on ten month appointments can occasionally gain clinical experience for one month. Clinical personnel rarely accomplish more than an occasional audit of a single class unless, of course, they return to campus for their own advanced degrees. In this instance true exchange is not accomplished because the very reason for the therapist's presence on campus is centered on immediate goals other than those of understanding student behavior and performance. True, some curricula are structured within the clinical setting but this is not the case in the majority of the thirty-two accredited schools. In large part the problem seems to have had no practical solution.

For this reason it seems pertinent to record impressions received by a therapist who recently moved quite unexpectedly from a position in a treatment center supervising affiliating students to a college campus supervising the undergraduate phase of occupational therapy education. As in all other participant experiences the individual received the greatest gain but a sharing of

thoughts will hopefully project the benefits and make it possible to spread the value gained.

The concepts presented are blatantly biased and colored by the setting of a small liberal arts campus experienced in a personal way by one individual. Other curriculum directors may rightfully take issue since their longer overview is undoubtedly more valid in many ways. This does not negate the impressions for our objective is to share generalizations with all who direct the young and inexperienced.

The Academic and Clinical Settings Compared

Certain elements of the academic setting are so distinctive from clinical practice as to require attention before comparison of counselling and instruction can be made. Fundamentally a student is a student on one campus or another, in one occupational therapy department or another. Certain traits become predominant in one setting over the other but for all practical purposes commonalities outweigh the differences. It is the setting itself which differs so markedly and is overwhelmingly notable to the newcomer. The clinical director must understand this difference if he is to understand how a faculty member functions and why he is prompted to hold the philosophies he holds.

The *purpose* is different. On campus all are concerned with the dissemination of knowledge, the development of creative thought, the growth of the individual. In the hospital (which we shall use as a broad reference for all clinical settings) all are concerned with the development or retention of the health of the patient. These needs preclude all others. The growth of the student assigned is not the purpose which alone justifies the existence of the hospital.

The *priorities* are different. On campus each student is the concern of all faculty either directly or indirectly and college services exist for his benefit. In the hospital the student merely has the privilege of using the facilities and he becomes the point of last and least concern. All thoughts are first directed to the patient, then to personnel in the order in which their service is of value to the patient. Students needs are subordinate to the critical and serious issues of life and death and rehabilitation.

The *atmosphere* is different. The social and philosophical elements of campus life and thought and their fusion with the purely academic and educational phases of education tend to equalize the status created by the structure of faculty appointments. Ingrained, rigid, pyramided and traditional as it is, it cannot compare with the status structure in a hospital where the doctor is the ultimate authority.

The *pace* is different. The time factor is markedly different. The academic setting is as clock conscious as the clinic yet there is a fluidity, a flexibility, an informality of programming which is unique. Campus and hospital are equally busy, their personnel bear equally heavy demands, each is equally overburdened in terms of things to be done and demands made on a given day's schedule, but the pace is different. True, courses are built in sequential steps. Pre-requisites must be met, but tomorrow comes after today and in somewhat different perspective; course outlines do permit the moving of one week's point of discussion into the following week, but the acute needs of today's patient cannot be circumvented until tomorrow. There is more freedom to teach in tune with the immediate interest of the student, to prolong one phase or pre-empt another, than is permissable in learning through experience in patient contact. There is a casualness persuasive to meditation and to free association of thought, an environment set to encourage question and answer, test and proof, which cannot always be created in the pressure of the clinical setting.

The *language* is different. The jargon of the clinical director is shared by all therapists and understood by all faculty members. The academic language is specific to campus rather than to therapy and is not familiar to directors unless they themselves are recent graduates or scholars. Clock hours, semester hours, credits, pre-requisites, the provost, honors, etc. are strange or forgotten to the clinical therapist and cause him to stop for interpolation when they are heard in joint discussions of curricular needs.

The *ratio of students* to instructor is inverted. One faculty member may be involved with forty or fifty students widely scattered geographically across campus, thus not always distinctive nor quickly identifiable. In the hospital a director is not permitted to accept more than two students per registered therapist hence almost a one-to-one relationship exists. This does not mean increased attention to a student since again patient need comes first.

The *role of personality* is different. A faculty is concerned with accepting a personality and molding the characteristics of that individual into a professional being. The director must inversely accept the professional being' and encourage the exercise of that personality in appropriate application of the student's raw professional skills. He is then asked to ignore the overlay of personality in completing the RPSA forms required for registration.

The *student psychology* differs. On campus students are a cohesive group and the very oneness of that group gives each individual student a different dimension. There is a mass psychology on campus not seen in the hospital even if it accepts groups of students. This is both a happy and difficult thing. There are strengths which come to a student from the s t u d e n t group. There are strengths which come to the faculty member in working through the group. The student body enthusiasms, the student leadership to set the pace, the support gained by a shy student, the interaction of question and answer, these are all of tremendous value and demand quite different instructional guidance than does work with a single student.

The *degree of instructor independence* is different. On campus one senses greater autonomy of action for each faculty member. In the hospital the patient is a potential legal and health risk and, in terms of the student, the director holds dual responsibility to administrator and president. The student is transient and holds allegiance to his faculty. Administratively there must be a different type of discipline and chain of command.

The *rewards* are different. A faculty member is in a position to see development and change and to witness the ultimate achievement of a goal. He sees a student move from one phase to another, sees him grow or fail to do so and can judge when and how to intrude to the point of correction or guidance or to allow freedom of self direction. The director sees only a wedge of the whole and struggles to project his vision.

These are some of the marked differences apparent in comparing the settings of clinical supervision and classroom instruction. Marked and numerous as they are the common motivation inspiring both faculty and director is a more unifying force than the differences a distracting one. The eagerness to share, to help, to give and to inspire are dominant in both settings. The difference in climate therefore becomes important only when we appreciate that certain traits of student behavior are apparent when he is seen in the security of the campus. There are paradoxes of behavior which are not obvious in the performance of one or a few students but are unmistakable in groups of students. No student loses these traits immediately as he moves from college to the hospital. The supervising director must recognize them if he is to be successful in guiding the student's attempts to adjust to the new demands of the new learning experience.

Paradoxes of Student Behavior

Students are *clannish*—they crave *individuality*. Just as we sometimes muse that beatniks deny their own resentment of society's controls and apparent subjection of the individual to the group demands through the very commonality of their bizarre living, so students deny their own readiness for complete independence in their strong desire for classmate support and acceptance. The student who goes to an affiliation is stripped almost entirely of the security he has had in the approval and understanding of his fellow students. He has moved away from his family control to a great degree but has assumed another type of dependency from which he must now again venture.

One of the symbols of this change is the cessation of competition in performance, in grades and in winning approval from a superior. Students freely express their wish to be free of the archaic system of grades, many faculties share their feeling, yet those guides continue to operate and the significance of grades and achievement of grade point averages cannot be denied. The Report on Student Performance in Affiliation rates a person on his performance without assigning a specific grade, the competitive element is removed and should be. Performance for performance's sake, achievement for the sake of employability and personal satisfaction are now factual. They are not repugnant, merely new in a student's experience. This behooves the one who rates and counsels to be aware that the removal of familiar grading may cause insecurity not sensed by the student. Wise rating and guidance can make it a very rewarding and interesting experience contributing amazing amounts to a student's sense of self security. Conversely it can be traumatic to the student, or if he is strong and the director is not, it can result in very harsh evaluations of the profession and misgivings on the student's part in his choice of his profession.

When a student finds himself in the clinical setting he finds he must assume a new stature, a new role. He is no longer a part of a tight knit group with the advantages of leadership, class spirit, the opportunity to challenge and equal, the freedom to share experience both painful and pleasant and the opportunity if he needs it to retreat into the class group from the very individuality he felt he wanted but was uncertain of assuming. This cannot be done with much success on affiliation for numbers are few and responsibilities many.

Moments of intimacy, sharing of similar experiences are now gone and suddenly the independence that has been assumed to be mandatory is found wanting. Roommates, classmates and fellow affiliates in the hospital lack the familiarity to fill the need. The clinical director who senses these things can guide a student through a difficult period. Not all students experience this, of course, and because many do not we tend to fail to see the ones who do.

Students are *ambitious*—but woefully *lazy*. Any faculty advisor who has once gone through the process of registering students is aware of their expressed eagerness to be involved with heavy demands. Their cry for difficult courses in some areas, their wish ofttimes to accelerate, to qualify by proficiency and to get on with the business of fulfilling requirements is constant. Every instructor is aware of the student quest for mature types of assignments, for classroom discussion, for debate, and aware too of their interest in issues and controversies and clamor for new and different presentations. Yet who among the faculty has not given what he felt to be a relatively easy assignment with a liberal time lapse prior to presentation, only ot hear the chorused groan and complaint. There is a freedom in voicing objection to assignment, complaints about deadlines and discontent with requests that clinical directors find difficult to understand. Undoubtedly this is in part due to sheer numbers of students but it is spontaneous in all kinds of situations on campus. The cry is frequently lifted against what the faculty felt was routine, yet the student viewed as an extra. This is commonplace among young people, not just therapists, and it will come with the student to the clinical level. An awareness of it often helps the clinical person realize that he is not at fault in his planning nor amiss in his requests but that time and responses change and respect for discipline and work is another facet of learning to be reinforced by clinical experience.

Student Guidance

Students are *independent thinkers*—they *seek guidance* in making decisions. Students want an opportunity to express thought, to think quietly and to voice opinion and counter opinion. They accept it as a mark of recognition if given the opportunity to function this way. Yet, withall, they sometimes quietly, sometimes openly, seek support and help in doing these things. They want the opportunity but it is best given in such a way as to build in available help, elected on student initiative if needed. This is difficult to do and is quite different from basic guidance and direction which must be offered by an instructor without request of the student. In other words, accommodating this need in the student does not free the director from his responsibility to insist on direction at appropriate times. It does not give the affiliate the privilege of designing and controlling his own clinical experience.

Sudents are *impervious*—they are *impressionable*. Occasionally it seems as though that which is valueless penetrates while that which is valuable is lost. Selectivity of emphasis is important and the persuasiveness of the individual director must be respected and channeled. Some personalities are so strong that they could lead a student to accept only one concept. We all use ourselves as tools of treatment. So too do we use ourselves as tools of instruction. The clinical director as the professor must use this tool wisely for it can be over-sharpened to the student's detriment. It can be underplayed too—the director must determine the balance.

Students are *mature*—they *lack many essentials of maturity*. Each of us is familiar through friend and family with young people and the paradox of maturity of manner and concept and the ingenue quality of performance. Academic courses today are accelerated. Course content has changed markedly. Basic mathematics, psychology, the sciences, philosophy—all are taught in much broader ways than they were even ten years ago. Elective course are supplied in a greater number of areas. A student therefore becomes informed in a very mature way. Thinking is accelerated because more information has been given. High schools are teaching what used to be included in college introductory courses. Yet the provision of factual material and thinking experiences does not negate the need for time in which to mature. Today's college student is a sophisticated young person who moves with a high degree of capability in a complex world. Ofttimes however, he is disarmingly simple, young and naive. The pace of current education does not always keep the individual well rounded in his personal development. Maturity of conduct may appear on the surface yet symptoms of immaturity are seen in a reluctance to accept correction, a sense of being imposed upon if things go against the student's will, and

an awkwardness in accepting the difficult and unwanted thing. Tolerance and patience are often a bit behind other phases of growth. Handling of money, a car, travel, a divorced family and college curriculum may be done with aplomb yet acceptance of that which is less than desirable in his own eyes or reprimand for some detail of performance may be impossible. The superficialities of manner may indicate maturity which is entirely lacking once the manner has been dented. If we recognize this we not only make the student more responsive to his learning situation but we also save ourselves a lot of anguish.

Student Attitudes

Students are *enthusiastic* about the profession—they are *disillusioned* by it. Students are inspired and awed by their new knowledge. They have gained many concepts woven through the experience in curriculum and in previous contact with therapists. The challenge of medicine, the urge to help those less fortunate than self, the stimulus of the unknown and glamor of hospital physician and patient have buoyed them through many a difficult or boring campus study hour. Intangible presentations and theories have a hollowness when divorced from practice and they are eager now to test their knowledge and prove their worth. Months of study acutely elongated by the pressures of graduation have, they feel, held them in bounds and they long to be important people free of restraints imposed by others. They are at once anxious and confident yet timorous, for the immediacy of the affiliation experience makes them feel strangely inadequate. The pre-clinical doubts and jitters are quite ripe.

Many however are fearful lest they will be disappointed. Rumor from the class immediately preceding has carried back to campus many stories of apparent injustice and inadequacies experienced in affiliation. The affiliate who has now completed all clinical assignments also has the jitters for he is concerned with the registration examination now confronting him and this reflects on his discussion of clinical experiences and permits him to present a distorted picture to upcoming affiliates. Or perhaps the circuitous route of the grapevine has diluted facts or lifted them out of context. This we must be ready to accept and expect. Faculty and directors must understand. The clinical people must be alert to being certain that those things they envision as vital to clinical experience are really being perceived by the student. In many ways it is far harder to instruct at this level than in the classroom. We must recognize that menial routines which are natural and insignificant parts of our own professional lives suddenly personify subordinate status to a new student. The experienced therapist puts such details in proper perspective with the far greater parts of his day's work. Thus they do not wrangle. The student lacks perspective and therefore is disturbed. The director must be sensitive, patient and observant of such reactions.

He must remember too that a student being new to the setting is quick to sense interpersonal relationships and innuendoes which old hands have failed to note. If superficial relationships have developed, if we have failed to relate well to our medical direction, if we are functioning on somewhat shallow performance, the student will quickly notice and draw his own conclusions, often deciding that we do not practice the vital service that we teach. A continuous self inventory of departmental and staff performance is a must for those who accept the responsibility of clinical teaching. The student has felt that occupational therapists play important parts and are fundamentally nice people. A clinical experience can make him feel that we are found wanting in measuring up to the standards of medically educated people providing essential service to patients.

Campus life protects the individual student from the paradoxes of his own behavior. It gives him a security which will not be duplicated in the hospital. On campus service is given to the student. In the hospital he must now begin to serve. On campus the student is learning about himself and how to live with himself and his peers. In the hospital he is learning not just to know himself, but to give of himself in relation to the needs and desires of others. These are two distinctly different learning situations. From their distinctions what implications can be drawn to improve the affiliation experience?

Implications for the Future

There are no profound points which should prompt immediate change, at least not now until the results of the Curriculum Study and its supportive data have been received. This year's experience has reconfirmed a high regard for the academic leaders of the profession and an understanding of the demands made on them has been enhanced. They as a group undoubtedly know the clinical problems far better than the clinical therapist will ever appreciate the academic problems. The clinical directors must therefore look forward to change in the educational pattern and prepare for acceptance of this change. Giving prior thought to possible development will help avoid needless trial and error, debate and discussion and enable the directors to give constructive evaluation and suggestions. A few major points should be our current concern.

Clinical personnel must be more aggressive.

Too often we reflect in our performance the very insecurity that we bewail in the student. We must somehow become more aggresive in representing our profession to our public, to our medical staff, to our patients and to our students. We must speak up and speak out. It is from us that the student learns how this is done acceptably. It cannot be taught in the abstract on campus. It cannot be taught at the clinical level unless it is practiced there.

Dual appointments for faculty and directors must be explored. This has been a stumbling block yet could conceivably be evolved. It would not be impossible for a faculty member to hold a part-time appointment with a college for classroom instruction and guidance and a part-time appointment in a nearby hospital for patient treatment and student instruction. This is constantly done in research and industry. He could perhaps treat patients two days a week and teach one class on campus. When the student was assigned to that hospital he could be apprenticed to the same therapist who was intimately familiar with his college program. A patient oriented-student oriented therapist would understand the idiosyncracies of both phases of instruction. This could not happen in all clinical affiliation centers but may portend of future planning.

Clinical affiliation may be *rescheduled completely*. It is quite possible that in order to meet our ever present problem of a five-year professional course much of the affiliation will have to be pulled down into summer sessions. This has frightening potentials for all clinical centers and perhaps disastrous ones for some centers. However, drastic measures are called for and will come. We in clinical practice will have to reorient or step down from the responsibility of contributing to professional education. Change is often traumatic. More frequently it is refreshing.

Clerkships must be strengthened. The practice of affiliating while studying on campus has merit but as long as many experiences consist primarily of observation without structure or inspiration it will be inadequate. Hospital departments have not been given specific guidelines. They in turn have functioned below the level of the student. The redesigning requires concessions from the clinical directors but will produce reward in the level of affiliation performance.

A Master's Degree in Occupational Therapy must become universal. Inevitably we must turn to incorporating an advanced degree into our educational framework. We ask a student to follow the custom of medicine in participating in internship experiences and he does so, but without the status that goes to the medical interne which helps him tolerate the situation financially and otherwise. We have no such prestige factor in our favor. Other disciplines offer the advantage of a masters—nursing, speech and social work. Our competition is becoming ever tighter but this cannot be our reason for adopting a master's program. It is instead a logical extension of current curriculum if we but increase the quality of some of our courses in order to produce a master's level of work. Today's college student thinks in terms of advanced degrees and has access to scholarship support. We must make our own decision before this is forced upon us.

Selection of Clinical Centers

Discriminate and limited selection of clinical centers must occur. Any proposed changes in our pattern of clinical education is a threat to those carrying affiliation programs. Changes in philosophy and needs may ultimately change our use of clinical centers a great deal. Our current scattered use of 250 centers for a small group of students is costly in terms of duplication of effort and may change completely. The prospect of losing an affiliation is very disappointing. Why? Because students are stimulating to our programs, student affiliation brings prestige, students help cover staff shortages; but what we really say is that we want students because we enjoy instructing students and if this were lost our position would be less interesting.

Perhaps there is another side too. We spread ourselves very thin in serving student, patient and research. The loss of an affiliation might prove to strengthen our program for we would give more attention and c r e a t i v e thought to strengthening our treatment skills, exploring new techniques and resetting our goals and plans of operation. Clinical affiliations may not be cut back but, if they are, let us be sure that as we raise the cry we really reflect our fundamental dedication to the patient. If readjustment of clinical experience makes it possible to produce a better therapist, shorter courses and more therapists, then we will solve even greater problems for each department by increasing supply and providing improved patient care.

One final thought. An opportunity to move from clinic to campus is a rich experience. A myriad of small new details are learned and broad concepts refreshed. An unending number of old ones are refocused. But perhaps the greatest gain is the realization that the profession is strong because of the high calibre of dedication and capability of its academic leaders, just as is true of its clinical instructors. As long as each respects the abilities and thoughts of the other and clues into those of all registered occupational therapists we shall continue to grow and to improve our profession and the service it gives.

Fieldwork Experience, Part II: The Supervisor's Dilemma

(students, occupational therapy; training, student)

Barbara A. Christie   Peggy Corcoran Joyce   Patricia L. Moeller

This paper examines the distinguishing characteristics of the effective and the ineffective supervisor and the role, responsibilities, problems, and current needs of the occupational therapy student supervisor. Data were obtained through questionnaires received from 188 therapists and 127 students in 65 fieldwork centers nationwide. Responses indicate a perceived lack of adequate preparation of occupational therapists for the role of student supervisor and provide evidence that the profession needs to assume a more active role in providing formal, standardized training programs for the occupational therapy student supervisor. The results demonstrate a need for greater accountability for the quality of the fieldwork experience and the supervisory process guiding that experience.

General guidelines for the Level 2 fieldwork experience have been formulated by the American Occupational Therapy Association (AOTA) (1) and by individual curricula. In practice, however, the specific objectives, content, and format of the fieldwork experience are determined by the individual supervisor.

For a registered occupational therapist to become a student supervisor, the only requirement is one year of experience. Usually the process of becoming an effective supervisor is evolutionary and based on trial and error.

To explore the issues of supervisor qualifications and preparation in greater depth, the following questions were addressed:

- What are the distinguishing characteristics of effective versus ineffective student supervisors?
- Are occupational therapists adequately prepared for the role and responsibilities of student supervisor?
- What are the major problems and needs experienced by student supervisors?
- What effect does experience have on the supervisor's perception of the supervisory process?

Review of Literature

While articles addressing the topic of clinical supervision are not abundant in occupational therapy literature or the literature of other health-related professions, each field has made some effort to explore this area.

In the field of social work, Kadushin (2) attempted to apply games theory to the supervisor-supervisee relationship. He also surveyed these two groups to define more clearly what was occurring in their interactions (3). Rosenblatt (4) also surveyed social work students to determine what kind of offensive types of supervision they had experienced during their training.

Stritter (5) surveyed medical students to determine their opinions on the most effective clinical teaching behaviors. He found that the

Barbara A. Christie, OTR, is Chief, Occupational Therapy and Educational Coordinator, Department of Rehabilitation Medicine, Peggy Corcoran Joyce, OTR, was Unit Head Occupational Therapist, Rehabilitation Unit; both at Michael Reese Hospital and Medical Center, Chicago, IL 60616. Patricia L. Moeller, MOT, OTR, at the time of this study was Assistant Professor and Community Coordinator, University of Illinois' Curriculum in Occupational Therapy, Chicago, IL. She is now Life Skills Supervisor, St. Joseph Hospital, Chicago, IL 60657.

most effective clinical teacher approaches teaching with enthusiasm and energy, is readily accessible to the student, encourages students to raise questions and practice their own problem-solving skills, and gives feedback in a constructive manner.

Irby (6) surveyed both medical students and faculty members about their views on the characteristics of the best and worst clinical teachers. The most important characteristics of the best clinical teacher were skillful interacting with students, accessibility, organized presentations, enthusiasm, enjoyment of teaching, and interest in students. The worst clinical teachers lacked the above attributes and instead displayed clusters of negative personal traits such as arrogance, dogmatism, lack of self-confidence, insensitivity, and belittling of others.

In 1978, the American Speech and Hearing Association (7) issued a special report on the status of clinical supervision within their profession. Many of their concerns are shared and have been expressed by other professions (e.g., the need for data to validate the supervisory process, role definition for supervisors, better quality of supervision, training of supervisors, and special standards for supervisors).

In the occupational therapy literature, as early as 1928, Bryan (8) outlined the importance of a harmonious relationship between the supervisor and the student. In the same year, Lermit (9) suggested that an effective supervisor should formulate a definite, concrete program of procedures; hold regular conferences with the student, and develop the ability to criticize gently. Brunyate (10–12) reviewed the general responsibilities of the

affiliation center, the important features of student supervisors, and the paradoxes of student behavior as they switch from academia to the clinics. Spelbring (13) questioned the quality of our clinicians as clinical educators and suggested that this area was being neglected. Schnebly (14) compared the roles of the clinician and the educator.

Method

Population

The research population was obtained through the cooperation of fieldwork centers recommended by occupational therapy curricula affiliated with Michael Reese Hospital and Medical Center in Chicago and from the *AOTA OT Fieldwork Centers Manual*. These centers represented all sections of the country and included large and small, traditional and nontraditional settings with established student programs. Table 1 summarizes population characteristics.

Instrument and Procedure

Open-ended questionnaires, specifically designed for this study,

were sent to 108 fieldwork centers for distribution to occupational therapy students and student supervisors in those settings. Students and supervisors were asked to define the respective roles of student and supervisor and to list the primary responsibilities of each, together with the distinguishing characteristics of the effective and the ineffective supervisor. Additional questions explored the perceived readiness of therapists for assuming supervisory responsibilities; current supervisory training practices; and students' and supervisors' opinions on whether special training was necessary, and if so, what the nature of that training should be. Supervisors were questioned about the major problems and needs confronting them as supervisors. Experienced supervisors were asked several questions to determine whether experience changed their perception of the supervisory process. Pilot questionnaires for both the student and student supervisor populations were field tested. A return of 66% from 108 centers resulted in a total of

Table 1
a) Demographic Comparisons of Student Supervisors (*N* = 188)

Sex	Age (years)		Years Experience		As OTR	As Supervisor	Area of Current Practice	
Male: 12	22–29:	114	Less than 1:		3	28	Phys. Dys.	74
Female: 176	30–39:	43	1–2		37	44	Psychiatric	64
	40–49:	22	3–5		65	56	Pediatric	21
	50–56:	7	6–10		50	34	Combination	8
	No Response:	2	11–15		19	11	Administration	10
			Over 15:		11	3	Clin. Spec. Area	4
			No Response:		3	12	No Response	7

b) Demographic Comparisons of Students (*N* = 127)

Sex	Age (years)		Current Fieldwork Experience	
Male: 5	20–22:	64	First:	48
Female: 122	23–25:	39	Second:	54
	26–30:	13	Third:	23
	31–39:	9	No Response:	2
	40–49:	2		

This population represents students from 38 occupational therapy curricula.

127 individual responses from students and 188 from student supervisors. Results were analyzed separately for students and supervisors.

Results and Discussion

Distinguishing Characteristics of the Effective Versus Ineffective Supervisor

Supervisors and students concurred in their responses; both consistently linked certain behaviors with certain attitudes to distinguish the effective from the ineffective supervisor. For example, the effective supervisor gave feedback (behavior) "in a supportive manner" (attitude), while the ineffective supervisor gave feedback "in a way that is demeaning to the student." Thus, the critical difference between effective and ineffective supervisors appears to be the attitude with which supervisors carry out their responsibilities.

The effective supervisor. The characteristics named by 90% of the students and 85% of the supervisors were interpersonal and communication skills. Active listening was the skill mentioned most frequently while openness and honesty were the attitudes most often associated with effective interpersonal and communication skills. One aspect of communication, feedback, received special attention. The effective supervisor provided feedback that was timely, constructive, consistent, and growth-promoting.

The effective supervisor was able to adapt his or her supervisory approach and also structure and grade the program to meet the student's individual needs. Flexibility and open-mindedness were the attitudinal qualities associated with effectively meeting the needs of the student.

Other significant characteristics of the effective supervisor were being available, being competent as a clinician and as an educator, and being a good role model. Supervisors included organizational and teaching skills as additional characteristics.

The purely attitudinal characteristics of being supportive and empathetic were most frequently attributed to the effective supervisor by both students and supervisors. Other important attitudes included open-mindedness, acceptance and nondefensiveness, concern for the students' growth, commitment to the supervisory role, sensitivity to students' needs, patience, objectivity, and enthusiasm.

The ineffective supervisor. Both students and supervisors perceived the ineffective supervisor as characterized primarily by poor interpersonal and communication skills, noting particularly the inability to effectively provide feedback. Two other major characteristics were not being available and not being qualified to be a supervisor because of a lack of clinical experience or supervisory skills.

Rigidity was cited by one-third of the supervisors as a primary characteristic of the ineffective supervisor. Students noted a related characteristic of "stifling originality, creativity, and independent problem-solving." Whereas flexibility and open-mindedness were the attitudes most closely associated with effectiveness in adapting a supervisory approach to meet students' needs, rigidity was associated with ineffectiveness as it inhibited the student's creativity and problem-solving. Students frequently associated controlling, dominating, smothering, and restrictive attitudes in the supervisor with lack of independence and creative problem-solving opportunities for the students. This corroborates Rosenblatt's finding (3), which cited "constrictive supervision," or supervision that does not give students opportunities to solve problems on their own, as one of the most objectionable supervision styles according to students.

In addition to rigidity, other attitudes frequently mentioned were being unsupportive, uncaring, and unconcerned. This corresponded to Rosenblatt's findings that being an "unsupportive" supervisor was considered another objectionable supervisory style (3).

Unsupportive supervisory styles have potentially far-reaching effects on the profession. As noted in Part I, 21% of the 131 respondents listed personal emotional responses during the fieldwork experience (depression, stress, anxiety, lack of confidence, discomfort) as being the primary factors contributing to the decision not to work in a particular area of clinical practice. If students do not feel they can discuss such problems with a supportive supervisor, their unresolved negative feelings may contribute to the future avoidance of a particular area of practice or compromise the future therapist's ability to provide optimal patient care.

In summary, a consistent picture emerges as to what constitutes an effective and an ineffective supervisor. The effective supervisor fulfills basic supervisory responsibilities with strong interpersonal skills and with attitudes of supportiveness, interest, flexibility, and enthusiasm. The ineffective supervisor lacks essential interpersonal and organizational skills and, furthermore, displays negative personal attitudes such as unsupportiveness, rigidity, lack of enthusiasm, and insensitivity toward others.

The American Journal of Occupational Therapy **677**

Education/Training

An examination of supervisor training revealed a major discrepancy between the current mode of preparing student supervisors and the way supervisors themselves felt they needed to be trained.

A major problem in supervisor training is the lack of a standardized approach. This was immediately evident not only in the data related to the current status of supervisor training, its format and content, but also in the lack of adherence to whatever standards do exist. Twenty-one percent of the supervisor respondents did not have the minimal requirement of one year clinical experience when they initially became student supervisors, and 90% of supervisor respondents felt that clinical experience alone was not enough to become a student supervisor.

Sixty-four percent of the supervisor respondents felt prepared to assume the role of student supervisor. Their confidence was founded primarily on their clinical expertise, motivation, and interest in supervising students. Another frequently mentioned factor was the positive influence of good supervisor role models present in current work settings or in earlier fieldwork experiences. Not one of these "prepared" supervisors cited confidence in supervisory skills as a reason for feeling prepared. Several commented, however, that they needed more training and guidance for developing specific supervisory skills.

Thirty-two percent of the supervisors stated that they did not feel prepared to supervise, citing the same facts that the "prepared" supervisors had cited for being prepared, but using a different perspective. They complained that

they had *only* their clinical experience or role models to rely on, and they felt more formal training was needed for their supervisory role.

Although 59% of the supervisors indicated that they had received some type of special training for supervisory responsibilities, the amount of training was variable: 25% had less than five hours of training; 25% had 5 to 25 hours; and 25% reported training "as needed." The method of training was more consistent. The majority of supervisors received their training through informal discussion in personal meetings with the occupational therapy director or another designated registered occupational therapist at their place of work. The content of these discussions varied from site to site, including anything from crisis intervention to a formal orientation to supervisory responsibilities. Some supervisors stated their training consisted primarily of reading materials, telephone contacts with the university, or audiovisual presentations.

The majority (78%) of supervisors indicated a preference for a different mode of training. Therapists desired greater involvement by universities and AOTA, as well as the opportunity to share ideas with other supervisors. Workshops and organized fieldwork supervisors' groups were the desired formats most often mentioned. Supervisors emphasized the need for standardizing supervisor training, using a variety of educational experiences with an experiential emphasis. The institution of supervised practica was also a popular suggestion. Sixteen percent felt that supervision content should be taught in the undergraduate occupational therapy curriculum. Less than 5% of supervisors felt no

training was necessary to become a student supervisor.

In summary, the nature and quality of supervisor training, when it exists, varies dramatically from site to site. Major discrepancies exist between the current mode of preparing student supervisors and the method by which the supervisors themselves would prefer to be trained.

Supervisors' Problems/Needs and Changed Perceptions

All supervisors were asked to identify the primary problems confronting them and to define their current needs for the further development of their supervisory skills. Only experienced supervisors were asked whether a supervisor's perception of the supervisory process changes with experience.

Problems. Student supervisors listed, in descending order of importance, the following major problems confronting them as student supervisors: 1. dealing with students' attitudinal and affective behaviors; 2. time management; 3. their own lack of supervisory problem-solving skills; and 4. the inadequate academic and theoretical preparation of students.

Problems with *attitudinal/affective behaviors* centered on students' immaturity, stress, and anxiety; negative student attitudes, such as defensive reactions to supervision; unprofessional student attitudes and resultant behaviors; lack of student interest and motivation in learning; and lack of student interest in a specific area of occupational therapy practice. It appeared that while new supervisors may feel prepared to guide the student in developing clinical competencies, they are not prepared for supervisory responsibilities relevant to the student's growth in the affective domain. Through experience supervisors realize they have more responsibility for guiding the student's personal, attitudinal, and professional behavior than they had originally anticipated.

The problems with *time management* appear to arise from a lack of preparation for the role of student supervisor. Most experienced supervisors felt they were neither prepared for nor aware of the variety of roles that would be demanded of them as student supervisors. As a result, beginning supervisors did not realize the need to reorganize their time to fulfill the responsibilities of this additional role. Supervisors stated that they had great difficulties in effectively integrating the various roles that are essential to being a student supervisor, balancing the responsibilities of those roles, and setting priorities among them.

Another major concern was *their own lack of supervisory problem-solving skills*. Supervisors were not always able to identify students' needs and problems in a timely fashion. Responses indicated difficulties in determining different learning styles; in developing basic supervisory observation skills; in objectively assessing students' affective behaviors; and in the formal evaluation of students' performance. Supervisors also noted difficulties in knowing when and how to structure or modify the program and supervision to meet individual student needs. Flexibility received particular emphasis as this quality was viewed as essential to effectively modifying the supervisory approach. Experienced supervisors indicated that their ability to recognize a student's individuality and to adjust their supervisory approach to that student's needs was developed through trial and error.

Finally, supervisors were concerned about the inadequate academic and theoretical preparation of students. They considered modifying the fieldwork program and their supervisory approach to meet the differences in students' academic preparation.

Needs. To more effectively and confidently manage the problems confronting them, supervisors expressed four major needs: 1. support; 2. growth in professional competency and currency; 3. supervisory skills development; and 4. teaching skills development. Only 9 of the 188 supervisors indicated that they have no current need for improving their supervisory skills.

Over 50% of the supervisors expressed a need for support (a need named more than twice as often as any other). On site, supervisors felt they needed more guidance, support, and feedback not only from their immediate supervisors, but also from students and other experienced supervisors in the fieldwork setting. Supervisors expressed a need for forming active, problem-solving support groups with other supervisors.

Increased, ongoing communication with universities was seen as being of critical importance. Specifically, supervisors wanted to be informed of curriculum changes and fieldwork expectations and receive guidance for handling students' problems. However, fewer than 10 of 188 supervisors felt that communication with the university was the responsibility of the student supervisor. This may indicate that there is a need to clarify the respective roles of the curriculum and the fieldwork center and to define the means whereby involved staff may fulfill those roles.

At the national level, supervisors wanted AOTA to assume more re-

sponsibility for the standardization and quality assurance of the fieldwork experience.

Being a student supervisor appears to challenge a therapist's level of personal confidence. This stimulates the need to keep abreast of current education and clinical practices to ensure *growth in professional competency* and thereby promote personal confidence when working with students.

To improve their *supervisory skills* supervisors felt a great need to develop competency in assessing the needs of the student, establishing performance objectives and expectations, evaluating student performance, structuring the experience, and adapting the supervisory approach to meet identified student needs.

The need to develop more effective feedback skills was also frequently mentioned. Over 23% of the supervisors expressed "difficulty in providing negative feedback and confronting students." The fact that poor feedback was identified as one of the major characteristics of the ineffective supervisor makes this particular need even more important.

To develop their *teaching skills*, supervisors asked for a theoretical understanding of the clinical teaching-learning process and for guidance in developing specific techniques to facilitate this process.

In summary, supervisors' responses concerning their problems and needs reinforced the impression that current supervisory training practices are inadequate. Supervisors felt a need for and asked for initial, as well as additional, formalized training in developing their supervisory skills. They felt that continuing education experiences should be predominantly multiexperiential, problem-solving experiences designed to meet the needs of supervisors at different stages of experience. Only 9 of the 188 supervisors indicated their needs in this area could be met by other means (i.e., reading, research, smaller patient loads, or more effective time management).

Changed perceptions. Supervisors' perceptions changed as a direct result of experience in the following three areas: 1. the role and responsibility of the student supervisor; 2. the role and responsibility of the student; and 3. the factors that contribute to effective supervision.

Through experience, and predominantly through a trial and error process, supervisors felt they were able to begin to differentiate between their responsibilities as supervisors and those of the student. Supervisors discovered there was much more to their role than clinical competence; certain additional skills, not initially anticipated, were necessary to effectively fulfill their role. This seemed especially true of the skills needed for dealing with the students' affective behavior. They also felt more confident and comfortable in their role as their supervisory skills became more clearly defined and developed.

Two-thirds of the experienced supervisors felt students should assume greater responsibility for the fieldwork experience, take more initiative in communicating their needs to the supervisor, and be more active in ensuring that their needs are met. Experienced supervisors also developed higher expectations for students with regard to independent functioning, particularly in the areas of independent learning, use of independent problem-solving skills, and creativity.

Responses seemed to indicate that the fieldwork experience should be a shared, collaborative process between the student and supervisor. A strong contrast existed, however, between these responses and responses earlier in the study where only 4 of the 127 students and 4 of the 188 supervisors mentioned that the fieldwork experience should be a shared, collaborative process. Supervisors seemed to place minimal emphasis on student initiative and responsibility when questioned earlier about their perception of student versus supervisor roles. This seems to indicate that supervisors are giving students "mixed messages" regarding expectations of their responsibilities. Supervisors strongly indicated that students should be more active in the fieldwork experience, yet they perceived the role of the student as being relatively passive.

Experienced supervisors felt that the two major distinguishing factors of effective supervision were effective interpersonal skills and a recognition of the impact of the attitudinal environment on the growth of the student.

Theoretical Growth and Development Sequence of the Occupational Therapy Student Supervisor

An analysis of experienced supervisors' changed perceptions, which was then related to findings throughout both parts of this study, indicated that the supervisor goes through a learning or growth process to become effective. This growth process appeared to be marked by the following specific stages of supervisory development.

New supervisors appear to feel totally responsible for the success or failure of the fieldwork experience. A rigid program is developed and applied to each student regardless of individual needs. New supervisors feel the need to control every aspect of the program and also seem to have a "self-centered" approach to the fieldwork experience (e.g., "Will I be able to answer all of the student's questions?"). This preoccupation with their personal performance seems to interfere with their ability to see beyond themselves to the needs of the students.

With experience, supervisors seem to realize that they are not totally responsible for the success or failure of the fieldwork experience and that the student also has a responsibility for learning. The supervisor gradually recognizes the student's individuality and the importance of assessing individual needs and learns to modify the overall fieldwork program and supervisory approach to meet those needs. The holistic concept, referred to in clinical practice as treating the "total patient," is gradually adopted in the supervisory process as the therapist begins to see the "total student." Parallel to this, the supervisor seems to lessen "controls" and becomes more flexible in adapting the supervisory approach and the program to meet the needs of the individual student. It appears that flexibility in the supervisor's approach increases with experience and is directly related to increased confidence levels in the supervisor.

With experience, therapists perceive the supervisory role as being more encompassing than they originally expected. They see themselves as a resource person, facilitator and guide, rather than as the person who gives or has all the answers, takes all the responsibility, directs, controls, or dominates.

As therapists reach this stage of development, they place greater importance on supporting and promoting students' individuality and creativity and increasing students' responsibilities and independence in the fieldwork experience.

Conclusion

This study examined the impact of the fieldwork experience on the professional development of the occupational therapist. Its findings underscore the importance of the role of the student supervisor.

The student supervisor was identified as a primary influence in the formation of a therapist's preference for a specific area of clinical practice. Both student and supervisor respondents perceived the supervisory process as the most critical element in distinguishing the good versus poor fieldwork experience.

Presently, it is primarily through trial and error experience that supervisors develop a clear perception of their responsibilities and learn to be effective. Few facilities or universities prepare prospective supervisors sufficiently for supervisory functions. Training programs which do exist are variable in quality because AOTA provides no standards or guidelines for their content. Because the supervisor's role in molding future practitioners is so very important, we conclude that formal, standardized training programs are needed to replace the current trial and error method.

ACKNOWLEDGMENT

The authors wish to acknowledge the increased attention that has been given to fieldwork education since the completion of this study in 1981. Research articles published after 1981 are not included in the references.

REFERENCES

1. Standards and guidelines for an occupational therapy affiliation program. *Am J Occup Ther* 25:313–315, 1971
2. Kadushin A: Games people play in supervision. *Social Work* 13:23–32, 1968
3. Kadushin A: Supervisor-supervisee: A survey. *Social Work* 19:288–296, 1974
4. Rosenblatt A, Meyer JE: Objectionable supervisory styles: Students' views. *Social Work* 20:184–189, 1975
5. Stritter F, Hain JD, Grimes DA: Clinical teaching reexamined. *J Med Educ* 50:876–882, 1975
6. Irby DM: Clinical teacher effectiveness in medicine. *J Med Educ* 53:808–815, 1978.
7. Current status of supervision of speech-language, pathology and audiology. *ASHA* 20:478–486, 1978.
8. Bryan WA: What should a hospital expect from pupil workers? *OT&R* 7:151–158, 1928
9. Lermit G: Practice training—What should a training school expect from a hospital for its pupils? *OT&R* 7:281–286, 1928.
10. Brunyate RW: Powerful levers in common little things. *Am J Occup Ther* 12:193–202, 1958
11. Brunyate RW: Clinical center: An integral part of the educational program. *Am J Occup Ther* 16:61–65, 1962
12. Brunyate RW: The student in pre-clinical education. *Am J Occup Ther* 17:181–186, 1965
13. Spelbring LM: Upheaval in clinical education. *Am J Occup Ther* 21:205–206, 1967
14. Schnebly ME: From clinician to educator. *Am J Occup Ther* 24:329–335, 1971

Fieldwork in Schools: A Model for Alternative Settings

Lou Ann Sooy Griswold, Beth Seybold Strassler

Key Words: education, occupational therapy

Objective. An exploratory study was conducted at the University of New Hampshire to increase the number of school-based fieldwork opportunities for occupational therapy students and to guide the development of a model for first-time fieldwork supervisors in schools.

Method. Responses to a questionnaire completed by 119 occupational therapists working in schools in northern New England provided a description of both school-based occupational therapy practice and of their needs as supervisors. Interviews with 12 occupational therapists who had supervised fieldwork students in schools provided qualitative information.

Results. Findings suggested that school-based practice issues such as working part time, traveling between schools, and using a variety of service delivery models created particular challenges for fieldwork supervisors in schools. A process of addressing fieldwork supervisors' concerns during recruitment and in a fieldwork supervisor seminar and providing ongoing support resulted in successful fieldwork experiences for occupational therapy students.

Discussion. This process of studying a practice setting in order to develop a model for fieldwork that addresses the uniqueness of the setting may be used to develop fieldwork opportunities in other practice settings as well.

Lou Ann Sooy Griswold, MS. OTR, is Assistant Professor in the Occupational Therapy Department, University of New Hampshire, Durham, New Hampshire 03824. At the time of this study, she was Project Director.

Beth Seybold Strassler, MHS. OTR, is an independent occupational therapy practitioner. At the time of this study she was Project Coordinator, Occupational Therapy Department, University of New Hampshire, Durham, New Hampshire.

This article was accepted for publication August 10, 1994.

Practice environments for occupational therapists have expanded beyond traditional medical facilities to include schools, work places, day care centers, technology centers, residential care facilities, and independent living centers (American Occupational Therapy Association [AOTA], 1991b; Baum, 1986). Entry-level occupational therapists must understand and prepare to work in the variety of practice settings that exist today and will increase in the future. Fieldwork experience is important in helping students to develop not only the clinical skills but also the interpersonal skills that they will need to work effectively in a particular setting. Because working relationships are not the same for all types of settings, Baum encouraged students to prepare themselves for potential employment settings by pursuing fieldwork experiences in the settings in which they are likely to eventually practice.

According to the most recent AOTA member data survey (1991b), of all types of facilities, public schools employed the largest percentage of registered occupational therapists. However, Royeen and Coutinho (1991) claimed that occupational therapists lack a basic understanding of special education issues within the school setting. Understanding the school setting enables occupational therapists to more effectively identify their roles in relation to teachers and other school staff members (Niehues, Bundy, Mattingly, & Lawlor, 1991). Niehues et al. suggested that occupational therapists need preparation before they begin working in schools. Coutinho and Hunter (1988) emphasized that occupational therapists must know the laws governing occupational therapy services in schools and understand how the school system operates in order to become part of that setting. They also indicated that occupational therapists who work in schools must have the interpersonal skills necessary to communicate effectively with teachers and parents. Communication difficulties created by the lack of a common language between occupational therapists and educators may preclude occupational therapists from understanding special education issues and from establishing effective working relationships (Coutinho & Hunter, 1988). Kaplan and Porway (1988) have urged occupational therapists who are planning to work in schools to obtain supervised, practical experience in the school setting before taking such a job. Fieldwork opportunities that prepare occupational therapy students for school-based practice are central to their educational needs (L. Jackson, personal communication, March 15, 1994; Whitworth, 1994). The Pediatric Curriculum Committee described pediatric Level II fieldwork as essential to preparing occupational therapists for entry-level practice (AOTA, 1991a).

Despite the emphasis in the literature on the need for preparation, the lack of fieldwork opportunities in the school setting limits the number of occupational therapy students who are able to gain the necessary experience.

In a random survey of 250 occupational therapists working in pediatrics, only 18.6% had completed a Level II fieldwork experience in a school system (AOTA, 1991a). Although the number of fieldwork sites in schools is increasing, the increase lags far behind projections for the number of occupational therapists who will be employed in schools (L. Jackson, personal communication, March 15, 1994; C. Rogers, personal communication, March 22, 1994).

Exploratory Study

To prepare to establish new fieldwork sites in schools for occupational therapy students at the University of New Hampshire, we conducted an exploratory study of occupational therapists who worked in schools within the university's primary fieldwork region. Through the study we obtained basic information about school-based occupational therapy practice and occupational therapists' fieldwork supervisory needs. We later used this information to develop components of a model that would be used to increase the number of school-based fieldwork opportunities for occupational therapy students.

Names of occupational therapists working in schools were obtained by contacting each school district in the state of New Hampshire as well as the area within a 100-mile radius of the University of New Hampshire that covered southwestern Maine and northeastern Massachusetts, including the greater Boston area ($N = 237$). An 8-page questionnaire was designed for the study to: (a) obtain an overview of school-based occupational therapy practice that we could use both to prepare students for practice and to help supervisors prepare for a fieldwork student, (b) identify the fieldwork supervisory needs of occupational therapists working in schools, and (c) identify occupational therapists who had experience supervising fieldwork students in schools. The questionnaire, along with a cover letter that explained how the data obtained would be used, was sent to the 237 occupational therapists working in schools; a reminder card was sent 2 weeks later. Of the 237 questionnaires sent, 119 were returned complete enough for analysis. We continued our exploratory study by interviewing 12 of the 23 occupational therapists in the region who indicated that they had supervised fieldwork students in schools. Our goal was to discover how they overcame obstacles to fieldwork in schools and how they juggled the responsibilities of fieldwork supervision with practice.

School-Based Occupational Therapy Practice

The questionnaire asked the respondents to provide (a) their employment arrangement with the school district (i.e., direct, independent, or agency contract), (b) the number of hours they worked in school districts, (c) their activities during a typical work week, (d) the number of

Table 1
Terms of Employment in School-Based Occupational Therapy Practice

Term of Employment	Number	Percent
Hired directly by school district	55	44
Independent contract (private practice)	30	24
Contract from outside agency	41	32

Note. $N = 126$. Some of the 119 respondents worked in more than one school district and answered questions for each district in which they worked.

children in their caseloads, (e) the sites for therapy, and (f) the frequency of their communication with other occupational therapists working in schools.

Analysis of the data (see Tables 1 through 3) revealed that the respondents were hired through a variety of arrangements and that they worked from a few hours to full time. Most worked the equivalent of 3 to 5 school days. Ninety percent of the respondents were not responsible for school duties such as lunch, bus, or recess. Most of their time was spent providing one-to-one treatment, group treatment, or assessment. Respondents reported seeing an average of 22 children per week (interquartile range: 13 to 30 children per week). Most of the respondents had weekly to monthly contact with other school occupational therapists.

Fieldwork Supervisory Needs

One section of the questionnaire contained a list of 20 perceived fieldwork supervisory need statements derived from studies by Christie, Joyce, and Moeller (1985) and Cohn and Frum (1988) as well as from concerns that we identified as specific to the school setting as a fieldwork site. Respondents indicated whether each item would be Very Helpful, Somewhat Helpful, or Not Necessary to becoming a fieldwork supervisor or to helping them become a better fieldwork supervisor. Fifteen of the 20 items were identified as Very Helpful or Somewhat Helpful by more than 60% of the respondents.

Table 2
Time Allotments in School-Based Occupational Therapy Practice

Factor	Range	Mean
Number of hours worked in school district	5–42	25
Number of children seen per week	0–99	22
Hours spent per week in occupational therapy activities		
Direct treatment: one-to-one	0–35	7.8
Direct treatment: group	0–21	4.5
Assessment	0–14	2.5
Consultation	0–8	1.1
Meetings	0–8	1.8
Travel	0–10	1.4
Documentation	0–9	2.1

Note. $N = 126$. Some of the 119 respondents worked in more than one school district and answered questions for each district in which they worked.

Table 3
Frequency of School-Based Occupational Therapists'
Communication With Other School-Based Occupational
Therapists

Frequency	Number	Percent
Daily	5	4
Twice per week	14	11
Once per week	21	17
Twice per month	29	23
Once per month	25	20
Seldom	32	25

Note. N = 126. Some of the 119 respondents worked in more than one school district and answered questions for each district in which they worked.

A panel of seven occupational therapy educators, three of whom had experience as academic fieldwork coordinators, analyzed and categorized the 15 items by the type of information that they addressed (see Table 4). This panel identified three categories of needs: (a) *general fieldwork needs*, which are common to most new fieldwork supervisors, included issues related to establishing and implementing a fieldwork program, (b) *administrative-logistical needs*, which are more specific to occupational therapists working in schools, included issues related to the school setting and to service delivery, and (c) *supervisory skill needs*, which are common to most new fieldwork supervisors, included issues related to the interpersonal communication involved in supervising a fieldwork student.

Occupational Therapists With Experience Supervising Fieldwork Students in Schools

Of the 119 respondents, only 23 (19%) had supervised

Table 4
School Therapists' Fieldwork Supervision Needs

Need	Percent
General fieldwork needs	
Outline learning tasks for a student	89
Grade/evaluate student performance	87
Organize objectives for a student's learning experience	86
Know what students are capable of doing during fieldwork in schools	82
Be able to judge when a student can work independently	72
Decide whether work setting would provide a good learning experience	66
Administration/logistical needs	
Acquire more time to supervise students	81
Know liability coverage for fieldwork students in schools	80
Budget time so I do not have more work to take home	76
Learn how to combine supervising a student with providing treatment	73
Supervisory skill needs	
Deal with student problems	85
Provide clear explanations to student's questions	77
Give constructive feedback to a student	75
Develop my own supervisory style	75
Be confident in my supervisory abilities	71

Note. Percent refers to respondents who reported that the item would be Very Helpful or Somewhat Helpful in their fieldwork supervisory preparation.

Level II fieldwork students in a school setting. Telephone interviews with 12 of them provided information about how they first began supervising fieldwork students in schools, how their supervisory needs were met, and what level of success they perceived in the experience.

Five of the 12 respondents worked part time. All described their work setting as "typical school-based practice," in which they traveled between schools, used a variety of service delivery models, and worked independently of other occupational therapists. They did not see themselves (or their work scenarios) as different from other school-based therapists.

Five of the 12 respondents had shared supervisory responsibilities for a fieldwork student, 7 had been the student's only supervisor, and 1 worked in a school in which other occupational therapists also supervised a fieldwork student. All felt successful in their fieldwork supervisory experiences. When asked how they began supervising a fieldwork student, most respondents said that they had not sought out a fieldwork student. Several respondents worked in a school district in which previously employed occupational therapists had scheduled fieldwork students; others had been asked to do so by an academic fieldwork coordinator at a nearby university.

Respondents identified a variety of benefits to fieldwork supervision. They said that fieldwork students had a positive effect on their school administrator's attitude toward occupational therapy. They also described their own professional growth that resulted from the experience, saying fieldwork students "had new ideas," "refreshed my own knowledge," and "kept me alert by their thought-provoking questions." Respondents expressed a strong motivation to continue supervising fieldwork students and a strong belief that fieldwork in a school setting is essential preparation for practice in that setting.

School Fieldwork Model

On the basis of the information obtained from the questionnaires and interviews, we developed a model designed to increase fieldwork opportunities in schools. The process of developing fieldwork sites in schools consisted of four key components: (a) recruiting occupational therapists, (b) preparing occupational therapists for fieldwork supervision, (c) preparing occupational therapy students for school settings, and (d) supporting supervisors and students.

Recruiting Occupational Therapists

To select potential fieldwork supervisors, we considered occupational therapists' interest in supervising a student (as expressed on the questionnaires), the school administration's willingness to support the supervisor and the student as needed, and the school's geographic location.

We contacted potential fieldwork supervisors by telephone and explored their concerns, their needs, and the administrative support available to them for fieldwork supervision. Respondents expressed concerns about four primary issues:

1. *Part-time work.* Several respondents questioned how they could supervise fieldwork students when they themselves only worked part time. We resolved this concern by helping them establish shared supervision responsibilities and offering them guidance in the selection of a colleague with whom they could share supervision tasks.

2. *Liability.* Several respondents expressed concern that they would be responsible for professional liability because fieldwork students would not have coverage to work in schools. We informed them that the students carried their own malpractice insurance through a university group policy and that practice liability was no different in schools than in other settings.

3. *Student learning opportunities.* Respondents who worked with children with a wide range of disabilities (from a mild learning disability to severe multiple impairments) were concerned about the lack of consistent caseloads for fieldwork students. They also were concerned because they did not see all the children on a regular basis, as frequency was determined by a child's individual education plan (IEP), thus students would lack continuity in learning. To address these concerns, we discussed the importance for fieldwork students to broaden their knowledge and skills by working with a greater number of children of different abilities and providing services to more children per week.

4. *Service delivery methods.* Many respondents, who consult with classroom teachers and work in classrooms with the teachers, expressed reservations regarding sufficient opportunity for fieldwork students to provide direct services with children. We helped occupational therapists recognize that experience using multiple service delivery models and skills in consulting and communicating with other staff members are precisely what fieldwork students need to become effective in working in schools.

Once their initial concerns were addressed, most respondents were interested in the possibility of supervising a fieldwork student. At this point we explained our school fieldwork model to them. We discussed the benefits that a fieldwork student might bring to them and their schools. We also sent written information about the fieldwork model to them and to their respective school administrators in order to help them make a final decision about whether to supervise a fieldwork student.

Preparing Occupational Therapists for Fieldwork Supervision

Twenty-nine occupational therapists agreed to become fieldwork supervisors for this project. Of these 29 participants, 27 completed a 2-day seminar before receiving a student for a fieldwork rotation. The 2 participants who were unable to attend either of the two scheduled seminars received seminar information during a 1-day meeting with a seminar faculty member. Through didactic learning, group discussion, and experiential activities, the seminar faculty members (the authors and guest presenters) provided theoretical and practical information to help participants develop and implement fieldwork programs in their schools.

We helped participants with their general fieldwork needs by providing them with guided practice in writing, help in organizing objectives and outlining learning tasks for their fieldwork students, and assistance in evaluating student performance. We also helped them define the role of fieldwork supervisor. We assisted participants with their administrative/logistical needs by helping them articulate the benefits that fieldwork students bring to children with special needs and to personnel in their schools. Participants explored creative ways to provide timely supervision to fieldwork students without disrupting service delivery in the schools. We helped participants with their supervisory skill needs by offering role-playing activities, in which they practiced providing clear explanations to possible fieldwork student questions, dealing with problems, giving constructive feedback, and developing effective supervisory styles.

During the seminar, participants examined the school-based occupational therapy practice activities in which they took part and used developmental learning theory to identify beginning, intermediate, and advanced level competencies for those activities. Participants then used these competencies to develop learning objectives for fieldwork students in their setting.

Preparing Fieldwork Students for School Settings

The 25 fieldwork students in this study had taken the courses required in the occupational therapy curriculum for pediatric practice. These courses provided information on social-emotional child development and neurodevelopmental evaluation and treatment. In addition, students who had requested a fieldwork experience in a school took a required half-semester seminar that was designed to prepare them for the school setting. This seminar emphasized communicating and working effectively in the school environment.

The seminar provided students with information about the unique features of the educational system, the laws governing occupational therapy services in schools, and the roles and limitations of occupational therapists in this setting (Coutinho & Hunter, 1988; Niehues et al., 1991; Royeen & Coutinho, 1991). Students examined the roles of other school staff members and the relationship between these staff members and the occupational therapist. The seminar emphasized the influence of the classroom environment on service delivery and program planning (Griswold, 1994). Consultation skills and communication in terms that educators could understand were highlighted as essential components of effective occupational therapy practice in schools.

The seminar included lectures, group discussions, and group activities. Parts of the videotape series, *Related Services in the Public Schools* (Gilfoyle, 1985), were used to broaden students' understanding of school-based occupational therapy practice. Student activities included a mock IEP meeting, a debate of the advantages and disadvantages of different service delivery models, the writing of an IEP, and the transcription of occupational therapy goals and activities into educationally relevant concepts.

Providing Support to Supervisors and Students

Support has been identified as a need by fieldwork supervisors (Christie et al., 1985). Responses to our questionnaire confirmed this need. In our fieldwork model, support for supervisors began with the initial contact for recruitment, in which we responded to participants' questions. Multiple contacts were made to confirm participation in and provide information about the supervisor seminar. After the seminar, we called supervisors to relay student information and answer their questions as they began to develop their fieldwork programs. Throughout the fieldwork experience, participating fieldwork supervisors and students were called several times. The telephone calls provided opportunities to answer questions that the supervisor or student had and to help them establish a better relationship with each other. We made fieldwork site visits to 16 of the 29 occupational therapists.

As part of the ongoing support offered during the fieldwork experience, supervisors and students attended a 1-day, midplacement seminar after completing 6 weeks of fieldwork. First, supervisors and students met in their respective groups to share experiences, formulate goals for the remainder of the fieldwork experience, and explore possible steps to meet these goals. Then, together, supervisors and students discussed how the fieldwork experience was influencing their views of school-based occupational therapy practice. Supervisors and students shared their assessments of the fieldwork experience up to this point and examined plans for the future on the basis of the goals each had written earlier in the seminar. The seminar also gave the fieldwork supervisors and students contact with their respective peers—an aspect which they claimed was especially helpful because alternative fieldwork sites, such as schools, generally provide

limited contact with other occupational therapists.

Outcomes

Both the fieldwork students and the fieldwork supervisors who participated in this model reported many benefits for themselves and for the school setting. The students reported that they gained clinical skills and a better understanding of the school environment as a practice setting. Students reported that this particular setting contributed greatly to their ability to organize their thoughts and actions while remaining adaptable and flexible. They said that they had more self-confidence because of the independence necessitated by the school setting. Students who had two supervisors believed they were at an advantage over students who had one supervisor because they experienced two different approaches to occupational therapy. Some students who had two supervisors were involved in two school districts, each with different personnel. These students reported that the experience broadened their perspective of school-based occupational therapy practice and enhanced their ability to identify an occupational therapist's role.

Several fieldwork supervisors said that helping the fieldwork students understand school-based occupational therapy practice aided in their own awareness of the setting. They said fieldwork students gave them a "fresh look at therapy in schools," provided new ideas for treatment activities, and enhanced their own knowledge base. As fieldwork students began to work independently with children, supervisors found they had more time for their own professional development, consultations with classroom teachers, and new program development. All supervisors agreed that fieldwork students asked thought-provoking, stimulating questions.

Supervisors also reported that a fieldwork student's presence had a positive effect on their school administrators' attitudes toward occupational therapy. Several special education directors wrote to the project faculty members to express their eagerness to continue offering fieldwork opportunities to students. They recognized the value in having an occupational therapy student offer creative ideas and enhance occupational therapy services. In several districts the students offered programming, such as developmental activities in a readiness classroom and a handwriting curriculum, that ended when they left the school. Administrators also saw the fieldwork students as potential employees who had entry-level skills specific to the school setting. Several special education directors requested the names of all the students who had completed fieldwork in schools for use in future job openings.

Discussion

This fieldwork model was developed for school systems

as an alternative to fieldwork settings that use a medical model. To establish fieldwork in this setting, we prepared students for fieldwork in the schools, recruited and prepared occupational therapists to serve as fieldwork supervisors, and supported supervisors during their first fieldwork supervision experience.

Although school-based occupational therapists had some fieldwork supervision needs specific to the school setting, most of their needs were identical to those previously identified by Christie et al. (1985) as typical of all first-time fieldwork supervisors. Because their fieldwork supervisory needs do not differ substantially from those of occupational therapists in other practice settings, we found it necessary to identify and address potential fieldwork supervisors' questions specific to their setting in relation to fieldwork and provide formal preparation. We went through a process of studying a practice setting and applying the information to a fieldwork model of supervisor recruitment and preparation, student preparation, and providing ongoing support. This process was viewed as successful by the fieldwork students, occupational therapy supervisors, and school administration. The process might be useful in expanding fieldwork opportunities in other alternative settings. ▲

Acknowledgments

We thank the occupational therapists and students who participated in this study, without whose risk-taking behavior the fieldwork model could not have been developed. We also thank Elizabeth Crepeau, PhD, OTR, former University of New Hampshire fieldwork coordinator, for her willingness to explore new fieldwork models and Maureen Neistadt, ScD, OTR, for editorial assistance and collegial support.

This project was funded by the U.S. Department of Education, Office of Special Education and Rehabilitation Services, Grant # G008730063. Portions of this paper were presented at the AOTA Annual Conferences in 1988 and 1989.

References

American Occupational Therapy Association. (1991a). *Guidelines for curriculum content in pediatrics.* Rockville, MD: Author.

American Occupational Therapy Association. (1991b). *1990 Member data survey.* Rockville, MD: Author.

Baum, C. M. (1986). "Stick to the knitting": Promoting performance through occupational therapy. In *Proceedings of Occupational Therapy Education: Target 2000* (pp. 66–71). Rockville, MD: American Occupational Therapy Association.

Christie, B. A., Joyce, P. C., & Moeller, P. L. (1985). Fieldwork experience, Part II: The supervisor's dilemma. *American Journal of Occupational Therapy, 39,* 675–681.

Cohn, E. S., & Frum, D. C. (1988). Fieldwork supervision: More education is warranted. *American Journal of Occupational Therapy, 42,* 325–327.

Coutinho, M. J., & Hunter, D. L. (1988). Special education and occupational therapy: Making the relationship work. *American Journal of Occupational Therapy, 42,* 706–712.

Gilfoyle, E. M. (Ed. & Producer). (1985). *Related services in the public schools* [videotape]. Fort Collins, CO: Colorado State University.

Griswold, L. A. S. (1994). Ethnographic analysis: A study of classroom environments. *American Journal of Occupational Therapy, 48,* 397–402.

Kaplan, L., & Porway, G. (1988). Letters to the Editor— Entry level education inadequate for practice in pediatrics. *American Journal of Occupational Therapy, 42,* 329–330.

Niehues, A. N., Bundy, A. C., Mattingly, C. F., & Lawlor, M. C. (1991). Making a difference: Occupational therapy in the public schools. *Occupational Therapy Journal of Research, 119,* 195–210.

Royeen, C. B., & Coutinho, M. (1991). The special education administrator's perspective. In W. Dunn (Ed.), *Pediatric occupational therapy: Facilitating effective service provision* (pp. 307–318). Thorofare, NH: Slack

Whitworth, J. E. (1994). The shortage of occupational therapy and physical therapy personnel in schools: Implications and actions. *American Journal of Occupational Therapy, 48,* 367–370.

Administration & Management

Special Interest Section Newsletter

Vol. 7, No. 1, March 1991
Published Quarterly by The American
Occupational Therapy Association, Inc.

Special Issue on Certified Occupational
Therapy Assistants

From the Editor

■ Marla Dittman, OTR/L

In addition to the American Occupational Therapy Association publications referenced elsewhere in this issue, there are five other Association publications that address the subject of certified occupational therapy assistants. They are as follows:

American Occupational Therapy Association. (1987). *Guidelines for occupational therapy services in home health.* Rockville, MD: Author.
American Occupational Therapy Association. (1989). Guide for supervision of occupational therapy personnel. In *Reference manual of the official documents of The American Occupational Therapy Association, Inc.* (pp. VII.1–VII.2). Rockville, MD: Author. (Original work published 1981)
American Occupational Therapy Association. (1989). *Guidelines for occupational therapy services in school systems* (2nd ed.). Rockville. MD: Author.
American Occupational Therapy Association. (1989). Standards of practice for occupational therapy. In *Reference manual of the official documents of The American Occupational Therapy Association, Inc.* (pp. IV.1–IV.3). Rockville MD: Author. (Original work published 1983)
American Occupational Therapy Association. (1990). Supervision guidelines for certified occupational therapy assistants. *American Journal of Occupational Therapy, 44,* 1089–1090.

This last paper summarizes the supervision requirements of a certified occupational therapy assistant as reflected in the existing Association documents.

In addition, I would like to remind you that your state Administration & Management Special Interest Section (A&MSIS) liaison can provide information about A&MSIS activities in your state and other states. Your state association president can identify your liaison if necessary. ■

Supervising the Occupational Therapy Assistant Student

■ Terry R. Hawkins, MPH, OTR

Why place an article on occupational therapy education in an administration and management newsletter? Perhaps the best reasons are that many managers and administrators receive their first exposure to certified occupational therapy assistants (COTAs) through an occupational therapy assistant student program, and that some managers reevaluate department job descriptions after working with occupational therapy assistant students. In this article, I assume that the reader knows basic supervision techniques, understands the basics of the supervision required for a student program, and knows the importance placed by our profession on fieldwork education. With these assumptions in place, this article will address some of the differences between programs for the occupational therapy student and programs for the occupational therapy assistant student.

Primary Role Differences

Before addressing the differences in the students, I will address the differences in the primary roles of those who have graduated from the different educational programs and have passed the certification examination. It is these differences that are the basis for the Essentials for Education on which education programs are either approved or accredited (American Occupational Therapy Association [AOTA], 1989a, 1989b). Just as the roles of the registered occupational therapist (OTR) and the COTA are different, the educational programs that train them are different, and the fieldwork components of their education must also be different. Table 1 shows the differences and similarities between the two levels of certified personnel in the profession of occupational therapy (Reed & Sanderson, 1983).

It is the differences within these roles that guide the student objectives that are used to define expectations during fieldwork. The new entry-level role delineation (AOTA, 1990) should help managers and administrators who previously experienced difficulty understanding the entry-level roles of the COTA and the OTR.

Writing the Objectives

Over the last few years I have found that fieldwork sites that were formerly reluctant to write objectives for students studying to be occupational therapists sometimes jump at the chance to write them for those studying to be occupational therapy assistants. In my opinion, this occurs because most fieldwork supervisors are OTRs and were educated as OTRs, and thus think they have a good idea of what the expectations are for future therapists. However, when providing a fieldwork experience for occupational therapy assistant students for the first time, it is the objectives that keep the supervisor and the students on track and prevent the blending of the professional roles. On two occasions I have had fieldwork supervisors tell me that after writing clear objectives for their occupational therapy assistant students they have gone back and rewritten the objectives for their occupational therapy students in a more complete and precise manner.

Managers of fieldwork centers that have only experienced COTAs on staff have reported difficulty writing fieldwork objectives for occupational therapy assistant students and job descriptions for entry-level COTAs. Their initial outcome objectives and job descriptions were geared to the experienced COTA rather than the entry-level COTA. Managers and administrators are acutely aware of the problems that occur when they write the same job description for both the entry-level staff member and the experienced staff member, whether it be a COTA or an OTR. The same applies to student objectives.

Another difficulty arises when student objectives for future occupational therapists are modified to fit a new program for future occupa-

2

Table 1
Performance Criteria[a]

Registered Occupational Therapist	Certified Occupational Therapy Assistant
Performs both as a team member and an independent practitioner	Performs as a team member
Organizes service programs in occupational therapy	Assists in the development of service programs
Performs assessments	Assists in assessments
Plans treatment	Assists in treatment planning
Implements treatment plans	Implements treatment plans under the direction of the therapist
Reassesses changes in performance	Reassesses changes in performance
Communicates results of intervention	Assists in communicating results of intervention
Participates in continuing education	Participates in continuing education

[a](Reed & Sanderson, 1983)

tional therapy assistants. In many cases, this modification works when the objectives are adjusted after study of the role delineation document; in other cases, incorrect assumptions are made about the duties and levels of expertise of different personnel because the objectives are modified without recourse to the role delineation document. I have found it interesting and somewhat discouraging to discover that many OTRs have not learned the differences between the role of the COTA and the role of the occupational therapy aide. (An aide is normally uncertified and is usually trained in-house by a clinician.) I have found it equally discouraging that there are still some OTRs who do not know the difference between the roles and educational backgrounds of the OTR and COTA. For assistance in writing student objectives, Crist's (1986) *Contemporary Issues in Clinical Education* is a valuable resource.

Inappropriate Expectations

During the 1988 Occupational Therapy Assistant Educational Program Directors' Meeting in San Antonio, Texas, a list of concerns was generated about the inappropriate expectations that the directors felt were being placed on their occupational therapy assistant students during Level II fieldwork experiences. The list has been greatly condensed for this article, but it shows problems that may be effectively eliminated by the use of appropriate objectives and job descriptions.

1. Two extremes are seen in the expectations of fieldwork supervisors regarding the testing of patients: (a) expecting occupational therapy assistant students to interpret tests, understand test design, and perform assessments for which they do not have the background, and (b) not allowing them to do any testing (and not respecting their skill level).
2. Occupational therapy assistant students are expected to develop an interview format for the patients and to do the interviews entirely by themselves.
3. Occupational therapy assistant students, with a minimum of 2 months' fieldwork, are expected to perform at the same level as occupational therapy students with 6 months of fieldwork. Problems arise in the areas of patient load, note-writing skills, presentations, and level of expertise on treatment plans.

4. Fieldwork supervisors tend to forget that an occupational therapy assistant student should have an assistant's entry-level knowledge base concerning functional skills, not an OTR's.
5. Supervisors often fail to understand that, for many, the occupational therapy assistant degree is a chosen terminal professional goal. Supervisors should respect this level of training, and should be careful with comments like, "You're smart; why are you just becoming a COTA?"
6. Inappropriate expectations are often placed on the occupational therapy assistant student when writing research papers and papers for presentations. The papers need to focus on functional symptoms, behaviors, and responses related to the patient, rather than on theory.
7. In the area of splinting, the expectations for occupational therapy assistant students should be competence with static splints only.
8. Expectations regarding neurodevelopmental treatment, proprioceptive neuromuscular facilitation, sensory integration techniques, and so on are at times inappropriate because the students do not have the necessary background.
9. Fieldwork supervisors should respect the activity background of students but should address activity in the universal sense, not just in the area of crafts.
10. Supervision of occupational therapy assistant students in sites where occupational therapy students are also being trained should be collaborative (e.g., occupational therapy assistant students could be responsible for administering functional evaluations, and occupational therapy students could be responsible for interpreting the results).
11. Occupational therapy assistant students are sometimes expected to not just run a group but to develop a group independently. This is not appropriate, especially if the group is theory based (as with a stress management group, for example).

Conclusion

In summary, it is important to remember that fieldwork objectives, as well as job descriptions, must be written at the level that is right for the person being trained or employed. A successful fieldwork experience or work experience is dependent upon this strategy. The manager's job is made easier, and thus more rewarding, when success is gained by the student or the employee. ∎

References

American Occupational Therapy Association. (1989a). Essentials and guidelines of an accredited educational program for the occupational therapist. In *Reference manual of the official documents of The American Occupational Therapy Association, Inc.* (pp. II.1–II.5). Rockville, MD: Author.
American Occupational Therapy Association. (1989b). Essentials and guidelines of an approved educational program for the occupational therapy assistant. In *Reference manual of the official documents of The American Occupational Therapy Association, Inc.* (pp. II.7–II.11). Rockville, MD: Author.
American Occupational Therapy Association. (1990). Entry-level role delineation for registered occupational therapists (OTRs) and certified occupational therapy assistants (COTAs). *American Journal of Occupational Therapy, 44,* 1091–1102.
Crist, P. A. (1986). *Contemporary issues in clinical education.* Thorofare, NJ: Slack.
Reed, K. L., & Sanderson, S. R. (1983). *Concepts of occupational therapy.* Baltimore: Williams & Wilkins.

Terry R. Hawkins, MPH, OTR, is Chair of the Occupational Therapy Assistant Program, Pueblo Community College, Pueblo, Colorado.

The Successful Fieldwork Student: Supervisor Perceptions

Georgiana L. Herzberg

Key Words: learning style

Qualitative research methodology was used to explore supervisor perceptions of learning style characteristics required for student success in fieldwork. A focus discussion group was used to elicit success themes identified by clinicians. These themes were compared to learning style themes previously identified in quantitative studies. Techniques of conversation analysis were used to assess congruence of verbalized themes with participant interactions during the discussion group. Themes that emerged were the importance of teamwork, active experimentation, flexibility, adaptability, and doing. Discussion participants actively modeled teamwork.

(Editor's note: At the time of publication of *The Fieldwork Anthology* in January 1998, the author is completing her PhD dissertation at the Center for the Study of Higher and Postsecondary Education at the University of Michigan, Ann Arbor, Michigan.)

Georgiana L. Herzberg, MA, OTR, is Senior Lecturer, Wayne State University, College of Pharmacy and Allied Health Professions, Department of Occupational Therapy, Detroit, Michigan 48202.

This article was accepted for publication October 12, 1993.

Supervisor perceptions of the successful fieldwork student are an important area for research. Supervisors are the gatekeepers who maintain the quality standards of the profession by providing professional socialization and by acting as role models. Student supervisors reinforce and operationalize the norms of inquiry and sphere of practice of the profession. Professional socialization enhances the *fit* of the person within a profession—the embracing of the values, norms, and interests of the profession—which contributes to the retention and personal satisfaction of that person. In occupational therapy, issues of increased retention and decreased burnout are of critical importance. With increasing demands for occupational therapy services, rising costs associated with the provision of services, and rising education costs, the fit of the person with the profession becomes more critical.

Quantitative research on the learning styles of clinicians and students has begun to explore the issue of fit (Baker & Marks, 1981; Barris, Kielhofner, & Bauer, 1985; Blagg, 1985; Cahill & Madigan, 1984; Fox, 1984; Hayden & Brown, 1985; Katz, 1990; Katz & Heimann, 1991; Markert, 1986; Stafford, 1986; Wilson, 1986). The qualitative study described in this article expands on the previous work by examining the clinical supervisors' perceptions of the learning characteristics of the successful occupational therapy student.

In this study, a focus discussion group with supervisors from the practice areas of physical disabilities and mental health was held at a large, urban medical center in the Midwest. Qualitative research techniques associated with ethnographic studies and conversation analysis were used to analyze the ensuing videotape for themes, frequency of characteristics mentioned, and interactive behavior among clinicians that reflected the themes. Recommendations are made for further study based on the hypotheses generated by this study.

Cultural Categories

In qualitative research, the cultural categories identified through a literature review and an examination of researcher foreknowledge provide a reference point for hypothesis generation in the analysis phase of the study. In this study, the terminology and concepts of Kolb's Learning Style Inventory (LSI) (Kolb, 1976, 1985) were used to identify learning characteristics expressed and demonstrated by the student supervisors. A review of the literature identified the LSI as the most commonly documented in research with occupational therapists and students. The learning style characteristics described in the LSI fall along two axes and allow some comparisons with the constructs of other learning style inventories. One LSI axis represents a continuum of behavioral preferences from concrete experience to abstract conceptualization. The intersecting axis represents a preferential continuum from active experimentation behaviors to reflective observation behaviors. Kolb (1984) found a strong correlation between career choice and expressed preferences for personal learning styles along these axes. He hypothesized that a person's learning style influences the initial selection of a profession and is accentuated as the person learns the profession's norms.

Literature Review

The Kolb (1976, 1985), Rezler (Rezler & French, 1975), and Canfield and Lafferty (Canfield, 1974) learning style and learning preference inventories have been used to categorize learning preferences in allied health programs. Kolb's LSI has been used in several studies with occupational therapy students. Katz (1990) concluded that occupational therapy students with learning styles compatible with faculty teaching methods did better on examinations with less study time than students whose styles were incompatible with those teaching methods. Katz and Heimann (1991) found that first-year students in occupational therapy programs had varied learning styles but that occupational therapists working in the field emphasized the active experimentation learning mode over reflective observation in the treatment setting. Stafford (1986) found that an active experimentation learning style was the single best predictor of occupational therapy student success in Level II physical disabilities fieldwork. Cahill and Madigan (1984), using the Kolb LSI and the Rezler–French Learning Preference Inventories at two points in time, systematically exposed students to different modes of instruction and identified no statistically significant differences in student learning preferences between the two times. They concluded that faculty members' efforts to provide varying methods of instruction were warranted because the individual learning styles of their students did not change significantly and because varying presentation methods maximized educational opportunities for all students.

The Rezler Learning Preference Inventory was used in two additional studies that included occupational therapy students as subjects. Rezler and French (1975) explored differences in learning styles of students in six undergraduate, preprofessional allied health programs and found that students of all of these professions indicated a preference for teacher-structured, practice-oriented learning experiences dealing with concrete, technical competencies rather than the abstract, theory-based aspects of course content. Rogers and Hill (1980) found preferences in both bachelor's and master's level occupational therapy students for teacher-structured, concrete, interpersonal learning activities. A preference for abstraction on the Rezler Learning Preference Inventory was consistently related to higher academic achievement in these student cohort groups. A similar preference for teacher-structured, experiential learning was identified by Llorens and Adams (1978), who used the Canfield–Lafferty Learning Styles Instrument with occupational therapy students at the University of Florida.

Role of Researcher Foreknowledge

Professional practice can be described as a normative enterprise with a goal of wise action in a specific situation. Occupational therapists use theoretical knowledge to focus on changing environments, skills, or attitudes to allow clients to function in ways that are considered normal or average. Occupational therapists minimize differences and dysfunction by making wise (theory-based) decisions. Consideration of the social contexts of treatment to improve functional performance forms the basis for our clinical reasoning and the rationale for our use of purposeful activity. Reflection on my own practice provides the basis for these statements and the foreknowledge for this study.

Swinehart and Meyers (1993), in their comparisons of clinician, student, and faculty member purposes for Level I fieldwork, provide empirical support for my intuitive perspective. Among all three groups, the purpose of fieldwork was described as "apply hands-on treatment" (clinicians), "apply theory to practice" (students), and "learn by doing" (faculty) (p. 69). With their clients, occupational therapists formulate and implement plans for the clients to maintain or regain functional independence and personal satisfaction. Occupational therapists create opportunities during the fieldwork experiences to allow students to learn the normative ways of occupational therapy in making theory-based treatment decisions.

Hypothesis Generation Based on Cultural Categories

From the literature and reflection on foreknowledge, themes related to active experimentation and doing were expected to emerge in this study. It was also expected that the clinicians would identify the learning characteristics of successful students as those characteristics that they themselves demonstrated in their interaction in the focus group.

Observation Design

Participants

A large, urban hospital was selected for this study to provide perspectives from supervisors of students in mental health and physical disabilities. The facility selected has a teaching mission, in addition to the mission of providing health care services, and has an active training program for occupational therapy students at both the technical and professional levels. Eight occupational therapists, whose experience ranged from 3 to 12 years, agreed to participate in the focus discussion group of this study. All had supervised students. As a registered and practicing occupational therapy educator, I led the discussion group; another researcher with no health care background videotaped the discussions. Of the discussion group members, 4 persons (including myself) represented the practice area of mental health, and 5 persons represented the practice area of physical disabilities.

Table 1 summarizes participant information in order of interaction in the subsection of text analyzed. The table identifies the current involvement of participants with the academic and the clinical preparation of students and the years of each participant's experience as an occupational therapist.

Setting

The discussion group was conducted during one lunch hour in the hospital's occupational therapy clinic where persons with physical disabilities are treated. Although the clinic itself is organized around the storage and use of functional equipment and illustrative charts, the single room providing staff member office space is crowded with personal objects, professional projects, and pictures of families, colleagues, and friends.

In the transcript of the videotape, a participant described this space by saying, "This is our home." Another stated, "It's your job, but I mean, you're here more than you're at home so you may as well enjoy it." Although client treatment is provided in the clinic and the clinic functions as a home base for the occupational therapists practicing in physical disabilities (who also provide services on various floors of the hospital), the clinic also serves as a meeting room and departmental home base for occupational therapists practicing in both mental health and physical disabilities. The personal and individually meaningful objects (e.g., photographs, small hobby projects, greeting cards, pictures, equipment uniquely adapted to address a client's need) that the participants have brought to the clinic office setting create a physical and psychological environment that reflects openness and willingness to share oneself with one's colleagues. The personalized, sharing nature of the physical environment supports and validates use of the word *home* to describe the setting. The use of *home* as a descriptive term carries with it the implicit assertion of family, which implies collaboration.

Discussion Structure

Discussion questions to provide focus and reflect the research question were constructed with a funnel sequence (moving from general to specific questions). These questions served as a guide, rather than as a rigid structure, for the discussion. The beginning focus was broad and was intended to gather information regarding participant perceptions of the work environment by asking about participants' current jobs. As the focus of the discussion narrowed, with questions such as, "What are the characteristics of students who have done well in your settings?", the researcher used probes such as, "Can you illustrate your point with a story about one of your students?" to encourage narrative accounts of specific examples. The group was videotaped and audiotaped to ensure adequate sound recording for transcription and verification of dialogue.

Analysis

Participants' speech behaviors were analyzed for themes about learning characteristics used by successful students and for themes of supervisor preferences. The identified themes were correlated with the word choices of the Kolb LSI on the abstract–concrete and the active–reflective continuua of response patterns (Kolb, 1985). In the LSI, a preference for concrete experiences is expressed in word choices that reflect a personal, involved, feeling response (e.g., "I am an intuitive person") whereas a preference for abstract conceptualization is expressed in word choices that emphasize an analytical approach (e.g., "I rely on logical thinking"). The active experimentation preference is expressed by action-oriented word choices (e.g., "I learn best from a chance to try out and practice"). Reflective observation is emphasized in an impartial, observational approach (e.g., "I take my time before acting"). (Examples given are representative of the choices available on the 1985 version of the LSI.) The frequency of the themes in the participants' speech was then tabulated.

A representational section of the transcript, selected

Table 1
Focus Discussion Group Participants

Subject	Practice Area	Experience as Occupational Therapy Practitioner (yrs)	Current University Involvement
G.H. — white woman	Psychiatry	27	Faculty member
A.J. — white woman	Physical disabilities	12	Guest lecturer
C.R. — black woman	Psychiatry	is certified occupational therapy assistant	Student
K.B. — white woman	Physical disabilities	3	None
A.C. — white woman	Physical disabilities	4	None
L.M. — white woman	Psychiatry	10	Guest lecturer
L.N. — white man	Physical disabilities	4	None
S.B. — black woman	Psychiatry	9	Guest lecturer
J.P. — Asian woman	Physical disabilities	3	None

Note. Presented in order of appearance in study subsection analyzed.

by its introductory question, was also analyzed for the turns and moves of interaction between the therapists. The transcript and videotape were used to examine and contrast participant speech acts with actual participant interactions. This analysis of participant interactions included evaluations of speaker sequence based on job role (occupational therapist, certified occupational therapy assistant, supervisory responsibility), length of experience, specialty area, and gender. It also included analysis of nonverbal communication indicating support or lack of support of the various speakers.

Results

Themes

The themes of doing, active experimentation, flexibility, adaptability, and teamwork first surfaced as the group identified the demands of occupational therapy practice in the urban medical center setting. These themes were reiterated in the narratives about students and in the narratives of the supervisor's role in facilitating student transition from the academic setting to the clinic. One participant stated, "That's what your clinical experience is for. It's to practice to learn new things — you know, practical things — on top of your theory," and the group members concurred nonverbally by nodding their heads. The participants emphasized this active experimentation learning style and discussed an effective, active experimentation learning style in terms of the resources required in this urban hospital setting: flexibility, adaptability, and teamwork. Participants stated that flexibility is required to do treatment ("Flexibility is the major demand . . . You have 30 seconds to get in there and make a splint in the operating room"). They also stated that it is required for team membership ("So we have to be flexible not only for [our] own time but respect each other's wishes and [help] out too"). Adaptability, according to statements, is required in structuring time ("You have to prioritize what you need to do"), setting ("The rest of the population is quite ill so they have to be seen bedside upstairs in the hospital"), and treatment approach ("We end up changing the whole total plan on what we intend doing with the group because of the [mental illness] level of the patients"). Teamwork is a way of life for these participants in both the physical disabilities and mental health practice areas. ("We try to team to do as much as we can for the patient while they are here"; "So we [occupational therapy staff members] have to have pretty open communication of what's going on and [communicate] with other staff members [psychiatrists and social workers] too.")

Expressed Preferences and Description of Turns and Moves

When participants were asked how they teach people to be occupational therapists in the clinic, their preferences

for specific learning characteristics clearly related to themes of doing, active experimentation, flexibility, adaptability, and teamwork. This section of the videotape was analyzed for turns and moves (initiation, exchange, and identification of preferred or nonpreferred goal-directed response patterns) of clinician interactions. Identification of these elements allowed evaluation of congruence between participants' verbally identified themes and participants' actions.

The section of the videotape begins, after a 7-sec pause in group discussion, with the discussion leader–researcher, G. H., acknowledging the effect of the wide variety and quantity of demands placed on clinicians in this setting and the effect of these demands on student training. The comment provoked appreciative laughter from the group and a response from the most senior clinician, A. J., who stated, "We had a wonderful discussion about this just recently amongst ourselves." She went on to describe her perception that students encounter difficulty when they make the transition from the structured and primarily passive learning of the academic setting to the active learning required in the clinical setting. She described the need for active experimentation by students and flexibility and adaptability in the often confusing, rapid-paced clinic setting, a setting that requires constant awareness of treatment objectives and willingness to reorganize treatment priorities. She identified the role of the clinical supervisor as promoting active involvement of the students ("We try to get the students to interact"), allowing the students to make mistakes ("They have to learn that way to see what they did wrong"), and watching carefully to maintain quality of care standards for patients ("We watch them very carefully so that patient care is not substituted [compromised] by that [mistake]"). All of these actions are part of a hypothesis of doing. She then checked for group consensus by looking around the room and asking, "Any of us feel any different on that?"

The most junior member of the group, C. R., responded immediately by establishing her credentials as the person most in touch with student issues. (She is both an employee and a student.) The group acknowledged this fact with supportive laughter. C. R. supported A. J., named her specifically (indicating teamwork), and stated, "Applying the knowledge is the most important thing."

K. B. responded, again without an obvious pause between speakers, to identify the theme of teamwork and the need to learn from other group members. She also talked about the decreased emphasis in the clinic setting on the common student focus of grades. She reiterated A. J.'s points by stating that there is no "spoon feeding in the clinic" and that students need to try to become more actively involved and to trust their supervisors to "pick up the pieces." She then identified and built on the idea of being open to new learning opportunities for information not taught in school by using the resources of other team members.

Participant A. C. immediately supported K. B. and clarified the role of the school as providing "background and theory" and the role of the clinic as a place "to learn new things—you know, practical things—on top of your theory" and restated A. J.'s hypothesis of doing. She concurred with K. B. that there is often a problem with student openness to new learning, stating, "They think that maybe something's wrong with them because they don't know that already." Participant L. M., the director of the occupational therapy department, followed up this statement with an elaboration of the different learning opportunities that have been available for staff members and students in the last year and the importance of "allowing yourself" to be open to new experiences.

An announcement was broadcast over the public address system at this time and, in typical hospital fashion, everyone ignored it after determining that it did not apply to them. During the announcement, eye contact did increase with the speaker, L. M., who stated that students sometimes "come in with an attitude—not wanting to let you know that they don't know . . . and that doesn't work in a setting like this." The clinicians, all of whom had been engaged at various times in nonverbal support of the various speakers, nodded vigorously at her statements.

Participant A. J. took the next turn and returned to K. B.'s statements about students' focus on grades and emphasized that the person with the best grades is not necessarily the best clinician. This again met with considerable nonverbal support from the group and a rapid response from L. N., the only man in the group. He supported A. J. by stating that worrying about grades detracts from what the student is really learning. He specifically identified K. B. as the originator of this idea. The group was strongly supportive of L. N. and provided several appreciative laughs and overlapping comments to his remarks.

For the first time, an identifiable pause of no longer than 1 sec occurred before the next speaker, S. B., began. She introduced the possible conclusion that the student may be psychologically uncomfortable in the clinic setting and that this is why he or she is unable to admit to gaps in knowledge. S. B. suggested that professional responsibility includes being able to admit that you do not know everything but that you are open to learning. S. B. recommended that this need be addressed in the classroom before students begin their clinical work. The group agreed nonverbally with this (by nodding, increasing eye contact, and smiling) and there was a 4-sec pause, which indicated closure to the current exploration of this topic. During this sequence J. P. did not speak, but the videotape revealed that, of all the group members, she communicated most extensively nonverbally to indicate agreement and support of the various speakers.

In the videotape, these participants come across as

so team-oriented that they appear almost able to finish each other's thoughts and sentences. The pauses apparent in the normal conversation of groups (Nofsinger, 1991) that would indicate opportunities to take turns did not exist for this group. At no point in the videotape do two or more persons overlap speech, although more than three group members overlap on four occasions in nonverbal and verbal concurrence with the speaker. Eye contact by the speaker or by the researcher does not appear to influence turn-taking, nor does proximity to the speaker. Turn-taking appears unrelated to practice area, status (based on length of experience), or the length or sequence of turns. The group's focus was on expressing jointly held beliefs as opposed to individual opinions. Such expression met with active, concurrent, nonverbal group support and verbal recognition by subsequent speakers. Participant behaviors in the focus discussion corresponded very closely with their expressed beliefs on the importance of teamwork.

Frequency of Themes

When the transcript was analyzed for concept frequency along the two LSI axes, active experimentation was overwhelmingly the preferred mode of behavior. Of 31 transcribed paragraphs that specifically addressed clinician roles, student roles, or descriptions of behaviors in the clinic, 18 paragraphs described active experimentation modes of behavior. When these paragraphs were analyzed for verbs associated with the LSI continuua, it was found that action verbs (e.g., *do, apply, practice, perform, give,* and *adapt*) occurred with much greater frequency (52% of the time) than verbs related to the concepts of concrete experience (29%), reflective observation (11%), or abstract conceptualization (8%).

Discussion

A limitation of qualitative research is that an in-depth analysis of a specific situation compromises the validity of generalizing the results to other populations and settings. The participants in this setting demonstrated behavior in the focus discussion group that was highly congruent with their verbally identified success themes for students.

The participants demonstrated, as well as discussed, the importance of teamwork by building upon each other's ideas, giving credit verbally to other team members, and using eye contact and body language to indicate recognition and support. Speakers never appeared surprised at the quantity, quality, or source of support. In fact, support was so accepted and expected that it appeared to require no acknowledgment. Teamwork appears to be the norm for this group.

The themes of doing, active experimentation, flexibility, and adaptability are also clearly supported by the content analysis. Although the analysis of turns and moves demonstrates teamwork and not the other themes, a logical assumption is that this demonstration of teamwork among group members would not exist without a previous history of actions to support the expressed beliefs in flexibility, adaptability, and active experimentation in job performance. The learning characteristics that the clinicians indicated they prefer in students are characteristics that the clinicians did, in fact, model. They interacted as a unit rather than as individuals to build upon the ideas presented; they gave credit to each other; and their focus was one of cohesive functioning to provide as much insight as possible from complementary perspectives. This required that they listen to each other and compare the input with their own experiences. The nonverbal communication of the clinicians indicated shared perceptions through the use of nods, eye contact, and facial responses. These therapists, regardless of years of experience or practice area, concurred verbally and behaviorally on the importance of teamwork, active experimentation, flexibility, adaptability, and doing as professional norms for the urban medical center setting.

Kolb (1985) hypothesized that a person's learning style influences the initial selection of a profession and is accentuated as one learns the profession's norms. It is unknown whether these clinicians demonstrated or expressed preferences for an active experimentation learning style before their professional training. They accentuate it now in words and actions. The degree of congruence between words and actions leads one to believe that they will express the importance of active experimentation and model it for their students.

Conclusion

This study triangulates content analysis of participant statements with observation of participant interactions and the findings of quantitative studies on learning characteristics of occupational therapists and occupational therapy students. Katz and Heimann (1991) found that clinicians emphasized an active experimentation learning style in the treatment setting. Stafford (1986) found that an active experimentation learning style was the best predictor of student success in Level II fieldwork. The working hypothesis generated in this study was that themes related to active experimentation and doing would emerge as normative, preferred learning characteristics for students. This hypothesis was supported by the analysis. An additional hypothesis was that the fieldwork supervisors would identify the learning characteristics of successful students as those characteristics that they themselves demonstrated in their interaction in the focus group context. This hypothesis was also supported. The themes that emerged from this analysis to provide a profile of preferred learning characteristics of a successful student were teamwork, active experimentation, flexibility, adaptability, and doing.

It is the extensiveness of these shared perceptions of desired characteristics in this clinic that provides insights into the occupational therapy profession and reinforces the need for research on professional socialization. In this clinic setting, the team is so valued that persons who do not share the norms, values, and interests related to doing, active experimentation, flexibility, adaptability, and teamwork would not be able to function there effectively. Future research on the importance of these themes in settings that do not carry the descriptors *urban* and *teaching hospital* would provide increased validity for generalizing the study's findings. Research on the fit of a person within the occupational therapy profession will also contribute to staff member retention and personal satisfaction.

Future directions for research include investigation of student perceptions of success characteristics and the comparison of therapist perceptions with student perceptions. Academic programs, which reinforce and reward abstract conceptualization and adherence to structure, may benefit from a reexamination of assignments and reward systems to facilitate the transition of the student to the doing, active experimentation demands of the clinic environment that require teamwork, adaptability, and flexibility. ▲

Acknowledgments

I thank the occupational therapy staff members at Detroit Receiving Hospital, Detroit, Michigan for their participation, enthusiasm, and support for this study, and Lea Allison, MA, for her assistance in data collection. ·

References

Baker, J. D., & Marks, W. E. (1981). Learning style analysis in anesthesia education. *Anesthesiology Review, 3*(7), 31–34.

Barris, R., Kielhofner, G., & Bauer, D. (1985). Learning preferences, values, and student satisfaction. *Journal of Allied Health, 14,* 13–23.

Blagg, J. D. (1985). Cognitive styles and learning styles as predictors of academic success in a graduate allied health education program, *Journal of Allied Health, 14,* 89–98.

Cahill, R., & Madigan, M. J. (1984). The influence of curriculum format on learning preference and learning style. *American Journal of Occupational Therapy, 38,* 683–686.

Canfield, A. A. (1974). *Manual for the Learning Styles Inventory.* Plymouth, MI: Experiential Learning Methods.

Fox, R. D. (1984). Learning styles and instructional preferences in continuing education for health professionals: A validity study of the LSI. *Adult Education Quarterly, 35,* 72–85.

Hayden, R. R., & Brown, M. S. (1985). Learning styles and correlates. *Psychological Reports, 56,* 243–246.

Katz, N. (1990). Problem solving ability and time needed to learn as functions of occupational therapy students' learning style and teaching methods. *Occupational Therapy Journal of Research, 10,* 1–15.

Katz, N., & Heimann, N. (1991). Learning style of students and practitioners in five health professions. *Occupational Therapy Journal of Research, 11,* 238–244.

Kolb, D. A. (1976). *The Learning Style Inventory: Technical manual.* Boston: McBer.

Kolb, D. A. (1984). *Experiential learning: Experience as a source of learning and development.* Englewood Cliffs, NJ: Prentice Hall.

Kolb, D. A. (1985). *Learning Styles Inventory.* Boston: McBer & Co.

Llorens, L. A., & Adams, S. P. (1978). Learning style preferences of occupational therapy students. *American Journal of Occupational Therapy, 32,* 161–164.

Markert, R. J. (1986). Learning style and medical students' performance on objective examinations. *Perceptual and Motor Skills, 62,* 781–782.

Nofsinger, R. E. (1991). *Everyday conversation.* Newbury Park, CA: Sage.

Rezler, A. G., & French, R. M. (1975). Personality types and learning preferences of students in six allied health professions. *Journal of Allied Health, 4,* 20–26.

Rogers, J. C., & Hill, D. J. (1980). Learning style preferences of bachelor's and master's students in occupational therapy. *American Journal of Occupational Therapy, 34,* 789–793.

Stafford, E. M. (1986). Relationship between occupational therapy student learning styles and clinic performance. *American Journal of Occupational Therapy, 40,* 34–39.

Swinehart, S., & Meyers, S. (1993). Level I fieldwork: Creating a positive experience. *American Journal of Occupational Therapy, 47,* 68–73.

Wilson, D. K. (1986). An investigation of the properties of Kolb's learning style inventory. *Leadership and Organization Development, 7,* 3–15.

To Fail or Not to Fail? A Course for Fieldwork Educators

Irene Ilott

Key Words: failure • fieldwork education, occupational therapy

Objective. *Assigning a failing grade to a student is one of the most important yet problematic responsibilities of a fieldwork educator, for it challenges both personal and professional values. This article describes and evaluates a 1-day course designed to prepare educators for this responsibility.*

Method. *The course was offered five times in 1989 and 1990 by the Derby School of Occupational Therapy, Derby, England, and was attended by 101 fieldwork educators. Surveys were administered to these educators immediately after the course and again 4 and 12 months later.*

Results. *Respondents reported increases in confidence and in their ability to differentiate between students' competence and incompetence. These changes were related to three factors: an understanding of the affective responses associated with a fail scenario, the reinforcement of effective methods of supervision, and the maintenance of professional standards.*

Conclusion. *It is recommend that the topic of failure be included in all fieldwork educator training courses.*

Irene Ilott, DipCOT, MEd, PhD, is Principal Lecturer, Derby School of Occupational Therapy, University of Derby, 138 Whitaker Road, Derby, DE23 6AP, United Kingdom.

This article was accepted for publication July 18, 1994.

Fieldwork educators are pivotal to the assessment of students' competence to practice. Their role as gatekeepers of the future quality of the occupational therapy profession is challenging under ordinary circumstances, but the demands that they face are exacerbated when a student's performance falls at the margins of competence. The process of judging that a student has not attained the required standard and should be assigned a failing grade is a costly, time consuming, and "emotionally taxing responsibility" (Meisenhelder, 1982, p. 348) that requires personal courage, professional integrity, and faculty member support. This article describes and evaluates a 1-day training course designed to prepare fieldwork educators for this responsibility.

Failure is a natural part of life, learning, and assessment—an expected outcome, albeit for a minority of students. It is inherent in the process of assessment, for the main function of the "teacher-as-judge" is differentiation of students' abilities to fulfill occupational roles (Geary, 1988, p. 242). Such assessments are particularly vital when they underpin licensure or registration that is intended to protect the public from incompetent, unsafe, or unscrupulous practitioners.

The difficulties associated with fail scenarios are well established in the literature. Retaining failing students and failing clinically unsatisfactory students were identified as the second and third highest stressors in a study of coping strategies among female baccalaureate nursing faculty members in Canada (Goldenberg & Waddall, 1990). Failing a student was ranked as the most problematic responsibility by two thirds of trained, experienced fieldwork educators in two surveys conducted at the Derby School of Occupational Therapy in 1988 and 1993 (Ilott, 1993). It is a responsibility that "presents an emotional struggle . . . and awareness of one's own fallibility" (Meisenhelder, 1982, p. 348) that can "debilitate those involved" (Carpenito, 1983, p. 32), as both student and educator feel "insufficient and powerless . . . like failures" (Turkett, 1987, p. 246). The fieldwork educator may also be "plagued with doubts" (Moeller, 1984, p. 208) if students are allowed to pass regardless of performance or if they secure passes through an inordinate amount of pastoral and academic support. Regardless of the outcome, an educator's decision-making process in regard to students who are at the margins of competence is characterized by "soul-searching" and self-interrogation (Ilott, 1990, p. 4). However, the process of assigning a failing grade has received scant attention. It seems to be a subject that is both taken for granted and taboo.

In response to these problems, the Derby School of Occupational Therapy planned a training course to prepare educators for this responsibility. The course aimed to challenge educators' negative assumptions about failure, to optimize the quality of their decision making during a difficult time, to reduce the incidence of their "failure to fail" students (Lankshear, 1990, p. 35), and to provide them with support during a "debilitating, emotionally draining experience" (Symanski, 1991, p. 18). The course supplemented existing supervisor training courses accredited by the College of Occupational Therapists. Its content was influenced by similar courses reported by Brozenec, Marshall, Thomas, and Walsh (1987) and Bradley (1990), and by additional suggestions from fieldwork educators and academic fieldwork coordinators.

The Derby School of Occupational Therapy offered the 1-day course five times in 1989–1990; a total of 101 fieldwork educators attended. After the course, these participants completed one immediate and two follow-up surveys that were designed to assess their opinions on the value of the course and on their incorporation of course material into their supervisory roles.

Course Aim, Objectives, and Program

The aim of the course was to explore the challenges and consequences—both personally and professionally—of failing an occupational therapy student on fieldwork practice.
This aim was supported by four objectives:

1. To identify criteria for student failure that educators could use in the assessment process.
2. To help educators appreciate a range of coping strategies.
3. To improve educators' understanding of the roles and responsibilities of the Derby School, the students, and themselves.
4. To provide educators with an opportunity to share experiences and exchange ideas.

The course simulated the natural sequence of an educator's decision making and action with a student whose performance falls at the margins of competence. It was divided into three sessions: morning and afternoon, in which participants were divided into small groups, and plenary.

The morning session began by placing the topic of failure within a personal, research context. The participants were then invited to react to a fieldwork educator's feelings about a fail scenario:

> It's been like a shadow hanging over me. It was 5 years ago and I still feel guilty. I felt awful—what had I ruined in just one afternoon; exhausted and put off having other students. All that effort, explaining to someone who was disinterested and making no effort to learn. I didn't gain anything.

Identifying the criteria for failure was the next part of the course. Participants were divided into groups that included participants both with and without experience in assigning a failing grade. Their tasks were to (a) introduce themselves and outline their experiences, and (b) compile a baseline—a minimum standard or checklist of behaviors, skills, and attitudes—that would constitute

student failure and differentiate between borderline and unsatisfactory performance.

After a 1-hr discussion, each group reported its criteria to the other participants. The opinions expressed in these presentations provided a springboard for the consideration of educational principles. These principles included the problems and benefits of subjective and objective aspects of assessment (Blomquist, 1985); the limitations of a causal theory of teaching, in which an educator accepts sole responsibility for learning outcomes (Ericson & Ellett, 1987); the contradictions in the dual role of counselor and assessor; the aspects of attribution theory related to the interplay between effort expenditure and ability level that influence feedback strategies and affective responses (Graham, 1984); and the conflicting values between the roles of educator and therapist. The morning session concluded with a comparison between the groups' criteria and the definition of unsafe practices in nursing, as defined by Darragh, Jacobsen, Sloan, and Sandquist (1986).

The afternoon session focused on strategies for coping with student failure. Participants returned to their groups to watch a video that was made by course organizers at the Derby School of three final evaluation meetings between educators and failing students. Each group was joined by an academic fieldwork coordinator and a lecturer who was skilled in group dynamics. The video illustrated three different students' reactions to receiving a failing grade: distress and regression, which was depicted through nonverbal behavior such as avoidance of eye contact, posture, and gestures; an angry confrontation between a female educator and a male student; and a student's attempt to manipulate the supervisor (who needed "to make everything better") into changing the grade from a fail to a pass. The emotional effects of each scenario were acknowledged by the participants before the situation was analyzed in order to identify alternative strategies. These strategies were considered along a continuum, from prevention to development of appropriate ways of dealing with the student's reaction and suggestions for follow-up support for the student and fieldwork educator. Suggestions ranged from simple, practical points (e.g., educators should provide tissues in anticipation of a tearful response from the student), to nonverbal methods of reinforcing the reality of a failing grade (e.g., educators should make eye contact and gestures for emphasis), to awareness of gender or generational issues between the supervisor and the student (e.g., definitions of professional behavior). Strategies that ensure due process and help maintain the dignity of both students and educators were highlighted (Wood & Campbell, 1985). Special emphasis was given to the importance for educators to document and provide students with unambiguous, honest formative and summative feedback on the basis of clear learning objectives.

In the plenary session, which followed the afternoon

session, participants were invited to pose questions related to student assessment, examination regulations, and appeal procedures to a panel composed of the Derby School's principal, assessment officer, and academic fieldwork coordinators. Professional responsibility and due process were reemphasized—in particular that "the failure to instruct properly (which includes passing a failing student or failing a passing student) may be a negligent act" (Goclowski, 1985, p. 108).

The fieldwork educators' right to make subjective judgments when appraising clinical behavior (if based on professionally accepted standards) was noted. This right was confirmed by the U.S. Supreme Court decision in the landmark case of *Board of Curators, University of Missouri v. Horowitz* (1977), in which an academically able, 4th-year medical student was expelled from the university (cited in Poteet & Pollok, 1981). The criteria for her dismissal included unacceptable personal hygiene, inappropriate bedside manner, and tardiness.

The plenary session concluded with a review of the positive consequences of failure for the student, the fieldwork educator, the Derby School, and the occupational therapy profession. This review reinforced both the educator's role as a gatekeeper of future practice and the value of a failing grade as a motivator for learning and change.

Each of the three sessions stimulated lively debate, and the whole course was well received. In recognition that such positive feedback might have been influenced by initial excitement and conformity effects that are unlikely to be sustained or transferred into practice, participants were surveyed at three points after the course.

Method: Data Collection and Analysis

Participants completed three single-page surveys: an initial survey that was given to all participants immediately after the course and two follow-up surveys that were mailed to 62 volunteers 4 and 12 months after the course. The first survey contained 9-point semantic differential scales to elicit their reactions regarding the helpfulness of each of the three sessions; a nominal format to evaluate the effectiveness of the course in meeting their expectations, needs, and objectives; and open-ended questions to probe for their reasons for attending the course and to ascertain whether the course had influenced their thoughts or feelings about assigning a failing grade.

The follow-up surveys focused on longer term appraisals and on applications of the course. Both of these follow-up surveys began with a closed-ended, biographical question (about whether they had experience with borderline or unsatisfactory students) to arouse interest (Youngman, 1978) and refocus attention on the topic of student failure. Open-ended questions requested examples of the influence of the course on their thoughts, behavior, and feelings when working with marginal stu-

dents. Participants were also asked to provide information about their practices as educators and to state the three most important points they learned in the course. The answers to the open-ended questions were subjected to a content analysis with coding categories based on the participants' language. On the 4-month follow-up survey, respondents were asked to rank statements on the basis of the aim, objectives, and elements of the course. On the 12-month follow-up survey, to aid retrieval of course information, more structured formats were used, including 4-point Likert scales about the value of the topics covered in the sessions, changes in confidence about the subject of failure, and the overall worth of the course.

All 101 participants who attended the course completed the initial survey. (Respondents were kept anonymous.) The follow-up surveys were circulated to the 62 participants who volunteered to complete them. Twenty-six participants (42%) returned the 4-month evaluation surveys and 37 participants (60%) returned the 12-month evaluation surveys.

Results

Initial Evaluation

In the survey administered immediately after the course, the majority of respondents reported that the course had met their needs (94%), their expectations (96%), and the course's objectives (91%). Table 1 contains the responses to session I (criteria for failure), session II (strategies for coping with failure), and session III (plenary).

Criteria for failure was rated extremely helpful by 90% of participants. Some added comments relating to the following three factors:

1. The reassurance and support gained from sharing experiences ($n = 47$)
2. The aspects of assessment including the complexity of criteria for student failure and increased awareness of the subjectivity or objectivity involved ($n = 27$)
3. The small group format that provided an appropriate introductory forum ($n = 16$).

Table 1
Semantic Differential Results Related to Perceived Helpfulness of Three Sessions (Initial Survey)

Session	Frequency of Rating on 9-point Scale[a]							M	SD
	3	4	5	6	7	8	9		
1: Criteria for failing a student	1	1	1	8	47	33	10	7.36	0.98
2: Coping with failing a student	1	1	3	12	33	44	7	7.33	1.04
3: Consequences of failing a student	—	6	24	52	55	20	7	6.49	1.12

Note. $N = 101$.
[a]1 = extremely unhelpful, 9 = extremely helpful.
No ratings below 3 were reported.

252   *March 1995, Volume 49, Number 3*

Research on Fieldwork Supervisor Learning and Training | 193

One participant wrote, "It was very helpful. It was good to pool ideas, see that people are feeling the same way about failing students and are using the same criteria." This statement reflects the assurance gained from a sense of universality (Yalom, 1985) and recognition of their expert role (Friedman & Mennin, 1991) in defining incompetence.

The session on strategies for coping with failure was rated extremely helpful by 84% of participants. The video was commended by 72 respondents. Their comments about the video included praise about its usefulness and performance ($n = 30$), its value for stimulating discussion ($n = 17$) and sharing experiences ($n = 9$), and its use as an enjoyable teaching tool ($n = 13$), which included specific examples illustrating the perspective of the student and fieldwork educator.

The plenary session on the consequences of failure, which elicited only 31 comments, was rated between neutral and extremely helpful. Responses noted the value of information about school procedures and the appeals policy ($n = 9$), reassurance gained from confirmation of the support networks available to students and educators ($n = 7$), and opportunities to ask questions and clarify points of personal interest ($n = 6$).

Follow-Up Evaluations

The positive perceptions of the course were sustained on both the 4- and 12-month follow-up surveys. On the 12-month surveys, all sessions were rated as valuable or highly valuable (see Table 2). Strategies for coping with student failure was most frequently rated as highly valuable on the Likert scale. This was followed by roles and responsibilities, criteria for failure, consequences of failure, and the objective and subjective aspects of assess-

ment. There is an interesting difference between these results and those of the 4-month surveys. The participants' 4-month surveys rated criteria for failure (which incorporated subjective and objective aspects of assessment) as the most helpful, followed by strategies for coping, and the plenary session. This difference may have resulted from the increase in the number of borderline students seen by the respondents (from 1 on the 4-month surveys to 11 on the 12-month surveys), which necessitated the use of coping strategies and clarity of roles.

Multifaceted Themes

The content analysis of the qualitative data obtained from the open-ended questions revealed three multifaceted themes that appeared in all of the surveys. These themes were affective responses; reinforcement of supervisory roles, responsibilities, and strategies; and obligation to maintain future standards of practice. These themes are considered along a temporal dimension to highlight continuities and variations in emphasis from the reasons given in the 12-month survey for attending the course. The percentages given refer to the number of responses, which was greater than the number of respondents.

Affective Responses

Respondents' affective responses confirmed the emotionally debilitating aspects of assigning a student a failing grade. They consisted of four elements:

1. Recognition of the feelings associated with assigning a failing grade, including guilt, isolation, personal failure, fear, and anxiety.
2. Support gained through sharing experiences (either through expression or through listening) that was related to the realization that such feelings are common responses.
3. Increases in confidence and conviction that accompanied confronting the prospect and process of assigning a failing grade.
4. Understanding of the widespread distribution of stress among those not involved in the assessment process and sources of support available for supervisors and students.

The affective responses theme accounted for two of the four reasons that participants cited for attending the course. These reasons were the opportunity to share or listen to others' experiences of failing a student (20%) and the opportunity to increase confidence and learn ways of supporting colleagues (16%).

On the initial survey, 90% acknowledged that the course had influenced their views about student failure in a positive direction. The most frequently mentioned reason for this change in view (30%) was the recognition of

Table 2
Likert Scale Results Related to Perceived Value of Topics Covered in Three Sessions (12-Month Survey)

Session and Topic	Rating			
	Highly Valuable	Valuable	Of Little Value	Of No Value
1: Criteria for failure	10 (30%)	23 (70%)	–	–
1: Objective and subjective aspects of assessment	7 (21%)	26 (79%)	–	–
2: Strategies for coping with failing a student	14 (42%)	17 (51%)	–	–
3: Roles and responsibilities of school, supervisor, student, and academic fieldwork coordinator	11 (33%)	21 (64%)	–	–
3: Consequences of failure on fieldwork practice	8 (26%)	23 (74%)	–	–

Note. $N = 33$.

the shared feelings of isolation, guilt, and fear that dealing with the fail scenario evokes. Increased confidence in dealing with borderline or unsatisfactory students was cited by 16% of the responses as the reason for this change in view.

On the 4-month survey, an understanding of the feelings associated with the fail scenario, which incorporated feelings of guilt, fear of failure, and personal feelings of failure, was the most frequently mentioned point learned (23%). Eight of the 26 respondents reported increased confidence in their ability and judgment related to their supervisory practices.

On the 12-month survey, 11 respondents who had had experience with marginal students noted an increase in confidence. These changes in affective responses were repeated on the Likert scale (see Table 3).

The course aim was sustained in the affective responses theme. Increased confidence provided educators with pragmatic, proactive supervision techniques and appropriate judgments that reduced the failure to fail students.

Reinforcement of Supervisory Roles, Responsibilities, and Strategies

The second multifaceted theme, reinforcement of supervisory roles, responsibilities, and strategies, was an unexpected spin-off from the course. It consisted of the following seven aspects:

1. The desire to learn about and therefore be prepared for dealing with students' failure
2. Recognition of the positive aspects of the process and outcome
3. Clarification of the criteria for students' incompetence
4. Increased awareness of objective and subjective aspects of assessment

Table 3
Perceived Changes in Awareness and Confidence (12-Month Survey)

Area of Change	Decrease	No Change	Increase	Large Increase
Awareness of personal consequences of failing a student	–	3 (8%)	22 (59%)	12 (32%)
Confidence in identifying borderline and unsatisfactory students	–	4 (11%)	23 (62%)	10 (27%)
Confidence in own ability to take appropriate action	2 (5%)	3 (8%)	16 (43%)	16 (43%)
Awareness of positive aspects of student failure	1 (2%)	2 (5%)	21 (57%)	13 (35%)

Note. N = 37.

5. Recognition of the importance of honest, regular, and documented feedback
6. Understanding that the students' responsibility to learn is underpinned but not determined by appropriate supervisory strategies
7. Knowledge of the Derby School examination rules, regulations, and appeal procedures.

Predictably, the two most frequently cited reasons for attending the course were to learn about the responsibility of failing students (35%) and to prepare for this responsibility (24%). Supervisory strategies accounted for one half the areas of change reported on the initial evaluation. These changes included an acknowledgment of the potential for positive outcomes from a fail scenario (15%); increased understanding of the complexity of failing students that would be shared with colleagues (13%); and reinforcement of supervisory strategies, including program planning, the student's responsibility to learn, and the need for objective assessment (9%).

The supervisory theme accounted for some of the most important points learned on the 4-month survey. These points included the need to give honest, objective, and timely feedback (15%); the recognition of positive outcomes (8%); the value of the criteria for students' failure (7%); the reinforcement of the student's responsibility to learn (7%); and the worth of subjective assessment (4%).

All of these points were also identified on the 12-month survey, in addition to two new points: coping strategies used by and for the supervisor, student, and department (15%) and an increased understanding of the Derby School's procedures (3%).

The difficulties associated with a fail scenario, including the possibility of a student's appeal, highlighted the importance of effective supervision (Christie, Joyce, & Moeller, 1985; Morgan & Knox, 1987; Nehring, 1990; Ogier & Barrett, 1985). The documentation of objective feedback on students' performance with guidelines for improvement is evidence that the fieldwork educators have fulfilled their responsibility and have made a fair, "expert evaluation of cumulative information" (Poteet & Pollok, 1981, p. 1890).

Obligation to Maintain Future Standards of Practice

The final theme is the most important because it makes explicit the purpose of assessment and licensure. The ability to place the immediate, personal trauma of the fail scenario within a longer term, professional perspective is a key mediating factor.

This underpinning theme provided the second most frequently cited reason on the initial evaluation for changed perceptions about failure. It included the reinforcement and reassurance at a personal and professional level of the obligation to assign a fail grade (17%). On the

4-month survey, 18% of the most important points learned were related to the acceptance of the obligation to maintain professional standards and assign a fail grade. On the 12-month survey, 10% of the statements noted the reinforcement of the role of fieldwork educators in maintaining professional standards.

Study Limitations

In small-scale studies, qualitative and quantitative data provide illuminative rather than generalizable results (Goulding, 1984). The lack of biographical details about the self-selected sample of fieldwork educators precludes comment about the applicability of the findings. Self-completion surveys, particularly those completed 1 year after attending a course, are subject to the vagaries of memory, recall bias, socially desirable responses, and spontaneous rather than salient answers. In addition, the failure to pursue those volunteers who did not return the surveys may have introduced a systematic bias, particularly with such a small sample.

Conclusion

The initial and follow-up surveys of a course designed to prepare fieldwork educators' for the responsibility of assigning students a failing grade supported the course's value for developing confidence, reinforcing supervisory skills, and maintaining professional standards. The success of the course seemed to be based on a simple formula: the opportunity to discuss this aspect of an educators' role increased awareness and acceptance and gave permission to take appropriate action. The subject of failure, presented by and for fieldwork and faculty staff members, has the potential to bridge the gap between these twin towers of academia and practice to obtain the shared goal of competency. ▲

Acknowledgment

I thank my colleagues and the fieldwork educators at the Derby School for sharing their experiences.

References

Blomquist, K. B. (1985). Evaluation of students—intuition is important. *Nurse Educator, 10*(8), 8–11.

Bradley, J. (1990). *The assessment of progress of student nurses in the clinical field.* Unpublished master's dissertation, University of Nottingham, England.

Brozenec, S., Marshall, J. R., Thomas, C., & Walsh, M. (1987). Evaluating borderline students. *Journal of Nursing Education, 26*(1), 42–44.

Carpenito, L. J. (1983). The failing or unsatisfactory student. *Nurse Educator, 8*(4), 32–33.

Christie, B. A., Joyce, P. C., & Moeller, P. L. (1985). Field-work experience, Part II: The supervisor's dilemma. *American Journal of Occupational Therapy, 39,* 675–681.

Darragh, R., Jacobson, G., Sloan, B., & Sandquist, G. (1986). Unsafe student practice: Policy and procedures. *Nursing Outlook, 34*(4), 176–178.

Ericson, D. P., & Ellett, F. S. (1987). Teacher accountability and the causal theory of teaching. *Educational Theory, 32*(3), 277–293.

Friedman, M., & Mennin, S. P. (1991). Rethinking critical issues in performance assessment. *Academic Medicine, 66*(7), 390–395.

Geary, A. (1988). Written judgements in school: A personal perspective. *Early Child Development and Care, 34,* 241–265.

Goclowski, J. (1985). Legal implications of academic dismissal and educational malpractice for nursing faculty. *Journal of Nursing Education, 24*(3), 104–108.

Goldenberg, D., & Waddall, J. (1990). Occupational stress and coping strategies among female baccalaureate nursing faculty. *Journal of Advanced Nursing, 15,* 531–543.

Goulding, S. (1984). Analysis and presentation of information In J. Bell (Ed.), *Conducting small-scale investigations in educational management* (pp. 230–251). London: Harper & Row.

Graham, S. (1984). Teacher feeling and student thoughts: An attributional approach to affect in the classroom. *Elementary School Journal 85*(1), 91–104.

Ilott, I. (1990). *Failure—The clinical supervisor's perspective.* Paper presented at 10th World Federation of Occupational Therapists Congress, Melbourne.

Ilott, I. (1993). *The process of failing occupational therapy students: A staff perspective.* Unpublished doctoral dissertation, University of Nottingham, England.

Lankshear, A. (1990). Failure to fail: The teacher's dilemma. *Nursing Standard, 4*(20), 35–37.

Meisenhelder, J. B. (1982, June). Clinical evaluation: An instructor's dilemma. *Nursing Outlook,* 348–351.

Moeller, P. (1984). Clinical supervision: Guidelines for managing the problem student. *Journal of Allied Health, 13*(3), 205–211.

Morgan, J., & Knox, J. E. (1987). Characteristics of 'best' and 'worst' clinical teachers as perceived by university nursing faculty and students. *Journal of Advanced Nursing, 12,* 331–337.

Nehring, V. (1990). Nursing clinical teacher effectiveness inventory: A replication study of the characteristics of 'best' and 'worst' clinical teachers as perceived by nursing faculty and students. *Journal of Advanced Nursing, 15,* 934–940.

Ogier, M. E., & Barrett, D. E. (1985). Sister/staff nurse and the nurse learner. *Nurse Education Today, 6,* 16–22.

Poteet, G. W., & Pollock, C. S. (1981, October). When a student fails clinical. *American Journal of Nursing,* 1889–1890.

Symanski, M. E. (1991). Reducing the effect of faculty demoralization when failing students. *Nurse Educator, 16*(3), 18–22.

Turkett, S. (1987). Let's take the 'i' out of failure. *Journal of Nursing Education, 26*(2), 246–247.

Wood, V., & Campbell D. B. (1985). The instructor, the student and appeals. *Nurse Education Today, 5,* 241–246.

Yalom, I. D. (1985). *The theory and practice of group psychotherapy.* New York: Basic.

Youngman, M. (1978). *Designing and analyzing questionnaires.* (Rediguide No. 12). Nottingham, England: Nottingham University.

Clinical Teaching: Fieldwork Supervisors' Attitudes and Values

Lisette N. Kautzmann

Key Words: adult • education, occupational therapy • fieldwork education, occupational therapy

The purpose of this study was to initiate the identification of fieldwork supervisors' educational needs by ascertaining their values and attitudes toward exemplary principles of teaching advocated by adult educators. Each principle was rephrased as an attitude or value associated with Level II fieldwork, matched with a Likert-type 5-point interval scale, and distributed to a convenience sample of 81 fieldwork supervisors. Ninety-two percent of the questionnaires were returned. The statement responses were tallied by frequency and were then summed and ranked. The range of scores indicated that the fieldwork supervisors' values and attitudes were congruent with the identified principles of teaching. The rankings revealed that the supervisors placed the highest value on providing a thorough orientation and the lowest values on individualization of the fieldwork experience and supervisor–student collaboration. The findings indicate a need for further education about ways to individualize learning and involve students in planning, implementing, and evaluating the learning experience.

Lisette N. Kautzmann, EdD, OTR/L, FAOTA, is Associate Professor, Department of Occupational Therapy, College of Allied Health and Nursing, Eastern Kentucky University, 109 Wallace Building, Richmond, Kentucky 40475-3133.

This article was accepted for publication February 10, 1990.

Fieldwork educators are faced with the dual challenge of coping effectively with the demands of the health care environment and providing learning experiences for students of increasingly diverse ages, interests, and abilities. Currently, 19.9% of the students enrolled in professional occupational therapy programs are 25 years of age or older (American Occupational Therapy Association [AOTA], 1989). These changes in the occupational therapy student population reflect current trends in higher education. The Carnegie Council on Policy Standards in Higher Education (1980) reported that the pool of traditional students (i.e., 18 years old) interested in attending a 4-year college is diminishing. As a result, colleges and universities are actively recruiting nontraditional students, including older students, women, and minorities. The pool of traditional students applying to programs in allied health and nursing has been reduced further by women's improved access to male-dominated schools of medicine, engineering, and business.

Although they are responding reactively (Strickland, 1987), the faculty and administrators of educational programs are learning to cope with adult students. Effective supervision of adult students presents new challenges to fieldwork educators. These challenges are superimposed on preexisting problems in fieldwork education, including the dearth of fieldwork supervisors and their limited knowledge of the teaching–learning process and adult development. Occupational therapy fieldwork supervisors need additional information and skills to improve their effectiveness and efficiency in educating both traditional and adult students. The purpose of the present investigation was to initiate the identification of fieldwork supervisors' educational needs by ascertaining their values and attitudes as related to Knowles's (1980) superior principles of teaching adults.

Literature Review

Authors representing a variety of health professions have documented the issue of clinicians' insufficient preparation for clinical teaching (Christ, 1986; Cohn & Frum, 1988; Daggett, Cassie, & Collins, 1979; Edwards & Baptiste, 1987; Irby, 1978; Karuhije, 1986; Meleca, Schimpfauser, & Witteman, 1981). Occupational therapy fieldwork supervisors' needs were investigated by Christie, Joyce, and Moeller (1985b) and Frum (1986). Christie et al. identified four major areas of need: (a) support, (b) growth in professional competency and currency, (c) supervisory skill development, and (d) the teaching of skill development. Additional findings from their study indicated that fieldwork supervisors look to academic curricula and to AOTA for assistance in preparing them for the role of fieldwork educator (Christie, Joyce, & Moeller, 1985a).

Frum (1986) surveyed fieldwork educators and academic fieldwork coordinators to identify training needs. Those persons surveyed preferred such workshop topics as analyzing and bridging the gap between classroom and clinic, evaluating student performance, linking theory to practice, solving fieldwork problems, and supervising students.

Gaiptman (1986) observed three major problems associated with fieldwork education: lack of attention to the supervisory skills of fieldwork educators, interpersonal difficulties between supervisor and student, and lack of consistency in therapists' perceptions of students' performance. Gaiptman postulated that differences in aptitudes and learning and teaching styles contributed to some of these problems.

Christie et al. (1985a) presented critical components of a fieldwork experience. Supervision, the most critical component, involved (a) the meeting of the student's needs through adaptation of the supervisory approach and program structure; (b) an organized, structured program with clear learning objectives and responsibilities; (c) ongoing, constructive feedback; (d) frequent, supportive, open communication in the development of skills and the application of knowledge; and (e) the availability of the supervisor.

Christie et al. (1985a) identified fieldwork supervisors as critical to students' selection of a practice preference. This finding was reaffirmed by Wittman, Swinehart, Cahill, and St. Michel (1989) in their study of variables affecting specialty choice. In contrast, the results of a study by Ezersky, Havazelet, Scott, and Zettler (1989) indicated that although the fieldwork experience was an influencing variable, fieldwork supervisors did not have a direct influence on specialty choice.

Differences between new and experienced supervisors were described by Christie et al. (1985b), who said that new supervisors feel responsible for the success or failure of the fieldwork experience and prefer to control all aspects of the program. They develop rigid structures that are applied to all students, regardless of individual differences. Preoccupation with their own performance clouds their ability to perceive and respond to students' needs. In contrast, experienced supervisors have learned to differentiate between supervisor and supervisee responsibilities. With experience, supervisors learn to recognize students as individuals, assess their individual needs, and modify the fieldwork program and supervisory approach. Flexibility in the supervisory approach increases with experience and seems to be directly related to the supervisor's increased level of confidence. Experienced supervisors support and promote

students' individuality and creativity and allow students increased responsibility and independence.

Strickland (1987) advocated individualization of the educational experience in his examination of planning for adult students. He suggested that adult students are a viable group for education and practice and that programs should develop options that accommodate their needs. Designers of educational programs also need to be cognizant of the developmental tasks and related responsibilities of older students.

Developmental approaches to student supervision have been presented by Schwartz (1984) and Frum and Opacich (1987). Schwartz proposed a developmental framework for individualizing the clinical learning experience and for student supervision. Frum and Opacich applied a counseling model developed by Loganbill, Hardy, and Delworth (1981) to student supervision. Frum and Opacich also suggested strategies and practice exercises that address the four essential elements of the supervisory process (i.e., the supervisor, the supervisee, the relationship, and the environment) identified by Loganbill et al.

Method

Instrument

A questionnaire was used to gather information on fieldwork supervisors' attitudes and values relative to principles of teaching adults. Likert's Method of Summed Ratings (Best, 1977) was used as a procedural guide to develop questionnaire statements and analyze data. Twelve of Knowles's (1980) 16 principles were rephrased into 13 statements of attitudes or tasks associated with occupational therapy Level II fieldwork. The 3 omitted principles—identification of the learner's problems due to gaps in experience, active participation in learning activities, and opportunities to apply new learning—were believed to be inherent in the Level II experience. The other deleted principle related to the classroom environment. Although it is assumed that occupational therapy settings are conducive to learning, students learn in a wide variety of environments. Because fieldwork supervisors may have little control over the environment, I predicted that answers to this statement would not be useful.

The individual statements were matched to a 5-point interval scale, with 5 representing the highest value and 1 representing the lowest value. The questionnaire was reviewed for clarity and content by a panel consisting of an adult educator and occupational therapy academic and fieldwork educators. The questionnaire was revised and field-tested by occupational therapy fieldwork supervisors who were not part of the identified sample.

Subjects and Procedure

The questionnaire was mailed to a nonrandom sample of 81 occupational therapy fieldwork supervisors. Responses to each statement were tallied by frequency and were then summed and ranked. The summed scores and rank order of the statements were used to determine fieldwork supervisors' values, attitudes, and educational needs.

Results

Seventy-five of the 81 fieldwork supervisors (92%) completed and returned the questionnaire. One questionnaire was unusable. Of the 74 remaining respondents, most were from the Midwest: 63% were from Wisconsin, and 15% were from Illinois, Minnesota, and Nebraska. Sixteen percent of the respondents were from the West, that is, Arizona, California, Colorado, New Mexico, and Washington. Six percent of the respondents were from the eastern seaboard states of New York, Georgia, and Virginia and from the District of Columbia. Although the results from all of the states were congruent, the findings can be generalized only to Wisconsin. Additionally, all Wisconsin facilities that, at the time of the survey, provided physical disability or psychosocial Level II fieldwork experiences for professional students were included in the convenience sample.

The summed scores and ranks for each questionnaire statement are presented in Table 1. An examination of the rankings provides information on fieldwork supervisors' perceptions of each questionnaire item. Statement 4, that students deserve a thorough orientation, received the highest ranking. Those statements ranked 2, 3, 5, 6, and 7a represent attitudes and assumptions about students or student supervision. In contrast, the items ranked 4, 7b, 9, 10, 11a, 11b, and 13 represent specific activities that require either student–supervisor collaboration or individualization of the fieldwork experience.

Discussion

The survey findings revealed that the fieldwork supervisors placed high value on Knowles's (1980) principles of teaching adults. In addition, the high range of summed scores indicated that the fieldwork supervisors' attitudes and values were congruent with Knowles's principles of teaching.

The highest ranked statement was related to the acknowledgment of students' need to be oriented to the facility and the fieldwork experience. Several factors may have contributed to this ranking. First, orientation has been a recommended component of fieldwork education since 1977 (AOTA, Commission on Education, 1977). Second, fieldwork supervisors are able to develop an orientation plan that can be ap-

Table 1
Fieldwork Supervisors' Summed Scores and Rankings for Questionnaire Statements

Statement[a]	Summed Score	Rank
1. Respect for learners' feelings and ideas.	347	3
2. Learning to function as a team member.	328	6
3. Supervisor is a resource person and provides feedback.	334	5
4. Students deserve a thorough orientation.	351	1
5. Students can identify learning needs.	322	7a[c]
6. Importance of assessing student's knowledge at start of fieldwork.	297[b]	11a[c]
7. Collaborative development of learning objectives.	312	9
8. Importance of adjusting instruction to student's learning style.	302[b]	10
9. Desirability of involving students in planning their learning.	297	11b[c]
10. Value of incorporating students' interests, skills, and experience.	348	2
11. Ability to adapt teaching to student's level.	335	4
12. Collaborative development of evaluation criteria.	269	13
13. Involving students in evaluating their performance.	322	7b[c]

Note. Possible range of summed scores is 74–370.
[a] Abbreviated for space considerations. [b] Transposed score. [c] Tied score.

plied efficiently and effectively to all students. Third, fieldwork supervisors may reflect on their own experiences as students and recognize the effect of the orientation process on their anxiety level.

It is encouraging to find a number of highly ranked statements related to attitudes and assumptions about students and student supervision. These rankings indicate that attitudes that facilitate learning and have a positive effect on the teaching–learning process are in place. Supervisors respect and value students' feelings, ideas, interests, skills, and experience. In contrast, the five lowest ranked items represent specific activities and methods related to either individualization of the learning experience or student–supervisor collaboration. Several authors have provided methods of individualization in the fieldwork experience, including the examination of students' and supervisors' learning styles (Gaiptman, 1986; Stafford, 1986), use of learning contracts (Windom, 1982), and strategies for the development of clinical reasoning skills (Cohn, 1989).

Although the occupational therapy literature related to fieldwork education strongly supports a collaborative supervisory relationship (AOTA, Commission on Education, 1977, 1984), findings from the present study indicate that in actual practice the existence of collaborative supervision may not be widespread. Retaining control of the fieldwork experience is a major issue for new supervisors (Christie et al., 1985b). Power and control may become central issues when fieldwork supervisors either are unwilling to allow students to function as active participants in the learning process or lack knowledge and skill in implementing a collaborative relationship. Insecurity and limited opportunities to observe role models of collaborative supervision appear to be the bases for this behavior (Christie et al., 1985b). As supervisors become more comfortable with their roles, however, they realize that it is healthy and growth promoting for students to take responsibility for their own learning (Christie et al., 1985b). Thus, topics for further investigation must focus on methods to accelerate and support this developmental process, because by helping fieldwork educators improve their supervisory skills, we benefit both traditional and adult students.

Conclusion

Although the survey findings in the present study indicate that fieldwork supervisors agree on the value of Knowles's (1980) principles of teaching adults for fieldwork education, it cannot be assumed that these principles are being applied appropriately. The survey results show that the greatest need for information is in methods to individualize fieldwork and involve students in planning, implementing, and evaluating the learning experience. ▲

Acknowledgments

Thanks to Malcolm S. Knowles, PhD, Jan Decker, MS, OTR, Carol Holmes, MS, OTR, FAOTA, Alice Punwar, MS, OTR, FAOTA, and Julia Van Deusen, PhD, OTR, FAOTA, for providing feedback on the survey questionnaire. Special thanks to L. Randy Strickland, EdD, OTR, FAOTA, for assistance in questionnaire development and for field testing.

References

American Occupational Therapy Association. (1989). *1989 education data survey: Final report.* Rockville, MD: Author.

American Occupational Therapy Association, Commission on Education. (1977). *Field work experience manual for academic field work coordinators, field work supervisors, and students.* Rockville, MD: Author.

American Occupational Therapy Association, Commission on Education. (1984). *Guide to fieldwork education.* Rockville, MD: Author.

Best, J. W. (1977). *Research in education* (3rd ed.). Englewood Cliffs, NJ: Prentice-Hall.

Carnegie Council on Policy Standards in Higher Education. (1980). *Three thousand futures: The next twenty years for higher education.* San Francisco: Jossey-Bass.

Christ, P. A. (1986). *Contemporary issues in clinical education.* Thorofare, NJ: Slack.

Christie, B. A., Joyce, P. C., & Moeller, P. L. (1985a). Fieldwork experience, part 1: Impact on practice preference. *American Journal of Occupational Therapy, 39,* 671–674.

Christie, B. A., Joyce, P. C., & Moeller, P. L. (1985b). Fieldwork experience, part II: The supervisor's dilemma. *American Journal of Occupational Therapy, 39,* 675–681.

Cohn, E. S. (1989). Fieldwork education: Shaping a foundation for clinical reasoning. *American Journal of Occupational Therapy, 43,* 240–244.

Cohn, E. S., & Frum, D. C. (1988). The Issue Is— Fieldwork supervision: More education is warranted. *American Journal of Occupational Therapy, 42,* 325–327.

Daggett, C. J., Cassie, J. M., & Collins, G. F. (1979). Research on clinical teaching. *Review of Educational Research, 49,* 151–169.

Edwards, M., & Baptiste, S. (1987). The occupational therapist as a clinical teacher. *Canadian Journal of Occupational Therapy, 54,* 249–255.

Ezersky, S., Havazelet, L., Scott, A. H., & Zettler, C. L. B. (1989). Specialty choice in occupational therapy. *American Journal of Occupational Therapy, 43,* 227–233.

Frum, D. C. (1986, July). Study shows fieldwork to be a high priority among occupational therapy educators. *Occupational Therapy News,* p. 7.

Frum, D. C., & Opacich, K. J. (1987). *Supervision: Development of therapeutic competence.* Rockville, MD: American Occupational Therapy Association.

Gaiptman, B. (1986). The application of cognitive style research to fieldwork education. *Canadian Journal of Occupational Therapy, 53,* 75–80.

Irby, D. M. (1978). Clinical teacher effectiveness in medicine. *Journal of Medical Education, 53,* 808–814.

Karuhije, H. F. (1986). Educational preparation for clinical teaching: Perceptions of the nurse educator. *Journal of Nursing Education, 25,* 137–144.

Knowles, M. S. (1980). *The theory and practice of adult education.* Chicago: Follett.

Loganbill, C., Hardy E., & Delworth, U. (1981). Supervision: A conceptual model [Monograph]. *Counseling Psychologist, 10*(1).

Meleca, C. B., Schimpfauser, F. T., & Witteman, J. K. (1981). *A comprehensive and systematic assessment of clinical teaching skills and strategies in the health sciences.* Bethesda, MD: National Library of Medicine.

Schwartz, K. B. (1984). An approach to supervision of students on fieldwork. *American Journal of Occupational Therapy, 38,* 393–397.

Stafford, E. M. (1986). Relationship between occupational therapy student learning styles and clinic performance. *American Journal of Occupational Therapy, 40,* 34–39.

Strickland, L. R. (1987). The ability of professional programs in occupational therapy to accommodate the older student. *American Journal of Occupational Therapy, 41,* 382–387.

Windom, P. A. (1982). Developing a clinical education program from the clinician's perspective. *Physical Therapy, 62,* 1604–1609.

Wittman, P. P., Swinehart, S., Cahill, R., & St. Michel, G. (1989). Variables affecting specialty choice in occupational therapy. *American Journal of Occupational Therapy, 43,* 602–606.

THE ISSUE IS

Alternatives to Psychosocial Fieldwork: Part of the Solution or Part of the Problem?

Lisette N. Kautzmann

Lisette N. Kautzmann, EdD, OTR/L, FAOTA, is Associate Professor, Department of Occupational Therapy, Eastern Kentucky University, Richmond, Kentucky 40475.

This article was accepted for publication January 8, 1994.

The recent increase in the number of occupational therapy programs, coupled with the limited number of fieldwork placements in mental health, has made it increasingly difficult to find placements for Level II fieldwork students in traditional mental health settings. Although some academic fieldwork coordinators have been able to continue placing students in typical in-patient and community-based mental health facilities, others have had to consider alternative strategies. One strategy is to place students at fieldwork sites, such as work hardening, pain management, and head injury programs, where psychosocial dysfunction is not the primary diagnosis. The problem is that, although psychosocial components are addressed in the daily interactions with the clientele in these programs, they are not the focus of assessment and treatment. The related issues are, what is being done to ensure that students placed in alternative sites are learning to apply psychosocial assessment and treatment methods and what will be the long-term impact of this type of placement on mental health practice?

It is clear that the diminishing number of Level II fieldwork sites in mental health is reflective of and interwoven with the decreased number of therapists practicing in mental health settings and in the reduced number of new graduates choosing mental health as a practice preference. The result of the reduced number of Level II fieldwork sites in mental health settings is that there are fewer opportunities for students to learn the occupational therapy interventions and skills traditionally practiced in mental health and to observe occupational therapy role models.

As a result, the likelihood of students choosing to work in mental health is reduced.

Literature Review

The influence of fieldwork and fieldwork supervisors on practice preference has been documented by several authors. Christie, Joyce, and Moeller (1985) examined the influence of three stages of professional development on practice preference. Overwhelmingly, respondents reported that fieldwork had a greater influence on their practice preference than did either their preprofessional experience or the academic curriculum. The fieldwork supervisor and the supervisory process were the most influential components of the fieldwork experience. Findings of Ezersky, Havazelet, Scott, and Zettler (1989) supported the conclusions of Christie et al. (1985) that fieldwork was the primary influence on specialty choice. Additionally, a poor fieldwork experience was a detractor in specialty choice for both psychosocial and physical dysfunction. Other factors influencing specialty choices included a sense of feeling effective in the specialty area, consistency of personal values with those of the specialty area, and availability of employment. Wittman, Swinehart, Cahill, and St. Michel (1989) surveyed recent graduates to determine which variables affected specialty choice. They concurred with Christie et al. (1985) and Ezersky et al. (1989) in concluding that fieldwork was the most important influence in specialty choice. Additionally, they found that within the fieldwork experience, the supervisor had the greatest influence on the student. Findings from a survey of Australian undergraduate occupational therapy students also indicated that fieldwork is a major factor in influencing practice preference (Cusick, Demattia, & Doyle, 1993). Other influencing factors included perceptions of the mental health work setting, the work role, and students' views of their own abilities.

In response to the decreased numbers of mental health clinicians and fieldwork sites, some have argued that mental health is no longer a viable practice option and should be dropped as a fieldwork requirement (Buckner, 1991). This view was challenged by Fine (1991) and Schwartzberg (1991). Prendergast (1991) and Jordan (1991) also refuted Buckner's suggestion and called attention to the need to address psychosocial issues in all areas of occupational therapy practice. The Mental Health Special Interest Section (SIS) Standing Committee's response (1991) pointed out that the *Essentials and Guidelines for an Accredited Educational Program for the Occupational Therapist* (American Occupational Therapy Association & American Medical Association, 1991) do not require one half of the academic and fieldwork content to be focused on mental health. The committee also stated that less training was not the way to combat the shrinking number of mental health therapists. More role models are needed and the psychosocial needs of all patients should be addressed, regardless of diagnosis or type of facility.

There is recognition of the value of the skills and interventions learned in mental health fieldwork. In an investigation of practicing therapists' perception of the value of mental health Level II fieldwork, Atwater and Davis (1990) found that the experience was perceived as highly valuable regardless of therapist or practice preference. Respondents indicated that they learned how to deal with mental health issues, to know themselves better, and to respond assertively to clients. Additionally, there is growing awareness of the applicability of skills and interventions learned in mental health fieldwork to other areas of clinical practice. In a study of occupational therapy managers' regarding therapists' use of psychosocial and physical rehabilitation interventions, Renwick, Friedland, Sernas, and Raybould (1990) reported that 44% of the respondents used physical rehabilitation interventions, 30% used psychosocial interventions, and 26% used a combined approach. In discussing the practice of psychosocial occupational therapy, Friedland and Renwick (1993) suggested that use of the traditional dichotomy of psychosocial and physical dysfunction is ineffectual in responding to current demands for health care from diverse populations and advocated a more holistic approach to the provision of occupational therapy services.

Classification of Fieldwork and Types of Sites Used

This holistic view that acknowledges the overlap of psychosocial and physical problems, needs, and interventions in many areas of occupational therapy practice has influenced the response of several professional occupational therapy curricula to the issue of diminishing mental health fieldwork sites. However, findings of a recent survey that I conducted on how baccalaureate level professional programs classify their Level II fieldwork experiences, how many are using alternative sites for mental health fieldwork, and what types of alternative sites are being used indicated that 19 programs (20%) do not classify their

Level II fieldwork experiences as physical and psychosocial dysfunction. Interestingly, 12 of these 19 programs (63%) were developed in the past 5 years. The remaining 72 (79%) of the baccalaureate level professional curricula continue to categorize their fieldwork experiences as physical and psychosocial dysfunction. Ninety-one of the 92 (98%) baccalaureate level academic fieldwork coordinators responded to the survey. Many reported extreme difficulty in finding sufficient sites for psychosocial fieldwork and indicated that they are actively searching for solutions to this problem. Although 28 of the 72 respondents (38%) who classify their Level II fieldwork experiences as physical and psychosocial dysfunction are able to place their students in traditional mental health settings, others have had to explore additional strategies. As a potential solution to the shortage of traditional mental health fieldwork sites, 61% of the 72 academic fieldwork coordinators who classified their Level II fieldwork experiences as physical and psychosocial dysfunction indicated that they are placing Level II fieldwork students in one or more of the following sites for their psychosocial experience: facilities for persons with developmental disabilities; work hardening, pain management, and head injury programs; hospices; and home health care.

Implications

One problem related to the use of these types of placements as alternatives to traditional mental health placements is that fieldwork educators in head injury, work hardening, and pain management programs originally may have developed their fieldwork education programs from a physical rather than a psychosocial dysfunction perspective. Fieldwork sites are required to develop goals, learning experiences, and evaluation criteria for the fieldwork experience. Do these differ when a student is placed in a fieldwork site for a psychosocial experience rather than a physical rehabilitation experience? When students are placed in these settings for a psychosocial fieldwork experience, they have the right to expect specific training in psychosocial assessment, treatment planning, and intervention. Academic fieldwork supervisors placing students in

alternative sites need to work closely with the fieldwork educators in developing goals, learning experiences, and evaluation criteria that are appropriate for the focus of the experience. If this occurs, then use of holistic sites for fieldwork experiences has the potential to expand and enrich professional practice. However, if students do not gain a level of comfort and mastery of psychosocial skills and interventions and observe effective role models who are willing to share their clinical reasoning, they probably will leave the fieldwork experience with an increased propensity to focus on the physical aspects of rehabilitation and without the necessary preparation to practice holistically. Furthermore, the likelihood that these students will choose mental health as a practice specialty is greatly diminished. Thus, although using alternative sites solves the short-range problem of finding sufficient student placements, without careful planning and recognition of the need to adapt the experience to fulfill the expectations and requirements of psychosocial fieldwork, it may contribute to the long-range problem of decreasing the number of students selecting mental health as a practice preference. ▲

References

American Occupational Therapy Association & American Medical Association. (1991). *Essentials and guidelines for an accredited educational program for the occupational therapist.* Rockville, MD: American Occupational Therapy Association.

Atwater, A. W., & Davis, C. G. (1990). The value of psychosocial level II fieldwork. *American Journal of Occupational Therapy, 44,* 792–795.

Buckner, M. K. (1991, July 11). A shrinking area of practice [Letter to the editor]. *OT Week, 5,* p. 54.

Christie, B., Joyce, P., & Moeller, P. (1985). Fieldwork experience, part 1: Impact on practice preference. *American Journal of Occupational Therapy, 39,* 671–674.

Cusick, A., Demattia, T., & Doyle, S. (1993). Occupational therapy in mental health: Factors influencing student practice preference. *Occupational Therapy in Mental Health, 12,* 33–53.

Ezersky, S., Havazelet, L., Scott, A. H., & Zettler, C. L. (1989). Specialty choice in occupational therapy. *American Journal of Occupational Therapy, 43,* 227–233.

Fine, S. B. (1991, August 22). Letter to the editor. *OT Week, 5,* p. 46.

Friedland, J., & Renwick, R. M. (1993). Psychosocial occupational therapy: Time to cast off gloom and doom. *American Journal* of *Occupational Therapy*, 467–471.

Jordan, R. (1991, August 22). Letter to the editor. *OT Week, 5*, p. 46.

Mental Health Special Interest Section Standing Committee. (1991, August 15). The future of mental health in the profession [Letter to the editor]. *OT Week, 5*, p. 54.

Prendergast, N. D. (1991, August 22). Letter to the editor. *OT Week, 5*, p. 46.

Renwick, R. M., Friedland, J., Sernas, V., & Raybould, K. (1990). Crisis in occupational therapy: A closer look. *Canadian Journal of Occupational Therapy, 57*, 279–284.

Schwartzberg, S. L. (1991, August 15). Letter to the editor. *OT Week, 5*, p. 54.

Wittman, P. P., Swinehart, S., Cahill, R., & St. Michel, G. (1989). Variables affecting specialty choice in occupational therapy. *American Journal of Occupational Therapy, 43*, 602–606.

THE ISSUE IS provides a forum for debate and discussion of occupational therapy issues and related topics. The Contributing Editor of this section, Julia Van Deusen, strives to have both sides of an issue addressed. Readers are encouraged to submit manuscripts discussing opposite points of view or new topics. All manuscripts are subject to peer review. Submit three copies to Elaine Viseltear, Editor.

Published articles reflect the opinion of the authors and are selected on the basis of interest to the profession and quality of the discussion.

Research on Fieldwork Supervisor Learning and Training | 203

Strategies In Clinical Teaching

LTC CORDELIA MYERS, AMSC*
MAJOR PHILLIP SHANNON, AMSC†
CAPTAIN CARL SUNDSTROM, AMSC‡

ABSTRACT

This article focuses on an appraisal of the educational concepts and teaching strategies employed in the thirty-six-week clinical affiliation conducted within a single center. Problem-solving group discussions and independent study are identified as basic strategies. A unit system of teaching designed to provide the student with sequential increments in theory and experience, and the problem-solving format for patient evaluation and treatment planning are presented as additional methods for the study and treatment of patients. Examples of essential treatment experience units are provided as is a clinical modification of the problem-solving method. Involvement of the student in the discovery of information with an emphasis on student responsibility for learning is considered vital to the teaching-learning process.

The clinical affiliations conducted by the Army Medical Specialist Corps consist of a sixteen-week phase with psychiatric patients, and two phases each of ten weeks referred to as the general affiliation. The latter may include treatment of all classifications of patients other than psychiatric patients. A higher degree of continuity exists if the two phases of the general affiliation are conducted in sequence, either preceding or following the affiliation with psychiatric patients.

An element basic to the three AMSC clinical affiliations is that the total thirty-six-week affiliation is conducted within a single center. One requirement for the medical center is a large general case load representing the major medical conditions and treatment classifications. To supplement the clinical experience of the student,

a week or more in specific treatment areas may be arranged at other local hospitals.

To therapists who conduct these programs, the advantages of a single center are clear. Supervising therapists know and understand the student far better at the conclusion of thirty-six weeks than at the end of the usual twelve-week period. His study and work habits, as well as his strengths as a potential therapist, are clearly revealed. Undue amounts of duplication in supervised clinical practice are eliminated. Perhaps the most important feature is that the student can be held responsible for the application of specific information which he has learned during this extended period. This feature is possible through the consistent supervision by the educational coordinator and staff.

In an earlier article by Myers[1] certain clinical teaching concepts were described. These concepts included (1) patient-centered problem-solving discussion groups and (2) independent study. Since that publication, twenty-five students representing seventeen occupational therapy curriculums have completed the clinical

*Editor, AJOT. Formerly Chief, Occupational Therapy Section, Letterman General Hospital.
†Supervisor, Occupational Therapy Clinic for Psychiatric Patients, Letterman General Hospital, San Francisco, Calif.
‡Educational Coordinator, Occupational Therapy Section, Letterman General Hospital, San Francisco, Calif.

affiliation under this program conducted at Letterman General Hospital. The practices as presented in the earlier published article have been effective; consequently, a follow-up appraisal appears to be timely. Therefore, during the intervening four or more years, certain developments and refinements have occurred which have been brought about through the study of teaching theories and through recognition of student problems.

One of the greatest sources of learning for instructors is through observing problem areas of the students. If the same areas present repeated problems for a noticeable number of students, these may denote either faulty instruction or lack of sufficient basic information on the part of the student. Such observations have been the basis for some of the changes within this program.

Basic Strategies

The two elements referred to above (problem-solving discussion groups and independent study), combined with clinical practice remain the basis for the thirty-six-week clinical affiliation conducted at Letterman General Hospital. The scheduled discussion periods, conducted by the student group and the educational coordinator, pertain to the medical and clinical problems of specific patients. Such discussions facilitate the transmission and application of theory to clinical practice. The depth of understanding on the part of the student is revealed through the discussion of topics such as symptomatology, involved anatomical systems or mental mechanisms, comprehensive medical measures, and the planning of the occupational therapy program. In turn, the application of occupational therapy concepts during the supervised clinical practice is accomplished with keener insight by the student as a result of these discussions. In this way, the student becomes a part of the teaching process and, to a considerable measure, takes an active part and responsibility for his learning.[2]

To support the supervised clinical practice and student group discussions, scheduled time for independent study[3,4] during the work day is a necessity. Such periods, which average about ten hours a week, may be spent in the medical library or in the clinic, the latter to improve a manual skill. Two special projects in the form of (1) a seminar presented to students in an occupational therapy curriculum and (2) the preparation of a professional paper written for publication also contribute to the need for scheduled periods of independent study in addition to study during off-duty time.

Staff members observe with interest the early reluctance of some students to effectively organize their use of time for independent study as well as their heavy reliance upon specific references for study. The average student demonstrates little skill in utilizing library facilities. Much depends upon the study habits formed earlier by each student as well as the amount of intellectual curiosity that he possesses. Gradually he grasps the concept that the organization of his duties and effective use of scheduled study periods are his responsibility and are for his benefit. Habits of continuing self-education are formulated through such practice; the characteristics of self-reliance and professional excellence are obtained as a practicing therapist.

One of the operating concepts stated in the earlier publication is that learning in depth should occur from the study of a few carefully selected representative cases rather than from a larger number of cases normally treated by a therapist. This concept remains in operation. The number of patients assigned to each student is controlled; he is expected to learn the maximum from the problem presented by each patient. Through discussion, clinical practice and reflection, both learning and maturation on the part of the student are expected.

Refinements in the program concerning the study and treatment of patients are the development of units of essential treatment experiences and the utilization of a treatment plan which is based upon the research format. These refinements resulted from the apparent inability of the majority of students to sufficiently benefit from a variety of complex cases presented simultaneously within the daily treatment schedule, and to organize pertinent information effectively. This was evident in both the psychiatric and the general phases of the affiliation.

Refinements of the Program

A series of six units of essential treatment experiences were devised to be implemented throughout the thirty-six-week period.[5] Consideration was given to the identification of those treatment experiences which (1) represent high frequency in clinical practice and (2) would provide the student the opportunity to identify and apply principles of treatment basic to occupational therapy.

Tables 1 and 2 indicate the scope of study and treatment in each of the units. Students in general who have been programmed in this manner have found the clinical experience to be less overwhelming and confusing because they are focusing upon a unit in which the majority of cases under consideration are related.

In devising the essential treatment experience units, the authors considered several educational concepts. Scheduled first were patients who represented conditions of lesser complexity, then patients with greater complexity. This progression is recommended by Brunner[6] and Gagné.[7] In this manner of teaching and practice, it is anticipated that the student will be able to more easily organize information and formulate treatment concepts, thereby increasing his rate of retention.

Essential Treatment Experience Units for the Psychiatric Phase

In organizing the units for the psychiatric phase, a growth and development model was used to provide the student with a consecutive series of treatment experiences. Accordingly, the sixteen-week psychiatric phase is divided into three units: Unit I—The Preadolescent (three weeks); Unit II—The Adolescent and Young Adult (eleven weeks); Unit III—The Older Adult (two weeks). As the student progresses from one unit to the next, sequential increments in both theory and experience are designed to strengthen and enrich his professional skills.

As an example of content, the adolescent components of Unit II are cited as an illustration in Table 1. In each unit the basic knowledge requirements are met through independent study, patient-centered problem-solving group discussions, and clinical practice. These requirements may take a new or review focus as is determined by the material studied during the academic years.

Evaluation of the patient is through review of the chart and through a history-taking questionnaire. This questionnaire pertains to the social adjustment, work, and free-time activities of the

TABLE 1
Essential Treatment Experiences:
Psychiatric Phase
Unit II—Eleven-Week Unit

Treatment of Adolescents	Basic Knowledge Required	Occupational Therapy Considerations

Mildly disturbed adolescent and Severely disturbed adolescent	1. Tasks of adolescent development
	  a. Emancipation
	  b. Occupational choice
	  c. Marital choice
	  d. Other
	2. Psychiatric problems of adolescence
	3. Psychology of mental disorders
	4. Personality theories
	5. Theories of work and play
	6. Theories of occupational choice
	7. Utilization of activity
	  a. As psychotherapeutic media
	  b. For work-play programming
	8. Interviewing techniques
	9. Observation techniques
		1. Evaluation of:
		  a. Developmental task level
		  b. Educational assets and deficits
		  c. Work and free-time activities
		  d. Social adjustment
		  e. Occupational choice tendencies
		2. Socialization aspects:
		  a. Family relationships (primary and secondary)
		  b. Relationships with peers and significant others
		3. Work-play aspects:
		  a. Creative free-time interests
		  b. Adolescent to adult play patterns
		  c. Development of play competencies:
		    1. Individual and group play
		    2. Cooperative and competitive play
		  d. Activities supporting occupational choice
		  e. Work experiences
		  f. Socio-economic factors
		4. Physical aspects:
		  a. Conditioning and reconditioning
		  b. Coordination
		5. Educational aspects:
		  a. Learning skills
		  b. Course work
		6. Other

patient and is given to ascertain the nature of the patient's daily living skills. Discussion of the patient's responses follows completion of the questionnaire. The student then designs the treatment program based upon his findings.

Essential Treatment Experience Units for the General Phase

The essential treatment experience units currently programmed for the two phases of the general affiliation are: Unit IV—Lower Extremity Injuries (four weeks); Unit V—Upper Extremity Injuries (eight weeks); Unit VI—Central Nervous System Disorders (eight weeks).

As an example of content, Unit IV is cited as an illustration in Table 2. Much of the basic knowledge within a given unit serves as a basis for the subsequent units. The patients studied and treated in Unit IV are primarily confined to bed rest; thereby the student becomes aware of the physiological problems of prolonged bed rest, as well as ward procedures and the ward environment. In addition this permits carry over to the physically disabled patient certain concepts that are emphasized in the affiliation for psychiatric patients, if this has preceded.

Examples of such concepts are the use of free time and educational pursuits. Units V and VI of the General Phase parallel the general structure of Unit IV.

There is not a complete break between units since the student may continue with the patients of the preceding unit, if appropriate. Concurrent with each of the units, patients with general medical conditions are scheduled. Surgical conditions considered are primarily orthopedic and neurological problems.

Treatment objectives, based on identified problems, must be supported with theoretical concepts from the literature. The problem-solving method utilized by the students in both the general and psychiatric phases appears to be one of the most reliable methods for evaluating the patient and planning his treatment program.

Clinical Modification of the Problem-Solving Method

The problem-solving method may be viewed as a procedure or series of steps through which an individual progresses to reach a solution. More succinctly, it is a way of organizing or assembling information within a logical or ordered

TABLE 2
Essential Treatment Experiences:
General Phase
Unit IV—Four-Week Unit

Treatment of Lower-Extremity and General Medical and Surgical Conditions	Basic Knowledge Required	Occupational Therapy Considerations

1. Fractures
2. Peripheral nerve injuries
3. Amputees
4. Conditions of the knee
5. Arthritis
6. Low back pain syndrome
7. Conditions of the hip
8. Tuberculosis of bones and joints
9. Circulatory disorders
10. Congenital deformities
11. Infections of bone, joints and tissue
12. Communicable diseases
	1. Physiology
	  a. Theory of exercise
	  b. Effects of bedrest
	2. Neuroanatomy
	  a. Lumbosacral plexus
	3. Anatomy
	  a. Bone and joint structures
	  b. Circulatory system
	  c. Muscles
	4. Healing processes
	  a. Peripheral nerves
	  b. Fractures
	5. Surgical procedures
	  a. Knee and hip conditions
	  b. Types of amputations
	  c. Peripheral nerve repair
	  d. Open and closed reduction of fractures
	6. Prosthetic devices
	  a. Fitting and training
	7. Gait training
	8. Kinesiology
	9. Psychological effects of illness
	10. Casting procedures
	11. Bracing methods
		1. Joint mobility
		2. Muscle strengthening
		3. Muscle balance
		4. Physical reconditioning and tolerance
		5. Work therapy
		6. Work-play balance
		7. Educational appraisal
		8. Social and economic problems
		9. Physical capacity evaluation
		10. ADL (transfer and ambulation)
		11. Other

TABLE 3
Modification of the Problem-Solving Method

Problem-Solving Method	Clinical Modification
1. Definition of problem	1. Identification of patient's problem(s)
2. Review of literature	2. Review of literature (medical records; medical, psychiatric, occupational therapy literature)
3. Research design	3. Occupational therapy design
4. Conduct experiment	4. Conduct therapy
5. Collect data	5. Observe and record performance
6. Analyze data	6. Analyze and summarize observational data
7. Interpret results	7. Interpret performance and adjust program as indicated
8. Recommendations	8. Projection of capabilities and recommendations
9. Report findings	9. Report findings

framework. Table 3 illustrates the steps characteristically inherent in the problem-solving method and the clinical modification used in the Occupational Therapy Section, Letterman General Hospital. The modification is a strategy used to assist the student in the process of organizing information for patient evaluation, treatment planning and follow-up. This procedure has been further organized into a form which the student utilizes to define the patient's problem, plan the treatment program, record observations and evaluate results.

The problem-solving method requires the student to identify the patient's problem before initiating treatment. Without such a process there is a tendency for the student to involve the patient in an activity before sufficient evaluation is completed or when the information is only partially collected.

Through the use of the clinical modified form the student learns to identfy the patient's problems and manifestations of symptoms, base the occupational therapy program upon authoritative sources within the literature, design and implement the program, observe and record patient performance, and prepare a summary of the treatment program.

The reliability of this method lies in its rejection of action based on isolated and unrelated data. It instead emphasizes the logical accumulation of data from which hypotheses can be developed and tested. The clinical environment of occupational therapy may be viewed as the setting in which the student develops and tests hypotheses and is thereby encouraged to develop the ability for critical analysis in the treatment process.[8]

Summary

A follow-up appraisal concerning clinical teaching strategies for twenty-five occupational therapy students has been discussed. These students completed the total clinical affiliation within a single teaching center where unified teaching methods were employed throughout the period. Examples of essential learning experience units and a clinical modification of the problem-solving method utilized for organizing information and basing treatment plans have been presented. These factors combined with involvement of the student in the discovery of information, in problem-solving, in assuming responsibility for learning have been the underlying strategies.

REFERENCES

1. Myers, Cordelia, "Teaching Method Concepts," *Amer J Occup Ther* XVII, 5 (Sept.-Oct. 1963), 187-189.
2. Hatch, Winslow R. and Bennet, Ann, "Effectiveness in Teaching," *New Dimensions in Higher Education* Number 2, US Dept of Health, Education, and Welfare (1964).
3. Hatch, Winslow R. and Richards, Alice L., "Approach to Independent Study," *New Dimensions in Higher Education* Number 13, US Dept of Health, Education, and Welfare (1965).
4. Kersh, B. Y., "The Adequacy of 'Meaning' as an Explanation for the Superiority of Learning by Independent Discovery," *J Educat Psychol* 49 (1958).
5. McDonald, Frederick, *Educational Psychology*, Second Edition, Wadsworth Publishing Company, Inc. (1966).
6. Bruner, Jerome S., *The Process of Education*, Knopf (1963).
7. Gagné, R. M., "The Acquisition of Knowledge," *Psychol Rev* 69 (1962).
8. Feinstein, Alvan R., *Clinical Judgement*, The Williams and Wilkins Co., (1967).

34

An Approach to Supervision of Students on Fieldwork

(administration, education, occupational therapy)

Kathleen Barker Schwartz

This paper describes a method for supervision of occupational therapy students on clinical affiliation. The approach is based on the assumption that students behave in ways that are consistent with Levels 3 through 4 of Jane Loevinger's stages of personality development. The most effective supervisory approach for students at each level of behavior is described. The model assumes that the level of student can be matched with a supervisory approach to result in a more satisfying experience for both student and supervisor.

Theories of Adolescent and Adult Development

Clinical supervisors need to have a way to evaluate and measure the growth of students on affiliation. Use of a developmental approach can help define a beginning and endpoint in a student's development during the three-month affiliation period. Recent theories in adolescent and adult development suggest, in part, how learning may take place. These theories offer a framework for supervisors to view the education process. Knowledge of a student's developmental level can aid the clinical supervisor in designing and fostering the learning experience.

Developmental theory seeks to map the individual's progress over time. The approach, using a biological model, assumes that development proceeds in an epigenetic pattern; that is, development proceeds through identifiable stages, with each stage increasing in complexity. At each new stage, qualities emerge that were not present at the previous stages (1). Recent theories of adult development provide models that describe the form that intellectual, moral, and personality development takes at specified stages. Since learning involves all three areas, clinical educators can benefit from understanding these current theories.

One of the most influential developmental stage theorists is Kohlberg (2). The model of moral development in adolescence and adults that Kohlberg describes draws heavily on Piaget's stages of intellectual development (3). Gilligan (4), an associate of Kohlberg's, expands the model by defining an element of morality not represented in Kohlberg's work, that of caring. Gilligan describes women's attempts to incorporate concern for justice with caring for others, and she hypothesizes that the stages of moral judgment are gender-related and may be based on self-definition.

Perry (5) formulated a developmental scheme based on his study of the intellectual and ethical development of college students. His work describes the transformation some students make: from an all-or-none, right-or-wrong construct, to one where many different perspectives are valid and where no single authoritative solution exists. Wilson (6), a British learning-theorist, presents a developmental model of student learning in higher education that incorporates

Kathleen Barker Schwartz, MS, OTR, is Academic Fieldwork Coordinator and Lecturer in Health Administration, Tufts University, Boston School of Occupational Therapy, Medford, MA 02115. She is also pursuing a doctoral degree in the Administration, Planning, and Social Policy Program, Harvard University Graduate School of Education, Cambridge, MA 02138.

research findings in such areas as cognitive processes, learning contexts, and academic achievement. Loevinger (7) defined a model of personality development, calling it a description of "ego development." She defines ego development as the way individuals make sense of the world. In this paper, Loevinger's model is applied to occupational therapy clinical education. It was chosen because the author thinks it aptly describes affiliating students' levels of intellectual and personality development.

Application of Loevinger's Developmental Model to Clinical Education

Loevinger and her associates have identified nine stages (six major and three transitional) that reflect a discrete and relatively stable pattern of cognitive, intrapersonal, and interpersonal functioning. Of the nine stages, Ego Stage Levels 3, 3/4, and 4 best describe behavior typical of occupational therapy students on affiliation. Levels 1 and 2 describe behavior that is less mature than is exhibited by most affiliating students, while Levels 5 and 6 describe highly autonomous and integrated behavior that goes well beyond students' capacity for functioning during fieldwork (see Table 1).

A discussion of student characteristics will help illustrate Loevinger's developmental stages. Students at Stage Level 3 usually obey the rules without asking questions. There is a need to belong to a group and gain approval from peers and authority figures. The student possesses a limited amount of self-awareness and is uncomfortable with the idea that a problem has several solutions.

Stage Level 3/4 shows a shift in complexity of thinking. Questions of causality arise, and the individual is able to see different possibilities and alternatives. Introspective ability increases as the student begins to differentiate individual responses to others. There is a tension between wanting to stand out in a group (to be an individual), yet a desire not to be outside the group. Although the student has the cognitive ability to understand the complexities of different viewpoints, the individual expresses his or her own beliefs and values with dogmatism and rigidity. The student does not want to discover anything that will confuse his or her configuration of the world.

Students at Stage Level 4 possess a high level of conceptual skill that includes an acceptance of multiple viewpoints and an ability to understand the complexities of problematic situations. Students internalize standards of performance, but are hypercritical and overly concerned with self-improvement.

Using Loevinger's model of ego stages, Lasker and deWindt (8) created a schema that correlates stage of ego development with a hierarchy of learning experiences that progresses from impersonal didactic situations to personal application situations. Table 1 is a

Table 1
Loevinger's Ego Stages Pertinent to Occupational Therapy Clinical Education

Ego Stage	Character Development	Interpersonal Style	Cognitive Style	What is Knowledge	The Learning Process
Level 3	Conformity to external rules, guilt for breaking rules	Belonging, superficial niceness	Conceptual simplicity, stereotypes	Necessary information in order to achieve the desired end. Takes the form of right or wrong, good or bad	Revelation of truth by an expert authority; if conflict between ideas is perceived, one element is dismissed as incorrect.
Level 3/4	Differentiation of norms, goals	Aware of self in relation to group, helping	Multiplicity	Information to be applied to situational problems, possibility of several correct solutions	Student questions information received from the expert authority and tries to align with own view.
Level 4	Self-evaluated standards, self-criticism, guilt for consequences, long-term goals and ideals	Intensive, responsible, mutual, concern for communication	Conceptual complexity	Skill in problem-solving	Discovery of solutions through logical analysis, multiple views acknowledged but simplicity sought

composite taken from Loevinger's description of behavior at Ego Stage Levels 3, 3/4, and 4, and Lasker's schema that describes how knowledge is perceived and how learning takes place at each level.

Lasker's schema for matching learner to learning experience supports the author's hypothesis that better clinical supervision can result from matching student level to supervisory approach. There is considerable research that correlates educational achievement with level of ego development (9-17). In addition, several prominent writers in the field of adult education (18-20) advocate matching student to learning experience by using developmental theory as one way to understand learners and how they might be taught more effectively.

A Method for Clinical Supervision

The clinic is the site for a minimum of six months of fieldwork Level II experience which, according to the "Essentials for an Accredited Educational Program" (21), provide the opportunity to apply theories and knowledge learned in the classroom. The clinic provides a structured educational experience with significant opportunity for rational analysis and practice where performance can be evaluated. The learning process is one of discovery through logical analysis where more than one solution is possible. The role of the teacher is as model and evaluator. The student role is to learn through doing and engage in frequent personal interaction with the teacher where behavior is analyzed and critiqued. It is presumed that the student will be able to perform as well as an entry-level therapist upon completion of the affiliation.

Supervision of affiliating students involves clinical teaching, administrative instruction, and counseling. Table 2 illustrates

Table 2
A Method for Clinical Supervision

Student Group	Teaching Approach	Supervision Sessions	Administrative Instructions	Counseling Intervention
Conscientious (Stage Level 3)	Assume student sees supervisor as "authority" and expert. Present information; show how several solutions can work. Lead toward student identification of problems, solutions.	Structure, with clear description of expectations. Make assignments to think about, bring to next meeting.	Delineate rules. Expect student to follow. Show disapproval if student does not.	Student desires acceptance, wants things to go well. Student will be upset with problems and look to supervisor for answers. Lead student to join supervisor in seeking answers.
Explorer (Stage Level 3/4)	Assume student in process of developing own system of problem solving. Discuss how student's view is worthwhile, problematic. Lead student toward accepting multiple viewpoints. Encourage exploration with clearly-defined limits.	Negotiate: Explain supervisor expectations, seek student input. Lead, but allow some flexibility in goals.	Delineate rules. Expect student will not follow if rules conflict with own ideas. Discuss implications if student chooses to follow own inclination.	Student will be dogmatic and upset when things do not work according to plan. Lead student to see several ways to be effective. Support student through confusion.
Achiever (Stage Level 4)	Assume student has developed systems of beliefs, problem solving. Challenge ideas. Discuss implications. Lead toward greater analytic competence in problem solving. Encourage exploration with feedback.	Discuss supervisor expectations and student's. Collaborate on discussing best method to achieve goals.	Delineate rules. Discuss origins where appropriate. Expect student to seek exceptions. Explain when supervisor can/cannot be flexible.	Student will be hypercritical of failures. Help student see when guilt is appropriate, when student is exceeding reasonable limit of responsibility.

a method for clinical supervision. The material cited under Teaching Approach is an extrapolation from Loevinger's description of behavior at Ego Stage Levels 3, 3/4, and 4, and Lasker's description of how individuals at those levels perceive the learning experience. Working from these descriptions of learner behavior, the table illustrates how a supervisor would conduct supervision sessions, administrative instruction, and counseling intervention. The supervisor can use the table first by identifying whether a student's behavior pattern fits into Loevinger's Ego Levels 3, 3/4, or 4 (see Table 1), and second, by matching the designated level to the teaching approach in Table 2. This proposed method enables a supervisor to match an individual student's behavior to a supervisory approach that is based on a description of how students at a particular level experience learning.

The teaching approach for the Conscientious group (Loevinger's Ego Stage Level 3) is based on the assumption that the student views the supervisor as an expert. So the student must be led through structured questioning to see that he or she can also provide viable solutions to clinical problems. A student in the Explorer (level 3/4) group is in the midst of developing his or her own system for problem solving. An effective teaching approach, then, is to guide the student through the problem to help him or her see which solutions are most effective and why they are viable. Students in the Achiever (level 4) group are able to define the problems and develop solutions to a clinical situation. They need a teaching approach that will help them examine the merit of their solutions and their problem-

solving procedure, and lead them to develop more sophisticated skills in interpretation.

In supervision sessions, the Conscientious student will predictably respond best to supervision where questions are highly structured with follow-up assignments given. Students in the Explorer group will benefit from limited exploration of a topic. To avoid confusion, the supervisor should watch for the point when the amount of data overwhelms the student. The student in the Achiever group will respond well to a discussion of why and how, and to an examination of any discrepancies between previously-acquired knowledge and new information given in the clinic.

For administrative instruction, the Conscientious student will not be bothered by the imposition of rules and will strive to obey them. The Explorer will challenge the rules if they do not fit within his or her value system. The Achiever will do best when the origin of the rules is explained so he or she can understand them better.

In counseling the Conscientious student, the supervisor should be aware that the student greatly desires acceptance and will tend to personalize criticism. The focus, then, would be on separating the student's view of personal worth and professional performance. The Explorer student may be inflexible when feedback contains a viewpoint that the student does not share. The supervisor needs to help the student gain perspective when it comes to comparing the merit of his or her own view with others' professional judgment. The Achiever student may need counseling to help set standards of performance that are realistic and achievable.

Discussion

The approach to supervision of occupational therapy students described in this paper is based on Loevinger's theory of adult development. Because adult development is a relatively new field, few of the theories have been tested to prove that they paint an accurate portrait of the way adults grow, change, and learn. Thus, Loevinger's description of ego stages might be criticized on the grounds that it is not a faithful portrayal of adult development. It could be argued, however, that Loevinger's theory is built on a strong foundation. Loevinger is a psychometrician who created her ego development construct from the results of a projective test (a 36-item sentence completion) that has been correlated with clinical observation. The test has been subjected to a number of reliability and validity studies and also used in a variety of research programs (15). While most of the adult development theories are based on empirical observation, Loevinger's is one of the few constructs created from the results of test data. Thus, the test can be used to replicate her research and examine her findings.

Developmental stage theory implies that "higher is better." To remove this hierarchical judgment, Ego Stage Levels 3, 3/4, and 4 were renamed in Table 2. The supervision approach in this paper is based on the assumption that each level has its strengths and potential problems, and that an effective supervisory approach should take both into account. There is research that shows a correlation between stage and years of education (15), and that education can stimulate development (22-24). Since professional standards for performance place heavy demands on students, it is desirable that they reach the developmental level that will enable them to best meet these demands. I believe that students at Level 3, 3/4, and 4 can meet the general fieldwork requirements. However, it may also be true that students at a certain level will have a better fit with a particular clinic. This match depends on the kind of demands placed on students within the different clinical programs.

Developmental stage theory could be accused of pigeonholing people into categories and levels. Probably no individual fits entirely into any one theorist's level. A construct such as Loevinger's has the additional problem of combining several areas of development, in this case cognitive, interpersonal, and intrapersonal. For example, the potential for discrepancy is greater than in Kohlberg's work where he only addresses the two areas of intellectual and moral development. However, the fact that many occupational theory clinical educators have found value in Loevinger's description cannot be dismissed and needs to be considered along with the potential for incorrect classification and stereotyping.

Conclusions
Research is needed to evaluate the validity of applying Loevinger's construct to occupational therapy clinical education. In addition to Loevinger, all of the adult developmental theorists mentioned in this paper provide theories that suggest patterns of learning behavior. Models based on these theories could provide supervisors with a methodology for clinical supervision. The method described

here is an example of such a model.

Acknowledgments
Thanks to Harry Lasker and K. Patricia Cross, faculty members at the Harvard Graduate School of Education; to Sharon Schwartzberg and Margot Howe, my colleagues at Tufts–Boston School of Occupational Therapy; and to Tuft's Clinical Associates, especially Sue Cleary Schwartz of Pacific Medical Center, for their support and enthusiasm. Special thanks to Ann Bonner, fieldwork assistant.

This paper was presented at the 1982 Annual AOTA Conference in Philadelphia; to clinical supervisors in June 1982 in Los Angeles and San Francisco; and in February 1983 in Providence, Rhode Island.

REFERENCES
1. Kitchener RF: Epigenesis: The role of biological models in developmental psychology. *Human Development* 21: 141-160, 1978
2. Kohlberg L: Continuities in childhood and adult moral development revisited. *Lifespan Developmental Psychology,* PB Baltes, KW Schaie, Editors. New York, NY: Academic Press, 1973
3. Ginsberg H, Opper S: *Piaget's theory of intellectual development.* Englewood Cliffs, NJ: Prentice-Hall, 1979
4. Gilligan C: *In a Different Voice.* Cambridge, MA: Harvard University Press, 1982
5. Perry WG: *Forms of Intellectual and Ethical Development in the College Years: A Scheme.* New York, NY: Holt, Rinehart and Winston, 1968
6. Wilson JD: *Student Learning in Higher Education.* New York, NY: Wiley, 1981
7. Loevinger J: *Ego Development: Conceptions and Theories.* San Francisco, CA: Jossey-Bass, 1977
8. Lasker HM, deWindt C: Implications of Ego Stages for Adult Education. Unpublished manuscript, Harvard University, 1974
9. Lasker HM: Ego development and motivation: A cross-cultural analysis of achievement. Unpublished doctoral dissertation, University of Chicago, 1978.
10. Lasker HM: Summative report on the ego development training program. Unpublished manuscript, Harvard University, 1978.
11. Jesness CF: *Report on the Youth Center Research Project.* Sacramento, CA: American Justice Institute, 1972
12. Broughton JM: The development of natural epistemology in adolescence and early adulthood. Unpublished doctoral dissertation, Harvard University, 1975
13. Chickering AW: Developmental change as a major outcome. *Experiential Learning: Rationale, Characteristics and Assessments,* MT Keeton, Editor. San Francisco, CA: Jossey-Bass, 1976
14. Weathersby R: A developmental perspective on adults' uses of formal education. Unpublished doctoral dissertation, Graduate School of Education, Harvard University, 1977
15. Hauser S: Loevinger's model and measure of ego development: A critical review. *Psychology Bulletin* 83: 928-955, 1976
16. Loevinger J, Wessler R: *Measuring Ego Development I: Construction and Use of a Sentence Completion Test.* San Francisco, CA: Jossey-Bass, 1970
17. Weathersby RP: Ego development. *The Modern American College,* AW Chickering, Editor. San Francisco, CA: Jossey-Bass, 1981
18. Chickering AW, Havighurst RJ: The life cycle. *The Modern American College,* AW Chickering, Editor. San Francisco, CA: Jossey-Bass, 1981
19. Cross KP: *Adults as Learners.* San Francisco, CA: Jossey-Bass, 1981
20. Knowles MS: *The Modern Practice of Adult Education.* New York, NY: Association Press, 1980
21. AOTA: The essentials of an accredited educational program for the occupational therapist. *Am J Occup* 37(12):817-823, 1983
22. Erickson VL: Psychological growth for women: A cognitive-developmental curriculum intervention. *Counseling and Values* 13:52-73, 1974
23. Erickson VL: Deliberate psychological education for women: From Iphigenia to Antigone. *Counselor Education and Supervision* 14(4):297-309, 1975
24. Kohlberg L, Mayer R: Development as the aim of education. *Harvard Education Review* 42(4):449-496, 1972

The American Journal of Occupational Therapy **397**

The clinician as student educator: Coaching vs educating

Judith Vestal, MA, OTR/L
Assistant Professor
Louisiana State University

Kristin Seidner, MSW, OTR/L
Program Director and Associate Professor
Occupational Therapy Department
Louisiana State University Medical Center
Shreveport, Louisiana

THE PROFESSION of occupational therapy requires that students complete a minimum of 6 months full-time fieldwork prior to taking the certification examination.[1] Although individual curricula, along with the American Occupational Therapy Association, provide general fieldwork objectives, the specific fieldwork experience is determined by the clinical supervisors.[2] Academic educators rely heavily on clinical supervisors to provide an environment in which the theoretic foundations of the occupational therapy profession can become integrated and blossom into effective practice. Yet many clinicians have minimal or no preparation to assume the role of clinical educator.[3,4]

The "Essentials and Guidelines of an Accredited Educational Program for the Occupational Therapist" state:

The purpose of Level II fieldwork is to provide an indepth experience in providing occupational therapy services to clients. Level II fieldwork shall

The authors gratefully acknowledge the assistance of Doris Ann Wart, a law student at Rutgers University, in preparation of the survey. The authors also thank Suzanne Poulton, MPH, OTR/L, and Debra Judd, PhD, OTR/L, for their critique of the manuscript.

Occup Ther Pract 1992; 3(3): 29–38
© 1992 Aspen Publishers, Inc.

be required and designed to promote clinical reasoning and reflective practice, to transmit the values and beliefs that enable the application of ethics related to the profession, to communicate and model professionalism as a developmental process and a career responsibility, and to develop and expand a repertoire of occupational therapy assessments and treatment interventions related to human performance.[1(p1,082)]

This document also states "Supervision shall be provided by a certified occupational therapist with a minimum of 1 year's experience in a practice setting."[1(p1,082)] Other requirements are dependent on the institution and/or occupational therapy department that is providing the fieldwork experience. Some hospitals do require training to become a student supervisor. However, many fieldwork supervisors, even though they may be novice therapists, are given the task of educating students in their clinics without any formal training in clinical supervision. Fieldwork educators have the task of questioning students to facilitate their reflective thinking on how theory translates into practice, but they must understand this process themselves before they can teach others.[5] It is ironic that often the clinical supervisors who usually have the least amount of training in educational theory are asked to perform the most difficult task in the education process.

The "Essentials" clearly reflect that clinical supervisors must teach technical skills—ie, assessments, treatment interventions—but the emphasis is placed on critical thinking. It is important that clinical supervisors understand their role as a coach who trains the student in technical skills and as an educator who facilitates the thinking process. Supervisors choose their role depending on the developmental level of the student and the specific clinical situation.

In an effort to define current practices in Level II fieldwork, a survey of clinical supervisors and students was conducted. The purpose of this informal survey was to examine to what extent supervisors used coaching and educating with their students; the response of students to the coaching and educating done by their supervisors; and the perceived effects of the supervisor-student relationship on learning.

LITERATURE REVIEW

Coaching and educating share some common characteristics. *Webster's Ninth New Collegiate Dictionary* defines the act of coaching as "to train intensively . . . instruct."[6(p253)] The word *educate,* on the other hand, is derived from the Latin word *educere,* meaning "to lead forth," and is synonymous with *teach,* meaning "to cause to know...to guide the studies of."[6(p1,209)] The clinical supervisor is in a position to train (coach) the student as well as guide the student in his or her studies (educate).

Contrasts between the two terms may be found by exploring the methods and philosophies of late football coach Paul "Bear" Bryant and educators Socrates and John Dewey. Coach Bryant was a well-known, popular coach from Alabama. He trained his players in the fundamentals of football without requiring that they be introspective.[7] Bryant's style in coaching brought his players to the game with a positive attitude as well as the skills to be good football players. However, he did not encourage independent exploration of ideas or expression of thought.

In contrast, Socrates encouraged independent thought and problem solving through a questioning process. "Genuine Socratic questioning . . . has to do with getting actual people, who have specific and often strong opinions, to examine carefully what they think they know. . . . Socrates wanted people to recognize and revere the limits of human knowing."[8(p21)] His approach is different from that of Bryant in that the process of learning comes from self-examination and decision making based on deep thought rather than from an external source (coach) who teaches the strategy to use in each situation. The questioning process offers the student an opportunity to explore options and to think more critically about what might or might not be effective and reasons why.

John Dewey, like Socrates, was an educator and philosopher. His major contribution to education was his emphasis on the thinking aspect of education, which is reflected in his statement, "Thinking is the method of an educative experience."[9(p239)] He was an advocate of "reflective thinking" and felt that "it differed from the looser kinds of thinking primarily by virtue of being directed or controlled by a purpose—the solution to a problem."[9(p37)] Dewey suggested that issues or solutions are related to choice, and "choice is always a matter of alternatives."[9(p262)] Some of Dewey's ideas are related to elements of coaching. He suggests that the ability of a student to analyze and synthesize the abstract situation may be extremely difficult unless the student has learned concrete skills. Similar to the coaching experience, the student needs to have the knowledge and skills (the concrete strategy of how to play the game) in order to begin the more abstract process of analyzing and synthesizing each individual case, which Dewey terms "reflective intelligence."[4(p240)]

In summary, coaching and educating share some common characteristics. The coach's role is one of directing the mastery of technical skills and instructing in specific strategy. The student has little role in directing what is being taught. The coach is responsible for designing and implementing the "lesson plan," whereas the student is responsible for absorbing information and following directions for utilizing such information. The educator guides the studies of the student to include the mastery of basic skills. In addition, he or she leads the student toward discovery of solutions to problems through reflective thinking. The student has an equal

responsibility for directing his or her learning. When presented with a problem, the student must analyze a thought, bring forth additional information, synthesize ideas, and develop a plan. Thus, the educator stimulates critical thinking.

Christie et al[10] determined supervision to be the most critical component of a "good" fieldwork experience. Specifically, they identified the following aspects of supervision to be most important:

- adapting the supervisory approach to meet student needs;
- having a structured program with clear objectives;
- providing feedback that is constructive and timely;
- promoting open communication and guidance; and
- being available to the student.

In addition to supervision, Christie et al found that open and honest communication, a supportive environment, and a variety of patient caseloads and experiences were also keys to a successful fieldwork experience.

Gjerde and Coble[11] identified teaching behaviors of family practice faculty that were perceived by students to be most or least effective. Again, the results of their survey suggested three factors that positively influenced clinical teaching: a positive attitude, a "humanistic orientation," and an environment in which the student could be an active participant. Emery,[12] in his review of physical therapy students, found communication skills to be most important. These included active listening and interactive teaching. Also important were interpersonal skills, which included such characteristics as demonstrating positive regard and empathy and establishing a "comfortable" environment. Stritter et al[13] surveyed medical students to determine effective clinical teaching behaviors. They found six factors to be most helpful: active student participation, preceptor attitude toward teaching, emphasis on applied problem solving, student-centered instructional strategies, humanistic orientation, and emphasis on content and research.

Pridham[14] and Henry[15] addressed more specifically the steps involved in the process of transforming classroom knowledge into clinical experience. Pridham proposed a series of questions that might support a student through the clinical reasoning process. These questions promote consideration of why the student might think something was occurring in a patient, what evidence the student had, what hypotheses were formulated, what alternatives there might be, and how results would be evaluated. By asking questions, the supervisor is able to facilitate the student's thought process in reaching clinical decisions. Slater makes the point that the thought process behind the action is what differentiates the technician from the therapist. She goes on to say that "learning requires time for reflection."[16(p4)] She suggests role modeling as a way in which the experienced therapist may promote clinical reasoning in the less experienced clinician or student.

Slater suggests role modeling as a way in which the experienced therapist may promote clinical reasoning in the less experienced clinician or student.

The literature supports the fact that clinical supervisors and students find an educational approach to learning (clinical reasoning) the most effective. However, that does not negate the need for the more obvious learning of technical skills and the training required to become a competent practitioner.

METHODS

The survey of clinical supervisors and students consisted of two questionnaires. Each contained four open-ended questions addressing current methods used in the supervisor–student educational process. A pilot survey was conducted with eight supervisors and five students to ensure the clarity and validity of the questions.

The questionnaire requested information on the following topics:

- methods used to facilitate clinical reasoning;
- the student–therapist relationship;
- methods used to facilitate the learning of technical skills; and
- teaching–learning styles.

The questionnaire was mailed to participants along with a stamped, self-addressed envelope and a cover letter explaining the purpose of the study. Participants were asked to return the questionnaire by a given time, which was 3.5 weeks from the time of mailing.

Responses to each question were analyzed in terms of key phrases or words representing similar concepts. These concepts were then grouped and analyzed for frequency of occurrence in order to determine current practices (supervisors) and perceived effectiveness of current practices (students).

Participants for the survey were obtained from a list of fieldwork sites affiliated with the Department of Occupational Therapy, School of Allied Health Professions, Louisiana State University Medical Center, and students who were currently affiliating and would graduate in 1991 or 1992 and former students who were 1990 graduates from the Shreveport campus. The sampling of former students was limited as a result of a lack of information on current addresses. The number of questionnaires sent to clinical supervisors was 255, and the number of questionnaires sent to students/former students was 42.

Sixty-four questionnaires were returned from clinical supervisors (25%), and 20 were returned from students/former students (48%). The sample of supervisors represents a variety of geographic areas and areas of clinical practice (Table 1). Table 1 also illustrates the number of years of practice, years of supervision, and the number of students supervised in the past 2 years by this sample. Characteristics of student participants are found in Table 2.

FINDINGS

Clinical supervisors' responses

Responses from clinical supervisors to the question on how they encouraged the *development of clinical reasoning* included giving feedback regarding problem solving; discussion with the student following treatment sessions to help the student process information; and verbally "walking through" situations so that there was immediate support for the students. Some supervisors indicated that they would question the student to determine how the student was thinking and the level of thought. There also seemed to be strong support for promoting and developing observation skills and for encouraging interaction with patients.

Responses by supervisors to the question on how the *student–therapist relationship* affected the ability of supervisors to facilitate growth and development of students reflected a common theme: the importance of a positive, open relationship with mutual respect and communication in order for the student to progress satisfactorily. Verbal reinforcement/feedback from supervisors was thought to be an important consideration in the formation of the relationship. Another common successful element was structuring a proper dual role of supervisor and coworker. Other characteristics mentioned that supervisors felt affected the relationship were degree of comfort, trust, and rapport; the supervisor's approachability and availability; and the student's level of motivation and

Table 1. Characteristics of sample of clinical supervisors

Characteristic	Description	%
Setting	Acute care rehab (n = 28)	37.5
	Psychiatric facility (n = 21)	32.8
	Pediatric rehab (n = 7)	10.9
	Work hardening (n = 3)	4.6
	Residential dev dis (n = 3)	4.6
	Outpatient rehab (n = 2)	3.1
Geographic distribution	Southeast (n = 35)	54.6
	Southwest (n = 6)	9.3
	Northeast (n = 5)	7.8
	Midwest (n = 5)	7.8
	Hawaii (n = 1)	<0.1
	Unknown (n = 3)	4.6
No of years practice	Range: 1–30	
	Mean: 9; median: 10; mode: 8,9	
No of years supervision	Range: 1–26	
	Mean: 4; median: 8; mode: 5	
No of students in past 5 years	Range: 1–30	
	Mean: 4; median: 8; mode: 4	

Table 2. Characteristics of student sample

Number	Educational status
15	Completed only psychiatric affiliation; currently enrolled in LSU program, Shreveport campus
2	Completed three affiliations; 1991 graduate
2	Completed three affiliations; 1990 graduate

assertiveness. Another description of the student–supervisor relationship was that of the supervisor "mentoring" the student.

The most frequent response to the third question, how supervisors facilitated the *learning of basic skills and independence,* was that responsibilities for the student were gradually increased. The second most frequent answer was to have the student observe therapists treating patients. Several supervisors provided opportunities for practicing clinical skills, and felt this was most important. Other responses received from several supervisors were (1) the therapist observes the student and provides feedback; (2) the therapist questions the student and assists in problem solving; (3) the therapist challenges the student; and (4) the therapist provides explanation/rationale. Some make the student responsible for his or her own learning through trial-and-error treatment, case analysis, use of protocols, and supervision of other students.

The fourth question asked supervisors to examine the dilemma that results when the *supervisor's teaching style and the student's learning style* are incongruent. Overwhelmingly, the supervisors responded that they adjust to the students' needs. One clinician noted, "I am here for the student's benefit and must be flexible enough to help him/her reach his/her greatest potential." In addition, clinicians seemed to strive to identify students' learning styles. Some administered learning style scales to the students. In some settings, supervisors were able to match the learning style of the student with the teaching style of the individual supervisor.

Students' responses

The first question asked students to describe which methods they thought were effective in helping them to develop *clinical reasoning ability.* Students described helpful supervisors as those who encouraged independent thought and creative problem solving, served as role models, and facilitated the exploration of alternative solutions to problems. Some students had the opportunity to maintain a journal that was used by the supervisor to explore the decision-making process, with the rationale given for each decision entered. One student made a very perceptive comment relative to clinical reasoning: "Clinical reasoning is an abstraction that should be fostered and nourished, not taught."

The second question asked students how the *relationship with their supervisor(s)* had a facilitatory or inhibitory effect on their learning and perception of the fieldwork. Facilitatory characteristics of the supervisor mentioned most often were kind, friendly, and respectful. Other characteristics included the use of positive reinforcement and constructive criticism. The positive supervisors were described as available, appreciative, comfortable, helpful, fostering a trusting and open relationship, utilizing a warm and accepting approach, and willing to listen. Some inhibitory characteristics were mentioned as sometimes having a positive effect; these included "pushing" a little at times; lack of respect, which one student reported caused him to be more assertive; and intimidation and humiliation, which were reported to make one student stronger.

The third question asked students to identify how the fieldwork experience facilitated their *learning of basic skills and ability to function independently*. Students felt that they learned basic skills and independence through being involved in the total occupational therapy process, including evaluation, setting goals and objectives, selecting activities, discharge planning, and documentation. They felt it was also helpful to represent the occupational therapy department and/or to speak at team meetings. Several students answered that they learned through a gradual increase in responsibilities, through interdisciplinary interactions, and through practice with supervision. Other, more infrequent answers were an open and honest relationship with supervisor, self-evaluation of treatment sessions, encouragement by the therapist to be creative, trust and support from the supervisor, and opportunities to observe staff members.

The fourth question asked students to identify their own *learning style*. The majority of responses indicated that students preferred a structured environment and a flexible style of supervision. Students indicated a preference for situations that were more directive initially but gradually moved toward allowing the student more independence. Again, students commented on the importance of being able to use their own clinical judgment with an appropriate level of supervision (interpreted as enough supervision to avoid major errors).

DISCUSSION

These responses reflected the essence of Level II fieldwork experiences from both the supervisors' and the students' perspectives. An analysis of responses indicates that there are more similarities than differences in the perceptions of supervisors and students of a "good" fieldwork experience. The answers to the question on clinical reasoning were similar, with some exceptions. Supervisors mentioned the promotion and development of observation skills and interaction with patients. Students commented on the importance of role models and the desire for supervisors to encourage independent thought through "creative" problem solving. Answers to the question on the supervisor–student relationship differed in that supervisors felt that a balance in the roles of supervisor and coworker was important to facilitate learning and that the student's level of motivation and degree of assertiveness were critical elements. Students emphasized the desire for a supervisor who was kind, friendly, warm, and accepting. Answers to the question on how learning and independence were best facilitated indicated both similarities and differences. Both groups overwhelmingly mentioned that a gradual increase in responsibility was critical to learning and independence, and that students needed to observe therapists "in action." Supervisors mentioned some methods to facilitate learning, whereas students mentioned more relationship factors—ie, open and honest relationship, trust, and support. Students also mentioned the importance of interdisciplinary interaction and involvement in team meetings. For the question on teaching/learning style, supervisors tended to take the major responsibility for adjusting to the student's need in terms of structure and flexibility. Students generally indicate a desire for a structured but flexible style of supervision in which they gradually gain independence and trust to use their own clinical judgment, with decreasing amounts of supervision.

It is evident that in a clinical teaching situation, there is the need to coach the student in skills and strategies. There is also the need to motivate and communicate with the student. However, that is not enough. Students must learn to think reflectively. This can be facilitated by questioning supervisors. Cohn points out that ". . . we are faced with the challenge of designing our fieldwork programs to teach technical skills and simultaneously provide a foundation for clinical reasoning."[4(p240)]

We propose that educational methods that encompass questioning and reflective thinking are essential to a good fieldwork experience. These methods take the student beyond the technical skills that were developed through coaching. Thus, the student not only develops basic skills but also learns the thinking process that is critical for the competent practitioner of today.

IMPLICATIONS FOR OCCUPATIONAL THERAPY

A clinical supervisor is responsible for providing an in-depth learning experience that encompasses elements of both coaching and educating. The supervisor has to know how to balance these two elements to best meet the learning needs of a particular student. To assist the supervisor in accurately assessing these needs, Schwartz[17] has proposed examination of Loevinger's developmental model for clinical education. This model is related to stages of ego development in students.

Loevinger and Wessler[18] described nine stages reflective of cognitive, interpersonal, and intrapersonal functioning. Schwartz[17] described how three of these stages (stages 3, 3/4, and 4) related to typical students in their clinical affiliation. At stage 3, the student is uncomfortable with the idea that several solutions to a problem are possible. At stage 3/4, the student realizes that various solutions to a problem are possible but experiences discomfort when the solutions confuse the student's "configuration of the world."[17(p394)] The student at stage 4 has a "high level of conceptual skill that includes an acceptance of multiple viewpoints and an ability to understand the complexities of problematic situations."[17(p394)] However,

these students are "hypercritical and overly concerned with self-improvement."[17(p394)]

These stages seem to parallel the three stages of stagnation, confusion, and integration described by Frum and Opacich.[19] They proposed that during a particular fieldwork the student progresses through three developmental stages. The first stage, stagnation, is characterized by the feeling of being "stuck" or being unaware but feeling a false sense of security. In the second stage, the student experiences confusion and instability as he or she searches for various solutions to problems. The third stage is one of integration in which the student becomes more comfortable with flexibility and creativity and sees the "whole" picture more clearly.

The role adopted by the clinical supervisor should reflect the developmental level of the student. As we have seen, the student who is developmentally youngest (Loevinger's stage 3 and Frum and Opacich's "stagnation" stage) may be overwhelmed, "stuck," or insecure when confronted with the expectations of clinical fieldwork. These students may need gentle guidance and carefully selected experiences that are geared for success to assist in the development of confidence in the clinical setting.

The role adopted by the clinical supervisor should reflect the developmental level of the student.

Students who have reached stage 3/4, or the "confusion" stage, may have difficulty appreciating the array of solutions to clinical problems that are available to them. They may feel uncertain about their ability to analyze clinical problems and select the most appropriate solution. Critical analysis of the pros and cons of each solution may be difficult. They may benefit from opportunities to explore these options, try various solutions, and, with support, evaluate the results.

The stage 4 student is beginning to integrate clinical experiences, to appreciate the array of options available, and to feel more comfortable exploring them. Such students need continued support while they analyze and synthesize data in preparation for problem solving. However, the need for support will lessen as the student begins to see his or her decision-making skills validated.

During any fieldwork a student may fluctuate through various stages of development. This draws on the supervisor's ability to be flexible and adapt his or her approach to each student's need at any given time. The supervisor's expectation of a student in a first fieldwork, as compared with a last fieldwork, will be different. The student will tend to progress through the stages more rapidly after more experience in the clinical setting.

Clinical supervisors responding to the survey indicated the use of a variety of techniques that seem to fall into a developmental framework. Supervisors suggested, for example, that they have the student observe the therapist treating patients as the therapist provides an explanation and rationale for the treatment. This approach may be comfortable for the student in an earlier stage of development. Other therapists indicated they used a questioning format to assist the student in problem solving. Students who need support to explore the options and critically analyze clinical problems may find this very helpful. Supervision of other students and case analysis were used by some to promote acquisition of independence and seem to be appropriate for the developmentally older student. Although clinical supervisors were not asked to relate their style and supervisory techniques to developmental levels in fieldwork students, the techniques reported can easily be viewed on a developmental continuum. This continuum is also supported by the supervisors' comments that they adjust to the students' needs.

Supervisors' comments not only related to a developmental sequence but also supported more forcefully the educational rather than the coaching aspect of clinical supervision. Supervisors reported the use of the Socratic method of questioning, reinforcement, and positive feedback. They referred to their roles as "facilitators" of learning. They also reported the importance of positive interactions and communication between student and supervisor. As facilitators of learning, clinical supervisors need to be flexible and willing to change their approach as needed for each student. In our survey, the majority of supervisors responded that they do adjust to student needs and that they attempt to match teaching style with learning style. If this is the case, then the structure and assistance provided will be flexible and personal rather than rigid and impersonal. Supervisors need to be aware that "good" academic curricula provide up-to-date theoretic concepts and technical information but provide limited skill application in labs and Level I fieldwork experiences. Students form the foundation for clinical reasoning in their academic programs; however, the situations, problems, and experiences necessary to continue the development of clinical reasoning occur during Level II fieldwork. It is here that the clinician engages in a process with the student, which facilitates growth in ego development and movement to an integration of the problem-solving abilities needed in the clinical environment. Extensive experience is a major factor in the development of clinical reasoning. Even in their final affiliation, students are at the beginning of the clinical reasoning "journey." Cohn points to the fact that "clinical reasoning is a complex process and is dependent upon years of experience."[4(p241)] Clinical reasoning is dependent on the student's knowledge of theory, concrete tasks, and skills. It is also dependent on the supervisor's ability to "educate" through questioning/probing, modeling, and incorporating methods of "coaching" to teach the best possible strategies for motivating the student and winning the "game" of improving quality of life for the patient.

•   •   •

A comparison has been made between coaching and educating as it relates to clinical education. Clinical supervisors need to be good educators and yet incorporate desirable traits of coaching—ie, the ability to motivate, communicate, and teach strategies. The educational role facilitates learning through questioning, reflective thinking, and problem solving. The outcome of a successful fieldwork is the student's progression through the developmental stages. When the educational process is effective, the result should be growth and development of the student in interpersonal skills (with patient, supervisor, and coworkers), increased degree of comfort in the therapeutic environment, ability to apply knowledge and technical skills to practice, and clinical reasoning ability.

The information gathered from the survey supported results found in the literature; however, there were limitations to the study. The student sample was small and consisted primarily of students on their first fieldwork, which was in psychiatry, and the return rate by clinical supervisors was small. Both factors limit the generalizability of the survey data.

Further research might address supervisory style as it relates to the various levels of ego development in students. It would be interesting to determine which methods are effective in facilitating a student's progression from Frum and Opacich's stagnation level to competence and from Loevinger's stage 3 to stage 4.

REFERENCES

1. American Occupational Therapy Association. Essentials and guidelines of an accredited educational program for the occupational therapist. *Am J Occup Ther.* 1991;45(12):1,085.
2. Cohn ES, Frum DC. The issue is fieldwork supervision: More education is warranted. *Am J Occup Ther.* 1988;42(5):325–327.
3. Crist PA. *Contemporary Issues in Clinical Education.* Thorofare, NJ: Slack; 1986.
4. Cohn ES. Fieldwork education: Shaping a foundation for clinical reasoning. *Am J Occup Ther.* 1989;43(4):240–244.
5. Stafford EM. Relationship between occupational therapy student learning styles and clinic performance. *Am J Occup Ther.* 1986;40(1):34–39.
6. *Webster's Ninth New Collegiate Dictionary.* Springfield, Mass: Merriam-Webster; 1984.
7. Smith ES. *Bear Bryant: Football's Winning Coach.* New York, NY: Walker & Co; 1984.
8. Sweers CJ. Teaching students to examine their lives. *Education Leadership.* 1988;May:20–22.
9. Hullfish HG, Smith PG. *Reflective Thinking.* New York, NY: Dodd, Mead & Co; 1961.
10. Christie BA, Joyce PC, Moeller PL. Fieldwork experience, part II: The supervisor's dilemma. *Am J Occup Ther.* 1985;39(10):675–681.
11. Gjerde CL, Coble RJ. Resident and faculty perceptions of effective clinical teaching in family practice. *J Fam Pract.* 1982;14(2):323–327.
12. Emery MJ. Effectiveness of the clinical instructor. *Phys Ther.* 1984;64(7):1,079–1,083.
13. Stritter FT, Hain JD, Grimes DA. Clinical teaching reexamined. *J Med Educ.* 1975;50:876–882.
14. Pridham KF. Why clinical field study? *Nursing Outlook.* 1990;38(1):26–30.
15. Henry JN. Identifying problems in clinical problem solving. *Phys Ther.* 1985;65(7):1,071–1,074.
16. Slater DY. A manager's role in shaping practice: The clinical reasoning process. *Special Interest Section Newsletter.* 1990;6:3,4.
17. Schwartz KB. An approach to supervision of students on fieldwork (administration, education, occupational therapy). *Am J Occup Ther.* 1984;38(6):393–397.
18. Loevinger J, Wessler R. *Measuring Ego Development I: Construction and Use of a Sentence Completion Test.* San Francisco, Calif: Jossey-Bass; 1970.
19. Frum DC, Opacich KJ. *Supervision: Development of Therapeutic Competence.* Baltimore, Md: The American Occupational Therapy Association, Division of Education; 1987.

SECTION FOUR | Research on Students' Perceptions and Attitudes Related to Fieldwork

Fieldwork revolves around the supervisor-supervisee relationship. The dynamics of this relationship include the student who comes to the facility with a variety of strengths and weaknesses, and who learns the strategies related to the job of occupational therapist or occupational therapy assistant. In this role, no two students are alike, yet they share some of the same issues and concerns.

Deborah C. Frum and Karin J. Opacich, authors of *Supervision: The Development of Therapeutic Competence* (1987), describe eight familiar issues that, according to supervisors, occur repeatedly with students:

1. Competence
2. Emotional awareness
3. Autonomy
4. Identity
5. Respect for individual differences
6. Purpose and direction
7. Personal motivation
8. Professional ethics.

Competence refers to the student's ability to implement an actual treatment or evaluation. It is the transition from classroom to clinic and involves taking "book-knowledge" to the next level. Fieldwork students typically are most nervous about this aspect of fieldwork because of the dependence on grades. Competence is also usually the most-important issue in beginning the supervisor-supervisee relationship.

Emotional awareness is the student's ability to recognize when their own personal reactions or behaviors are emotionally attached to the client or supervisor. A student who is aware of their emotional status will be able to distinguish the client's and supervisor's needs and assess the situation more objectively.

Autonomy refers to the students being responsible for their own decisions and functioning independently (within the framework of fieldwork and supervision). Here the student begins to learn that ideas may originate with themselves and not necessarily with others. The student who has been dependent in the classroom and who is experiencing his or her first training may need prompting to develop this attribute.

Identity is the student's ability to identify and integrate various theories of practice during the fieldwork experience. The issue is whether the student (and often the supervisor) has an understanding of what guides practice in the particular setting. There may be an eclectic approach to practice; however, a student who has trouble linking theory to practice will have difficulty establishing a plan of care and treatment appropriate for the client. Progress in the clinic often correlates with the student's ability to identify the theories of practice.

The next issue is the *respect for individual differences,* which means respect not only for the fieldwork staff but for the clients as well. Understanding and respecting others' values and individual styles is vital to the delivery of quality care, to the transition from student to practitioner, and to the relationship between supervisor and supervisee.

Of major concern to students on fieldwork is *purpose and direction* in the treatment planning, implementation, and theoretical approaches to practice.

Both occupational therapy and occupational therapy assistant students should be able to demonstrate levels of clinical reasoning and be able to reflect on their treatment/activity choice. This issue also involves the ability of the student to distinguish the purpose of occupational therapy approaches compared to interdisciplinary service delivery.

Motivation is an issue that both students and supervisors face throughout their careers. The motivation to deliver occupational therapy services was crucial to the choice of the profession in the first place. Personal motivation becomes an issue with students who come to the fieldwork experience with different expectations, especially when the supervisor is questioning their role within the clinical set-ting or the profession at large. Personal motivation often can determine whether a student or supervisor will continue with the relationship and the fieldwork experience.

Finally, there are *professional ethics*. A notion of ethics often begins by observing others in their professional roles and a students, feeling of worth in a clinical environment. A fieldwork supervisor should always strive to be a role model for the student in learning and honing professional ethics in the clinic.

This section of the anthology will hopefully provide both students and supervisors more information regarding the above eight issues.

The Student Speaks

Field Work Experiences in Nursing Homes

Judy Doerfler, *Student*
Bernadette Wiemer, *Student*
Ohio State University
Columbus, Ohio

As students on a field work affiliation, we discovered that we had expeiences in common in working with the elderly in nursing homes. One of us had been employed as a nurse's aide and activities director; the other had completed a three-month affiliation in an urban nursing home. In addition, we both encountered negative attitudes expressed by our classmates toward working in such settings and we were concerned that such attitudes could have an affect on the quality of care received by the geriatric client and thus deprive the students of an experience conducive to professional and personal growth. Therefore, we decided to share our perceptions of the value of occupational therapy in the nursing home with the hope that such students will come to view working in this setting as both challenging and satisfying.

The nursing home provides an excellent opportunity for treating the total person. The therapist assesses patient needs and implements treatment in the following areas: increasing independence in activities of daily living, improving physical and cognitive abilities, developing avocational interests, and facilitating adjustment to institutional living.

In our experiences, nursing staff priorities for providing medical care do not allow time for restoring independence in dressing and feeding. General activity programs often need to be adapted so that

therapists can prescribe specific activities to meet individual patient needs. Moreover, since the nursing home is usually the patient's permanent living environment, it is readily accessible to therapists for making adaptations.

Consideration of the resident's emotional needs is of primary importance. Many of our clients suffered from depression due to the inevitable aspects of aging: decreasing physical capacities, increasing dependency on others, inadequate financial resources, and loss of family and friends. Emotional needs are likely to take precedence regardless of the patient's physical problems.

Working in a nursing home fostered an appreciation of the needs and the predicament of the elderly in all living situations. In becoming more aware of our responsibilities for improving the quality of life for the aged, we began to examine our feelings toward our own aging and eventual death. This self-exploration heightened our appreciation of the work experience. Because we feel enthusiasm and commitment are of utmost importance in providing quality care, we hope students and therapists will re-evaluate their attitudes toward caring for the elderly.

The Self-Fulfilling Prophecy in Supervision

Bonnie L. Gschwend, *Student*
Ohio State University
Columbus, Ohio

There is a phenomenon described in the psychological literature called the "self-fulfilling prophecy," which

simply refers to the idea that an individual who is expected to perform at a certain level will perform at that level without regard to his actual abilities. The implications of this phenomenon in therapist/patient interactions seems obvious. It may be detrimental to the development of the patient's potential if a therapist enters the initial contact with a preconceived notion regarding the patient's performance.

What are the implications in supervisor/affiliate interactions? As a student in my third field work experience, I have looked retrospectively at how supervision affected my performance as an affiliate. When I was expected to perform as a student, I did, often refusing opportunities for more responsibility. When I was expected to perform as a therapist, taking more initiative and responsibility for my actions, I did. The difference is one's attitude in these two situations.

Usually, affiliates have been students for more than three fourths of their lives. They have been indoctrinated into the student role. I believe affiliates need the opportunity to practice the new role of therapist, the role they will move into abruptly once their field work experience is completed and they pass the registry exam. It seems an injustice to the affiliate, the prospective employer, and the profession not to have affiliates perform occasionally as therapists while in training. They need opportunities to begin to develop a healthy professional role and to be weaned from the more dependent student role.

Yet, valuable qualities can be developed in students that need to be maintained as they move into the therapist role, qualities such as good listening skills, the desire to learn, inquisitiveness, empathy, and a respect for both experience and new research. In speaking with an occupational therapy administrator who deals directly with the problems of supervisor/affiliate (new therapist) interactions, the need for these qualities become evident. Too often, it appears, an affiliate or new therapist is initially "turned off" by or in some way resents supervision. This can result in an unhealthy pattern of interaction and its becoming established. The affiliate or new therapist is unable to maintain the qualities mentioned above and thus is unable to benefit from the supervisor's experience.

The affiliate or new therapist often *expects* supervision to be a negative, nonvaluable experience; and because of this expectation, it is. In a similar fashion the supervisor may be unable to benefit from the affiliate's or the new therapist's recent formal educational experiences. Everyone loses, and again, because of attitudes.

Supervision is necessary and extremely important for the therapist in quality performance and in attaining professional competence. Yet, there can be a fine line between supervision that is beneficial and supervision that is stifling to one or both parties involved. The

difference can be in attitude. Affiliates, new therapists, and supervisors may need to look introspectively at their expectations of supervision. Once these attitudes are conscious, communication between supervisor and affiliate (new therapist) should include an open, honest, and direct discussion of these attitudes. Through this communication common objectives, methods, and goals can be reached that could improve the supervisory process.

The profession needs to put an end to the negative implications of the "self-fulfilling prophecy" in supervisory interactions.

AN INVESTIGATION OF THE RELATIONSHIP BETWEEN COLLEGE GRADES AND ON-THE-JOB PERFORMANCE DURING CLINICAL TRAINING OF OCCUPATIONAL THERAPY STUDENTS*

HELEN V. ENGLEHART

INTRODUCTION TO THE STUDY

Occupational therapy has been a recognized major objective of college students for about twenty-five years. During this time one of the chief problems of teachers in the field and the American Occupational Therapy Association, which coordinates all phases of the work, has been to determine whether or not the courses being taught were critically related to successful on-the-job performance. Up to the present time no systematic investigation of the relationship between performance in required courses and performance on-the-job has been reported.

The American Occupational Therapy Association made an investigation of the relationship between college grades and registration examination scores during 1947 and 1948. However, the problems of reliability of grades and variations between the various schools resulted in discontinuance of the study.

Statement of the problem. It was the purpose of the present study to (1) investigate the predictive value of performance in required college courses for performance on-the-job during clinical training; (2) investigate the predictive value of performance in required courses for the national registration examination; (3) investigate the predictive value of performance on-the-job during clinical training for the national registration examination.

SAMPLE TESTED AND INSTRUMENTS USED

The data for the study consisted of the grades earned in required college courses, the numerical scores on the occupational therapy student clinical training report, and the decile score earned on the registration examination. Grades were recorded from the college registrar's records, and the other data from the occupational therapy department files.

Subjects. The subjects for the present study were 104 students who graduated from San Jose State College, San Jose, California, during the college years 1945 through 1951. Ages ranged from 20 to 45, with 97 ranging from 20 to 29 and 7 from 30 to 45. Marital status was un-

known. Social and economic status varied but were similar to the extent that all were college graduates. Ninety-nine of the subjects were women and five were men.

College grades. For the present study college grades were translated into numbers as follows: A = 4; B = 3; C = 2; D = 1; F = 0.

Table 1 presents the means and standard deviations of all course grades used in the study. It will be noted that the mean grade in the social recreation course was found to be 3.41, or almost as high as the highest grade possible. However, the means for the other required courses are nearer the middle of the grade range, which is 2. The lowest mean found was in the sociology course where 2.38 was found. The standard deviations varied from .25 to .88.

Means and standard deviations for all course grades. (N = 101 to 104.)

Course	Mean	Standard Deviation
OT. crafts	3.05	.25
OT laboratory	2.87	.35
Social recreation	3.41	.55
Biological science	2.41	.88
Medical information	2.44	.79
Sociology	2.38	.83
OT theory	2.47	.71

Table I

The subject of grades is one about which much has been written and about which considerable differences in opinion exist. Ross[6] feels that teachers marks (grades) are lacking in both reliability and validity and that the principal reason for this is that teachers allow various extraneous factors to enter into the determination of grades. Carter[2] in a study of the non-intellectual variables entering into teachers grades found evidence to support the conclusion that personality, socio-economic status and intelligence seemed to be factors in the assignment of grades, but that grades represent more than chance estimates of student achievement. Kelley[14] states the opinion that whatever capacity it is that a

*An abstract of a thesis presented to the faculty of the department of psychology at San Jose State College, California, in partial fulfillment of the requirements for the degree of Master of Arts.

grade in any given subject stands for, it is a fairly accurate estimate of that capacity when the grade represents several estimates from more than one teacher.

Most of the grades used in the present study were based on written work, even in courses such as occupational therapy laboratory and social recreation. These courses are largely performance courses but the instructor for each stated that course grades were based largely on written work.[5, 8] Written work in the form of case

---

The relationship found between ratings in the four fields of clinical training. (N=101 to 102.)

	Tuberculosis	Orthopedics	Pediatrics..
Psychiatry	.23*	.26**	.22*
Tuberculosis		.29**	.37**
Orthopedics			.28**

*Significant at 5% level
**Significant at 1% level

Table II

---

histories of patients, written reports of patients' treatment and progress, library research projects, and quizzes on the outside reading are the basis for grading in the laboratory course. Grades in social recreation are based largely on written plans for group entertainment, a card file of various types of group projects, and written tests covering these materials.

No estimate of the reliability or validity of the grades used in the present study was attempted. The possibility of various kinds of error from these sources will be considered in evaluation of the results.

Ratings. The total score received by each student was used in the study of the occupational therapy student clinical training report. A measure of over-all performance during clinical training in the four fields was obtained by giving the ratings in each field equal weight and adding them to yield a single score. The office of the American Occupational Therapy Association advises that no studies of the reliability of the rating form have been made.

It will be noted, as shown in Table II, that the relationships found between ratings during clinical training in psychiatry and tuberculosis was $r=.23$, and between psychiatry and pediatrics $r=.22$, both of which are significant at the 5% level. All other relationships found were significant at the 1% level, as indicated by correlation coefficients of $r=.26$ between psychiatry and orthopedics; $r=.29$ between tuberculosis and orthopedics; $r=.37$ between tuberculosis and pediatrics; and $r=.28$ between orthopedics and pediatrics.

The level at which a rating scale is considered reliable varies from one authority to another.

However, it is generally agreed that a correlation coefficient of $r=.70$ is necessary for a scale to be acceptable. The self-correlation for orthopedics, $r=.81$, falls well above this lower limit of acceptability. Consequently, statistical results indicate that the rating scale has high reliability for the field of orthopedics. The low but significant relationships found between ratings in orthopedics and ratings in the other three fields of clinical training might suggest that the scale is not measuring the same things in the different fields of training. In spite of these low intercorrelations it is still possible that self-correlations in the other fields of training, if data were available to make such a test, would not be significantly different from the self-correlation in orthopedics. In this event the scale could be considered reliable for the other clinical training affiliations, as well as for orthopedics.

Table III shows the means and the standard deviations of the ratings for each of the four fields of clinical training as obtained from the occupational therapy student clinical training report. It will be noted that the means for orthopedics, 76.3 and pediatrics, 76.8, are very nearly the same but the standard deviations 8.81 and 10.10, show the greatest variation of the four sets of ratings. The greatest variation between means was found between tuberculosis, 83.6, psychiatry, 73.7, but the standard deviations were very nearly the same, 9.90, and 9.78.

Means and standard deviations for the four fields of clinical training. (N=103 to 104.)

	Mean	Standard Deviation
Tuberculosis	83.6	9.90
Psychiatry	73.7	9.78
Orthopedics	76.3	8.81
Pediatrics	76.8	10.10

Table III

The variation between the four sets of means is 9.9, or about one standard deviation. The variation between the means for orthopedics and the other training fields was found to be .5 to 7.3. This seems to substantiate the suggestion made above, that possibly the results of a test of reliability of the scale for the three fields of training for which data were not available to make such a test might produce results similar to that found in orthopedics. The low relationships between the ratings in the different fields of training and the similarity of the means and standard deviations suggest that the scale measures different fields of training, but may not suggest that the reliability of the scale is not similar.

Prior to 1950 the numerical scoring on the rating form was not the same as that which is used at the present time. In order to have just one set of scores to work with the scores prior to 1950 were statistically converted to the new scoring.

The registration examination. Information regarding the registration examination is limited due to the fact that it was constructed at the office of the American Occupational Therapy Association. Only enough copies for one for each student taking the examination are sent out to the colleges where it is administered, and immediately upon completion of the examination the questions as well as the answer sheets are returned to the association office. The examina-

Standards for reliability of tests seem to vary from one authority to another. Ross[6] states that a reliability coefficient of .94 is necessary if a test is to distinguish between individuals, but that .70 is sufficient for group prediction. Greene, Jorgensen, and Gerberich[3] hold that test reliability of .80 is evidence of marked reliability. With the lack of any specific standard, the coefficients reported (.75 to .85) seem to be high enough to indicate that the examination may be regarded as probably reliable.

The association reports that no studies of the validity of the examination have been made. The

THE RELATIONSHIP BETWEEN REQUIRED COLLEGE COURSES AND PERFORMANCE
ON* THE JOB COLLEGE COURSES AND REGISTRATION EXAMINATION AND
PERFORMANCE ON THE JOB AND REGISTRATION EXAMINATION (N=104)

Clinical Affiliations			College Courses					
	O.T. Crafts	Science Bio	Lab. O.T.	Theory O.T.	Info. Med.	Rec. Soc.	Socio.	Registration Examination
Tuberculosis	.02	.01	—.01	—.01	—.07	—.08	—.10	.06
Orthopedics	.33**	.07	.17	.21*	.22*	.07	.14	.23*
Psychiatry	.06	.27**	.15	.10	.16	—.07	.02	.34**
Pediatrics	.28**	.14	.12	.11	.19*	—.07	—.02	.08
Composite Ratings	.17	.21*	.09	.06	.14	.01	.10	.23
Registration Examination	.16	.45**	.37**	.46**	.64**	—.04	.40**	

*Significant at the 5 per cent confidence level
**Significant at the 1 per cent confidence level

Table IV

tion is composed of two parts. Each part contains 150 questions and two hours are allowed for completion of each part. The questions are all objective type, multiple-choice items. It covers all of the fields of clinical training and the required college subjects, i.e. occupational therapy crafts, biological science, occupational therapy theory, medical information, social recreation, and sociology.

The association reports that the scores on part I and part II of the examination are correlated against each other at every administration, February and June of each year. The reliability coefficients reported have ranged from .75 to .85. Means and standard deviations for the examination have not been reported but the association states that it has shown considerable stability, even though there has been the deletion and addition of new items, sometimes running as high as 25% or more for a single administration.

Whether or not the reliability coefficients of the registration examination as reported by the association have been corrected by the Spearman-Brown formula was not indicated. If not, the reliability coefficients reported would be stepped up by its use to a point where the examination would be considered quite reliable.

examination may or may not be valid, but whether or not it is valid, it is necessary to achieve a passing score on it before becoming a registered occupational therapist.

After the examinations are scored at the association office the decile and quartile scores are forwarded to the colleges for dissemination to the individuals concerned. The decile scores were used in the present study. The mean of the decile scores used was found to be 4.66 and the standard deviation was 2.51.

Statistical treatment. Scatter diagrams were plotted from the date of the study and examined to determine linearity. The bi-variant distributions appeared satisfactory and Pearson product-moment correlations were computed. As indicated by Table IV the following relationships were obtained:

1. Performance in required college subjects, as measured by course grades, and performance on-the-job during clinical training, as measured by the standard rating scale, for each of the four fields of clinical training.

2. Performance in required college subjects, as measured by course grades, and over-all performance on-the-job during clinical training, as measured by the standard rating scale, when the ratings for the four fields of clinical training were combined.

3. Performance in required college subjects, as meas-

ured by course grades and performance on the registration examination, as measured by score received.

4. Performance on-the-job during clinical training, as measured by the rating scale, for each of the four fields of clinical training, and performance on the registration examination, as measured by score received.

5. Over-all performance on-the-job during clinical training, as measured by the rating scale, with a composite rating for the four affiliations, and performance on the registration examination, as measured by score received.

RESULTS

Table IV presents the intercorrelations obtained. The relationships between required college courses and performance on-the-job, college grades and the registration examination, and performance on-the-job and the registration examination are given. The results obtained will be presented in three parts; on-the-job performance and the registration examination.

On-the-job performance and college grades. Grades in occupational therapy craft courses predict performance on-the-job during clinical training in orthopedics as indicated by a relationship $r = .33$, and during training in pediatrics where the relationship was found to be $r = .28$, both of which are significant at the 1% level. Grades in crafts courses do not predict performance during training in tuberculosis where the relationship was found to be $r = .06$, or over-all performance where the relationship found was $r = .17$, none of which is significant.

Grades earned in required biological science courses predict performance on-the-job during the psychiatric affiliation where a relationship of $r = .27$, significant at the 1% level, was found, and over-all performance where a relationship of $r = .21$, significant at the 5% level, was found. Biological science course grades do not predict performance during clinical training in tuberculosis where a relationship of $r = .01$ was found, or during pediatrics where a relationship of $r = .14$ was found. Neither of these relationships is significant.

Grades earned in occupational therapy laboratory courses do not significantly predict on-the-job performance for any of the four clinical affiliations, or over-all performance. Table IV shows the low relationships which are found, none of which are significant.

Grades in occupational therapy theory were found to be significantly related to on-the-job performance in one field of clinical training. For orthopedics a correlation coefficient of $r = .21$, significant at the 5% level, was found. In tuberculosis, psychiatry, pediatrics and over-all performance, the relationships found were not significant.

Grades in medical information courses were found to predict performance on-the-job at the 5% level for two affiliations of clinical training; for orthopedics $r = .22$ and for pediatrics $r = .19$. For tuberculosis, psychiatry, and over-all performance the relationships to medical information courses were not significant.

Grades earned in the social recreation course do not predict on-the-job performance for any of the four affiliations or over-all performance during clinical training. All relationships found were not significant.

Sociology grades do not predict performance for any of the clinical training affiliations, or over-all performance during training. No relationship of significance was found.

College grades and registration examination. Performance on the registration examination is significantly related to most of the required college courses. However, two courses do not predict performance on the examination as will be noted from Table IV. The relationship between occupational therapy craft grades and performance on the registration examination is not significant, nor is the relationship between grades in social recreation and registration examination score significant.

The college courses which predict performance on the registration examination with correlations which are significant at the 1% level are: biological science, $r = .45$; occupational therapy laboratory, $r = .37$; occupational therapy theory, $r = .46$; medical information, $r = .64$; and sociology, $r = .40$.

On-the-job performance and registration examination. Performance on-the-job in two of the clinical training affiliations significantly predict performance on the registration examination and two do not. Clinical affiliations which do not predict performance on the registration examination are tuberculosis and pediatrics. Clinical affiliations which do predict performance on the registration examination are orthopedics, where $r = .23$, significant at the 5% level, was found; psychiatry, where $r = .34$, significant at the 1% level, was found; and over-all performance, where $r = .23$, significant at the 5% level, was found.

DISCUSSION OF RESULTS

The predictors used in the present study, college course grades, should be viewed from the perspective of only partial cues to performance on-the-job. Thorndike[7] made the statement, "It must be recognized that performance during training and grades as an index of that performance, are only partial cues to eventual success in that job." This statement may very well be applied to the results of the present study and perhaps it might indicate that the grades used as predictors of on-the-job performance are of more importance than indicated by the results

100

obtained. That more than knowledge goes into performance on-the-job is accepted without question. No attempt to determine other ingredients of on-the-job performance was made. Burt[1] holds that it is not only what an individual can do but what he will do that determines to a large extent the relationship between performance on-the-job and any predictor. This is certainly applicable to college grades and on-the-job performance. Then, of course, the fallibility of grades, as predictors, and of rating scales, as performance indexes, must not be overlooked. The many possible sources of error and the assumptions that had to be made will be discussed later.

The results obtained indicate that on-the-job performance can be predicted from grades in some required college courses and cannot be predicted from grades in other required courses. The results for the registration examination are the same. Grades in some courses predict performance and some do not. Likewise performance on the registration examination may be predicted from performance on-the-job during some clinical training affiliations, but for some clinical affiliations no significant relationship was found.

CONCLUSIONS AND SUMMARY

From the results of the present study it is concluded that on-the-job performance during clinical training, and performance on the registration examination for occupational therapy students may be predicted from performance in some required college courses. However, performance in other required college courses does not predict on-the-job performance or performance on the registration examination. Likewise, on-the-job performance during some clinical training affiliations does not predict performance on the registration examination, but performance during other clinical training affiliations does predict performance on the registration examination.

For the subjects of this study it is concluded:

1. On-the-job performance during clinical training in tuberculosis cannot be predicted from performance in college courses.

2. On-the-job performance during clinical training in orthopedics may be predicted by low but significant relationships from college grades in occupational therapy crafts, occupational therapy theory and medical information courses.

3. On-the-job performance during clinical training in psychiatry may be predicted from biological science course grades by low but significant relationships.

4. On-the-job performance during clinical training in pediatrics may be predicted by low but significant relationships from craft and medical information courses.

5. Over-all performance during clinical training, as measured by combined ratings, may be predicted by low but significant relationships from biological science course grades.

6. Performance on the registration examination may be predicted from biological science, occupational therapy laboratory, theory, medical information and sociology grades, and from performance on-the-job during clinical training in orthopedics, psychiatry and over-all performance. The relationships between the examination and course grades were low but significant. The relationships between the examination and on-the-job performance were low to moderate.

The purpose of the study being reported was to (1) investigate the predictive value of performance in required courses, as measured by college grades, for on-the-job performance during clinical training, as measured by the standard rating scale used by all institutions approved for training students; (2) to investigate the predictive value of performance in required courses, as measured by college grades, for the national registration examination, as measured by score received on the examination; (3) to investigate the predictive value of performance on-the-job during clinical training, as measured by the standard rating scale, for the national registration examination, as measured by score received on the examination, for occupational therapy majors.

Subjects for the study were 104 graduates of San Jose State College majoring in occupational therapy. 99 were women and 5 were men. College course grades were translated into numbers and correlated with total score received on the rating scale and the decile score received on the registration examination. Total scores on the rating scales were correlated with the decile scores of the examination.

Under each of the three conditions noted in the first paragraph, certain course grades were found to be significantly correlated with the criteria. Some course grades were found to have correlations with the criteria which were so low as to be of no value in prediction.

ACKNOWLEDGMENTS

The helpful suggestions, criticisms and constant encouragement of Dr. J. T. Rusmore, under whose direction this study was carried on, is gratefully acknowledged.

Sincere thanks are also extended to Dr. E. W. Minium and to Miss Mary D. Booth, O.T.R. for their assistance and cooperation.

(Continued on page 107)

In direct contrast, self-spoon feeding could only be accomplished with the prostheses and the experimental infant hand. Since self-feeding appeared to elicit more purposeful prosthetic performance than other activities, and because of its importance in activities of daily living, the training schedule was revised so that prosthetic activity would be incorporated into the eating schedule. The new schedule firmly established the prosthetic routine into the mother's busy day. Ample time for the subject to engage in other activities was permitted either before or after the meal.

Self-feeding by means of the experimental infant hands attaches value to the prostheses. This may lead to early acceptance of the prostheses into the body image and place the subject in a good position to gradually incorporate the limb substitutes into his self concept.

Neither the broad palmar surface of the experimental infant hand nor the rigid point contact of the revised UCLA infant hand was utilized for body support when the subject assumed crawling or sitting positions. Instead, weight was placed on the flexed prosthetic forearms. The subject was observed to support some of his body weight on one palmar surface of the experimental infant hand when he reached for something with the other hand. This occurred in both the prone and sitting posture. Perhaps this form of support would have been more useful to the subject if it had been available when he was developmentally ready to support himself with his arms.

The developmental examinations revealed an equal motor performance in bilateral clasping of objects with the revised UCLA infant hands and the experimental infant hands. Both demonstrated improvement with maturation.

REFERENCES

1. Aitkin, George T., and Charles H. Frantz. "Prostheses for the Juvenile Amputee." *American Journal of Diseases of Children*, LXXXIX, February, 1957, 137-143.
2. Artificial Limbs Project, University of California at Los Angeles. Personal interview with Robert Jones, engineer, November, 1955.
3. Bechtol, Charles C., "Artificial Limbs for Child Amputees." *Children*, I, March, 1955, 92-99.
4. Child Amputee Prosthetic Project. First Annual Report prepared by the Department of Engineering and School of Medicine, University of California, Los Angeles, December, 1955.
5. Child Amputee Prosthetic Project, University of California at Los Angeles. Personal interview with Harry E. Campbell, prosthetist, March 10, 1956.
6. Ibid. Personal interview with Jeannine Dennis, occupational therapist, November, 1955.
7. Ibid. Personal interview with Murray Kahane, psychologist, 1956.
8. Chittenden, Rea F. "Problems Related to Prosthesis in Childhood." *Clinical Orthopedics*. To be published.
9. Gottlieb, M. "Force and Excursion Requirements for the Child's Prehension Device." Department of Engineering, UCLA, Special Technical Report No. 21, July, 1954.
10. Kessler, Henry J. "The Management of Congenital Amputations." *Kessler Institute of Rehabilitation*, I, 1953, 28-35.
11. Child Amputee Prosthetic Project. Medical records, University of California, Los Angeles, 1954-1956.
12. Tayback, Matthew. "Congenital Disorders, a Problem for Research." *Public Health Report*, LXX, September, 1955, 928-929.

Clinical Training . . .

(*Continued from page* 101)

BIBLIOGRAPHY

1. Burtt, H. E., *Principles of Employment Psychology*, Second Edition, Harper and Brothers, New York, 1942, 431 pp.
2. Carter, Robert S., "Non-Intellectual Variables Involved in Teachers' Marks," *Journal of Educational Research*, Vol. 47, No. 2, October, 1953.
3. Greene, H. A., Jorgensen, A. N., Gerberich, J. R., *Measurement and Evaluation in the Secondary School*, New York, Longmans, Green and Company, 1943, 670 pp.
4. Kelley, T. L., *Educational Guidance*, New York, Teachers College, 1914, 363 pp.
5. Mann, Eleanor P., O.T.R., Private communication with the writer, May, 1954.
6. Ross, C. C., *Measurement in Today's Schools*, New York, Prentice-Hall, Inc., 1947.
7. Thorndike, Robert L., *Personnel Selection*, New York, John Wiley and Sons, 1949, 358 pp.
8. Wilson, Sarah, B. S., Private communication with the writer, May, 1954.

A GUIDE TO PLANNING

● And Measuring Growth Experiences in the Clinical Affiliation

GAIL S. FIDLER, O.T.R.*

Perhaps at no time since its inception has occupational therapy been more concerned with its educational process. Change and growth in scientific knowledge and skill has had an impact on all areas of medicine. Along with medicine, related professions have become increasingly aware of the need to reassess and evaluate roles, functions, areas of focus and thus methods and concepts of professional education.

This process of reassessment has inevitably brought more sharply into focus questions concerning the purpose of professional education in order that its nature and quality may be more clearly defined. The search for a more succinct delineation of the nature of our profession and the relationship of its definition to educational methodologies and curriculum content has been evident in a number of studies and workshops during the past ten years. The American Occupational Therapy Association's Psychiatric Study Project which culminated in the Allenberry Conference[1] placed considerable value on the interpersonal relationship and thus on the therapeutic use of self. This study project and conference emphasized the need for the occupational therapist to work toward increased self-awareness and understanding as a means of enhancing capacities in therapeutic relationships. Surveys from the curriculum study[2] point up similar interest and concern in relation to occupational therapy practice and student education. Proceedings from the Highland Park Curriculum Study Workshop[8] seem to support the impression that occupational therapists have become increasingly concerned with the need to enhance interpersonal skills and thus the understanding of self and others. Further evidence of interest in this area may be found in reports from psychiatric institutes sponsored by the American Occupational Therapy Association, educational committees, clinical affiliation councils and numerous other meetings and discussion groups throughout the country.

This paper will explore some concepts related to professional learning and growth, suggesting a frame of reference for the clinical affiliation experience which may be perceived as both basic to and essential for such growth. Although these emanate from the clinical area of psychiatry, they would seem to be germane to other areas.

Concepts

If professional education for the occupational therapist has as its ultimate objective the "making of a therapist," then one may expect that the focus of such education will be on those experiences which provide impetus toward growth, increase capacity for maturation, and augment such growth. Such a goal recognizes the essential relationship between the educational process and the development of the learner as a professional person.[4] When we make these assumptions, we must inevitably acknowledge the relativity of self-understanding to the understanding of others and thus to being a therapist. Understanding of one's own conscious and unconscious feelings and attitudes is inextricably related to the use of self in treatment. A recent paper dealing with the education of the occupational therapist[5] explains that "the rationale for such emphasis (i.e., self-awareness and self-understanding) is predicated upon the awareness that relationships are at least two dimensional and one cannot fully understand another's behavior without first having some specific knowledge concerning the object (person) to which the other is responding. If one-to-one and group relationships are to attain the position of prominence we seem to be pressing for, then the occupational therapy student must be helped to work toward an increased understanding of his own conscious and unconscious feelings and behavior to provide some assurance against their interference in treatment, to heighten skill and knowledge in relationships, and to develop capacities for objective evaluation and understanding of others." Such insights are inherent in the development of a professional person and thus become an intrinsic part of professional education.

Within this context, the clinical affiliation is conceptualized as a continuity of integrated experiences directed toward maximizing growth in:

1. *Self-concept and personal identity*
2. *Self-awareness and self-understanding*
3. *Receptivity to learning and growth*

*Director, professional education, department of occupational therapy, New York State Psychiatric Institute; associate in occupational therapy, College of Physicians and Surgeons, Columbia University; clinical director, masters degree program in psychiatric occupational therapy, New York University.

Research on Students' Perceptions and Attitudes Related to Fieldwork | 235

4. *Flexibility, objectivity and judgment*
5. *Interpersonal relationships*
6. *Communication skills*
7. *Problem solving and decision-making skills*
8. *Observational and evaluative skills*
9. *Treatment planning and implementation skills*
10. *Group process skills*

Growth is always specifically related to the integration of a new function or the expansion of a function or capacity.[6] Pearce and Newton[6] state that in order for learning to be integrated into the personality, it must be clearly in awareness at the time of integration, include the synthesis of prior and current experiences, a conscious recognition of this synthesis and a validation of the new function or capacity. This theory underlines the significance of self-understanding in the process of integrating learning.

The clinical affiliated experience then needs to be structured in such a way that learning include opportunities for bringing the process of synthesis into awareness and making validation possible. Such an expectation emphasizes the importance of supervision and places a high premium on the nature and quality of such supervision. Supervision is a collaborative relationship committed to the growth of the supervisee. As such, it provides guidance and counsel for the student in the process of analyzing and evaluating his own involvement and his learning for the purpose of developing a definable set of constructs related to his own and other's conscious and unconscious motivations and behavioral responses.

Learning Expectations

One important requirement in approaching these goals and objectives is that the immediate learning expectations need to be within the student's current level of capacity. One cannot integrate new learning if the preliminary growth necessary for such learning has not been previously acquired. Thus, the nature and quality of supervision needs to begin at a level which makes integration possible for a given student. While our definition of growth and its purpose in the development of a professional person remains constant, it is evident that the structural quality of each learning experience and the expectation of these must necessarily vary with each learner. Some prior knowledge about the student's current functional capacities therefore becomes one of the first concerns in structuring an affiliation experience. The following form was devised for the use of schools referring students to us for clinical affiliation as a first and essential step in planning appropriate opportunities for learning and increasing the probability of integration of new learning.

Recognizing that one's receptivity to learning is influenced by many factors, we feel that some prior knowledge of the student as a person enables us to plan program implementation and growth experiences more accurately in terms of the individual's abilities and readiness, and thus contributes immeasurably to his capacities to use constructively such experiences. Therefore, your impressions with regard to the student in the following areas will be extremely helpful.

1. *Relationships*

How is the student seen by peers and authority and, in turn, how does he perceive each of these and act upon such perceptions?

What seems to be the quality and nature of his self-concept, and how does this seem to influence relationships with others?

What qualities are most characteristic of the student, i.e., flexibility, warmth, passivity, aggressivity, guardedness, spontaneity, rigidity, assurance, hesitancy, compliance, compromise, etc.? Explain.

2. *Function*

What is the nature of the student's integrative capacities, i.e., how does he react to change, uncertainty, challenge, responsibility?

Is he self-determining, self-assertive? In what way and to what extent?

What is his capacity to think with creativity and originality, and to then act productively on such conceptualizations?

What is the nature of his ability to analyze, synthesize, and draw conclusions?

Are there discrepancies between basic intelligence and performance? What is the nature of this?

3. *Capacity for Personal Growth*

What is the extent of the student's self-awareness and self-understanding?

To what degree is he able to look at his feelings and behavior? What blocks are evident?

In what ways has the student demonstrated a willingness to increase self-awareness and an ability to use such toward growth and understanding?

Such information about the student makes a higher correlation possible between presentation of material and the student's capacity to integrate such material thus diminishing anxiety and eliminating some blocks to growth.

The educational patterns of occupational therapy require that periodic assessments be made of a student's learning and growth. Ongoing evaluation and assessment is inherent in supervision and is thus an integral part of the clinical experience. However, problems arise when, within the context of the clinical affiliation as it has been defined here, one attempts to use the RPSA either as a rating form or as a counselling guide. It has been our experience that both student and supervisor find it difficult to reconcile the focal points of supervision and clinical affiliation with the frame of reference and focus of the RPSA.

In an attempt to resolve this dilemma and provide a more meaningful guide to evaluation and counselling, the following outline was developed. The content and structure of this outline seemed to more accurately represent both the purpose and quality of the clinical affiliation experience and more clearly define appropriate areas of emphasis. In addition, it can be expected that its use will provide the means for a more accurate measure of student growth, delineating more succinctly those areas of minimal and maximum development. Furthermore, we expect that the use of this evaluation over a period of time will make possible a truer estimate of the assets and limitations of our program as a learning experience, providing some index to the nature and extent of our successes and failures.

GUIDE TO THE EVALUATION OF STUDENT FUNCTIONING

Scale equals 1 (minimal) to 7 (maximum)

1. SELF-CONCEPT AND INTEGRITY
Tolerance for error and/or failure
Capacity to constructively integrate criticism
Ability to make decisions
Ability to act upon decisions—to implement
Capacity to act on own perceptions
Capacity for compromise
Consistency between words and actions
Appropriate self-expectations
Self-determining—self-directed
Self-assurance—belief in self—self-respect
Right of self to be different
Appreciation of common factors between self and others
Courage of convictions—values own judgment and perceptions
Integrative capacities—ability to withstand frustration, anxiety, disagreement

2. FLEXIBILITY
Ability to change—to adjust to change
Capacity for spontaneous response
Ability to respond appropriately to a simultaneous variety of experiences
Adaptiveness—capacity to modify behavior—to have alternative patterns available for varying circumstances

3. OBJECTIVITY AND JUDGMENT
Perception of common denominators among persons and groups
Appreciation of individual differences
Acceptance of rights of others to be different
Appropriate emotional control—frustration tolerance
Capacity to establish appropriate relative values
Tolerance
Ability to appraise situations realistically and objectively
Ability to reach sound conclusions
Appropriateness of timing
Sees things in proper proportions
Establishes appropriate priorities

4. SELF-AWARENESS AND UNDERSTANDING
Sensitivity to own needs and feelings
Ability to work toward increased self-understanding
Understanding of how own needs and feelings influence others
Capacity to distinguish own needs from those of others
Realistic assessment of own assets and limitations

5. RELATEDNESS TO OTHERS (PATIENTS AND STAFF)
Capacity to use increased awareness concerning self and others
Capacity to give to others
Capacity to receive
To be direct and forthright
Spontaneity
Empathy—sensitivity to needs and feelings of others
Capacity for warmth and tenderness
Ability to demonstrate warmth
Appropriate expectations of others
Respect for others
Capacity to allow others to be self-directive—independent
Capacity for engagement in collaborative problem-solving and decision-making

6. RESOURCEFULNESS AND CREATIVITY
Self-starting
Self-reliant
Enterprising
Capacity to formulate and develop independent ideas and theories
Capacity for invention—initiation—original ideas—to see beyond
Capacity to enlarge upon and develop existing fact and knowledge
Ability to act upon—implement creative thought

7. LEARNING CAPACITIES
Ability to analyze, synthesize, and draw conclusions
Ability to assimilate new facts and concepts
Ability to use old knowledge as a bridge to the new—inductive, deductive thinking
Capacity for experiencing a perception
Translating perceptions into concepts
Capacity for interpreting concepts into theories
Functions in keeping with potential

8. COMMUNICATION SKILLS
Effectively makes one's self understood (ability to translate ideas and concepts into forms readily understood by others)
Ability to communicate in an organized manner
Ability to focus on appropriate and essential points

9. MOTIVATION
Curiosity and drive to learn
Demonstrates active interest and enthusiasm
Incentive derived from inherent belief in concept of occupational therapy
Inducement derived from concern with patient welfare
Patient care and treatment pre-empt status needs, pleasing authority, grades, etc.
Contributes beyond requirements

10. RESPONSIBILITY
Ability to perceive responsibility
Capacity to accept responsibility for own actions and decisions
Dependability
Predictability

11. ORGANIZATION
Ability to do many things simultaneously
Follow-through in logical sequence and order
Appropriate use of structure and flexibility
Ability to interrelate and coordinate
Appropriate organization of time

12. THEORETICAL KNOWLEDGE
Basic dynamic psychiatry
Normal growth and development
Dynamics of pathology
Theories of the unconscious
Symbolism

Theory of occupational therapy—meaning of activities

Dynamics of the one-to-one relationship—transference—countertransference

Group process

Concepts of milieu as a therapeutic agent

13. *OBSERVATIONAL AND EVALUATIVE SKILLS*

Ability to focus on essentials—to know what to look for

Ability to perceive interrelationships

Ability to translate perceptions into useful data

Interpret validly

Relate observations and evaluations to a defined purpose

Skill in using evaluation outline

Skill in communicating these to others

Capacity and efficiency in locating and identifying problems

Ability to make sound and valid observations and evaluations

14. *TREATMENT PLANNING AND IMPLEMENTATION SKILLS*

Ability to delineate those patient needs and problems with which occupational therapy can deal

To establish on this basis reasonable and pertinent treatment goals

Make reasonable predictions—anticipate results

Plan on basis of treatment goals and theory: interpersonal experiences, activity experiences

Ability to use knowledge of symbolism and meaning of activities in planning and implementation

Capacity for sustaining an empathic interpersonal relationship related to patient needs and treatment goals

Skill in handling transference and countertransference

Degree of security in treatment planning and implementation

Ability to use concepts of milieu in treatment

15. *GROUP PROCESS SKILLS*

Ability to perceive interaction

Ability to associate content with feeling

Ability to define problem areas

Ability to help others move toward solution

Help others to define limits, structure and clarify expectations

Awareness of needs of individual and group

Skill in communicating needs

Capacity to move others toward satisfaction of needs

Ability to allow leadership to develop

Capacity to contribute to mutual interdependence

Capacity to support and protect others

Degree of security and integrity

16. *RELATIONSHIP TO THE TOTAL INSTITUTION*

Capacity for perceiving the broad aspects of patient care

Ability to contribute to the use of milieu as a therapeutic agent

Knowledge and understanding of the significance of others in treatment and patient care

Capacity to work collaboratively with others, share thinking and elicit contributions from others

Perceives occupational therapy as one of many valuable experiences

Reflects a strong professional image

Students entering the program are asked to rate themselves on each item, using a scale 1 (minimum) through 7 (maximum), on the basis of their perceptions of their current capacities. The completed rating is kept on file and is not seen by the student's supervisor at this time. Midway through the affiliation, the student is again asked to complete a rating of himself and at this time the supervisor also rates the student. The supervisor and student compare and discuss these two ratings, and these are then compared with the student's original assessment of himself. Supervisor and student ratings are again made at the end of the affiliation and compared with the earlier ones.

This procedure, in addition to measuring evidence of growth, makes it possible for both persons to become aware of agreements and discrepancies between the student's concept of his own functioning and growth and the supervisor's perceptions about these, to explore some of the biases which may be involved and to arrive at a consensus.

Summary

Certainly, the use of this outline is only one aspect of a series of interrelated growth experiences. The development of the learner as a professional person, as an emotionally mature human being with self-respect and understanding sufficient for understanding and respecting others, and thus for being able to contribute significantly to their health and welfare, can be realized to the extent that our education provides a variety of integrated experiences directed toward such maturation. In the last analysis, our education must have as its primary commitment the development within the learner of: an awareness of his potential, an incentive to grow and the ability to realize potential. As our educational experiences are structured within such a frame of reference, we may hope to achieve our goal of professional growth.

REFERENCES

1. West, Wilma L., O.T.R. (Editor) *Changing Concepts and Practices in Psychiatric Occupational Therapy,* American Occupational Therapy Assn., 1959.

2. *Curriculum Study Reports,* American Occupational Therapy Assn., 1963.

3. *Highland Park Curriculum Study Workshop,* American Occupational Therapy Assn., 1963.

4. Towle, Charlotte, *The Learner in Education for the Professions as Seen in Education for Social Work,* University of Chicago Press, 1954.

5. Fidler, Gail S., "Educational Experiences for the Occupational Therapist," *Jour. South African Occupational Therapy Assn.,* Sept. 1963.

6. Pearce, Jane, M.D. and Saul Newton, "The Conditions of Human Growth," New York: The Citadel Press, 1963.

Occupational therapy programs seek to integrate classroom theory and clinical reality. Early introduction of clinical contacts, concurrency of theory and practice, and coordinated program planning is directed to orderly growth and change in the occupational therapy student. It was hypothesized that, with complete integration of theory and practice, no sharp belief changes would occur during the first full-time field experience. Data from responses to social psychological instruments by one group of 28 occupational therapy seniors supported the hypothesis. There were no statistically significant changes in authoritarianism, dogmatism, or Machiavellianism during the first full-time field experience.

CHANGES IN BELIEFS

Held by

Occupational Therapy

Students

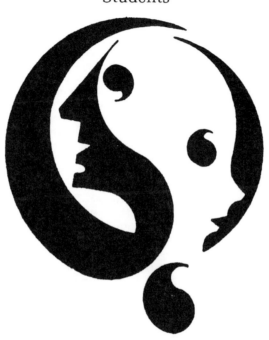

Before and After

the First Field Experience

Lillian R. Greenstein

Professional programs, such as education and occupational therapy, follow approximately four years of university-based study with a period of on-the-job supervised practice in which the individual is a step higher than a student, but not quite a graduate professional. The supervised working experience is the crucial period the student has been anticipating with a mixture of enthusiasm and apprehension. Here is the ultimate opportunity to demonstrate the academic learning, the theory, and the ideals accumulated during the past years of study.

Are attitudes and beliefs held by the student following the didactic program implemented during the practitioner period? In one investigation, education students changed beliefs sharply during the practice teaching. Data from a Central Michigan University study indicated a significant increase in authoritarianism and manipulative tendencies with a general loss of ideals during the student teaching experience.[1]

Do beliefs change sharply during the practitioner period of the occupational therapy curriculum? Is there a dichotomy between beliefs held at the completion of the academic program and beliefs accepted after the student has experienced supervised practice? More specifically, what belief change can be expected in a class of occupational therapy students who are the product of a curriculum based upon the philosophy of complete integration of classroom theory and clinical reality?

Literature Review

In the occupational therapy literature, investigations of student attitudes and personality traits are concerned with predictive factors of success in field experience performance,[2,3] screening instruments for program admissions,[4] behavioral patterns of occupational

Lillian R. Greenstein, M.A., O.T.R., was a graduate student at the University of Alabama, Birmingham, at the time of this study. She is presently continuing her graduate program at the University of Alabama, Tuscaloosa.

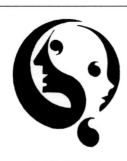

BELIEFS

therapy students,[5] student attitudes toward a client group,[6] and student attitudes toward the curriculum.[7] No data are available concerning attitude and belief change in occupational therapy students during the first field experience.

A number of investigations involved studies of changes in education students during the student or practice teaching experience.

In the Central Michigan University study, an experimental group of 117 subjects entering the student teaching experience completed opinion questionnaires that contained social-psychological scales. The experimental group consisted of all the students assigned to the Southeastern Michigan Student Teaching Center and the Flint Student Teaching Center. The primary consideration in the assignment area was the choices made by the student. In examining the data at the two centers, the investigators found the results so similar that they were pooled for analysis. There was no reason to believe that students assigned to the other centers throughout the state were any less similar. At the same time, 56 control group subjects who were not participating in student teaching also completed the questionnaires. The control group and the experimental group were equivalent except for the student teaching experience. Sixteen weeks later, following the teaching experience, posttest questionnaires were administered. Mean change data indicated a significant increase in the endorsement of authoritarianism, measured by the F Scale, and manipulative strategies, measured by the Mach IV Scale, by the experimental student-teacher group. The control group showed no significant mean change in responses to the instruments.[1]

Several other investigations corroborate an increase in authoritarianism and loss of idealism during the student or practice teaching experience. Walberg et al used a battery of semantic differential scales and items from the Minnesota Teacher Attitude Inventory (MTAI) to examine self-concepts and attitudes in practice teaching and tutoring by education students in a New England university. The sample of practice teachers included 64 college senior women enrolled in a practice teaching course, whereas the tutoring group included 77 college junior women enrolled in core education and methods courses. During the 14-week period of practice teaching, the students became more controlling and less pupil-centered. The opposite was true of the tutoring group, which became more pupil-centered and more egalitarian. Variables implicated included the program level, the concurrency of didactic classes in the junior tutoring group, and the number of pupils handled at one time. Pertinent to this study was the significant increase in controlling attitudes and decrease in egalitarian attitudes among the full-time practice teachers.[8]

Jacobs, in a study covering five teacher-edu-

cation institutions, explored multifaceted questions dealing with attitudes, perceptions of cooperating teachers, number of placements, socio-economic level of the schools and the students, age, and grade-point average. The student group of 1,007 included 550 enrolled in education courses and 457 in student teaching. Attitudes were measured in pre-tests and post-tests, using the Valenti–Nelson Survey of Teaching Practices, an inventory of attitudes ranging from rigid authoritarian to very liberal and democratic. Significant attitude changes occurred in both groups: the didactic group becoming more liberal and democratic, and the student teachers more rigid and formalized.[9]

Changes in attitudes, values, and dogmatism were studied by Greene in a University of Nebraska sample of 66 elementary education juniors and 116 elementary education seniors on a 16-week student teaching assignment. The Minnesota Teacher Attitude Inventory, The Dogmatism Scale, and The Study of Values measured pre-test and post-test changes. Greene found no significant changes in either direction among the student teachers. The junior students showed no significant change in values or dogmatism, but showed a desirable change in attitudes at a .05 level of significance.[10]

Although the University of Nebraska study found no significant attitude changes during the student teacher assignment, data from the Greenstein, Walberg, and Jacobs investigations showed significant belief change during supervised student teaching; but this data cannot be generalized to other teacher-education institutions.

The Occupational Therapy Curriculum

The *Essentials of an Accredited Educational Program* stipulates that "Supervised field work experience shall be an integral part of the educational program."[11] A primary goal of many occupational therapy programs has been to provide for the integration of the field experience with the didactic program, in accordance with this requirement.

As a supervisor of clinical education, the author has seen occupational therapy faculty, clinicians, and students in three different geographical areas labor with curriculum revision during the past decade. The following discussion of measures to systematically coordinate didactic classroom learning with clinical experience is based on personal experience with these universities and may be equally characteristic of other occupational therapy programs.

Orientation to the reality of occupational therapy starts in some schools during the freshman or sophomore years. Lower level classes include visits to a diversity of treatment centers as well as observation of the clinician at work. Thus the student has a realistic basis for reexamining original interests in occupational therapy and can either implement this interest or select a different course of study.

In the junior and senior years the practicum or preclinical courses bridge the classroom instruction and the full-time field experience (clinical affiliation). The practicum courses coordinate theory and practice and offer clinical contacts that progress from observation to assisting the clinician and possibly to treating selected patients under the direct supervision of the occupational therapist. By the time students enter their first full-time field assignment, they have already experienced a participatory role in patient treatment.

In addition to the integration of theory and practice early in the occupational therapy curriculum, other procedures provide program coordination. Conferences between university faculty and clinic supervisors offer mutual awareness and feedback. University-associated clinic directors provide an environment for observation, theory, demonstration, practicum, and field experience, thereby ensuring program continuity. Some universities limit the geographical dispersement of the field experience to assure direct contacts among the faculty coordinator, the occupational therapy clinician, and the affiliating student.

The goals of these multidimensional procedures are to provide program continuity—a melding of theory and practice to avoid a sharp split in beliefs held after the university-based program and beliefs adhered to as a result of the clinical affiliation. Because of the integration of theory and practice, the student is expected to enter the field experience with observed assurance that classroom theory is a true basis for clinical practice and clinical practice is based upon classroom theory.

Has the occupational therapy curriculum as described above achieved its goal? Has the integrated program avoided a dichotomy between classroom theory and clinical reality that produces sharp changes in student beliefs?

Hypothesis

To explore this latter question, it was hypothesized that no significant change in the beliefs of occupational therapy students would occur as a result of the first full-time field experience. If classroom theory and clinical practice are coordinated, one does not expect sharp changes in opinions, attitudes, and beliefs following the first clinical affiliation. The student entering field experience is expected to be prepared for clinical realities so that beliefs will not be sharply altered during these experiences.

Instruments

The Central Michigan University study, using social-psychological measures, found significant changes in belief systems after the student teaching experience.[1] By replicating this study in part, the significant changes found after the occupational therapy field experience can be compared with those found in the student teachers. Instruments of the social-psychological type that are replicated in this investigation include: (1) The California F Scale, forced-choice short form, to measure authoritarianism;[12] (2) The Dogmatism Scale, short form, to measure open- and closed-mindedness;[13] (3) The Mach IV Scale to measure Machiavellianism or manipulative tendencies.[14]

Authoritarianism   Adorno and associates developed the F scale to measure the political "right" and the extent of authoritarian-based convictions.[15] On the authoritarian extreme (the high scorer) is an individual concerned with adherence to conventional values, rejection of people who violate these values, uncritical acceptance of the leader–follower dimension, and opposition to the tender-minded. In the other direction is the permissive, egalitarian, affectionate individual.

It is foreseeable that a student might meet a situation in the field experience that provides the necessary conditions for a latent verbal expression of authoritarian convictions. With increasing responsibility, the need to establish control may shift beliefs in an authoritarian direction. On the other hand, increasing participation in staff planning may shift beliefs in an egalitarian direction; increased understanding of patients and their problems may change beliefs toward the more tender-minded end of the scale.

This study uses the Berkowitz and Wolkon Short-Form Forced-Choice F Scale.[12] It combines reversals with positively worded items in a forced-choice format, indicating to the respondent the choice of opposites. Thus it avoids the acquiescent response set that may detract from validity in the original, positively worded F Scale. Although some reliability may be sacrificed in the short form (reliability .58), it is especially useful for field studies as part of a battery.

Dogmatism   One of the limitations of the F Scale was its original concern with authoritarianism on the "right" and therefore a political form of authoritarianism. Rokeach developed his Dogmatism Scale to measure general authoritarianism.[16] Where the F Scale is concerned with the content of a belief, the Dogmatism Scale is concerned with the adherence to a belief, the degree of open- and closed-mindedness.

The *high dogmatic* or closed mind views the world as threatening and authority as absolute, strongly rejects beliefs he does not adhere to, and bases response on irrelevant internal and external pressures. The *low dogmatic* views the world as friendly and authority as not absolute, has a low magnitude of rejection of disbeliefs, and responds to information on its own intrinsic merit.

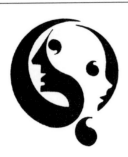

BELIEFS

The degree of adherence to a belief may differ among students as they select modes of treatment or procedures. Some students may become more dogmatic as they adhere strongly to a belief in a selected treatment procedure and reject alternative choices. With other students, a diversity of procedural choices may contribute to an understanding and acceptance of alternate methods, an open mind, and a lowered dogmatism score.

Troldahl and Powell viewed the Dogmatism Scale as a potentially useful social-psychological instrument, but felt that its 40-item length was a deterrent to its practical use.[13] They developed a 20-item form that could be more useful for field surveys. Reliability of the Troldahl and Powell Short Dogmatism Scale is .79. Their reliability findings on the 40-item scale was .84. The short form was used in the present study.

Machiavellianism Christie noted that the F Scale appeared to be more reliable in tapping authoritarianism in the lower socio-economic classes than in the upper socio-economic groups.[14] His search for a construct to define the man at the top, the big operator, led to the development of his Machiavellianism or Mach Scales. Using items congruent with statements from *The Prince and The Discourses,* the Mach IV Scale attempts to measure a person's general strategy for dealing with others.[17] At the scale's extremes, the *high Mach* is viewed as an emotionally detached realist with orientation to cognitions and manipulative strategy rather than to goals. The *low Mach* is an affectively involved idealist with orientation to persons and ideology rather than to strategy.

Christie cautions against pejorative attachments to the concept of Machiavellianism. It would appear that the more complex the role relationship with others, the greater the endorsement of manipulative tactics. Data on a sample of Washington lobbyists indicated that those lobbyists who served more than one client were *higher Machs* than those who had only one client. Field studies show that, in the medical specialties, psychiatrists score the highest and surgeons the lowest on the Mach scales.

What changes might be expected in the degree of students' endorsement of Machiavellian statements? It is possible that increasing clinical responsibility may induce some acceleration in manipulative strategy and agreement with strategic principles. Toward the *low Mach* change is the effect of increasing affective involvement with people—patients, families, staff.

The Mach IV Scale includes 20 items—ten positively worded and ten reversals to minimize acquiescent response set. The instruments in this study combine Dogmatism and Mach Scale items in a 6-point Likert format. Split-half reliability on Mach IV samples averaged .79.

Procedures

All accredited occupational therapy programs were surveyed to determine the availability of students entering their first field experience in January 1974. Five programs responded with lists of students. The number of students on four of the lists ranged from 5 to 14. It was decided to limit this phase of the study to the fifth curriculum, Indiana University, which had 37 seniors starting clinical affiliation on January 2, 1974, a larger and probably more representative group.

Pre-test self-report instruments were mailed to the students at their clinical centers, and they were requested to complete the questionnaires during the first week of affiliation, prior to any heavy involvement with clinical activities.

Three months later, on April 1, 1974, the subjects entered their second field experience. Post-test instruments were mailed to them during the first week in April.

Responses were hand-scored and hand-calculated by the author.

Results

A 76 percent response of usable instruments was received. Twenty-eight of the class of 37 seniors responded to both the pre-test, prior to field experience involvement, and the post-test, following the first full-time field experience. Three of the questionnaires had scales with incomplete items. Scoring on these responses were prorated according to procedures described by Christie for scoring scales

TABLE 1

Changes in Authoritarianism, Dogmatism, and Machiavellianism Scores
Before and After the First Three-Month Field Experience

Scale	Mean Change	t	DF	Significance
Authoritarianism	− .96	−1.02	26	> .30 NS
Dogmatism	1.18	.71	27	> .40 NS
Machiavellianism	−1.64	− .98	27	> .30 NS

with three or fewer omissions.[18] One F Scale was not usable. Questionnaires available for data analysis included 28 Dogmatism and Mach Scales and 27 F Scales.

Differences were calculated for the paired pre-tests and post-tests and mean change scores were tested for significance with two-tailed t tests for correlated groups.[19] Table 1 summarizes the group change data.

The mean changes in authoritarianism (F), dogmatism, and Machiavellianism (Mach) were not statistically significant. In the F and Mach Scales there was more than a 30 percent probability that the mean change could be attributed to chance fluctuation; in the Dogmatism Scale ($p > .40$), almost 50 percent of the change could have occurred by chance.

Data analysis indicates support for the hypothesis that no significant change in the beliefs of occupational therapy students would occur as a result of the first full-time field experience. During the period measured, the group as a whole showed no significant change in directions of authoritarianism or egalitarianism, closed-mindedness or open-mindedness, manipulative tendencies or affective involvement. Beliefs as reported in the three scales were evidently stabilized in a curriculum continuum process prior to the clinical affiliation or at an earlier level of learning. It appears that the students were generally well prepared for the realities of their first clinical affiliation. Because of the previous integration of classroom theory and clinical practice, the students, as a group, showed no sharp changes in beliefs during the three-month period measured.

In contrast, the Michigan students were entering the student teaching experience directly from didactic classes. There had been no previous exposure to teaching practice, and the first opportunity for practical experience resulted in a significant increase in the endorsement of authoritarian and Machiavellian be-

liefs. Table 2 compares the scores of the student teachers and the student occupational therapists on the three scales.

In authoritarianism, the student teacher scores increased with an $< .02$ level of significance. The increase in the student teacher Mach Scale was significant at the $< .001$ level. The changes in the occupational therapy students' mean scores were not significant in any of the three scales.

In discussing the student teacher increase in Machiavellianism and authoritarianism, the Michigan investigators pointed out the need for concern among educators.[1] They show that the high Mach increase on the post-tests suggests that, as a result of the student teacher experience, the students viewed the effective teacher as a manipulator and as aloof in interpersonal relationships. Moreover, they state, the increase in the F Scale mean score suggests that the education students surveyed may be unprepared for classroom management and resort to authoritarian methods to gain control.

Similar concerns for undesirable changes during the student teacher experience are expressed by other researchers. A possible schism between classroom theory and practice in the teacher training curriculum is implicated, and the educators raised questions concerning the need for coordination of professional education courses with the realities of teaching;[8] dialogue between teacher education institutions and cooperating school systems;[9] and concurrency of field experiences with method courses preliminary to student teaching.[10]

Concern for the coordination and concurrency of theory and practice has guided curriculum planners in occupational therapy for some time. Nedra Gillette included this concern in introductory remarks to the 1963 Second Curriculum Study Workshop.[20] In a recent Eleanor Clarke Slagle lecture, Alice Jantzen discussed the inclusion of the concurrency

TABLE 2

A Comparison of Authoritarianism, Dogmatism, and Machiavellianism Scores of Occupational Therapy and Education Students

	N	Pre-test Mean	SD	Post-test Mean	SD	Change Mean	Sig.
Authoritarianism							
Occupational Therapy	27	38.70	7.67	37.74	7.06	− .96	NS
Education	102	35.83	8.35	37.70	8.41	1.87	<.02
Dogmatism							
Occupational Therapy	28	61.86	10.31	63.04	13.24	1.18	NS
Education	103	66.21	12.52	66.05	11.69	− .16	NS
Machiavellianism							
Occupational Therapy	28	86.46	12.73	84.82	13.69	−1.64	NS
Education	103	89.00	12.18	93.00	13.53	4.00	<.001

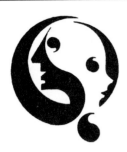

BELIEFS

concept in the early stages of curriculum planning, prior to 1960.[21] Data in the present study suggest that these goals of a coordinated program have been achieved, at least in the curriculum surveyed. There were no sharp changes in the students' beliefs during the first field experience and no dichotomy of beliefs were present after the university-based program and after the first full-time field experience.

Limitations and Implications

The occupational therapy subjects (28) were considerably fewer in number than the group of student teachers (102). With larger numbers, smaller changes attain higher *t* ratios and significance levels. Since enrollment in occupational therapy programs is much smaller than that in teacher education schools, it may require responses from a number of occupational therapy programs in order to attain the larger numbers needed for comparable results.

The generalizability of this study is limited. The absence of sharp belief changes described in this report is characteristic of one group in one curriculum. Studies of other curriculums and of multiprogram levels may corroborate or refute these findings. More decisive changes in beliefs may occur during the first clinical participation, which is usually on an earlier level than the affiliating experience.

Similarly, the generalizability of the teacher education investigations cited in the literature review is limited to the programs studied and is not representative of all education programs.

Social-psychological instruments are one type of measure of change. The avoidance of the personally evaluative type of measurement in which a number of different supervisors rate the subjects is an advantage. However, other types of measurement could supplement self-report instruments and contribute to incremental validity.

The absence of statistically significant belief changes found in this study suggests that a coordinated curriculum may have been instrumental in avoiding a dichotomy between beliefs learned in the university-based program and beliefs accepted after the first field experience. It does not evaluate the pattern of beliefs that is desirable for occupational therapy students. It does not answer questions such as: Do occupational therapy students with high Machiavellianism scores function better than students with lower Mach scores? Also, this study does not explore the presence of a continuum of belief change. Hopefully, the limitations of this study will be a heuristic impetus to further investigations. In the 1965 Eleanor Clarke Slagle lecture, Fidler pointed out the need to include change in beliefs, attitudes, and values as part of learning and growth.[22] It may now be time to identify the presence of such change with measurable units.

Summary

Previous studies of education students pointed to significant belief change with a general loss of idealism during student teaching. It was hypothesized that no significant change in beliefs of occupational therapy students would occur as a result of the first field experience since they had had an early introduction to concurrent theory and practice. Pre-tests and post-tests, using social-psychological instruments, support this hypothesis. The mean belief change in 28 students before and after the first full-time field experience was not significant in any of the three scales. Limitations of the study are discussed, including generalizability and instrumentation. ∎

REFERENCES

1. Greenstein J, Greenstein T: Belief system change in student teachers. In *Association of Teacher Educators Research Bulletin 12: Alternative Approaches to Student Involvement in Teacher Education,* Three Research Studies, Washington, D.C., 1973
2. Bailey JP, Jr., Jantzen AC, Dunteman GH: Relative effectiveness of personality, achievement and interest measures in the prediction of a performance criterion. *Am J Occup Ther* 23: 27–29, 1969
3. Lind Al: An exploratory study of predictive factors for success in the clinical affiliation experience. *Am J Occup Ther* 24: 222–226, 1970
4. Crane WJ: Screening devices for occupational therapy majors. *Am J Occup Ther* 16: 131–132, 1962
5. Patterson TW, Marron JP, Patterson NB: Behavioral patterns of occupational therapy students on the FIRO-B. *Am J Occup Ther* 24: 269–271, 1970
6. Mills J: Attitudes of undergraduate students concerning geriatric patients. *Am J Occup Ther* 26: 200–203, 1972
7. Pang D: A Survey of Differences in Attitudes and Career Expectations of Occupational Therapy Students Enrolled at San Jose State College in 1970–71. Unpublished master's thesis, San Jose State College, 1972
8. Walberg JH et al: Effects of tutoring and practice teaching on self-concept and attitudes in education students. *J Teacher Educ* 19: 283–291, 1968
9. Jacobs EB: Attitude change in teacher education. *J Teacher Educ* 19: 410–415, 1968
10. Greene G: A comparison of attitudes, values, and dogmatism of college juniors and seniors. *J Teacher Educ* 23: 343–347, 1972
11. AOTA, Council on Education: *Essentials of an Accredited Educational Program for the Occupational Therapist.* October 1972
12. Berkowitz N, Wolkon G: A forced-choice form of the F scale—free of acquiescent response set. *Sociometry* 27: 54–65, 1964
13. Troldahl VC, Powell FA: A short-form dogmatism scale for use in field studies. *Social Forces* 44: 211–214, 1965
14. Christie R, Geis F: *Studies in Machiavellianism,* New York, Academic Press, 1970
15. Adorno TW et al: *The Authoritarian Personality,* New York, Basic Books, 1950
16. Rokeach M: *The Open and Closed Mind,* New York, Basic Books, 1960
17. Machiavelli N: *The Prince and the Discourses,* New York, Random House, 1950
18. Christie R, Geis F: *Studies in Machiavellianism,* New York, Academic Press, 1970, p 27
19. McCall RB: *Fundamental Statistics for Psychology,* New York, Harcourt Brace & World, 1970, pp 208–209
20. Gillette NP: Guest editorial. Occupational therapy education and the curriculum study project. *Am J Occup Ther* 19: 351–353, 1965
21. Jantzen AC: 1973 Eleanor Clarke Slagle Lecture: Academic occupational therapy—a career specialty. *Am J Occup Ther* 28: 73–81, 1974
22. Fidler GS: 1965 Eleanor Clarke Slagle Lecture: Learning as a growth process: A conceptual framework for professional education. *Am J Occup Ther* 20: 1–8, 1966

AN EXPERIMENT IN CLINICAL AFFILIATION FOR OCCUPATIONAL THERAPY STUDENTS IN A MENTAL HOSPITAL[1]

PRELIMINARY REPORT

L. B. HILL, M.D.

Worcester State Hospital

Implicit in the term School of Occupational Therapy is the idea that there is a technique which can be taught and learned, whereby certain abnormal conditions may be treated with a view toward cure or amelioration. This technique involves the application of occupation or directed activity on the part of the patient. Occupational therapy is then a means to an end. A school proposing to graduate professional therapists would appear obligated to teach more than the technique or means. It must explain the ends in view, and the processes by which a disordered condition may again become orderly.

To students who are not familiar with the general discipline of the medical arts and sciences, there are being taught today in various schools a considerable variety of more or less technical therapeutic procedures. One thinks of physiotherapy, hydrotherapy, occupational therapy, psychotherapy, and a host of less clearly justified modalities. In the production of groups of ambitious therapists who are not quite clear what it is they are to treat with their so carefully acquired technique, there lies a real danger. It is a medical axiom that diagnosis is very difficult; once diagnosis is correct, therapy is relatively simple.

Recognizing this dangerous situation, the Boston School of Occupational Therapy has come to believe that technical training in therapy is but one step, and that that therapist only is safe

[1] Read at third annual conference of Massachusetts Association for Occupational Therapy, held at Boston February 17–18, 1928.

107

OCCUPATIONAL THERAPY AND REHABILITATION, VOL, VII, NO. 2

who has taken another step, namely, toward understanding of the conditions to be treated, and of the modus operandi of the affliction and of its relief. The school curriculum accordingly includes instruction concerning the physical conditions which will commonly be referred for treatment. Therapy being an art, this instruction is preliminary only to actual experience in hospitals treating such conditions. This actual contact, under experienced supervision, with patients being treated for the conditions previously studied develops the art of occupational therapy.

Now remembering that each of the physical disorders referred for treatment exists in the presence of a patient, that is, of an individual with a personality, and not forgetting that half the hospital beds in this country are devoted to patients suffering from disorders which are not localized and physical in nature, but are generalized and mental, we are not surprised to find in the curriculum instruction in psychology. I wish to emphasize that whereas not over half our available patients are in need of treatment directed toward physical diseases, all of our patients are in possession of personalities which must be considered and to some extent understood as we apply our therapy. Those in the mental hospitals are primarily treated from the viewpoint of psychology, the other half in general hospitals are frequently equally in need of adjustment as individuals to their unfortunate situations.

The next logical step, of course, is the inclusion in the curriculum of the school of a period of practical training in a mental hospital where under experienced direction may be practiced the art of applying occupational therapy to the problem of the straightening out of a disordered personality.

Without any further preamble, the experience of an affiliation whereby students from the Boston School of Occupational Therapy receive clinical experience and instruction in the Worcester State Hospital seems worthy of a preliminary report. In September, 1927, a group of eight students were received into the occupational therapy department of the hospital for a period of three months. They became working members of the department, living within the hospital, and in general under the same regulations and with similar duties as the regular personnel of the department. In addition, they were offered and required to pass examinations on a course of instruction.

The work of these students may be summarized as follows:

Observation, i.e., before actual duties were assigned....	46 hours	46
Duty with classes of patients:		
a. Newly admitted females.........................	66 hours	
b. Continued care—female or male..................	66 hours	
c. Habit training—female...........................	66 hours	
d. Physical education and special case-work..........	66 hours	
	264 hours	264
Preparation for above class work......................	171 hours	171
Didactic work:		
1. Neurologic and Psychiatric Theory...............	45 hours	
2. Mental Nursing.................................	10 hours	
3. Habit Training..................................	9 hours	
4. Play-ground Therapy............................	10 hours	
5. Application of Crafts............................	24 hours	
	98 hours	98
		579

This program contemplates 579 hours of duty in twelve weeks— meaning five days of $8\frac{3}{4}$ hours each and a sixth of $4\frac{1}{2}$ hours. On time taken from the above schedule, each student also had a brief experience of assigned duty with patient groups for evening entertainments, including dances, moving pictures, athletics, etc. Each student also was excused from the regular schedule in order to attend for a time the regular hospital staff meetings and ward walks. There was conducted each Saturday morning a conference of the students with the superintendent of the hospital, wherein could be discussed any problems related to the work which the students wished to present.

The didactic work was rather difficult to plan as there were few precedents by which to go. For this very reason, it was an interesting experience. The neurologic and psychiatric theory was presented under the following titles on next page.

I. Introductory
    1. Hospital Organization and Rules
    2. Precautions and Advice
II. Neurology
    1. Comparative Neurology
    2. Embriology
    3. The Neuron
    4. Gross Anatomy
    5. Structure and Function
    6. Special Senses
    7. Review
III. Psychiatry
    1. Historical Orientation
    2. } Modern Schools
    3. } of Psychiatry
    4. Review
    5. The Organic Syndrome
    6. Organic Psychoses
    7. Paresis
    8. Clinic—Organic Psychoses
    9. Alcohol and Drug Addiction
    10. Review
    11. Affective Psychoses
    12. } Psychoneuroses
    13. }
    14. Review
    15. Clinic
    16. Primitive Thought
    17. }
    18. } Dementia Praecox
    19. }
    20. Clinic
    21. Involutional Melancholia
    22. Psychopathic Personality
    23. Epilepsy
    24. Mental Deficiency
    25. Clinic
    26. }
    27. } Review
    28. }
    29. Clinic—Mental Hygiene
    30. } Mental Hygiene
    31. }
    32. Examination.

There were included four discussions of social service, these being presented by that department.

Mental nursing included the following:

1. Mental Hospitals
2. Admissions to Mental Hospitals
3. Care of Patients
4. Restraint and Seclusion—Parole
5. ⎫
6. ⎬ Hydrotherapy with demonstrations
7. ⎭
8. Hospital Industries
9. Occupational Therapy
10. Psychotherapy of ward details.

This first class was, so far as we know, the first to be sent from an extramural school of occupational therapy to take up residence for a considerable period of experience in a mental hospital. We observed the following: One of the eight students dropped out early in the course, apparently for personal reasons. The remaining seven came to us in the spirit of doubting adventure. At first they were counting the days, because for most of them it was a first experience with mental patients, with all the emotional disturbance which that implies, and for most of them also the hardest work they had undertaken. It is one thing to be a visiting student and another thing to be a regular soldier in the line of duty. Later the students generally expressed the opinion that three months was not long enough to absorb the value which was in the experience. At the end of the three months they felt, as did we, that they were just ready to begin to assume responsibility and acquire that experience which comes in no other way.

That this expression was genuine and not related to impending examinations is attested by the fact that we have received applications from some of these students for further undergraduate training or for graduate employment.

The speaker, who was responsible for the psychiatric teaching of this group felt strongly that three months is not sufficient for any remarkable change in emotional attitude, for the acquisition of even the rudiments of the art of dealing with the mentally ill, and for an intelligent introduction to the underlying theory of personality and its disorders.

It is better not to talk of the future. However, this much is necessary to state, that as a result of our experiences the present arrangement has been made to permit of six months' service in a mental hospital to include the same didactic work and considerably more clinical teaching in ward walks and conferences. Furthermore, there has been a slight rearrangement of the psychology instruction in the school so that a part of it continues to be preparatory to an understanding of technical problems in craft work and another part is preparatory to the abnormal psychology to be taught in the hospital. Upon this better integrated foundation, it is expected that the student will erect a better understanding of personality problems. It is perhaps appropriate here to state that the psychiatric teaching has been presented largely in terms of individual or dynamic psychology.

IN CONCLUSION

1. The hospital has found this experiment, like similar experiments with student nurses and social workers who affiliate, to be valuable in that it lifts morale, combats institutionalization, and stimulates patients and workers alike. Further, it is good mental hygiene propaganda.

2. The school has found the experiment so satisfactory as to justify its extension and continuation.

3. The students, admitting that it is vigorous, have expressed satisfaction with the experience.

4. It has made possible the extension of occupational therapy to a large number of patients in the hospital.

5. The experiment as made has suggested obvious improvements which are being made, chiefly in better correlation of schedule of teaching in the two institutions and in the extension of time of service in the hospital.

6. We do not hope that these students will, because of this experience, all specialize in mental hospital work. We do hope that mental work will be presented in a fairer light to those who have hitherto rejected it without trial, and particularly that those who work in other fields will take with them a sympathetic

understanding of human nature, a knowledge of sound mental hygiene.

7. The foregoing is a preliminary report of an endeavor which we like and wish to develop further. However, we would caution that for its successful outcome there must exist certain conditions which are not as yet universally found. The result of the endeavor will depend upon the physical possibilities of the school and the hospital, and chiefly upon the personnel and coöperation available.

CASE REPORT

Approaches to Improving Student Performance on Fieldwork

Paula Kramer, Karen Stern

Key Words: education • fieldwork, occupational therapy

Paula Kramer, PhD, OTR, FAOTA, is Professor and Chair, Department of Occupational Therapy, Kean College of New Jersey, 311 Willis Hall, Union, New Jersey 07083.

Karen Stern, MS, OTR, is Assistant Professor, Department of Occupational Therapy, Kean College of New Jersey, Union, New Jersey.

This article was accepted for publication July 17, 1994.

Fieldwork is an important aspect of occupational therapy education. It provides an opportunity for students to demonstrate their understanding of didactic classroom material by applying their knowledge in a controlled practice setting with supervision. Students must demonstrate an acceptable level of clinical skill by meeting preset behavioral objectives in order to complete their occupational therapy education and become eligible to take the certification examination. It would seem logical that students who do well in their academic studies would do well in their clinical performance. However, in numerous studies, no correlation between academic and clinical performance has been found (Anderson & Jantzen, 1965; Englehart, 1957; Ford, 1979; Katz & Mosey, 1980; Lind, 1970; Mann & Banasiak, 1985).

Our experience as educators has concurred with this research. Although most students who demonstrate good academic performance succeed in the clinical setting, the few who have had problems on their fieldwork experiences tended to stand out. To gain further insight into problems encountered by the students who experienced difficulty on fieldwork, we used a case study approach as suggested by Mann and Banasiak (1985) to examine several cases. One theme surfaced consistently: students who had difficulty engaging in the supervisory process encountered problems more frequently than other students during their fieldwork experiences. These students generally did not accept responsibility for their behavior and did not respond well to feedback. Supervision plays an important part in the continuing growth and development of all occupational therapists (American Occupational Therapy Association, 1994; Haiman, 1992). Hughes and Opacich (1990) reported that the ability to take responsibility for one's own behavior is an important aspect in developing appropriate professional behaviors.

In this article we present two case studies that illustrate the type of problems encountered by students on fieldwork and the intervention process used by academic and clinical supervisors to handle the problems. Each demonstrates a different outcome to intervention. As background information, our program requires three Level I experiences and two Level II experiences with an optional third Level II experience.

Case Study 1: Susan

Susan was identified by faculty members as a potentially difficult student during her first semester in the junior year of the occupational therapy program. She was argumentative with faculty members regarding tests, assignments, and grading. She frequently complained that test questions were unfair and ambiguous and that grading on assignments was subjective. Peer evaluations from classroom activities indicated that she had difficulty reaching consensus with the group and did not work well on team-oriented activities. These behaviors were evident during the following semesters in the classroom. Her faculty advisor and course instructors discussed Susan's behaviors with her several times. Susan's response was that she had a right to her opinions and that she did not think that her behavior was inappropriate.

During her first Level I fieldwork experience, Susan's evaluation indicated that her performance was satisfactory but that her ideas and viewpoints were rigid. The Appendix includes excerpts from the fieldwork evaluation form that relate to self-awareness and participation in supervision, as well as the rating scale used.

Susan's supervisor suggested that she needed to become more flexible and to listen to other alternatives presented to her. This suggestion was echoed by her faculty advisors. She repeated that she thought her behavior was appropriate. It was pointed out by the faculty advisors that although she was entitled to her opinions, her supervisors were also entitled to their opinions and that it might be helpful for her to try to see another perspective. In essence, her responses validated the comments made about her behaviors on fieldwork. It was also suggested that increased flexibility might help her to better understand persons with values and life experiences that were different from her own.

Typically in our program, the faculty members meet at the end of each semester to discuss students who have been identified as having problems with fieldwork. Initially, Susan's situation was viewed by the academic supervisors as an isolated incident, but as time progressed, it became apparent that this was not the case.

During the next semester, similar behaviors were noted both in class and on her second Level I fieldwork evaluation. Two faculty members met with Susan, discussed the importance of engaging in the supervisory process, and pointed out that using feedback could promote her professional growth. The faculty members expressed their concerns to Susan that these recurring problems might interfere with her Level II fieldwork experience unless they were addressed.

During the midterm evaluation of Susan's first Level II fieldwork, her supervisor contacted the school to report problematic behaviors, including lateness, lack of preparation for the clinical activity, and lack of adequate participation in the supervisory process. Susan, her clinical supervisor, and the fieldwork coordinator met again to discuss the situation. Objective examples of her performance were given, with alternative behaviors suggested. Susan blamed her supervisor for the problems and claimed that the faculty members were being unfair to her. She did not accept any responsibility for the negative evaluation or for the specific behaviors ascribed to her.

In the next meeting of academic faculty members, Susan's fieldwork difficulties were placed on the agenda. First, areas of difficulty and behaviors cited by the clinical supervisor were identified. Then, her Level I fieldwork evaluations were reviewed and similarities were noted

with her Level II performance. Because students who encounter problems on their fieldwork experiences often report a personality conflict with their supervisor, we believed that it was important to make certain that this was not the case. As there were clear similarities between Susan's Level I evaluations and behaviors reported during her Level II fieldwork, the faculty members determined that the evaluation probably was based on performance, not on an interpersonal conflict. Finally, the student's responses to the supervisor's feedback were examined.

After this review, the fieldwork coordinator and a faculty member met with Susan to develop an individual plan. They reviewed the clinical evaluations and the similar behaviors identified from all fieldwork experiences. In addition to the inability to be flexible and responsive to supervision, Susan's specific problems noted on both fieldwork experiences included being late, being unprepared, and not handing in assignments on time. Behavioral objectives were established, with stated performance criteria and a time line for review.

Susan insisted that she had many responsibilities outside of her fieldwork that prevented her from meeting the necessary deadlines. She stated that her supervisors had not been sensitive to her needs, even though she had discussed them. The faculty members reminded her of the need for timeliness in clinical settings and the requirements of documenting treatment promptly for third-party payers. They also pointed out that although a supervisor should try to be sensitive to a student's educational needs, it is not necessarily appropriate for the supervisor to be sensitive to personal needs. The suggestion was made that Susan reexamine some of her priorities to see how she could adjust her schedule to meet the demands of a clinical setting. Susan was asked to develop her own plan for modifying her behavior. This request proved to be unsuccessful, because Susan insisted that both supervisors were rigid and inflexible with their suggestions for improving performance. She was asked to consider the validity of her supervisor's feedback and try to identify ways in which she could meet the stated expectations of the fieldwork center.

Similar behaviors continued during her final fieldwork placement. Although meetings and problem-solving sessions with Susan continued, she made little progress in changing her performance. She managed to complete all Level II fieldwork placements with a minimally passing grade. This was of great concern to the faculty members, because we thought that continual problems with supervision and failure to meet previously set objectives should not be rewarded with a passing grade.

Case Study 2: Sally

Sally did not encounter any academic problems until her first Level I fieldwork experience, when she received a marginally passing grade. Comments on her evaluation indicated that she was frequently unprepared, did not raise questions during her observations of clinical interventions or during supervision, and appeared to lack a clear understanding of theory or treatment principles. During her meeting with the faculty representatives, she blamed her clinical supervisor for her own behaviors, claiming that the supervisor was not supportive and tended to put her down and that she therefore did not feel comfortable enough to ask questions or demonstrate her knowledge. She indicated that she and the supervisor had a personality conflict. Similar comments appeared on her second and third Level I fieldwork.

During the midterm evaluation of her first Level II fieldwork placement, similar comments were expressed again. The academic fieldwork coordinator met with Sally, pointed out the similarity between the comments on her three Level I evaluations and the comments being made by her current supervisor, and suggested ways that Sally could change her performance. Sally reluctantly agreed to try some of the strategies.

Three weeks later, at a follow-up meeting, Sally no longer blamed her problems on personality conflicts with supervisors. She was able to see the patterns of behavior that her supervisors had identified and to make use of their feedback. She found that some of the suggestions from the past meeting had worked well for her. Sally successfully completed the affiliation with significant improvement noted on her final evaluation. She subsequently wrote a letter to the faculty members thanking them for being so persistent and supporting her even when she had been hard to deal with. She stated that she had finally understood the feedback she had been receiving. Sally completed her next two Level II experiences without a problem.

Suggested Courses of Action for Academic Faculty Members and Fieldwork Coordinators

Our experience in analyzing several cases, including those presented here, has taught us several things. The primary concern of faculty members and fieldwork coordinators is to identify whether the student is able to apply theoretical material in practice and perform competently in the clinical environment. The coordinator must therefore determine whether the fieldwork problems are general or specific to the student's performance in one clinical site. On the other hand, students need to develop a sense of personal responsibility for their actions and a willingness to accept feedback. If a student is unable to engage in supervision, he or she is likely to encounter problems in any setting.

The following is a suggested template for approaching problematic fieldwork issues. First, it is important to identify what really is the problem — not by placing blame, but by listening to both the student and the supervisor and hearing the stated concerns of each party. Often, it is

difficult to tell whether a personality conflict exists, unless the coordinator has prior knowledge of the behavior of both the student and the supervisor. Second, trends and patterns of student behavior can help to identify whether the problem is specific to the fieldwork center, the chemistry between student and supervisor, or the student. Third, sometimes awareness can bring about change. Once students become aware that they have some control and can make a change in behavior that can result in a change in the outcome, they may be motivated to try other behaviors. Fourth, repeating the feedback can be helpful. As Sally pointed out to us, she finally understood the feedback, which indicated that repeating it to her several times, in different ways, was valuable. Finally, specific suggestions about changes in behavior can be useful to some students. If the student is receptive to the idea of change, this can be a collaborative process.

Suggested Courses of Action for Clinical Supervisors

When a student is identified as having a problem during the fieldwork experience, the clinical supervisor is concerned with the immediate problem and the student's ability to function within the particular clinical experience. Certainly, this problem may have implications for the student's overall performance and ability to work effectively as an occupational therapist, but the concern at first is more immediate. The following are some suggested steps for clinical supervisors to take when addressing student problems.

First, the supervisor should depersonalize the situation. It is important that the student understand that constructive feedback is not a personal attack, but an attempt to improve performance. If the supervisor can facilitate the student's investment in the supervisory process, he or she will have made a major contribution to the student's professional development. Second, the supervisor should identify specific objective behaviors that could be changed or modified. It might be helpful to make specific suggestions about change or identify resources that could be used or people who could serve as role models. Third, if the student remains unresponsive, the supervisor could involve the academic fieldwork coordinator. Together, the supervisor and coordinator can determine specific behavioral objectives, criteria for successful performance, and a time frame for evaluation of this plan.

Conclusion

Problems encountered during fieldwork experiences do not occur often; however, when they arise, these issues can be difficult and time consuming. It is important to attempt to identify potential problem areas during Level I fieldwork to avoid repeated difficulties during Level II placements. By helping students to understand the need to openly engage in supervision, learn from their supervisors' feedback, and take responsibility for their own behavior, supervisors and faculty members can foster positive learning experiences. Assessing the problematic situation objectively and developing strategies for intervention is critical to successful outcomes. This will foster an ongoing collaborative relationship between the clinical supervisors and the academic faculty members. If we are able to facilitate a positive resolution together, the student will be able to grow and learn. ▲

Appendix
Excerpt of Items From the Kean College of New Jersey Level I Fieldwork Evaluation Form

Self Awareness
1. The student is able to recognize his/her own feelings, attitudes and behavior.
2. The student is able to discuss his/her own feelings, attitudes and behavior.
3. The student is aware of his/her reactions in a clinical setting.

Participation in the Supervisory Process
1. The student is able to articulate learning needs and issues of concern.
2. The student is able to utilize feedback from supervisor and staff.
3. The student is able to give feedback to supervisor and staff.
4. The student shows a positive attitude towards and is actively engaged in problem-solving.
5. The student is actively involved in the supervisory process.
6. The student asks appropriate questions.

The following 5-point rating scale is used for each of the above questions:

Rarely	The student displayed this behavior less than 40% of the time.
About half the time	The student displayed this behavior 40% to 65% of the time.
Frequently, with prompting	The student displayed this behavior 75% to 89% of the time.
Frequently	The student displayed this behavior 75% of the time.
Consistently	The student displayed this behavior 90% to 100% of the time.
Not applicable	

Note. Reprinted with permission of the Department of Occupational Therapy, Kean College of New Jersey, Union, New Jersey.

References

American Occupational Therapy Association. (1994). Career exploration and development: A companion to the occupational therapy roles document. *American Journal of Occupational Therapy, 48,* 844–851.

Anderson, H. E., & Jantzen, A. C. (1965). A prediction of clinical performance. *American Journal of Occupational Therapy, 19,* 76–78.

Englehart, H. V. (1957). The investigation of the relationship between college grades and on the job performance during the clinical training of occupational therapy students. *American Journal of Occupational Therapy, 11,* 97–101.

Ford, A. L. (1979). A prediction of internship performance. *American Journal of Occupational Therapy, 33,* 230–234.

Haiman, S. (1992). Directing. In J. Bair & M. Gray (Eds.), *The occupational therapy manager.* Rockville, MD: American Occupational Therapy Association.

Hughes, C., & Opacich, K. (1990, April). *Academic assessment beyond the cognitive domain.* Paper presented at the 70th Annual Conference of the American Occupational Therapy Association, New Orleans, LA.

Katz, G. M., & Mosey, A. C. (1980). Fieldwork performance, academic grades and preselection criteria of occupational therapy students. *American Journal of Occupational Therapy, 34,* 794–800.

Lind, A. I. (1970). An explanatory study of predictive factors for success in the clinical affiliation experience. *American Journal of Occupational Therapy, 24,* 222–226.

Mann, W. C., & Banasiak, N. (1985). Fieldwork performance and academic grades. *American Journal of Occupational Therapy, 39,* 92–95.

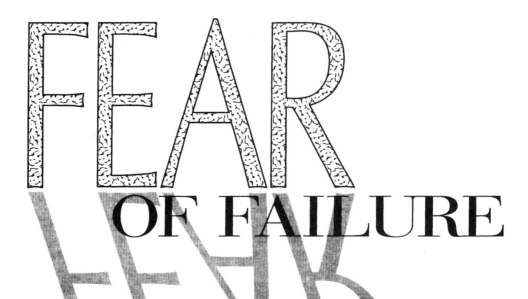

FEAR OF FAILURE

Many OT students doing their Level II fieldwork may face ethical dilemmas.
Fear of failing their placement or jeopardizing their future makes confrontation frightening

By Penny Kyler-Hutchison, MA, OTR/L

"KNUCKLE UNDER OR DIE." What a feeling! This fear may occur to some students when doing their Level II fieldwork. The students see their supervisor do something unethical and possibly illegal. The students during fieldwork are asked to perform a task for which they have had no preparation and feel totally incompetent. Good patient outcomes are at stake. Some students feel as if their careers as OT practitioners are at stake. These questions and concerns are dilemmas many students have voiced.

It is rare that a student will ever be told directly to do something or fail Level II fieldwork. There is, however, the perception by some students regarding fear of raising concerns to the fieldwork supervisor or coercion placed upon them by the fieldwork supervisor during the fieldwork experience to participate in activities for which they do not feel prepared or fail the fieldwork placement.

Fieldwork is a time of transition. Role models and clinical practice values are still in the formative stage. According to AOTA Commission on Education's "Guidelines for an Occupational Therapy Fieldwork Experience-Level II," "the fieldwork placement recognizes that the primary objective of the fieldwork experience is to benefit the student's educa-

> The fieldwork placement recognizes that the primary objective of the fieldwork experience is to benefit the student's educational experience.

tional" experience. The value of fieldwork is education, not a primary extension of occupational therapy services.

If fieldwork is truly seen as an extension of education and continued preparation for entry-level practice, the role expectations for students are such that their fieldwork supervisors offer guidance and

encouragement to try new tasks and experiences. Fieldwork educators responsible for training and educating students should be cognizant of and apply the 1994 revised occupational therapy code of ethics. Principle 3-E of the 1994 revised code states that "occupational therapy practitioners shall protect service recipients by ensuring that duties assumed by or assigned to other occupational therapy personnel are commensurate with their qualifications and experience." This does not mean that students are not to try and learn new tasks or work with new types of service recipients. It does mean that when students are asked to assume a role or do a new task, guidance and guidelines are provided. This guidance can be in the form of role modeling, observation, reading policies and procedures or a combination of these different methods.

In keeping with the general concepts of Principles 1, 2 and 3 of the 1994 revised occupational therapy code of ethics, students have raised questions concerning how patients are addressed and treated by OT practitioners. Unfortunately, the fieldwork students are not always comfortable or capable of asking their fieldwork supervisor for the rationale behind the supervisor's actions or verbal communication style. Students have mentioned the demonstrated lack of respect by OT practitioners for service recipients and students of different cultures, religions, sexual orientation and age. This lack of respect has been demonstrated by failure to abide by dietary restrictions for service recipients of different faiths and cultures during cooking groups, failure to provide privacy in some ADL training activities for older patients, failure to provide needed accommodations to some students with disabilities or religious restrictions.

Other examples cited by students are the obvious change in attitudes regarding approaches to treatment when the OT practitioner realizes the recipient of service is engaged in a lifestyle or other practice strongly opposed to the practitioner's belief system. As examples, students noted changes by OT practitioners when their service recipient is homosexual, elderly or an atheist. Also noted is a change in level of respect and outcome expectations for individuals of lower socioeconomic status, and changes in quality of service provided when the recipient of service is nearing the end of their life expectancy.

What do you do when faced with one or more of the above mentioned scenarios? Students should seek the high ground. Open communication between yourself and your supervisor may ease the problem. Caution in this approach should be taken by commenting on just facts. Divorce yourself from the emotion of the situations. A giant step forward in the moral development of all is the recognition of an ethical dilemma and moving forward to seek resolution of that dilemma. Ethical dilemmas and ethical resolution don't just occur, we have been prepared for dilemmas and resolution by our daily lives. Interest in different things, our role as members of society, increased knowledge of medical, social and political events have all helped formulate our thoughts on ethical issues and our concept of what type of resolution to a dilemma we would prefer.

In each of the examples cited the student should gather all facts regarding the situation. The second step is to take some time for introspection. What do you feel about the situation and why? The third step is to marshal your argument as to why something or someone should change. You may seek information regarding the treatment philosophy of the facility and the philosophy underlying fieldwork to help you in marshaling your argument. This is the development of the concept of justice. Justice is the overarching principle behind Principle 4 of the occupational therapy code of ethics. The principle of justice allows for mutual respect and the development of moral au-

A giant step forward in the moral development of all is the recognition of an ethical dilemma and moving forward to seek resolution of that dilemma.

tonomy. When mutual respect and moral autonomy occur, one is well on his or her way to becoming a good OT practitioner. When mutual respect and autonomy are present it allows participants in the discussion to actively listen, decrease defensiveness and work toward resolution. These concepts are needed not only in practice but also in daily life.

The fourth step is usually the hardest. Here you need to have a fruitful discussion with the fieldwork supervisor. At this point OT students and practitioners are bringing feelings and their individual value systems to the conversation. Since value systems are individualized, each party has a different interpretation of the issue to be discussed. If this does not go well, you may wish to seek guidance from the clinical coordinator at your school, a mentor, or someone neutral— someone not involved in the situation but knows the situation. Some fieldwork supervisors are overly paternalistic and seek to control the student. Some fieldwork supervisors are laissez faire and look upon the student with benign neglect.

Some fieldwork supervisors are too busy and under the gun to increase productivity. Hopefully, most fieldwork supervisors will respond to the student's concern. It is helpful for all to remember that each type of supervisor was at one point a student going through the same process.

The last step is resolution. Resolution can take on several forms. Competing, accommodating, avoiding, collaborating, or compromising. Each type of conflict-management approach has good points and bad points. When you are competing you stand up for your position, and one person is a winner and the other person is the loser. When you are accommodating you may neglect your position to satisfy the wishes of your supervisor. Accommodating is demonstrated by keeping silent regarding an issue when you prefer not to. Avoiding is when you sidestep an issue or withdraw from the situation. When you are collaborating you attempt to work together and to satisfy the concerns of both parties. Collaboration helps us learn from one another. Compromising is not as good as collaborating but better than avoiding. When you compromise you seek some resolution that partially satisfies both parties.

The above-cited concept of conflict management is based on the Thomas-Kilman Conflict Mode Instrument (K. Thomas, *Academic Management Review,* July 1977). It is important for all parties to recognize that not all dilemmas are solvable by a win-win solution. Students on fieldwork and fieldwork coordinators and educators should all work together to provide for a well-rounded entry-level therapist.

The values of the profession as a whole supersede the values of an individual OT practitioner. The educational and philosophical concepts behind fieldwork experiences are to train a new generation of practitioners, instill a sense of obligation to practice ethically and promote these same ethical standards among their colleagues.

The quality and consideration of values that students and educators share with one another only strengthen our profession and the services we provide. Fieldwork is a time of transition and it should be enjoyable. ∎

Penny Kyler-Hutchison is AOTA's ethics program manager.

Learning Style Preferences of Occupational Therapy Students

Lela A. Llorens

Sandra P. Adams

Lela A. Llorens, Ph.D., OTR,
FAOTA, is Professor, Chairperson,
and Graduate Coordinator, University of Florida, Gainesville, Florida.

Sandra P. Adams, M.O.T., OTR,
is Assistant Professor, University of
Florida, Gainesville, Florida.

Fifty-five undergraduate and 22
graduate students in occupational
therapy were surveyed by using the
Canfield-Lafferty Learning Styles
Inventory. The results of the study
indicate that their learning style
preferences favor the learning conditions that permit knowing and
liking the instructor personally, setting one's own objectives, and working alone and independently. The
highest content and mode
preferences for learning were working with people and engaging in
direct experience, respectively. The
lowest content and mode
preferences were for working with
numbers and for reading. Achievement expectations for grades were
A and B. The findings are discussed.

Interest in learning style preferences and their impact on the teaching-learning process is a recent phenomena in Allied Health Education. The recognized need for innovative approaches in teaching and the demand by students for relevance in learning experiences have motivated educators to consider individualized approaches to teaching and learning. Individually paced and programmed instruction have been accepted by some educators as innovative methods and as viable alternatives to the lecture method. However, these methods as well as the traditional lecture method may not be the most preferred by all students. Planning effective learning experiences requires the educator to possess knowledge of students as individuals as well as knowledge of them in groups. Specific knowledge of each student is necessary to both individualize and diversify instruction (1). This knowledge should be available and understandable to both the educator and the student, and should increase the students' awareness of themselves as learners as well as the teacher's awareness of the individual similarities and differences among students.

Research into learning style preference in Allied Health Education has focused on identifying the personality types and learning style preferences of students by professional disciplines, on comparing students of different disciplines, and on comparing students with experienced workers in their fields.

Studies reported by Bancroft and Collins (2), Fiel and Ways (3), and Sullivan and Lorenz (4) have *recognized* that there are individual differences in students. Brown (5), McCaulley (6), and McCaulley and Smith (7) have *identified* individual differences in students through testing. In a study by Rezler and French (8) that identified personality types and learning preferences of students in six allied health professions, the results specifically pointed to the value of studying individual differences of students within a profession as being of more importance for teachers who wish to adjust their teaching styles to student preferences

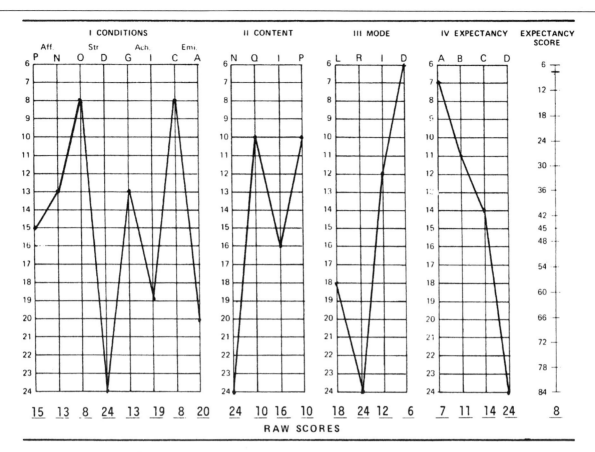

	I CONDITIONS							II CONTENT				III MODE				IV EXPECTANCY				EXPECTANCY SCORE
	Aff.		Str.		Ach.		Emi.													
	P	N	O	D	G	I	C	A	N	Q	I	P	L	R	I	D	A	B	C	D	

RAW SCORES

15 13 8 24 13 19 8 20   24 10 16 10   18 24 12 6   7 11 14 24   8

---

in learning than identifying differences among the professions.

The purpose of this paper is to report the use of the Canfield-Lafferty Learning Styles Inventory in determining the learning style preferences of undergraduate and graduate occupational therapy students at the University of Florida.

Description of the Study

A study of learning style preferences of 55 undergraduate and 22 graduate students in occupational therapy was conducted over a 3-year period. Determining and examining learning style preferences were considered an important initial step in evaluating the feasibility of instituting multifaceted learning experiences to meet the learning needs of students.

The students were administered the Canfield-Lafferty Learning Styles Inventory (LSI) (9). The undergraduate juniors were given the test during the fall quarters of 1974 and 1976. The graduate students were given the test during the fall or winter quarters of the 1974, 1975, and 1976 academic years. The tests

were scored and the raw score profiles were plotted.

The Canfield-Lafferty Learning Styles Inventory focuses on four affective variables in the teaching-learning situation—conditions of learning, content, mode, and expectation. The conditions of learning concern the dynamics of affiliation with others, structure, achievement, and eminence in the learning situation. *Affiliation* refers to the student's preference for peer or teacher relationships for learning. Students who prefer teacher affiliation like knowing the teacher personally; whereas those who prefer peer affiliation enjoy working in student teams. *Structure* refers to the student's preference in study plans. The student who prefers the organization dimension likes logically, clearly organized course work with assignments and a sequence of activities that are meaningful to the student; whereas the student who prefers detail likes specific information on assignments, requirements, and rules. *Achievement* refers to independence of action and the pursuit of his or her own study plan.

Eminence refers to the student's perception of him or herself in relation to other students and to authority. Students who prefer the competition dimension desire comparison with others and need to know how they are doing in relation to others; whereas students who prefer the authority dimension desire classroom discipline and order maintained by knowledgeable teachers.

Content concerns the major areas of interest in learning. These include numeric, qualitative, inanimate, and people dimensions. *Numeric* refers to working with logic and numbers, computing, and solving mathematical problems. *Qualitative* refers to working with words or language, writing, editing, or talking. *Inanimate* refers to working with things—building, repairing, designing, or operating objects. The *people* dimension refers to working with people—interviewing, counseling, selling, or helping. Students who indicate a high preference for one of these dimensions will prefer learning activities that involve that content area.

Mode concerns the general

RAW SCORE PROFILE

Table 1
Learning Styles Inventory Data

	Undergraduate N = 55		Graduate N = 22	
Rank	**Conditions**	**Percentage**	**Conditions**	**Percentage**
1	N (Instructor)	(.890)	N (Instructor)	(.954)
2	G (Goal Setting)	(.781)	I (Independence)	(.772)
3	I (Independence)	(.672)	G (Goal Setting)	(.681)
4	P (Peer)	(.472)	O (Organization)	(.590)
5	O (Organization)	(.454)	C (Competition)	(.409)
6	C (Competition)	(.381)	P (Peer)	(.363)
7	A (Authority)	(.127)	A (Authority)	(.181)
8	D (Detail)	(.018)	D (Detail)	(.045)
Rank	**Content**	**Percentage**	**Content**	**Percentage**
1	P (People)	(.981)	P (People)	(.954)
2	Q (Qualitative)	(.454)	I (Inanimate)	(.454)
3	I (Inanimate)	(.381)	Q (Qualitative)	(.409)
4	N (Numeric)	(.127)	N (Numeric)	(.136)
Rank	**Mode**	**Percentage**	**Mode**	**Percentage**
1	D (Direct Experience)	(.654)	D (Direct Experience)	(.636)
2	L (Listening)	(.581)	I (Iconics)	(.590)
3	I (Iconics)	(.545)	L (Listening)	(.545)
4	R (Reading)	(.072)	R (Reading)	(.181)
Rank	**Expectancy**	**Percentage**	**Expectancy**	**Percentage**
1	B	(1.00)	A	(1.00)
2	A	(.745)	B	(.954)
3	C	(.181)	C	(.045)
4	D	0	D	0

modality through which the student prefers to learn. Mode includes listening, reading, iconics, and direct experience. *Listening* refers to the student's preference for hearing information such as lectures, audiotapes, and speeches. *Reading* refers to the student's preference for examining the written word through reading texts, pamphlets, and other materials. *Iconics* refers to the student's preference for viewing illustrations, movies, slides, pictures, or graphs. *Direct experience* refers to the student's preference for handling materials or performing—shop, laboratory, on field trips, or in practice exercises.

Expectation concerns the student's anticipated level of performance. These levels are designated as outstanding or superior, above average or good, average or satisfactory, and below average or unsatisfactory. An expectancy score is also computed.

The statistical reliability for Conditions is .59-.71; for Content and Mode, .67-.83; for Expectancy Level; .46-.72; and for Expectancy Score, .92. The LSI inventory produces data that is profiled as shown in Figure 1. Low scores indicate high preference. High scores indicate low preference.

Data and Findings

The profile results of the Canfield-Lafferty Learning Styles Inventory were analyzed in accordance with the student's preference scores. The highest four of the eight possibilities for Learning Conditions, and the highest two of the four possibilities for Content, Mode, and Achievement Expectation were considered to represent the student's preference in each area. These data were tabulated for all students and ranked by percentage preference. A 60 percent cut off was established as indicating high preference; whereas below 20 percent was considered low preference. This left a range between 20 percent and 60 percent that is neither high nor low. The tabulations thus ranked indicated that both the undergraduate and graduate students showed a high preference in the Conditions of Learning for 1. knowing the instructor personally, having mutual understanding, and liking one another (N); 2. for setting their own objectives, using feedback to modify goals, and making their own decisions on objectives (G), and 3. for working alone and independently, determining their own study plan, doing things for themselves (I), and a low preference for classroom discipline, maintenance of order, having authoritarian instructors (A), and for specific information on assignments, requirements, and rules (D). The items reflecting competitiveness (C), working with peers in groups (P), and organization of course work (O) fell in the middle range.

In the Content area both groups showed a high preference for people and low preference for numbers. Inanimate and qualitative content fell in the middle range.

In Mode, both groups showed a high preference for direct experience, with a low preference for reading. Listening and iconics fell in the middle range.

All students showed high preference for As and Bs with low preference for Cs and Ds in their level of achievement expectation (*see* Table 1).

Discussion of the Findings

The findings of this study were used to increase the sensitivity of faculty members and students to learning style preferences. The findings have been generalized for application by the authors and their faculty colleagues to increase or reinforce faculty responsiveness in planning the presentation of course material and in student advisement.

In response to the learning mode data, increased emphasis has been placed whenever possible on experiential learning and has been reinforced by listening, iconics, and reading through the use of videotapes, slide tape programs, audiotapes, films, discussion, lectures, and readings. The need for the use of multiple methods for presenting specific information has been acknowledged. Reading, although least preferred of the four modes, is necessary and considered desirable because a great deal of the needed content for learning is available only in written form. Students are advised of this necessity.

In the Content area, the findings supported the emphasis that has been present in this curriculum for many years on simultaneous involvement in practice and academic components of learning because the ma-

jority of the students indicated a high preference for working with people. The low preference indicated by students for working with numbers was of particular concern to the authors. This finding led to the question of how to effectively involve students, particularly graduate students, who indicate low preference for working with numbers in statistics and research. With graduate students, collaboration with statisticians and researchers who have expertise in their area of low preference has been used as a technique for assisting the student in developing knowledge and skill in this content area.

The findings relative to conditions of learning pointed to the use of informal teaching conditions, with independence and goal-setting permitted as high preferences, and the authority and detail dimensions as low preferences. The awareness of the students' preferences has aided the authors to better understand the students' learning needs and has supported the goal of achieving positive learning climates in classroom and laboratory settings.

Individual students who have had problems in learning specific course material have been advised in terms of their learning modes by using data from their Learning Styles Inventory. For example, individual students who have a high preference for the listening mode have been advised to tape record material for learning through listening. More elaborate individualized student programming is not possible nor advisable with the limited data available from the LSI.

Summary

This study was undertaken to determine the learning style preferences of undergraduate students in occupational therapy. The Canfield-Lafferty Learning

Styles Inventory was administered to 55 undergraduate and 22 graduate students at the University of Florida. The findings indicate that students in this study prefer the conditions of learning that permit informal teaching conditions in which the student has a personal relationship with the instructor; that allows individual setting of one's own objectives and opportunities to work alone and independently. These students show a high preference in the content area for working with people, in their learning mode for direct experience, and in achievement expectation for grades of A and B.

REFERENCES
1. Llorens LA, Adams SP: Entering behavior—student learning styles. In *Teaching in the Health Professions*, CW Ford, MK Morgan, Editors. St. Louis: CV Mosby, 1976
2. Bancroft JA, Collins K: Instructional design team. *Nurs Outlook* 20: 4, 1974
3. Fiel NJ, Ways PO: Development and evaluation of self-instructional materials. *J Med Educ* 47: 10, 1972
4. Sullivan AM, Lorenz RB: Designing an audio-tutorial learning experience in medical technology. *Am J Med Technol* 39: 3, 1973
5. Brown PU: *Career Development and Satisfaction of Occupational Therapists in Florida*, Doctoral Dissertation, University of Florida, Gainesville, Florida, 1973
6. McCaulley MH: The Myers-Briggs type indicator and health occupations education. In *Cognitive and Affective Dimensions in Health Related Education*, MD Morgan, CS Broward, DM Filson, Editors. Gainesville: Center for Allied Health Instructional Personnel, 1974
7. McCaulley MH, Smith AB: The use of the Myers-Briggs type indicator to describe the characteristics of the University of Florida freshman and transfer students, 1972-73. *Office of Instructional Resources Newsletter*, No 3, 1974
8. Rezler AG, French RM: Personality types and learning preferences of students in six allied health professions. *J Allied Health* (Winter), 1975
9. Canfield AA, Lafferty JC: *Learning Styles Inventory*, Plymouth, MI: (now called the *Canfield Learning Styles Inventory*)

Stereotypes, Stigma, and Mental Illness: Learning From Fieldwork Experiences

Michael Lyons, Jenny Ziviani

Key Words: fieldwork education • mental disorders • students

Objectives. *A phenomenological study explored occupational therapy students' experiences in psychiatric fieldwork. Of particular interest were students' experiences with and perceptions of persons using psychiatric services.*

Method. *Data were gathered from 16 informants, via in-depth interviews and participant observation, on multiple occasions throughout the students' fieldwork affiliations in hospital and community psychiatric service settings. Triangulation of data gathering methods and member checking were used to strengthen the interpretive validity of the study.*

Results. *Informants manifested stereotyped preconceptions and associated anxiety regarding persons labeled as mentally ill, though the strength of such beliefs and feelings was found to diminish as fieldwork progressed. Sensationalized popular images of mental illness (e.g., that it is linked with malevolence) and some aspects of academic and clinical education (e.g., a deficit focus) seemed to adversely affect students' perceptions.*

Conclusions. *Assisting students to acquire a sound appreciation of the humanness of persons with psychiatric disorders is an educational imperative. There is a need to critically appraise academic and fieldwork practices in psychiatric occupational therapy.*

(Editor's note: At the time of publication of *The Fieldwork Anthology* in January 1998, Michael Lyons is at the University of Newcastle, Australia.)

Michael Lyons, PhD, is Lecturer, Department of Occupational Therapy, The University of Queensland, Brisbane Qld 4072, Australia.

Jenny Ziviani, PhD, is Senior Lecturer, Department of Occupational Therapy, The University of Queensland, Brisbane, Australia.

This article was accepted for publication December 23, 1994.

During their fieldwork in psychiatry, occupational therapy students come face-to-face—in many cases for the first time—with persons identified as having a psychiatric disorder. Dormant or unconscious beliefs and feelings about such persons are likely to manifest themselves at this time (Lyons, 1991).

In a study of occupational therapy students' perceptions of persons with disabilities, Lyons and Hayes (1993) expressed concern about the students' diminished regard for persons with psychiatric disorders, relative to those with other disabling conditions. Furthermore, the finding that freshman and senior students did not differ in their attitudes raised questions about the professional education of occupational therapists. What sorts of beliefs and feelings about persons with disabilities, particularly those with psychiatric disorders, are being fostered during occupational therapy students' professional education? This article presents some findings of a phenomenological study of occupational therapy students' experiences of persons with psychiatric disorders during fieldwork.

Stigma and Mental Illness

A substantial body of research over the last three decades has unequivocally supported claims about a mantle of negative attitudes that envelops persons with disabilities (e.g., Chubon, 1982; Gordon, Minnes, & Holden, 1990; Shears & Jensema, 1969; Yuker & Block, 1986). What is more, persons with mental illness have consistently been identified as among the most devalued of all persons with disabilities. The stigma of mental illness is such, it seems, that other members of society wish to distance themselves socially from persons so identified (Bowman, 1987; Socall & Holtgraves, 1992; Steinwachs et al., 1992).

Research has shown that the term *mental illness* suggests images of persons who are unpredictable, unreliable, unlikable, incompetent, and bizarre (Bhugra, 1989; Mansouri & Dowell, 1989; Socall & Holtgraves, 1992). Most pervasive and damaging of all, perhaps, is the image of persons with psychiatric disorders as being violent and dangerous (Dowbiggin, 1988; Link, 1987; Steinwachs et al., 1992). These images persist despite evidence that they are highly inaccurate; such is the nature of stereotypes (Retzinger, 1990; Townsend, 1990).

Postulates about the stigmatizing effects of the label *mentally ill* on the etiology of psychiatric disorders are known collectively as *labeling theory* (Link, Cullen, Frank, & Wozniak, 1990).The extent to which the label itself is the genesis of negative societal reactions, rather than any deviant behaviors the labeled person might exhibit, has been a contentious issue (Gove, 1990; Link, Mirotznik, & Cullen, 1991; Weinstein, 1983). Regardless of a person's behavior, however, it seems that a mental illness label has its own effect in evoking negative societal reactions (Link et al., 1990; Socall & Holtgraves, 1992).

Professional Views of Mental Illness

Health professionals, like the general population, may be quite susceptible to stereotypes about persons with psychiatric disorders (Townsend, 1990). Indeed, the use of medical diagnoses has itself been conceptualized as a form of stereotyping, in the sense that diagnoses provide "conceptual packages" (Townsend, p. 417) for identification and ordering of patients, which define the essential characteristics of the case and help shape the treatment process (Griffiths & Hughes, 1993).

The use of diagnoses per se is not problematic; rather, it is their misuse. This is apparent in the interpretation of diagnostic categories as evidence of homogeneity. For example, Steinwachs et al. (1992) noted how many research studies, based on this assumption, have failed to take account of differences in service needs of persons with psychiatric disorders on the basis not only of diagnosis and functional level but also of other factors such as gender, ethnic background, and age. Diagnostic labeling has also been found to contribute to a mindset where almost any behavior of psychiatric patients may be perceived by hospital staff members as a symptom of psychiatric disorder. That is, once persons have been labeled mentally ill, perceptions of their actions may be distorted to adhere to the label or to fulfill the prophecy (Mansouri & Dowell, 1989).

With regard to occupational therapists in particular, Elliott, Hanzlik, and Gliner (1992) studied the attitudes of occupational therapists and occupational therapy assistants toward colleagues with disabilities in the workplace. They found that occupational therapy personnel generally expressed positive attitudes toward working with peers with disabilities, with the exception of persons with drug dependency problems and psychiatric disorders.

Students' Attitudes

Students in human service professions such as occupational therapy do not differ substantially from their counterparts outside the human services (e.g., business students) in their general attitudes toward persons with disabilities (Lyons, 1991; Tringo, 1970). From their study of students in six health professions including occupational therapy, Westbrook, Adamson, and Westbrook (1988) expressed concern about the narrow and pessimistic beliefs regarding persons with disabilities in evidence among their cohort of student health professionals. They speculated that this situation might be attributable to the unrepresentative samples of persons with disabilities with whom students come into contact on clinical placements. For example, students tend to encounter persons who are currently experiencing problems rather than those who are functioning well.

Where research has attempted to differentiate among categories of disability, there is evidence that students in occupational therapy and related professions regard persons with psychiatric disabilities as among the least favorable of all, in the company of persons such as those who have a criminal record (Lyons & Hayes, 1993; Tringo, 1970). In this sense, students appear to reflect patterns of prevailing community attitudes.

In summary, psychiatric illness carries considerable stigma and persons with psychiatric disorders are generally perceived in extremely negative terms. Health professionals and students may be susceptible to prevailing stereotypes, with implications for their judgments about persons labeled as mentally ill. The views of health professionals and students warrant further examination in light of their ramifications for service delivery. This article explores the fieldwork experiences of a cohort of occupational therapy students and addresses two questions: (a) How did informants experience those persons accessing psychiatric services, whom they encountered in fieldwork settings? (b) How did these experiences find expression in students' perceptions of persons labeled as mentally ill?

Method

Informants

This study employed a qualitative methodology to investigate these questions with 16 occupational therapy undergraduates, all of whom were women and were either juniors or seniors. Twelve of the 16 were undertaking fieldwork in hospital settings. These figures reflect a situation where the majority of psychiatric fieldwork places currently available to students are within hospitals (i.e., where supervising therapists work).

Informants were selected by "stratified purposeful sampling" (Patton, 1990, p. 174). The purpose of this strategy is to capture and describe the central themes that cut across several major strata of informant or program variation. Students were stratified on the basis of the type of setting in which they were undertaking their fieldwork. Setting types identified included public versus private hospital, hospital versus community clinic, and short-stay versus medium- to long-stay psychiatric unit.

These facilities differed somewhat in their stated goals and anticipated outcomes for service users and, hence, differed in terms of their processes of intervention. We reasoned that they might constitute substantially different learning environments for occupational therapy students. By including in the sample informants who we considered might have quite different fieldwork experiences, we hoped to understand variations in experiences while at the same time identifying major shared elements of their experiences.

Data Collection

The primary technique used for collecting data on informants' experiences was unstructured (and later semi-structured) interviewing (Bogdan & Biklen, 1992). The aim of the interviewing was to have informants talk about issues of most relevance to them in a manner that allowed them to use their own concepts and terms (Stainback & Stainback, 1989).

Typically, informants were interviewed on four or five occasions, each lasting approximately 1 hr. With permission, almost all interviews were audiotaped to provide for increased accuracy in capturing informants' words: the essence of what Maxwell (1992) has termed the *descriptive validity* of their accounts. To maximize the *trustworthiness* of data gathering, the interviewer regularly engaged in *member checking* (Krefting, 1991). That is, questions were raised with informants about the interviewer's interpretations of their fieldwork experiences discussed in prior interviews. Before the final interview with each informant, all prior transcripts were reviewed in search of any gaps in understanding of that informant's perspectives. These gaps were then addressed in the final interview.

In an effort to strengthen what Maxwell (1992) has termed *interpretive validity* (or the accuracy of interpretation of informants' perceptions), this research drew on participant observation as an additional means of data gathering. Used in conjunction with interviewing, observation assisted in discerning more of the meaning of what informants were saying in interviews, as well as the congruence between what they were saying and what they were doing in given situations (Tebes & Kraemer, 1991).

Most of the participant observations were conducted around groups of persons with whom the informants were interacting on a regular basis during their fieldwork affiliations. They were typically groups of persons using the services of the psychiatric fieldwork sites. For example, observations occurred in a social group at a neighborhood center, in discussion groups on topics as diverse as self-esteem and leisure options, in exercise and relaxation groups, and in cooking groups where persons prepared, ate, and cleaned up after a meal. Typically, one participant observation session was undertaken with each informant. These lasted from 30 min to 3 hr, depending on the nature and duration of the activity being observed. Detailed field notes about the event observed were then prepared within 24 hr of leaving the setting.

Data Analysis

The narrative data from interviews and observations were analyzed inductively. "Inductive analysis means that the patterns, themes, and categories of analysis come from the data; they emerge out of the data rather than being imposed on them prior to data collection and analysis" (Patton, 1990, p. 390). Analysis began while data collection was still underway. As data were gathered through interviews and observations, they were subjected to preliminary inspection and comparative analysis for the

emergence of themes (Henwood & Pidgeon, 1992). After data collection had been completed, a full thematic analysis was undertaken with the assistance of a computer package, The Ethnograph (Seidel, Kjolseth, & Seymour, 1988).

Results and Discussion

The results under discussion here are part of a theme concerned with the students' expectations and typological understandings of persons with psychiatric disorders. Several aspects of this theme are outlined: anxieties regarding persons labeled as mentally ill; changes in conceptions as fieldwork progressed; and sources of perceptions of persons with psychiatric disorders, particularly sensationalized images and educational influences. Pseudonyms are used for informants throughout.

Anxiety

Almost all informants registered considerable anticipatory anxiety at the beginning of their fieldwork, as they contemplated contact with persons with psychiatric disorders. For example, informants expressed fear of the unexpected as they anticipated persons who would be unpredictable in their behavior:

> I think [psychiatric patients] are the biggest unknown group of reactions and they can come out with the absolutely unexpected — break down and cry. All that sort of thing is a lot more frightening than just treating someone with a physical problem who's going to talk to you anyway. So their actions are a lot more unexpected and more difficult to cope with (Karen).

It is a common human experience to approach new situations with a certain amount of anxiety — even more so in the case of students who must prove their competence to assessors who will judge their fitness to become practitioners. For these students, however, the label of *psychiatric disorder* prompted further anxiety because of the connotations of erratic and difficult behavior — a point raised in the literature (e.g., Bhugra, 1989; Socall & Holtgraves, 1992). A host of preconceptions about someone whose condition is diagnosed as mental illness will be activated merely by use of the label (Mansouri & Dowell, 1989).

Informants commonly evaluated persons with psychiatric disorders unfavorably against those who have disorders of a physical nature. As suggested previously, there is a great deal more stigma attached to persons with psychiatric disorders than to persons whose disorders have physical origins (Bowman, 1987; Lyons & Hayes, 1993). One student recounted a personal experience of this phenomenon:

> I was shocked to see someone I knew in a group: the mother of a girl that went to school with me . . . and then I thought later "If I'd seen her in a [general hospital] ward, it probably wouldn't have shocked me so much" . . . probably because of mental illness. I meant in a ward where it was a physical condition (Silla).

Hackett (1991), writing as a person who has encountered discrimination as a result of her psychiatric disorder, questioned why society cannot view a person hospitalized for treatment of a psychiatric illness with tolerance and understanding, as it does when someone receives treatment for a physical illness. She speculated that someone who had recently had a heart attack, for example, would be treated with concern and gentleness in the period following discharge from hospital. On the other hand, "people tend to have a fear or an anger or an impatience" (Hackett, 1991, p. 19) with a person hospitalized for a psychiatric condition.

Fieldwork can bring students face-to-face with a mix of fears about persons with psychiatric disorders. For example, one informant commented:

> You are a bit worried about whether you'll know what to do with them or what you'll do if they suddenly attack you or ask you some strange questions or something like that (Sophie).

One feature of the public face of mental illness that is often projected in the popular press is the association of mental illness with criminal and violent acts (Gartner & Joe, 1987; Steinwachs et al., 1992). It is hardly surprising to find that, for some informants, coupled with their fear of the unexpected was at least a hint of fear for their personal safety. However, whatever difficulties students experienced in their dealings with persons with psychiatric disorders during their fieldwork, these were typically not of the magnitude expected.

Changing Conceptions

Many of the informants' fears diminished with continuing contact with persons during fieldwork. One informant expressed that it took her 4 to 5 weeks to "get used to the patients." With their worst fears about persons with psychiatric disorders not realized as they progressed through their fieldwork placement, most students relaxed somewhat.

Analogous with the findings of Westbrook and Adamson (1989), many of the informants expressed surprise at the relative ordinariness of the persons with whom they were dealing— something that they began to appreciate with their ongoing association during the placement. In some cases, informants began to attribute to these persons not only a semblance of normalcy but even positive attributes such as pleasantness—in stark contrast with the negative connotations of their psychiatric label. This changed view might be prompted, for example, by a word of encouragement or other forms of positive feedback given to a student by a persons using the service.

> You just get little bits of feedback from them that what you've said has counted and that they've listened to you and that maybe you've helped them in one way or another (Nancy).

In stark contrast with their negative expectations,

several informants identified their dealings with persons with psychiatric disorders as having been one of the most positive aspects of the placement experience. Feedback from service users, in the form of supportive words or gestures, was rewarding for students. Yet some students found this awkward to deal with, as the notion of receiving support from service users did not sit comfortably with these students' image of being a competent professional (e.g., being self assured and emotionally insulated from service users).

For those informants who sensed the normalcy of persons with psychiatric disorders, it is notable that this view was confined not only to situations where pleasantries were being exchanged. On occasions, even while these persons were exhibiting what were regarded as undesirable symptoms of a disorder, students still identified positive human qualities within them:

> These people are so different when they're ill; and it's not their real person, it's just the illness; and then when the illness is controlled, you can see a different side of them. Basically they're fairly normal people, apart from their illness. I think that's something that you realize when you're on prac[tice] too: that these people are human (Sophie).

It has been noted that medicalization of various forms of deviant behavior as *mental illness* has been helpful in shifting blame from persons with this condition when they exhibit deviant behavior (McLean, 1990). Their behavior is regarded as a symptom of illness and, therefore, as something beyond the person's own control and responsibility. For Sophie, this separation was used to reconcile her observations of substantial (and possibly alarming) variations in persons' behavior with her acceptance of this as part of the human condition. Schwartz and Struch (1989) have postulated that a sense of shared humanity with members of a stigmatized group is fundamental to their being treated with dignity and respect by other, more powerful persons.

It is apparent that, among the expectancies with which students approached the psychiatric fieldwork placement, there were many negative preconceptions of persons with psychiatric disorders. It is also apparent that some of these negative expectations were altered over the course of fieldwork. Other preconceptions might have persisted, in some form, throughout the placement and beyond. At this juncture, therefore, we will consider some of the sources of informants' preconceptions.

Sensationalized Images of Mental Illness

The origins of informants' preconceptions are understandably varied. First, it would seem reasonable to expect that students are susceptible to the negative images of persons with psychiatric disorders that pervade our society. For example, one student said:

> I haven't seen [the film] *One Flew Over the Cuckoo's Nest* and I've been told I shouldn't if I'm going to work in psych. There's things

like that. I've seen parts of it and it's pretty horrendous; and things keep popping up like the Townsville 10B thing [a hospital psychiatric unit about which there was a public outcry and, eventually, an official inquiry in Australia], that really makes such an impression on the public. It reinforces stereotypes so much. I guess you can't help it but relate it back to something like that (Rosie).

The media and entertainment industries often sensationalize psychiatric disability (e.g., linking it with malevolence). Some journalists, like film scriptwriters, have been accused of not letting truth get in the way of a good story. Even where concern for the well-being of the subjects of the story is present, the reader may be misinformed due to the writer's ignorance, so that negative impressions persist. Students, already uneasy about an upcoming psychiatric placement, were perhaps even more susceptible to the negative undercurrent within such stories.

Furthermore, students themselves may contribute to their fellow students' fears through their own stories of experiences on psychiatric fieldwork. For example, one student stated

> I've heard stories from other people doing their psych placements, who talk about all these really psychotic people, really in very ill sort of stages. The people here are surprisingly normal (Rosie).

It is hardly surprising that students would share stories of their placement experiences with each other. Because students typically have some choice about where they undertake fieldwork, it would be in their best interests to sound out their fellow students before making decisions. Students undoubtedly put this informal information network to good use.

Psychiatry has that additional ingredient, however, of the powerful stereotype surrounding the person with a psychiatric disorder. The quest for information, therefore, may be mixed with a morbid fascination for astonishing stories of persons' behavior. Existing stereotypes may help to fuel listener interest, making an otherwise ordinary story a more memorable one for the storyteller to relate. Add to this a certain thrill for the storyteller in titillating others:

> I've always liked the idea of working in an area where other people are scared to work in. . . . I like to be able to say "I work in psychiatry" and have people say "Oh do you really!" . . . yeah, a bit of shock value and then it's an education thing too because I like being able to say "It's not as bad as it sounds" (Chia).

The menacing aura surrounding mental illness plays out its influence on students in various ways including, as already mentioned, their choices of fieldwork placements:

> I think community unawareness still affects you. Some [students] don't want psych because they haven't got over psych having a bad reputation in the community (Jane).

In synchrony with societal fear and ignorance, students may vote with their feet in choosing among fieldwork options. They may make a conscious decision to avoid fieldwork involving persons with psychiatric disorders.

Academic and Clinical Influences

Another source of students' negative preconceptions may lie with the style of their education. Teaching about reasoning processes in occupational therapy is often structured around *problems* linked with diagnoses, reflective of the clinical perspective of persons with disabilities (Cocks, 1989):

> Well, I suppose it comes from the lectures: "You're going to come across patients who have this problem. They're going to be poor to motivate. They're going to withdraw and prefer to be by themselves." . . . I mean the whole list of negative symptoms which, to me, I'd expect to find in a really acute setting (Chia).

One likely consequence of the preoccupation with *deficits* is the tendency for students to acquire a pessimistic view of persons with psychiatric disorders, as Chia has indicated. What is more, the primacy of diagnostic labels as the means of identifying persons and as the basis for discussion about them does nothing to dispel ignorance and fear:

> You tend to be a bit scared of them when you're at Uni[versity] because you label them as schizophrenic and that type of thing. But when you get to meet them, they're very normal. I mean, apart from their illness, they're just people (Sophie).

University teaching, in other words, may inadvertently support students' adherence to negative stereotypes rather than fostering greater appreciation of persons' normalcy. Additionally, because occupational therapy services are mostly located within hospitalized settings, students have little or no opportunity to meet and come to know persons with psychiatric disorders in more normal surroundings associated with community life (e.g., homes, acquaintances, neighborhoods, daily routines), to the detriment of their understanding of the normalcy of persons (Westbrook & Adamson, 1989). As has been proposed, students are also most likely to encounter persons only during those times when, as patients, they are experiencing substantial problems in their lives; this situation contributes further to a jaundiced view of persons with psychiatric disorders.

By way of contrast, several students on fieldwork in a community clinic commented on how contact with persons outside the clinical setting had influenced their perceptions markedly. For example, two students attended a week-long camp where they lived alongside some persons with psychiatric diagnoses. From this experience and hearing these persons' stories of their lives, the students reported a growing sense of respect for them as survivors against a backdrop of considerable trauma and hardship.

What can be inferred from informants' comments, then, is that they gleaned a mixed bag of perceptions of persons with psychiatric disorders from their fieldwork experiences. Although negative overtones pervaded students' expectations before and at the commencement of fieldwork in psychiatry, these tendencies were challenged and modified substantially in some students with fieldwork experience. Yet positive attitudinal shifts were not apparent among all informants. What is more, the existence of such overtones of devaluation of persons with psychiatric disorders, among students entering and leaving fieldwork, is surely cause for concern as an educational issue in a profession that professes social justice for, and activism in the interests of, disadvantaged persons (Joyce, 1993; Townsend, 1993).

Conclusion: Toward Appreciating Human Value

An issue of concern arising from this research is the propensity of informants to diminish the personhood of those labeled as mentally ill, somewhat akin to that described by Peloquin (1993). This raises the question of whether a sound appreciation of the humanness and individuality of persons with psychiatric disorders is being propagated within occupational therapy students.

The informants of this study live in a society that cloaks mental illness in malevolence and devalues persons so labeled. There is every reason to believe that occupational therapy students do not escape the insidious influence of these societal perceptions — insidious in the sense that they are pervasive, lifelong, but largely unconscious (Mitchell, 1990). Although some students may become aware of their stereotyped preconceptions, this is apparently not so for all.

This tendency toward depersonalization gives rise to an educational issue of how information about persons with psychiatric disorders is conveyed to students. Are students being schooled in psychiatry in a way that places too much emphasis on medical diagnoses (e.g., etiology, symptomatology) as the essence of understanding the experience of mental illness, the needs of persons, and the formulation of a professional response?

The formulation and use of psychiatric diagnoses are matters of substantial controversy (Landrine, 1987; Szasz, 1993). These are issues that a proactive education of analytical practitioners should incorporate (i.e., a critical understanding of the limitations and possible misuse of diagnoses). Whatever the opinion of the diagnostic system in psychiatry, however, it is unlikely that any mental health professional would suggest that diagnoses define persons. Yet findings from this study indicate that the principal means by which students are given to understand the meaning and consequences of mental disturbance for persons is via teaching to diagnoses.

If this is so, educators need to rethink the information being presented to students, in favor of a more balanced view. Unintentionally, we may be offering a one-sided view of all that can be "wrong" with persons who have a specified diagnosis, without conveying a sense that there is much that can be "right" and "whole," or anything of the uniqueness of experience of mental disturbance to different persons. The starting (and finishing) points in students' learning must be the person rather than the

diagnosis. Diagnostic information must be understood as, at best, telling only one part of each person's story rather than being presented as the core or central plot around which everything is arranged and understood.

As much as we educators might see this in our mind's eye as desirable educational practice, we should recognize the importance of the way in which we frame and present information to students. Whatever means we use in our teaching must attempt to present students with a well-rounded view of persons with psychiatric disorders at all times, just as we would want to convey a complete sense of the qualities of any client, to be true to our holistic heritage. With all persons who have disabilities, we may be insufficiently attuned to recognize their giftedness in the face of deficiencies — not by intent but by the largely unconscious influence of a reductionist clinical gaze. Some informants in this study began to recognize this tendency on their fieldwork. All students should be well aware of it by virtue of a sound professional education. There are consumer groups keen to help us and our students address this issue. We should draw on them more as educational consultants and teachers.

It is our belief that most occupational therapy students (as therapists themselves) are persons with a positive commitment to the well-being of their fellow humans. Our experience of students is that most are keen to put their considerable talents to work for the benefit of persons who will use their professional services. The collective *we* in the occupational therapy profession have a responsibility as educators and mentors to help these students channel their capabilities, enthusiasm, and idealism into high-quality professional practice in the service of persons who are disadvantaged. Doing so requires that we foster the development of not only their skills and knowledge (to enable them to act proficiently in practice) but also their attitudes and values (to enable them to act justly and humanely in their dealings with service recipients). ▲

Acknowledgments

This article is based on research conducted by the first author, in partial fulfillment of the requirements for the degree of Doctor of Philosophy at The University of Queensland. The first author thanks his dissertation committee — Jenny Ziviani, PhD, and Alan Hayes, PhD, — for their support.

References

Bhugra, D. (1989). Attitudes towards mental illness. *Acta Psychiatrica Scandinavica, 80,* 1–12.

Bogdan, R., & Biklen, S. (1992). *Qualitative research for education. An introduction to theory and methods* (2nd ed.). Boston: Allyn & Bacon.

Bowman, J. (1987). Attitudes toward disabled persons: Social distance and work competence. *Journal of Rehabilitation, 53,* 41–44.

Chubon, R. (1982). An analysis of research dealing with the attitudes of professionals toward disability. *Journal of Rehabilitation, 48,* 25–30.

Cocks, E. (1989). *An introduction to intellectual disability in Australia*. Canberra: Australian Institute on Intellectual Disability.

Dowbiggin, I. (1988). French psychiatric attitudes towards the dangers posed by the insane ca. 1870. *Research in Law, Deviance and Social Control, 9*, 87–111.

Elliott, D., Hanzlik, J., & Gliner, J. (1992). Attitudes of occupational therapy personnel toward therapists with disabilities. *Occupational Therapy Journal of Research, 12*, 259–277.

Gartner, A., & Joe, T. (1987). Introduction. In A. Gartner & T. Joe (Eds.), *Images of the disabled, disabling images* (pp. 1–6). New York: Praeger.

Gordon, E., Minnes, P., & Holden, R. (1990). The structure of attitudes toward persons with a disability, when specific disability and context are considered. *Rehabilitation Psychology, 35*, 79–91.

Gove, W. (1990). Labelling theory's explanation of mental illness: An update of recent evidence. In M. Nagler (Ed.), *Perspectives on disability* (pp. 75–85). Palo Alto: Health Markets Research.

Griffiths, L., & Hughes, D. (1993). Typication in a neurorehabilitation centre: Scheff revisited? *Sociological Review, 41*, 415–445.

Hackett, C. (1991). Positive role models. *Australian Disability Review, 3*, 17–20.

Henwood, K., & Pidgeon, N. (1992). Qualitative research and psychological theorizing. *British Journal of Psychology, 83*, 97–111.

Joyce, L. (1993). Occupational therapy: A cause without a rebel. *British Journal of Occupational Therapy, 56*, 447.

Krefting, L. (1991). Rigor in qualitative research: The assessment of trustworthiness. *American Journal of Occupational Therapy, 45*, 214–222.

Landrine, H. (1987). On the politics of madness: A preliminary analysis of the relationship between social roles and psychopathology. *Genetic, Social, and General Psychology Monographs, 113*, 341–406.

Link, B. (1987). Understanding labeling effects in the area of mental disorders: An assessment of the effects of expectations of rejection. *American Sociological Review, 52*, 96–112.

Link, B., Cullen, F., Frank, J., & Wozniak, J. (1990). The social rejection of former mental patients: Understanding why labels matter. In M. Nagler (Ed.), *Perspectives on disability* (pp. 212–237). Palo Alto: Health Markets Research.

Link, B., Mirotznik, J., & Cullen, F. (1991). The effectiveness of stigma coping orientations: Can negative consequences of mental illness labeling be avoided? *Journal of Health and Social Behavior, 32*, 302–320.

Lyons, M. (1991). Enabling or disabling? Students' attitudes toward persons with disabilities. *American Journal of Occupational Therapy, 45*, 311–316.

Lyons, M., & Hayes, R. (1993). Student perceptions of persons with psychiatric and other disorders. *American Journal of Occupational Therapy, 47*, 541–548.

Mansouri, L., & Dowell, D. (1989). Perceptions of stigma among the long-term mentally ill. *Psychosocial Rehabilitation Journal, 13*, 79–91.

Maxwell, J. (1992). Understanding and validity in qualitative research. *Harvard Educational Review, 62*, 279–300.

McLean, A. (1990). Contradictions in the social production of clinical knowledge: The case of schizophrenia. *Social Science and Medicine, 9*, 969–985.

Mitchell, R. (1990). A liberation model for disability services. *Australian Disability Review, 3*, 31–36.

Patton, M. (1990). *Qualitative evaluation and research methods* (2nd ed.). Newbury Park, CA: Sage.

Peloquin, S. (1993). The depersonalization of patients: A profile gleaned from narratives. *American Journal of Occupational Therapy, 47*, 830–837.

Retzinger, S. (1990). Mental illness and labeling in mediation. *Mediation Quarterly, 8*, 151–159.

Schwartz, S., & Struch, N. (1989). Values, stereotypes, and intergroup antagonism. In D. Bar-Tal, C. Graumann, A. Kruglanski, & W. Stroebe (Eds.), *Stereotyping and prejudice: Changing conceptions* (pp. 151–157). New York: Springer-Verlag.

Seidel, J., Kjolseth, R., & Seymour, E. (1988). *The ethnograph*. Corvallis, OR: Qualis Research Associates.

Shears, L., & Jensema, C. (1969). Social acceptability of anomalous persons. *Exceptional Children, 35*, 91–96.

Socall, D., & Holtgraves, T. (1992). Attitudes toward the mentally ill: The effects of label and beliefs. *Sociological Quarterly, 33*, 435–445.

Stainback, W., & Stainback, S. (1989). Using qualitative data collection procedures to investigate supported education issues. *Journal of the Association for Persons with Severe Handicaps, 14*, 271–277.

Steinwachs, D., Cullum, H., Dorwart, R., Flynn, L., Frank, R., Friedman, M., Herz, M., Mulvey, E., Snowden, L., Test, M., Tremaine, L., & Windle, C. (1992). Service systems research. *Schizophrenia Bulletin, 18*, 627–669.

Szasz, T. (1993). Crazy talk: Thought disorder or psychiatric arrogance? *British Journal of Medical Psychology, 66*, 61–67

Tebes, J., & Kraemer, D. (1991). Quantitative and qualitative knowing in mutual support research: Some lessons from the recent history of scientific psychology. *American Journal of Community Psychology, 19*, 739–756.

Townsend, E. (1993). Occupational therapy's social vision. *Canadian Journal of Occupational Therapy, 60*, 174–183.

Townsend, J. (1990). Stereotypes of mental illness: A comparison with ethnic stereotypes. In M. Nagler (Ed.), *Perspectives on disability* (pp. 102–117). Palo Alto: Health Markets Research.

Tringo, J. (1970). The hierarchy of preference toward disability groups. *Journal of Special Education, 4*, 295–305.

Weinstein, R. (1983). Labelling theory and the attitudes of mental patients: A review. *Journal of Health and Social Behavior, 24*, 70–84.

Westbrook, M., & Adamson, B. (1989). Knowledge and attitudes: Aspects of occupational therapy students' perceptions of the handicapped. *Australian Occupational Therapy Journal, 36*, 120–130.

Westbrook, M., Adamson, B., & Westbrook, J. (1988). Health science students' images of disabled people. *Community Health Studies, 12*, 304–313.

Yuker, H., & Block, J. (1986). *Research with the Attitudes Toward Disabled Persons Scales (ATDP) 1960–1985*. Hempstead, NY: Center for the Study of Attitudes Toward Persons with Disabilities, Hofstra University.

Student Coping Strategies and Perceptions of Fieldwork

Marlys M. Mitchell, Charlene M. Kampfe

Key Words: fieldwork education, occupational therapy • stress

A questionnaire, the revised Ways of Coping Checklist, was sent to all professional (entry-level) graduate students in the United States in one academic year during their second fieldwork level II experience to determine what coping strategies they used during their fieldwork experience. Information was also gathered regarding their perceptions of this clinical experience. Responses from 101 students showed that they used Problem-Focused and Seeks Social Support strategies more than Wishful Thinking, Blamed Self, or Avoidance strategies. More than half of the students found the experience to be stressful, and almost all agreed that it was important. Most agreed that they had control over their present circumstances in the fieldwork experience.

Marlys M. Mitchell, PhD, OTR/L, FAOTA, is Professor, Division of Occupational Therapy, Medical School Wing E, CB-7120, University of North Carolina at Chapel Hill, Chapel Hill, North Carolina 27599–7120.

Charlene M. Kampfe, PhD, is Adjunct Associate Professor, Department of Special Education and Rehabilitation, University of Arizona, Tucson, Arizona. At the time of this study, she was Assistant Professor, University of North Carolina at Chapel Hill, Chapel Hill, North Carolina.

This article was accepted for publication August 24, 1992.

The purpose of this study was to identify the coping strategies used by professional (entry-level) occupational therapy graduate students during their second fieldwork level II experience and to determine their perceptions of the experience. Making the transition from an academic to a clinical setting requires an adjustment to different settings, activities, and responsibilities. Literature has suggested that making this transition can be stressful (Butler, 1972; Cole, Kolko, & Craddick, 1981; Frum, 1986; Gold, Meltzer, & Sherr, 1982; Goplerud, 1980; Greenstein, 1983; Kampfe & Mitchell, 1990; Mitchell, 1985; Mitchell & Kampfe, 1990; Punwar & Decker, 1986; Snow & Mitchell, 1982; Solway, 1985; Wiemer, 1984). Although some stress may facilitate growth and learning (Whitman, Spendlove, & Clark, 1986), high levels of stress may be related to loss of productivity and effectiveness (Colford & McPhee, 1989). Stressors may be acute or chronic, and work-related or non–work related (Cooper & Marshall, 1976; Greenhaus & Parasuraman, 1987; Ivancevich & Matteson, 1980; Pelletier, 1984). They may be personal, job-related, or environmental (Holmes & Rahe, 1967) and may be seen as a problem of person–job–environment fit (Martin, 1988).

In occupational therapy, several authors have addressed fieldwork-related topics such as stress (Butler, 1972; Greenstein, 1983; Mitchell & Kampfe, 1990) and applied them to supervision (Christie, Joyce, & Moeller, 1985a, 1985b; Frum & Opacich, 1987; Yerxa, 1984a, 1984b; Yuen, 1990), course work (Delworth, 1972; Wise & Page, 1980), and collaboration (Mitchell, 1985; Snow & Mitchell, 1982). Underlying these discussions is a basic concern for providing a successful fieldwork experience for the student.

Coping is a mechanism used to reduce stress (Spierer, 1977). It is related to how people perceive an event (Aldwin & Revenson, 1987; Folkman, 1984; Folkman & Lazarus, 1980). Mor-Barak (1988) stated that social support also can be beneficial when there are stressful life events. He referred to this proposition as "the Buffering Hypothesis" (p. 664), because the social ties to others provide protection for a person. Mor-Barak suggested that intervention to prevent adversity (or stress) can involve focusing on stressors or social support, because the context of the adversity or a person's vulnerability to stress are more difficult to change. Veninga (1986) stated that to cope with the pressures of life, we must stay physically and mentally healthy. The stronger the pressure, the greater the need to rely on the strength of friends.

In an exploratory study of coping strategies and perceptions of fieldwork level II students in occupational therapy, Mitchell and Kampfe (1990) found that students expended more percent effort (%E) on health-promoting, adaptive coping strategies (Problem-Focused and Seeks Social Support) than on less desirable, less adaptive strategies (Blamed Self, Wishful Thinking, and Avoidance). Additionally, students perceived the transition from an academic to a clinical setting as important, controllable, and stressful. In Madill, Hagler, and Mitchell's (1990) survey of 167 occupational therapy, physical therapy, and speech therapy students in Canada, the 51 undergraduate occupational therapy student respondents used two coping strategies, Problem-Focused and Seeks Social Support, more than the others. They also perceived the transition from an academic to a clinical setting as stressful. Kampfe and Mitchell (1990; 1991a; 1991b) reported similar results with graduate students in rehabilitation counseling; as did Hagler, Madill, Kampfe, and Mitchell (1990) with undergraduate students in speech therapy.

The present study is a national replication of the exploratory study to verify results and permit generalization. It differs from the exploratory study in sample size ($n = 101$ vs $n = 24$) and geographic distribution (national or 15 occupational therapy schools vs local or 1 occupational therapy school). The research questions were: "What are the coping strategies employed by students in transition from academic learning to clinical internship?" and "How do students perceive the transition from academic learning to clinical internship?"

Method

Subjects

Subjects in this study were students from all 15 professional graduate occupational therapy programs in the United States who were in their second fieldwork level II experience in one academic year. A total of 207 questionnaires was sent and 104 were returned for a response rate of 52%. Three questionnaires were unusable. Subjects were 88 women and 13 men; 29% were in the 21–25 year age group, 38% were in the 26–30 year group, 28% were in the 31–40 year group, and 5% were over 41 years of age.

Instruments

Revised Ways of Coping Checklist (WCCL). The revised WCCL (Vitaliano, Maiuro, Russo, & Becker, 1987; Vitaliano, Russo, Carr, Maiuro, & Becker, 1985) was used to determine coping strategies used by subjects. It is reported to have "respectable internal consistency, reliability, and construct and criterion-related validity" (Vitaliano et al., 1985, p. 24). The 42 Likert items have five scales: Problem-Focused, Seeks Social Support, Blamed Self, Wishful Thinking, and Avoidance. The instructions were modified for this study by specification of the transition to the fieldwork experience as the stressful event under consideration. Subjects indicated the degree to which they used each coping strategy on the revised WCCL in relation to the transition from being an academic student to being a full-time intern. In two exploratory studies (Kampfe & Mitchell, 1990; Mitchell & Kampfe, 1990), the

revised WCCL took about 20 min to complete and it discriminated among students.

Transition Questionnaire. A questionnaire was developed for the study based on a literature review and on a previous questionnaire developed by the investigators (Mitchell & Kampfe, 1988). The questionnaire asked subjects to rate their perceptions of the transition from an academic setting to a fieldwork experience on a 5-point Likert scale from strongly disagree (0) to strongly agree (4). These perceptions were importance, disruption, control over transition, control over present circumstances, and stress.

Procedure

Letters were sent to directors of all 15 accredited professional graduate occupational therapy programs to explain the study and request participation of their students. All existing programs participated. Questionnaires were sent to students 1 month before the end of their 3-month fieldwork experience. Each questionnaire was coded by school. No follow-up of nonrespondents was conducted because of timing constraints.

Analyses

Analyses involved describing the distribution of all the variables. Continuous variables were described with means and standard deviations. The percent effort (%E) attributed to each scale was computed by calculating a mean effort for each scale and dividing the mean effort for each scale by the sum of the mean efforts of all scales. No comparisons among graduate programs were made because of the disparity in numbers of students from each program ranging from 2 in small programs to 13 in larger programs.

Results

Coping Strategies

Means and standard deviations of the percent effort of the five coping scales are shown in Table 1. Problem-Focused (PF) and Seeks Social Support (SS) strategies were used more frequently than Blamed Self (BS), Wishful Thinking (WT), or Avoidance (AV). T-tests showed a significant difference in scores at the .0001 level between all coping strategies except WT/AV which was not significant ($p \leq$ .06).

Perception of Transition

Results of subject ratings of perceptions of transitioning are shown in Table 2. The perception of importance (statement 1) was strongly weighed toward agreement. Disruption was moderately directional, but women tended to agree that the transition and the fieldwork expe-

Table 1
Students' Percentage of Effort Scores on the Five Coping Scales of the Revised Ways of Coping Checklist (N = 101)

Scale	Number of Items	X (%E)	SD
Problem-Focused	15	28	.07
Seeks Social Support	6	25	.05
Blamed Self	3	18	.07
Wishful Thinking	8	15	.06
Avoidance	10	13	.05

Note. %E = Percentage of Effort. Relative scores (%E) were computed by calculating a mean effort for each scale and dividing the mean effort for each scale by the sum of the mean efforts of all scales. Due to rounding, %E does not equal 100%. %E score is the proportion of effort of each coping scale in relation to all of the scales of the revised Ways of Coping Checklist.

riences were disruptive, whereas men were less likely to perceive the experience as disruptive. Having control over the transition was somewhat directional for women who tended to agree with this perception; men showed no directionality of perception. The perception of control over present circumstances was strongly directional and received strong agreement by subjects. The perception of stress was strongly agreed to by women and moderately agreed to by men.

Discussion

This study of 15 graduate programs confirmed the results of the exploratory study (Mitchell & Kampfe, 1990) in regard to coping strategies used by professional occupational therapy graduate students in fieldwork settings and the students' perceptions of the transition. However,

because the response rate was low (52%), due, perhaps, to the lack of follow-up from the initial mailing, or to the timing of the receipt of the questionnaire by the subjects near the end of their fieldwork experience, these results are limited in their generalizability.

Coping Strategies

Results of the current study showed percent effort expended on various coping strategies to be virtually identical to those of the exploratory study and to follow the same rank order. Students expended significantly more effort on positive than on negative strategies, verifying healthy coping skills for dealing with fieldwork transition and stress. Also, these results of positive coping strategies corroborate those of a study of graduate students in rehabilitation counseling (Kampfe & Mitchell, 1991a) and those of a study of undergraduate occupational therapy students in Canada (Madill et al., 1990).

The Problem-Focused strategy is considered to be health-promoting and adaptive, and related to good mental health (Vitaliano et al., 1987). Similarly, Seeks Social Support implies that seeking outside help acknowledges an outside support system that may promote maintenance of good mental health. The less frequent use of the negatively regarded strategies, Blamed Self, Wishful Thinking, and Avoidance, implies that occupational therapy students have healthy strategies available to them to cope with fieldwork transitions and stress.

Perception of the Transition

The perception of importance of the transition into the clinical site is a positive result and is similar to results with

Table 2
Subjects' Agreement With Statements of Perception of the Transition (N = 88 Women, 13 Men)

Statement	Strongly Disagree (0)	Disagree (1)	Agree and Disagree (2)	Agree (3)	Strongly Agree (4)	X Raw Score
The change was important to me[a]						3.63
Women	0 (0%)	0 (0%)	6 (7%)	23 (26%)	58 (67%)	
Men	0 (0%)	0 (0%)	0 (0%)	2 (15%)	11 (85%)	
The change has been disruptive to my life						2.17
Women	10 (11%)	16 (18%)	23 (26%)	23 (26%)	16 (18%)	
Men	2 (15%)	4 (31%)	3 (23%)	2 (15%)	2 (15%)	
I had control over whether or not to make this transition						2.18
Women	10 (15%)	15 (17%)	20 (23%)	20 (23%)	20 (23%)	
Men	3 (23%)	2 (15%)	3 (23%)	3 (23%)	2 (15%)	
I have control over the present circumstances of my internship						2.48
Women	3 (3%)	8 (9%)	35 (40%)	29 (33%)	13 (15%)	
Men	1 (8%)	0 (0%)	5 (38%)	5 (38%)	2 (15%)	
The transition has been stressful						2.69
Women	5 (6%)	6 (7%)	21 (24%)	30 (34%)	26 (30%)	
Men	0	3 (23%)	5 (38%)	3 (23%)	2 (15%)	

Note: Mean scores range from 0 to 4. Percentages have been rounded.
[a]One subject did not respond to this statement.

subjects in rehabilitation counseling (Kampfe & Mitchell, 1992). Such attribution can be anticipated because fieldwork is an expected culmination of a long-awaited experience leading to a professional credential. The perceived importance of the fieldwork experience may suggest to academic and clinical educators that fieldwork level I experiences be planned early and frequently in students' academic programs.

The fact that women and men differed in their responses regarding the disruptive nature of the transition (44% and 30% respectively) suggests that some other factor may have led to this disparity. Perhaps the necessity to relocate, which has been reported to be stressful (Goplerud, 1980; Kaslow & Rice, 1985; Solway, 1985) accounts for differences in these results. The necessity to relocate and the desire to relocate may lead to different perceptions of disruption. Loss of a social network (Solway, 1985) may also affect the sense of disruption differentially.

The perception of control over whether or not to make the transition confirmed the results of the exploratory study, but this perception was more strongly felt by women than by men. Generally, the perception of control has been judged (Kampfe & Wedl, 1989) to be related to the level of stress, that is, the perception of little control leads to more stress, which leads to greater use of Problem-Focused and Seeks Social Support behaviors.

Perceived control relates positively to physical and mental health (Butler, 1972; Wolk & Kurtz, 1975). The finding that 50% of the subjects perceived that they had control over their present circumstances explains their increased use of positive strategies such as Problem-Focused and Seeks Social Support behaviors.

The majority of respondents perceived stress, but women felt it more strongly than men. This difference could be attributed to a number of variables such as marital status, relocation, finances, or individual circumstances. Because sample size for men is small, interpretation must proceed with caution.

Implications

This study indicates that occupational therapy students generally choose healthy strategies to cope with stress generated by moving from an academic setting into a fieldwork experience. Problem-focused strategies, healthy strategies, generally involve doing something about a situation or about oneself and call for self-initiated action. Such actions imply possession of a sense of control over one's life. This sense can reduce destructive forms of stress and enhance both physical and psychological health. The results of the study imply that students are proactively functioning in ways that can increase their sense of control and empowerment and thus reduce stress.

Social support strategies used by occupational ther-

apy students can buffer their stress. This was borne out in two studies. As Mor-Barak stated (1988), social ties to others protect a person by supporting the person in adversity. Students can align themselves with supportive groups or persons including faculty, clinicians, families, or student peers to buffer their stress. Goplerud (1980) found that supportive peers were emotionally and professionally helpful to graduate students and Whitman et al. (1986) found that such peers help mediate stress. Choice of coping strategies is also of concern to academicians and clinicians because they can offer guidance to those needing to learn new coping strategies. Such guidance can be given in formal and informal classroom groups or through individual conferences.

In the clinical setting, an environment in which open communication is fostered, close supervision is gradually decreased as autonomy is gradually increased. Planned time for discussion and feedback is provided, leading to positive interaction and stress reduction. As the student experiences more autonomy, a sense of control or empowerment evolves, which can lead to better performance and less stress. Intervention strategies for supervisors to assist students in making transitions appear elsewhere (Mitchell & Kampfe, 1990).

Meetings of clinical councils involving academicians, clinicians, and students provide a forum for addressing many fieldwork issues. Perhaps the most important benefit of any discussion in any setting is transmission of the feeling of support, which can lead to greater satisfaction and fewer emotional problems (Goplerud, 1980) and reduce student stress. Indeed, students' responses to their individual positive perceptions of a situation may lead to acceptance of their own success, thus keeping their perceptions positive and under their own control and reducing stress. Discussions that convey the notion that thinking positively and focusing on solutions will lead to more experiences of success. Another point for discussion is that the fieldwork experience is a time to apply new learning, gain new skills, test what has been learned, and learn from errors.

Among students, a common anxiety-producing belief is that they must demonstrate skill and knowledge without error—certainly not an expectation of academicians or clinicians. To the extent that academicians and clinicians are skillful in the use of reflection, confrontation, and empathy in discussions with students, they can provide an atmosphere in which students can learn and grow. Most students are resourceful in seeking help from peers, therapists, or families when in anxiety-producing situations. Joint viewing of videotapes followed by discussion of scenarios viewed can be helpful for academicians, clinicians, and students. These tapes may be made onsite, or purchased, such as the recently developed Self-Paced Instruction for Clinical Education and Supervision (SPICES) materials (Crepeau & LaGarde, 1991).

Because students use more positive than negative

coping strategies, their time and energy can be devoted to the major focus of the internship, learning, rather than to managing less positive strategies. Clinicians and academicians can recognize the suggested relationship between perceptions of an event and coping strategies and can provide students with opportunities to experience personal control, less disruption, and less stress in their respective settings. Experiences might include more preinternship opportunities, seminars that focus on strategies for working in clinical settings, and time management discussions.

A situation unique to professional master's entry programs is the students' previous work experiences following their baccalaureate degree. Such experiences might result in reduced stress and more fully developed coping strategies. This study did not address such relationships in a statistical analysis because of the small sample size, but they could be explored in future research. Another question for investigation is the effect of coping strategies used in fieldwork experience on the future use of strategies in the first and second year of clinical practice. A additional question is how academicians and clinicians can help new therapists with coping strategies meet the demands of being new therapists. As new therapists assume clinical roles, experienced occupational therapists should consider the potential stresses of making such a transition and plan strategies to smooth the way. ▲

Acknowledgments

This research was supported in part by a grant from the Health Promotion/Disease Prevention Program, University of North Carolina, Chapel Hill, North Carolina, and by funds to the Biostatistics Laboratory from the School of Medicine, University of North Carolina, Chapel Hill, North Carolina.

References

Aldwin, C. M., & Revenson, T. A. (1987). Does coping help? A reexamination of the relation between coping and mental health. *Journal of Personality and Social Psychology, 53,* 337–348.

Butler, H. F. (1972). Student role stress in education for the professions. *American Journal of Occupational Therapy, 26,* 399–405.

Christie, B. A., Joyce, P. C., & Moeller, P. L. (1985a). Fieldwork experience, Part I: Impact on practice preference. *American Journal of Occupational Therapy, 39,* 671–674.

Christie, B. A., Joyce, P. C., & Moeller, P. L. (1985b). Fieldwork experience, Part II: The supervisor's dilemma. *American Journal of Occupational Therapy, 30,* 675–681.

Cole, M. A., Kolko, D. G., & Craddick, R. A. (1981). The quality and process of the internship experience. *Professional Psychology, 12,* 570–577.

Colford, J., & McPhee, S. J. (1989). The ravelled sleeve of care: Managing the stresses of residency training. *Journal of the American Medical Association, 261,* 889–893.

Cooper, C. L., & Marshall, J. (1976). Occupational sources of stress: A review of the literature relating to coronary heart disease and mental health. *Journal of Occupational Psychology, 49,* 11–28.

Crepeau, E. B., & LaGarde, T. (Eds.). (1991). *Self-paced instruction for clinical education and supervision.* Rockville, MD: American Occupational Therapy Association.

Delworth, U. M. (1972). Interpersonal skill development for occupational therapists. *American Journal of Occupational Therapy, 26,* 27–29.

Folkman, S. (1984). Personal control and stress: A theoretical analysis. *Journal of Personality and Social Psychology, 46,* 839–852.

Folkman, S., & Lazarus, R. S. (1980). An analysis of coping in a middle-aged community sample. *Journal of Health and Social Behavior, 21,* 219–239.

Frum, D. (1986). *Fieldwork education specialist report. Commission on Education proceedings.* Rockville, MD: American Occupational Therapy Association.

Frum, D., & Opacich, K. J. (1987). *Supervision: Development of therapeutic competence.* Rockville, MD: American Occupational Therapy Association.

Gold, J. R., Meltzer, B. H., & Sherr, R. L. (1982). Professional transition: Psychology internships in rehabilitation settings. *Professional Psychology, 13,* 397–403.

Goplerud, E. N. (1980). Social support and stress during the first year of graduate school. *Professional Psychology, 11,* 283–290.

Greenhaus, J. H., & Parasuraman, S. (1987). A work-nonwork interactive perspective of stress and its consequences. *Journal of Organizational Behavior Management, 8(2),* 37–60.

Greenstein, L. R. (1983). Student anxiety toward level II fieldwork. *American Journal of Occupational Therapy, 37(2),* 89–95.

Hagler, P., Madill, H. M., Kampfe, C., & Mitchell, M. M. (1990, November). *Students' coping strategies and prediction of practicum performance.* Paper presented at the American Speech and Hearing Association Annual Conference, Seattle, WA.

Holmes, T. H., & Rahe, R. H. (1967). The social readjustment rating scale. *Journal of Psychosomatic Research, 11,* 213–218.

Ivancevich, J. M., & Matteson, M. T. (1980). *Stress and work: A managerial perspective.* Dallas: Scott, Foresman.

Kampfe, C., & Mitchell, M. M. (1990). Rehabilitation counseling internships: Students' perceptions and coping strategies, *Rehabilitation Education, 4(1),* 13–22.

Kampfe, C., & Mitchell, M. M. (1991a). Coping strategies of master's degree students during internships: A national study. *Rehabilitation Education, 5(1),* 1–12.

Kampfe, C., & Mitchell, M. M. (1991b). Relationships among coping strategies and selected variables in clinical internships. *Rehabilitation Education, 5(1),* 29–41.

Kampfe, C., & Mitchell, M. M. (1992). Students' perceptions of master's level rehabilitation internships: A national study. *Rehabilitation Education, 6(2),* 89–98.

Kampfe, C., & Wedl, L. C. (1989, March). *Coping strategies and life satisfaction of older persons in residential relocation.* Paper presented at the annual meeting of the American Association of Counseling and Development, Boston, Massachusetts.

Kaslow, N. J., & Rice, D. G. (1985). Development stresses of psychology internship training: What training staff can do to help. *Professional Psychology, 16,* 253–261.

Madill, H. M., Hagler, P., & Mitchell, M. M. (1990, October). *Student's coping strategies: An extension of the Chapel Hill project.* Paper presented at the Great Southern Occupational Therapy Conference, Nashville, TN.

Martin, W. T. (1988). *Motivation and productivity in public sector human service organizations.* New York: Quorum Books.

Mitchell, M. M. (1985). Professional development: Clinician

to academician. *American Journal of Occupational Therapy, 39,* 368–373.

Mitchell, M. M., & Kampfe, C. M. (1988, October). *Coping strategies associated with the transition from academic learning to clinical internship: A pilot study.* Paper presented at the Great Southern Occupational Therapy Association Conference, Orlando, FL.

Mitchell, M. M., & Kampfe, C. M. (1990). Coping strategies used by occupational therapy students during fieldwork: An exploratory study. *American Journal of Occupational Therapy, 44,* 543–550.

Mor-Barak, M. E. (1988). Social support and coping with stress: Implications for the workplace. In R. C. Larsen & J. S. Felton (Eds.), *Occupational Medicine, 3,* 663–676.

Pelletier, K. R. (1984). *Healthy people in unhealthy places.* New York: Dell.

Punwar, A., & Decker, J. (1986, November). Problems and failures in level II fieldwork: Impressions of academic coordinators and fieldwork supervisors. *Occupational Therapy News,* pp. 14–15.

Snow, T., & Mitchell, M. M. (1982). Administrative patterns in curriculum-clinic interactions. *American Journal of Occupational Therapy, 36,* 251–256.

Solway, K. (1985). Transition from graduate school to internship: A potential crisis. *Professional Psychology, 12,* 415–419.

Spierer, H. (1977). *Major transitions in the human life cycle.* New York: Academy for Educational Development.

Veninga, R. L. (1986, April). *The work/stress connection: How to remain hopeful in changing times.* Professional Development Seminar, Proceedings of the Commission on Education of the American Occupational Therapy Association. Rockville, MD: American Occupational Therapy Association.

Vitaliano, R., Maiuro, R., Russo, J., & Becker, J. (1987). Raw versus relative scores in the assessment of coping strategies. *Journal of Behavioral Medicine, 10,* 1–18.

Vitaliano, R., Russo, J., Carr, J., Maiuro, R., & Becker, J. (1985). The Ways of Coping Checklist: Revision and psychometric properties. *Multivariate Behavioral Research, 20,* 3–26.

Whitman, N. A., Spendlove, D. C., & Clark, C. H. (1986). *Increasing students' learning: A faculty guide to reducing stress among students.* ASHE-ERIC Higher Education Report No. 4. George Washington University.

Wiemer, R. B. (1984). Student transition from academic to fieldwork settings. In Commission on Education of the American Occupational Therapy Association (Ed.), *Guide to fieldwork education* (pp. 155–161). Rockville, MD: American Occupational Therapy Association.

Wise, B. L., & Page, M. S. (1980). Empathy levels of occupational therapy students. *American Journal of Occupational Therapy, 34,* 676–679.

Wolk, S., & Kurtz, E. (1975). Positive adjustment and involvement during aging and expectancy for internal control. *Journal of Consulting Psychology, 43,* 173–178.

Yerxa, E. J. (1984a). Duties and responsibilities of fieldwork educators in the educational process. In Commission on Education of the American Occupational Therapy Association (Ed.), *Guide to fieldwork education* (pp. 161–168). Rockville, MD: American Occupational Therapy Association.

Yerxa, E. J. (1984b). Techniques of supervision. In Commission on Education of the American Occupational Therapy (Ed.), *Guide to fieldwork education* (pp. 168–176). Rockville, MD: American Occupational Therapy Association.

Yuen, H. K. (1990). The Issue Is — Fieldwork students under stress. *American Journal of Occupational Therapy, 44*(1), 80–81.

Coping Strategies Used by Occupational Therapy Students During Fieldwork: An Exploratory Study

Marlys M. Mitchell,
Charlene M. Kampfe

Key Words: adaptation, psychological •
fieldwork education, occupational therapy •
stress, psychological • students,
occupational therapy

This exploratory study examined the coping strategies and perceptions of 24 graduate students in occupational therapy who were participating in their second Level II fieldwork experience. The instruments used were the revised Ways of Coping Checklist (WCCL) (Vitaliano, Russo, Carr, Maiuro, & Becker, 1985) and a questionnaire developed by the authors. The results showed that of the five coping scales of the WCCL, the students used the Problem-Focused and Seeks Social Support strategies more than the Blamed Self, Wishful Thinking, and Avoidance strategies. Most of the students perceived the fieldwork experience as important, controllable, and stressful, but not disruptive to their lives.

Marlys M. Mitchell, PhD, OTR/L, FAOTA, is Professor, Division of Occupational Therapy, Department of Medical Allied Health Professions, The University of North Carolina at Chapel Hill, CB 7120, Medical School Wing E, Chapel Hill, North Carolina 27599-7120.

Charlene M. Kampfe, PhD, is Assistant Professor, Division of Rehabilitation Counseling, Department of Medical Allied Health Professions, The University of North Carolina at Chapel Hill, Chapel Hill, North Carolina.

This article was accepted for publication January 25, 1990.

A variety of professions require that students complete at least one internship or fieldwork experience in preparation for employment. These experiences vary among professions, but they all include work at a clinical site, with emphasis on practical application of the knowledge and skills learned in the classroom. The purpose of the present study was to identify the coping strategies used by entry-level graduate students in occupational therapy during their fieldwork and to determine their perceptions of the fieldwork experience.

Literature Review

The literature suggests that the transition from academic learning to a clinical setting can be stressful (Cole, Kolko, & Craddick, 1981; Gold, Meltzer, & Sherr, 1982; Greenstein, 1983; Hohaus & Berah, 1985; Kaslow & Rice, 1985; Mitchell, 1985; Punwar & Decker, 1986; Shows, 1976; Snow & Mitchell, 1982; Solway, 1985; Wiemer, 1984). This stress can reduce students' effectiveness and productivity at the clinical site (Colford & McPhee, 1989; Hohaus & Berah, 1985). Variables that might contribute to or mediate stress associated with fieldwork, therefore, need to be identified. Many authors believe that student guidance during fieldwork is needed to alleviate stress or to help students cope with it (Christie, Joyce, & Moeller, 1985a, 1985b; Frum & Opacich, 1987; Greenstein, 1983; Wiemer, 1984; Yerxa, 1984a, 1984b). Others have suggested the need for collaboration between academic and clinical sites to ensure a successful fieldwork experience (Mitchell, 1985; Punwar & Decker, 1986; Snow & Mitchell, 1982).

The supervisor, as a role model, is often the most influential factor in a student's success and enthusiasm for the profession. The supervisor plays a major part in allaying or alleviating a student's stress. Christie et al. (1985a) reported that recurring interpersonal and attitudinal influences emanating from the student–supervisor relationship during the fieldwork experience are critical components of a good fieldwork experience. Christie et al. (1985b) also reported a need for a formal, standardized training program for supervisors, because they play a crucial role in the development of future practitioners.

On the basis of eight issues judged important in fieldwork supervision (Loganbill, Hardy, & Delworth, 1982), Frum and Opacich (1987) summarized their general intervention strategies and related them to occupational therapy students. One of these issues is students' personal motivation, including awareness of a sense of power or control in their lives. The supervisor can assist or channel the student's energy toward development of autonomous behaviors. Frum and Opacich suggested a workshop format to alert supervisors to issues related to fieldwork, so that they can meet students' needs effectively.

Yerxa (1984a, 1984b) pointed out the pressures and the responsibilities of the fieldwork supervisor, including his or her role in helping the student develop an appropriate self-concept as a professional and an appropriate concept of the profession. Notably, communication is identified frequently as the major force behind successful completion of any experience. Thus, the supervisor can help a student with problem-solving and coping strategies in various situations. Wiemer (1984) described the complex nature of the fieldwork experience. Variables such as purposes and goals of the student and the supervisor as well as physical, emotional, intellectual, academic, ethical, moral, and economic forces all influence and shape the fieldwork experience. Students must adjust to new purposes, moving from a student-centered to a patient-centered role and environment. Wiemer stated that success in fieldwork is as much related to a student's philosophy, or attitude, as it is to specific talents. These philosophical, or attitudinal, variables will affect the coping, stress, and success involved in the fieldwork experience.

Stress in fieldwork was specifically addressed by Greenstein (1983), who reported that before their Level II fieldwork experience, students had high anxiety levels, but this anxiety was reduced when the students reported for fieldwork. Butler (1972) also reported that the clinical experience was stressful to graduate students and that these students may need new behavioral strategies, but the literature offers little information regarding strategies to help students deal with such stress. Butler suggested that socialization techniques, the perception of relatedness and belonging, and a guided move from dependence to independence can aid a student in overcoming stressful conditions. Further, she cited ambiguity regarding expectations, evaluations, and rewards as critical sources of stress in students, who then react to this stress with coping and defensive behaviors. Delworth (1972) described a 12-hour workshop offered to occupational therapy students before fieldwork that focuses on interpersonal and communication skills. This type of workshop may provide an opportunity for the dissemination of information about positive coping strategies to deal with stress in the internship.

Researchers in related professions have expressed concern about students' stress in their training programs. Hohaus and Berah (1985) described the stressful nature of first-year medical training and suggested it as a cause of impairment in first-year medical students. They assessed issues of role conflict, role support, role confidence, stress, and depression and reported that the burden of academic work was very stressful and that students had difficulty

establishing and maintaining close, supportive relationships. Colford and McPhee (1989) reported that stress affects residents' attitudes, professional behaviors, and job satisfaction. Pediatric interns under stress had negative attitudes toward patients, poor physician–patient relationships, and decreasing positivity about life. The residents were seen to lose compassion for their patients and were prone to cynicism. Sleep deprivation and financial burdens contributed to their fatigue and stress.

Solway (1985) stated that psychology graduate students face unexpected turmoil as they make the transition from graduate school to a professional internship. He discussed three types of stressors created by this transitional period—clinical, institutional, and personal—with the latter being the most important, because it involves the loss of meaningful relationships due to relocation. He believed that this transition leads to interpersonal and professional changes that are emotionally hazardous. The clearest source of stress is the adoption of the role of the professional (Gold et al., 1982; Shows, 1976; Solway, 1985). Solway (1985) identified institutional stressors resulting from the new status of service provider and professional. He stated that such a person's stressors include moving to a new city, developing new social networks, changing residences, and earning little money. Lamb, Baker, Jennings, and Yarris (1982) identified five passages of an internship: (a) preentry preparation, involving prearrival apprehension; (b) early intern syndrome, in which the intern finds a place in the agency; (c) intern identity, involving a realization of strengths and weaknesses and a period of self-doubt; (d) an emerging professional, which involves an increased sense of competence and independence; and (e) resolution, which involves ways of separating from the agency. Lamb et al. suggested that anxiety and stress decrease as the intern moves through these passages. In addition, Kaslow & Rice (1985) listed some of the major stressors of the internship period to be the adjustment to a new program, the development of a sense of trust in the staff, the questioning of one's competence, the taking of risks to learn new skills with different patient groups, the accurate assessment of one's strengths and weaknesses, and the planning of one's professional life after the internship.

Aldwin and Revenson (1987) suggested that the well-being of a person under stress is related to how that person appraises and copes with stress. Several researchers have categorized coping strategies as problem focused (i.e., strategies used to manage or alter a stressful situation) and emotion focused (i.e., strategies used to manage or control emotions) (Folkman & Lazarus, 1980; Lazarus & Folkman, 1984). Problem-focused strategies are most often found to relate positively to measures of psychosocial well-being, whereas emotion-focused strategies are most often found to relate negatively to these measures (Aldwin & Revenson, 1987; Felton & Revenson, 1984; Kampfe & Wedl, 1989; Vitaliano, Maiuro, Russo, & Becker, 1987). Given these relationships, the kind of coping strategies students use to adapt to the requirements of internships might influence the degree of distress they experience. According to the cognitive phenomenological theory of stress (Lazarus, 1966), "observable threat and stress reactions are reflections or consequences of coping processes intended to reduce threat" (p. 152). Lazarus further stated that "coping processes depend on cognitive activity" (p. 152). Coping, then, depends on a person's perception of a threat and cognition involved in the threat, thus leading to individual behaviors (Lazarus, 1981; Lazarus, Kanner, & Folkman, 1980). Folkman (1984) believed that appraisal, or the perception of an event, is influenced by both the situation and environment and a person's unique characteristics. This cognitive phenomenological theory seems to apply to occupational therapy students in the fieldwork experience, yet no empirical studies have examined this. In the present study, we explored students' perceptions of the transition to the fieldwork experience and their coping strategies during this experience.

Method

Subjects

Twenty-four entry-level graduate students in occupational therapy participated in this study. All of these students were in their second full-time Level II fieldwork experience and were enrolled in their final semester of study at a major southeastern university. Ten of these students (42%) were aged 21 to 25 years, 9 (38%) were aged 26 to 30 years, and 5 (21%) were aged 31 to 40 years. All were women. The fieldwork experience consisted of 12 weeks in either a physical disabilities or a psychosocial setting. The sample group completed the first Level II fieldwork experience, followed by a semester of course work, followed by the second Level II fieldwork experience. Fifteen (62%) of the sample students, upon their request, relocated to another city for fieldwork.

Instruments

Coping strategies were measured with the revised Ways of Coping Checklist (WCCL)(Vitaliano, Russo, Carr, Maiuro, & Becker, 1985). This checklist was originally developed by Folkman and Lazarus (1980) to examine a broad range of cognitive and behavioral strategies that may be used in response to specific stressful events. The revised WCCL comprises 42 items, to which subjects respond on a 4-point Likert

scale, yielding scores on five coping scales: Problem-Focused, Seeks Social Support, Blamed Self, Wishful Thinking, and Avoidance.

Problem-Focused strategies involve management of the sources of stress. This scale includes such statements as "Made a plan of action and followed it." *Seeks Social Support* strategies involve efforts to obtain information, advice, or emotional support. Statements in this category include "Talked to others and accepted their sympathy." *Blamed Self* strategies are passive, that is, they are directed inward rather than outward toward the problem. "Felt responsible for the problem" is a statement from this category. *Wishful Thinking* strategies are emotion-focused and include such statements as "Hoped a miracle would happen." *Avoidance* strategies include such statements as "Slept more than usual." These scales were based on a factor analysis of the results of 425 medical students and were reexamined with separate samples of 83 psychiatric outpatients and 62 spouses of persons with Alzheimer disease. The revised WCCL was found to have "respectable internal consistency, reliability, and construct and criterion-related validity" (Vitaliano et al., 1985, p. 24), and its scales were found to be more reliable and to have considerably less variance than the original WCCL (Folkman & Lazarus, 1980) across the three samples.

In previous uses of the WCCL, the subjects were asked to identify an event that was stressful to them and to respond to the items based on the strategies they used to cope with that event. For the present study, we modified the instructions by specifying the stressful event: the movement from an academic setting into a 3-month fieldwork experience. By holding the stressful event relatively constant (e.g., using only a fieldwork experience, as opposed to a variety of events), it is thought that one can better assess coping strategies (Folkman & Lazarus, 1980).

On the basis of our clinical experience, we believed that the revised WCCL may not include the broad array of coping strategies used by occupational therapy interns. The subjects in the present study, therefore, upon completion of the revised WCCL, were given the opportunity to add strategies not stated in the instrument.

Because perceptions may influence coping strategies, we developed a questionnaire, The Transition from Being an Academic Student to Being a Full-Time Intern, to gather information regarding perceptions of the transition and demographic variables. Five statements were developed from information found in a review of the literature regarding perceptions of life events (Aldwin & Revenson, 1987; Folkman & Lazarus, 1980; George, 1980; Lazarus, 1966, 1981). The subjects were to appraise this transition with regard to degree of importance, disruption, control over the

Table 1
Subjects' Agreement With Statements of Perception of the Transition (N = 24)

Statement	Strongly Disagree	Disagree	Agree and Disagree	Agree	Strongly Agree
1. "The change was important to me."[a]	0 (0%)	0 (0%)	2 (9%)	11 (48%)	10 (43%)
2. "The change has been disruptive to my life."	5 (21%)	9 (38%)	5 (21%)	2 (8%)	3 (13%)
3. "I had control over whether or not to make this transition."	2 (8%)	1 (4%)	7 (29%)	5 (21%)	9 (38%)
4. I have control over the present circumstances of my internship."	0 (0%)	0 (0%)	8 (33%)	10 (42%)	6 (25%)
5. "The transition has been stressful."	1 (4%)	6 (25%)	4 (17%)	8 (33%)	5 (20%)

Note. Statements 2, 3, and 5 are moderately directional; Statements 1 and 4, strongly directional. Percentages have been rounded.
[a] One subject did not respond to this statement.

decision to make the transition, control over present circumstances in the fieldwork experience, and stress associated with the transition. These appraisals were reported on a 5-point Likert scale from *strongly disagree* (0) to *strongly agree* (4) and yielded a separate score for each perception.

Procedure

Twenty-five occupational therapy graduate students were sent the revised WCCL and the transition questionnaire at their fieldwork sites at the beginning of the ninth week of the fieldwork experience. This timing allowed the subjects to accrue a range of experiences requiring coping and an opportunity to use a range of responses. At 9 weeks, the subjects had passed through the initial phases of an internship (Lamb et al., 1982) but were not yet in the final flurry of activity typical of the last days of a fieldwork experience and therefore could respond to the questionnaire. Such timing also minimized the problem of memory and retrospective reporting on clinical experiences. Each questionnaire was coded to maintain anonymity; the codes were used only for follow-up purposes for nonrespondents.

The second fieldwork was chosen because the initial design of the study included a comparison with another academic discipline, and in both disciplines, the second fieldwork followed completion of all course work.

Data Analysis

Relative scores for each scale were calculated. These scores represent the percentage of effort expended on each scale. Frequency tables and the percentage of subjects who agreed or disagreed with perceptions of the transition were constructed to answer the research questions. Means and standard deviations were computed to measure the five coping strategies used.

Results

Twenty-four of the 25 students completed the survey, a 96% response rate. The results are presented in

the sequence in which the research questions were presented.

Perception of the Transition

Table 1 shows the level of agreement or disagreement among the subjects for each of the five statements in the transition questionnaire. Two of the statements showed strong directionality of responses: 91% of the respondents agreed or strongly agreed with the statement, "The change was important to me," and 67% agreed or strongly agreed with the statement, "I have control over the present circumstances of my internship." Three statements showed moderate directionality: "The change has been disruptive to my life," "I had control over whether or not to make this transition," and "The transition has been stressful" (see Table 1).

Coping Strategies

As shown in Table 2, all of the coping strategies were used, however, there was considerable variation among the subjects. The Problem-Focused and Seeks Social Support strategies were used more than the Blamed Self, Wishful Thinking, and Avoidance strategies. Of the identified coping strategies not listed on

Table 2
Students' Percentage of Effort (%E)[a] Scores on the Five Coping Scales of the Revised Ways of Coping Checklist[b] (N = 24)

Scale	No. of Items	X (%E)	SD
Problem-Focused	15	.30	.06
Seeks Social Support	6	.28	.05
Blamed Self	3	.18	.05
Wishful Thinking	8	.13	.06
Avoidance	10	.12	.05

Note: Relative scores (%E) were computed by calculating a mean effort for each scale and dividing that number by the sum of the mean efforts of all scales. Due to rounding, %E does not equal 100%.
[a] The proportion of effort of each coping scale in relation to all of the scales of the revised Ways of Coping Checklist. [b] (Vitaliano, Russo, Carr, Maiuro, & Becker, 1985).

the questionnaire, the two most frequently cited strategies were exercise (cited 10 times) and support from friends and family (cited 6 times).

Discussion

Perception of the Transition

The results show that students perceived the transition to the fieldwork experience as important, which is not surprising, because such an experience is viewed by the academic institution, the clinical site, the profession, and the student as the culmination of the training program. Fieldwork experience recognizes accomplishment and provides students with an opportunity to apply and integrate what they have learned; it is the fulfillment of a long-term expectation.

The subjects thought they had control over their present circumstances. This is a critical result, because the literature suggests that perceived personal control relates positively to good physical and mental health (Butler, 1972; Langer & Rodin, 1976; Pelletier, 1977; Reid & Ziegler, 1980; Wolk & Kurtz, 1975). This result is substantiated by the subjects' frequent use of Problem-Focused coping strategies, which are seen as action oriented and indicate efforts to control the environment.

Over one half of the subjects thought they had control over whether or not to make the transition, and approximately one third were ambivalent, yet the fieldwork experience is a requirement, not an option. Perhaps this perception of control can be attributed to the practice of allowing students to state their preferences for placement at specific sites. The subjects may also have thought they had control because it was their decision to enter the program, which included a commitment to complete a fieldwork experience.

The finding that few of the subjects indicated that the internship was disruptive suggests that the internship was generally a positive experience. The sense of disruption has been reported to relate positively to less adaptive coping strategies and negatively to psychological well-being (Kampfe & Wedl, 1989). The perception that the internship was not disruptive, therefore, may have influenced the subjects' greater use of the Problem-Focused and Seeks Social Support strategies.

The finding that over one half (53%) of the respondents perceived the transition as stressful suggests that stress occurs even when the transition is generally not perceived as disruptive and is thought to be controllable. Twenty-nine percent of the subjects, however, did not perceive the transition as stressful. This variability in responses might be attributed to individual circumstances. For example, because relocation is stressful (Butler 1972; Solway 1985), the perception of stress may have been heightened in those students who had to relocate to their fieldwork site.

Most of the perceptions measured in this study were positive. Perhaps this was due to the time at which the questionnaire was administered (9 weeks into the 12-week fieldwork experience). As Greenstein (1983) pointed out, anxiety is reduced as a student begins the fieldwork experience. Lamb et al. (1982) suggested that students pass through phases of an internship, which implies that perceptions change with this passage. Perhaps the subjects in our study would have perceived the transition differently if they had been contacted earlier in their fieldwork experience.

Coping Strategies

The finding that greater effort was expended on the Problem-Focused and Seeks Social Support strategies than on the Blamed Self, Wishful Thinking, and Avoidance strategies suggests that occupational therapy students more often use healthy approaches in dealing with the fieldwork transition.

Theoretically, the Problem-Focused strategy is expected to be negatively related to depression (Abramson, Seligman, & Teasdale, 1978; Coyne, 1976a, 1976b; Coyne, Aldwin, & Lazarus, 1981). Persons who use a Problem-Focused strategy will have less depression than those who do not use this strategy, that is, this strategy is considered to be health promoting and adaptive (Vitaliano et al., 1985; Vitaliano et al., 1987). Research findings have supported, in part, this theoretical notion. Researchers have reported that a Problem-Focused strategy relates negatively to depression and anxiety in spouses of patients with Alzheimer disease (Vitaliano et al., 1985) and in medical students (Vitaliano et al., 1987). It also relates negatively to psychological symptoms in adults (Aldwin & Revenson, 1987). Although some researchers have not found a positive relationship between all dimensions of Problem-Focused strategies and good mental health, general findings appear to support a positive relationship between these two variables (Vitaliano et al., 1987).

The Seeks Social Support strategy is considered to be adaptive and has been reported to be significantly related to anxiety but not to depression (Vitaliano et al., 1985). This implies that persons who are more anxious are more likely to seek outside help and that this activity may promote maintenance of good mental health (Butler, 1972). Thus, students in fieldwork experiences who use this strategy appear to acknowledge an external support system that they believe can be helpful to them. In the present study, besides the revised WCCL items identified as Seeks

Social Support strategies, 6 students (25%) cited obtaining support from friends and family as a coping strategy. Apparently, support from significant others was perceived as different from the kind of social support described in the items on the revised WCCL. In addition, the Seeks Social Support strategies may be perceived as internal to the fieldwork site, whereas support from friends and family may be perceived as external to the fieldwork site.

The Blamed Self, Wishful Thinking, and Avoidance strategies, which were used less frequently than the Problem-Focused and Seeks Social Support strategies, are considered to be negatively related to mental health (Aldwin & Revenson, 1987, Vitaliano et al., 1987). Thus, occupational therapy students appear to be using active, salutary strategies more often than they are using less adaptive strategies to cope with fieldwork stress.

Besides the strategies identified in the revised WCCL, exercise was cited by 10 subjects (42%) as a coping strategy, which suggests that the WCCL may not fully explore the range of positive coping strategies available to students. The identification of additional coping strategies by 57% of the subjects leads one to question whether this revised WCCL offers students enough options. Irion and Blanchard-Fields (1987) raised a similar question for an older adult sample using Folkman & Lazarus's (1985) revised WCCL.

The results of the present study show a pattern similar to that of medical students (Vitaliano et al., 1987) and rehabilitation counseling students (Kampfe & Mitchell, 1990), who were found to use Problem-Focused and Seeks Social Support strategies most frequently, followed by Wishful Thinking, Blamed Self, and Avoidance strategies. These three groups of students, therefore, generally use the same coping strategies, with occupational therapy students producing the highest number of responses on the Problem-Focused and Seeks Social Support strategies.

It should be noted that in the present study, all of the subjects used a variety of strategies, and there were variations within each of the strategies used. This supports the findings of Folkman and Lazarus (1980), who stated that individuals respond in unique ways to a specific situation or event.

Implications

Curriculum directors, faculty members, academic fieldwork coordinators, clinical supervisors, and students can facilitate the process of transition from an academic to a clinical status and a positive experience in the fieldwork setting by being aware of the various coping strategies used in the transition and proactively creating an environment conducive to the student's personal and professional growth. Such an environment could include the opportunity for open communication, counseling, or both; a clear definition of expectations; a balance between supervision and autonomous behavior; and positive and timely reinforcement.

Awareness of adaptive strategies, perceptions of the transition, and the potential interactions among these two variables will sensitize faculty to factors that might affect students but might otherwise be ignored. Curricula could include the discussion and development of health-promoting coping strategies, such as Problem-Focused and Seeks Social Support behaviors, to reduce stress. A student could use these strategies, for example, to cope with stressors such as those identified by Solway (1985), that is, moving to a new residence, instituting new social networks, and adjusting to limited finances.

Clinical supervisors can assist students by acknowledging the difficulties and stressors both at the clinical site and in concurrent external situations. Sensitivity to such issues can facilitate a positive professional relationship, reduce the stressful quality of the experience, and influence the type of coping strategies used by students. For example, supervisors can address conflicts between student and professional roles by providing clear written and verbal role definitions and expectations. Supervisors can also identify students who are more likely to use maladaptive strategies and encourage them to use adaptive coping strategies, such as seeking social support and problem solving. Training programs for supervisors could include information about perceptions of a transition, coping strategies, and their potential relationship within the fieldwork experience.

Loganbill et al. (1982) suggested five categories of interventions that supervisors can use to promote effective transitions for students: (a) facilitative interventions, including warmth, like, respect, and empathy, which give the student a sense of personal security; (b) confrontational interventions, which can positively highlight discrepancies between the student's feelings and emotions, attitudes and beliefs, and behaviors and actions; (c) conceptual interventions, which can help the student apply theories and principles pertinent to the internship site, thereby linking experience and theory; (d) prescriptive interventions, in which the supervisor provides the student with a specific plan of action, such as treatment plans or goals for a specific patient; and (e) catalytic interventions, such as role modeling, which promote change and activate a process or movement.

Students should be aware of potential stressors in the transition, both external and internal to the site, and plan to control variables that might increase stress. They should be aware that Problem-Focused and Seeks Social Support strategies are health promoting and should therefore develop the skills needed to use such strategies. Students should seek a clear understanding of expectations, request ongoing evaluation, and identify sources of support. They must also recognize that their perceptions of an event will influence their response to that event, thus they have the power to determine the coping strategies they use to help them in their transition.

Future Research

Due to the small sample size used in this exploratory study, definitive conclusions cannot be drawn. The results, however, appear to be worthy of further investigation. A larger sample would permit study of potential relationships among variables. Additional questions for future study may address (a) differences in stressors and coping strategies used by undergraduate and entry-level graduate students; (b) differences in perceptions and the use of coping strategies based on the administration of instruments in first and second internships, early and late phases of an internship, and concurrent and spaced internships; (c) variables not explored in this study, for example, work history, marital status, geographic relocation, personality factors, cognitive style, and familial predisposition; and (d) coping mechanisms not included in the revised WCCL, for example, exercise. Studies examining the efficacy of coping strategies might be planned as well as studies analyzing intervention strategies. The use of raw scores versus mean effort scores on the revised WCCL could also be examined. ▲

References

Abramson, L. Y., Seligman, M. E., & Teasdale, J. P. (1978). Learned helplessness in humans: Critique and reformulation. *Journal of Abnormal Psychology, 87*, 49–74.

Aldwin, C. M., & Revenson, T. A. (1987). Does coping help? A reexamination of the relation between coping and mental health. *Journal of Personality and Social Psychology, 53*, 337–348.

Butler, H. F. (1972). Student role stress in education for the professions. *American Journal of Occupational Therapy, 26*, 399–405.

Christie, B. A., Joyce, P. C., & Moeller, P. L. (1985a). Fieldwork experience, part I: Impact on practice preference. *American Journal of Occupational Therapy, 39*, 671–674.

Christie, B. A., Joyce, P. C., & Moeller, P. L. (1985b). Fieldwork experience, part II: The supervisor's dilemma. *American Journal of Occupational Therapy, 39*, 675–681.

Cole, M. A., Kolko, D. G., & Craddick, R. A. (1981). The quality and process of the internship experience. *Professional Psychology, 12*, 570–577.

Colford, J. M., & McPhee, S. J. (1989). The ravelled sleeve of care—Managing the stresses of residency training. *Journal of the American Medical Association, 261*, 889–893.

Coyne, J. C. (1976a). Depression and the response of others. *Journal of Abnormal Psychology, 85*, 186–193.

Coyne, J. C. (1976b). Toward an interactional description of depression. *Psychiatry, 39*, 28–40.

Coyne, J. C., Aldwin, C., & Lazarus, R. S. (1981). Depression and coping in stressful episodes. *Journal of Abnormal Psychology, 90*, 439–447.

Delworth, U. M. (1972). Interpersonal skill development for occupational therapists. *American Journal of Occupational Therapy, 26*, 27–29.

Felton, B. J., & Revenson, T. A. (1984). Coping with chronic illness: A study of illness controllability and the influence of coping strategies on psychological adjustment. *Journal of Consulting and Clinical Psychology, 52*, 343–353.

Folkman, S. (1984). Personal control and stress and coping processes: A theoretical analysis. *Journal of Personality and Social Psychology, 46*, 839–852.

Folkman, S., & Lazarus, R. S. (1980). An analysis of coping in a middle-aged community sample. *Journal of Health and Social Behavior, 21*, 219–239.

Folkman, S., & Lazarus, R. S. (1985). If it changes it must be a process: Study of emotion and coping during three stages of college examination. *Journal of Personality and Social Psychology, 48*, 150–170.

Frum, D., & Opacich, K. J. (1987). *Supervision: Development of therapeutic competence.* Rockville, MD: American Occupational Therapy Association.

George, L. (1980). *Role transition in later life.* Monterey, CA: Brooks/Cole.

Gold, J. R., Meltzer, B. H., & Sherr, R. L. (1982). Professional transition: Psychology internships in rehabilitation settings. *Professional Psychology, 13*, 397–403.

Greenstein, L. R. (1983). Student anxiety toward Level II fieldwork. *American Journal of Occupational Therapy, 37*, 89–95.

Hohaus, L., & Berah, E. F. (1985). Impairment of doctors: Are beginning medical students psychologically vulnerable? *Medical Education, 19*, 431–436.

Irion, J. C., & Blanchard-Fields, F. (1987). A cross-sectional comparison of adaptive coping in adulthood. *Journal of Gerontology, 42*, 502–504.

Kampfe, C. M., & Mitchell, M. M. (1990). Rehabilitation counseling internships: Students' perceptions and coping strategies. *Rehabilitation Education, 4*(1), 13–22.

Kampfe, C. M., & Wedl, L. C. (1989, March). *Coping strategies and life satisfaction of older persons in residential relocation.* Paper presented at the annual meeting of the American Association of Counseling and Development, Boston.

Kaslow, N. J., & Rice, D. G. (1985). Development stresses of psychology internship training: What training staff can do to help. *Professional Psychology, 16*, 253–261.

Lamb, D. H., Baker, J. M., Jennings, M. L., & Yarris, E. (1982). Passages of an internship in professional psychology. *Professional Psychology, 13*, 661–669.

Langer, E. J., & Rodin, J. (1976). The effects of choice and enhanced personal responsibility for the aged: A field experiment in an institutional setting. *Journal of Experimental and Social Psychology, 34*, 191–198.

Lazarus, R. S. (1966). *Psychological stress and the coping process.* New York: McGraw-Hill.

Lazarus, R. S. (1981). The stress and coping paradigm. In C. Eisdorfer, D. Cohen, A. Kleinman, & P. Maxim (Eds.), *Models for clinical psychopathology* (pp. 177–214). New York: Spectrum.

Lazarus, R. S., & Folkman, S. (1984). *Stress, appraisal, and coping.* New York: Springer.

Lazarus, R. S., Kanner, A., & Folkman, S. (1980). Emotions: A cognitive-phenomenological analysis. In R. Plutchik and H. Kellerman (Eds.), *Theories of emotion* (pp. 189–217). New York: Academic Press.

Loganbill, C., Hardy, E., & Delworth, U. M. (1982). Supervision: A conceptual model. *Consulting Psychologist, 10,* 3–42.

Mitchell, M. M. (1985). Professional development: Clinician to academician. *American Journal of Occupational Therapy, 39,* 368–373.

Pelletier, K. R. (1977). *Mind as healer, mind as slayer.* New York: Delta.

Punwar, A., & Decker, J. (1986, November). Problems and failures in Level II fieldwork: Impressions of academic coordinators and fieldwork supervisors. *Occupational Therapy News,* pp. 14–15.

Reid, D. W., & Ziegler, M. (1980). Validity and stability of a new desired control measure pertaining to psychological adjustments of the elderly. *Journal of Gerontology, 35,* 395–402.

Shows, W. D. (1976). Problems of training psychology interns in medical schools: A case of trying to change the leopard's spots. *Professional Psychology, 7,* 205–208.

Snow, T., & Mitchell, M. M. (1982). Administrative patterns in curriculum–clinic interactions. *American Journal of Occupational Therapy, 36,* 251–256.

Solway, K. (1985). Transition from graduate school to internship: A potential crisis. *Professional Psychology, 12,* 415–419.

Vitaliano, R., Maiuro, R., Russo, J., & Becker, J. (1987). Raw versus relative scores in the assessment of coping strategies. *Journal of Behavioral Medicine, 10,* 1–18.

Vitaliano, R., Russo, J., Carr, J., Maiuro, R., & Becker, J. (1985). The Ways of Coping Checklist: Revision and psychometric properties. *Multivariate Behavioral Research, 20,* 3–26.

Wiemer, R. B. (1984). Student transition from academic to fieldwork settings. In Commission on Education of the American Occupational Therapy Association (Eds.), *Guide to fieldwork education* (pp. 155–161). Rockville, MD: American Occupational Therapy Association.

Wolk S., & Kurtz, E. (1975). Positive adjustment and involvement during aging and expectancy for internal control. *Journal of Consulting Psychology, 43,* 173–178.

Yerxa, E. J. (1984a). Duties and responsibilities of fieldwork educators in the educational process. In Commission on Education of the American Occupational Therapy Association (Ed.), *Guide to fieldwork education* (pp. 161–168). Rockville, MD: American Occupational Therapy Association.

Yerxa, E. J. (1984b). Techniques of supervision. In Commission on Education of the American Occupational Therapy Association (Ed.), *Guide to fieldwork education* (pp. 168–176). Rockville, MD: American Occupational Therapy Association.

Multiple Mentoring Relationships Facilitate Learning During Fieldwork

Terrie Nolinske

Key Words: fieldwork education, occupational therapy • mentor

Fieldwork provides a means by which students are socialized into their profession and their careers. During Level I and Level II fieldwork, students acquire and apply the knowledge, skills, and attitudes that will enable them to achieve entry-level competence. The experiences that students have during Level II fieldwork influence their subsequent career choices. To support these experiences, students form a variety of helping relationships with faculty members, clinicians, peers, family, and friends. This article examines the role and responsibilities of the student as protégé and of the clinical educator as information peer, collegial peer, special peer, and mentor. In light of the challenges faced by most clinicians secondary to health care reform, an alternative to the one-to-one supervision model is presented. The multiple mentoring model of fieldwork supervision has several advantages: (a) fieldwork educators work with students according to their strengths and interests; (b) the model promotes collegiality and clinical reasoning skills because students use each other as resources and observe different fieldwork educators approaching similar situations; and (c) the model allows a fieldwork site to accept more students at one time, while minimizing stress on any one fieldwork educator. A framework defining the functions of the mentor–protégé relationship is provided, with an emphasis on the effect that clinical educators have in their roles as mentors, guides, role models, and teachers who provide opportunities for the student to develop entry-level competency in a chosen profession.

Terrie Nolinske, PhD, OTR/L, CO, is President, TNI: Consultants in Professional Development, 930 North Boulevard, #402, Oak Park, Illinois 60301, and Fieldwork Coordinator and Associate Professor, Department of Occupational Therapy, Rush University, Chicago, Illinois.

This article was accepted for publication June 24, 1994.

The collective fieldwork experience in occupational therapy provides a means by which students are socialized into the profession and into a career. Early work experiences are important to future career success; experiences students have during fieldwork influence subsequent career choices (Christie, Joyce, & Moeller, 1985; London & Stumpf, 1986).

Traditionally, one student is paired with one occupational therapy practitioner to work together for the duration of Level I or Level II fieldwork placement. However, due to health care reform, the shortage of occupational therapy practitioners, staffing and productivity issues, and the paucity of fieldwork sites, the one-to-one model of fieldwork supervision may no longer be realistic. There are simply not enough occupational therapy practitioners available to support the fieldwork education needs of students in academic programs.

Another model of supervision may make it easier for occupational therapy practitioners in various settings to supervise and provide fieldwork students with a successful learning experience. This article introduces two concepts—peer relationships and multiple mentoring—and compares them to the traditional concept of one-to-one mentoring. It also explores the role of fieldwork educator as mentor, the role of fieldwork student as protégé, and the functions inherent in the mentor–protégé relationship.

The Mentor–Protégé Relationship

For this article, the mentor–protégé relationship is defined as the "pairing [of] a more skilled or experienced person [mentor] with a lesser skilled or experienced one [protégé], with the agreed-upon goal of having the lesser skilled person grow and develop specific competencies, skills and attitudes" (Murray, 1991, p. xiv).

The fieldwork educator, or mentor, and the fieldwork student, or protégé, work together to foster the protégé's knowledge, skills, and attitudes. Both mentor and protégé are concerned with applying academic theory and knowledge to practice situations. By design, fieldwork experience fosters entry-level competency in assessment, planning, intervention, problem solving, administration, and professionalism. How protégés perform in these areas is paramount to their future career success. The mentor at the fieldwork site plays a critical role in contributing to that success by shaping the protégé's attitudes and behaviors. But how realistic is it to assume that one mentor can meet all the needs of the protégé?

Traditional One-to-One Mentoring Model

The traditional one-to-one mentoring relationship assumes that the mentor is an expert who has all the answers. The literature suggests that the traditional mentor nurtures a person 8 to 15 years younger and with less experience. The mentor provides information, wisdom, and emotional support to the protégé in an interactive relationship that includes political and socialization experiences (Carden, 1990; Hunt & Michael, 1983; Merriam, 1983; Noe, 1988; Robertson, 1992). Mentoring is a nurturing, supportive process that includes information giving, role modeling, teaching, and counseling, to open doors that provide protégés with as many opportunities as possible (Rogers, 1986). The mentor takes a personal interest in the protégé and offers leadership, guidance, and advice on issues encountered during fieldwork.

To develop mutual admiration, trust, and respect, the one-to-one mentor–protégé relationship requires the time and effort of both parties. The relationship typically lasts a long time, and it is marked by emotional commitment from both sides. The *Dictionary of Titles* ranks mentoring as the highest and most complex level of functioning in the person-related hierarchy of skills (Alleman, 1982). The emotional intensity between mentor and protégé sets the relationship apart from role modeling, training, counseling, coaching, or sponsorship — functions subsumed under any type of helping relationship.

The literature also suggests problems with the one-to-one model of mentoring. First, it is unlikely that any one mentor can possibly be all things to the protégé (Horgan, 1992; Kram & Bragar, 1992). Second, due to the intense interaction between mentor and protégé, personality conflicts may arise. Third, the mentor may develop varying degrees of favoritism for the protégé that make the mentor biased and less effective as a fieldwork educator. Fourth, because the mentor has the authority and power of an expert, the pressure rests primarily on the mentor to ensure the protégé's success. Fifth, some mentors give poor advice or incomplete information, or they exhibit a style that is idiosyncratic or inappropriate for a particular protégé (Horgan, 1992).

All mentors are not equal and do not provide consistent role modeling, training, and information to their protégés. The protégé's needs may be better met through peer relationships or multiple mentoring relationships.

A Continuum of Peer Relationships

As students enter their roles at a fieldwork site, they strive to create a professional identity and gain a sense of who they can become. They struggle to reconcile concerns about themselves, their professional competence, their careers, their families, and their personal relationships. Students address these concerns by developing relationships with other students, friends, family members, supervisors, and professional and technical staff members, as well as academic and clinical faculty members. Developing these relationships allows students to work on their concerns while they gain confidence from having

developed skills and competency during fieldwork (see Figure 1).

Members in this continuum of relationships may play one or more roles including information peer, collegial peer, special peer, and mentor (Kram, 1985). *Information peers* might include fellow students in the academic program, academic advisors, and faculty members who are primary sources of information. During fieldwork, information peers might include students from other schools as well as department staff members who provide information about the department's operations, policies, and procedures. *Collegial peers* might include friends, family members, academic faculty members and advisors, academic and fieldwork educators, and occupational therapy practitioners at the fieldwork site. They offer emotional support and encouragement on personal and professional issues. Collegial peers may give advice about which fieldwork site to choose and how that experience might affect the student's career plans. This advice continues, as collegial peers provide feedback to students regarding their performance, judgement, and attitudes on a variety of tasks and issues that arise throughout the fieldwork experience.

Special peers generally form enduring interpersonal bonds. Such relationships can develop between the student and an academic or research advisor, a special faculty member, or a fieldwork educator — anyone with whom the student establishes a special rapport, trust, or mutual admiration. They provide intimacy, honest feedback, and a personal confirmation of worth (Kram, 1985). Due to the rapport and emotional connection between the student and the special peer, feedback is often focused more on personal issues than on job-related performance and skills. It is at this level that the relationship between special peer and student may approach that of mentor and protégé — especially on a Level II placement, where experiences tend to be more intense than those on a Level I placement.

The Multiple Mentor Experience

Engagement in a mentor–protégé relationship often fol-

Information Peer	Collegial Peer	Special Peer
Primary Function	Primary Functions	Primary Functions
Information Sharing	Career Strategizing Job-related feedback Friendship	Confirmation Emotional Support Personal Feedback Friendship

Figure 1. Kram's Continuum of Peer Relationships supports development at every career stage. Reprinted with permission from Kram, K. E. (1985). *Mentoring at work: Developmental relationships in organizational life.* Glenview, IL: Scott, Foresman.

lows entry-level education as the next phase of professional socialization (Robertson, 1992). This relationship often begins while on Level II fieldwork. One fieldwork student paired with one fieldwork educator will learn one perspective and assume the risks previously described. However, a situation in which several mentors collaborate with several protégés stimulates learning from many perspectives, while minimizing the risks incurred in an exclusive relationship.

Multiple mentors can give a protégé access to several experienced, knowledgeable occupational therapy practitioners who will fulfill a variety of needs for the protégé during the fieldwork placement (Horgan, 1992). Multiple mentoring allows each mentor to contribute to the protégé on the basis of the mentor's particular interests and strengths. Having multiple mentors as role models gives the protégé a chance to observe how different occupational therapy practitioners approach similar situations. Multiple mentoring decreases the likelihood that personality conflicts will occur because protégés divide their time between several mentors rather than spending an extended period of time with one. In addition, protégés are likely to find a role model among the multiple mentors who shares their particular style. Multiple mentoring also creates an awareness of diversity and sensitivity between mentors, protégés, and consumers (Horgan, 1992). Multiple mentoring tends to balance the protégé's overall fieldwork experience.

How might this multiple mentoring model work? Occupational therapy practitioners in any given setting may have a fieldwork educator who is the liaison with the fieldwork coordinator of the academic program. The fieldwork educator may be responsible for making reservations and, alone or with occupational therapy practitioners at that setting, supervising students at any given time. One mentor working in a setting that uses a model of multiple mentoring might supervise several protégés, or several mentors might supervise several protégés. Each occupational therapy practitioner may assume a particular role with or responsibility to fieldwork students. Some might share with students their developed expertise with a particular frame of reference or in orthotic fabrication. Other mentors might share tips for preparing lectures and methods of instruction to apply to either consumer education or inservices to other professionals. The practitioner as manager–mentor might share information on budgets, staffing, and productivity. The practitioner as researcher–mentor might show students how something they do every day can yield data that provide information on the efficacy of a particular intervention or support efforts in continuous quality improvement.

In the multiple mentoring model, no one occupational therapy practitioner has the sole responsibility for the education of any one fieldwork student, although one practitioner may coordinate the process. The overall responsibility is shared by practitioners working within that setting, unless there is only one occupational therapy practitioner within the setting. One mentor supervising several protégés may not necessarily require more of the mentor's time and work, because protégés working together tend to support each other, share information, and answer each other's questions.

Formal or informal supervision can take several forms. One-to-one meetings between mentor and protégé should be held as necessary. Ongoing group meetings of all protégés should also be held, guided by one or more mentors. Protégés bring their questions and concerns to this peer group for joint problem solving. They exercise clinical reasoning and critical thinking skills as they collaboratively analyze problems and provide feedback. In this way, protégés learn from their own experiences as well as each other's. They also learn from the experiences of their mentor or multiple mentors. Protégés learn how occupational therapy practitioners think and come to realize that there are different approaches rather than one correct answer. With several protégés offering daily mutual support, they often answer questions for each other, thus saving the time of any one mentor. The multiple mentoring model encourages protégés to assume responsibility for their own learning and professional development by reaching out to their resource network.

Evaluation of student performance can be done in various ways, although any mentor who has interacted with a particular protégé should contribute feedback on that protégé's fieldwork evaluation form. This feedback from multiple mentors might then be synthesized by a fieldwork educator who shares the feedback with each protégé as part of a formal meeting.

The multiple mentor–protégé relationship uses the team approach and encourages active involvement to focus on what the protégé learns from the mentor rather than from the relationship itself. The relationship between mentors and protégés addresses many functions, depending on the fieldwork setting and the protégé's needs.

Although the concept of one or more mentors supervising multiple protégés is one solution for easing the strain of time pressures on occupational therapy practitioners, it is not without risks. These risks can be minimized if appropriate measures are taken by both mentors and protégés. For example, fieldwork students supervised by and responsible to multiple mentors must be careful not to play one mentor against the other. If students have problems, they may tend to blame them on the inconsistency of supervision provided by multiple mentors rather than assuming responsibility for those problems themselves.

Occupational therapy practitioners who assume a multiple mentorship role must establish clear lines of communication with each other as well as with each fieldwork student. A mechanism for providing feedback to the protégé must be established early on in the fieldwork experience. Expectations must be clearly defined and understood by all involved in the process to minimize mixed messages about performance. Practitioners must avoid putting the fieldwork student in the middle of their differing points of view. Occupational therapy practitioners as mentors need to be flexible, modifying their supervisory styles and approaches to intervention as appropriate. Differences between mentors do exist and may even be healthy, as long as the student is made aware of the reasons for some of these differences.

Roles of Mentor and Protégé During Fieldwork

As academic faculty members instruct and motivate students in the classroom, so fieldwork educators must instruct and motivate students in various practice arenas and encourage them to apply the techniques and skills learned in the classroom. Equally important, fieldwork educators as mentors must support student protégés as they struggle to further develop and apply skills in critical thinking and clinical reasoning (Cohn, 1989). It is the fieldwork educator who ultimately shows the student how successful practice depends more on the ability to reflect before taking action than on simply applying theory and factual knowledge (Schön, 1987).

Gray (1988) proposed a mentor–protégé relationship model for moving protégés from passive to active learning. Applying Gray's model to clinical education, the fieldwork educator as mentor can move through the following continuum: (a) imparting information needed by the protégé (b) coaching the protégé to learn new skills, (c) making decisions and solving problems together, (d) providing support while the protégé takes the lead, and (e) stepping back as the protégé achieves relative independence from the mentor (see Figure 2)

Occupational therapists at Rush-Presbyterian-St. Luke's Medical Center in Chicago receive formal training in preparation for becoming fieldwork educators. They have found Gray's model helpful for visualizing the de-

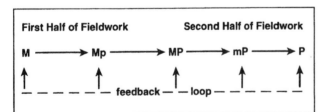

First Half of Fieldwork **Second Half of Fieldwork**

M ——→ Mp ——→ MP ——→ mP ——→ P

↑ —— ↑ —— ↑ —— ↑ —— ↑
feedback — loop — — — —

Figure 2. Gray's Mentor–Protégé Relationship Model (© 1984) shows varying levels of help by mentors. M = fieldwork educator as mentor, P = student as protégé. Reprinted with permission from Gray, W. A. (1988). Developing a planned mentoring program to facilitate career development. *International Journal of Mentoring*, 2(1), 9–17.

gree of shared responsibility that should occur during the fieldwork experience, regardless of the length of the placement. In most cases, the protégé comes to the mentor knowing next to nothing about that setting and leaves with some degree of competence and expertise. As a therapist instructs and motivates the patient, and as a fieldwork educator instructs and motivates the student, so the mentor encourages the protégé to learn and then apply higher level thinking skills to new situations.

Responsibilities of Mentor and Protégé During Fieldwork

The functions addressed in multiple mentor–protégé relationships may not be extremely different from the functions in a one-to-one relationship, because it is the mentoring process itself that fosters growth of both career and psychosocial functions. The mentoring process has the potential to facilitate career advancement and psychosocial development in early and middle adulthood (Kram, 1985). Career functions are enhanced through such functions as sponsorship, exposure-and-visibility, coaching, protection, and challenging work assignments. *Sponsorship,* the most often observed career function, involves the mentor's actively nominating the protégé for opportunities. The fieldwork coordinator sponsors the protégé and creates opportunities for the protégé to work with other occupational therapy practitioners and gain a variety of experiences. *Exposure-and-visibility* allows the protégé to develop relationships with other practitioners and professionals in the immediate practice area in addition to meeting persons in other parts of the organization. This process begins during the fieldwork orientation, when the protégé is asked to meet with professionals from other disciplines to determine his or her role on the team, and continues as the protégé attends rounds, care conferences, or organizational inservices.

Coaching is used by the mentor to suggest specific strategies for achieving goals. It is an important function of the relationship throughout the fieldwork experience. The mentor *protects* the protégé at appropriate times from untimely or potentially damaging contact with others, yet does so judiciously, because so doing can both support and smother the protégé. Finally, *challenging work assignments* from the mentor provide opportunities for learning time management, responsibility, and professional and technical skills. Protégés may be responsible for such assignments as case studies, intervention plans, patient notes, in-services, and independent projects or study during the fieldwork placement. Career functions are important because they enhance the protégés' visibility within the area of practice while contributing to their career growth and development.

Mentoring enhances fieldwork students' psychosocial development through role modeling, acceptance-

and-confirmation, counseling, and friendship (Kram, 1985). *Role modeling* is the most often used psychosocial function, because mentors model attitudes, values, behavior, and skills for protégés to emulate. *Acceptance-and-confirmation* aid in the development of mutual admiration, trust, and respect and provide an underlying support to help protégés learn to tolerate differences and ambiguity and to take risks. As any fieldwork educator knows, mastery of this function is critical to the success of the would-be occupational therapy practitioner in any health care delivery system. Mentors use *counseling* skills as they discuss such personal concerns as clarifying one's relationship with self, with the organization, and with others. The protégé shares doubts, concerns, and fears—trusting the mentor to maintain confidentiality. The mentor's ability to communicate in an effective and timely manner is of utmost importance in fostering the protégé's trust. Finally, *friendship* is developed through social interaction between mentor and protégé and results in informal exchanges about work and personal experiences. The more that the protégé and the mentor can relate to each other as human beings, with personal dreams and concerns, the better understanding each will have of the other. Awareness and mastery of psychosocial functions can enhance the protégé's sense of confidence, competence, identity, and effectiveness in a work-related role.

Summary

Students form a variety of developmental relationships between entering an academic program and successfully completing Level I and Level II fieldwork placements. Whether these relationships are formed with information peers, collegial peers, special peers or mentors, these relationships have the potential to enhance the capabilities of the protégé in functions related to career and psychosocial development.

Use of the multiple mentoring model in the supervision of fieldwork students has distinct advantages over the one-to-one model of supervision often used. The multiple mentoring model allows a fieldwork site to accept more students at a time while minimizing the stress on any one fieldwork educator. It encourages students to use each other as resources and thus minimizes time spent by a fieldwork educator. Multiple mentoring also spreads the responsibility for supervision and dissemination of information among several practitioners within an area of practice or across practice areas. It promotes collegiality as protégés meet with multiple mentors to discuss clinical reasoning related to professional issues. In addition, the process of multiple mentoring offers support and direction while placing the responsibility for learning on the protégé.

The mentor–protégé relationship, whether match-ing one mentor with multiple protégés or multiple mentors with multiple protégés, offers benefits to all who are involved, including the mentor, the protégé and the organization itself (Nolinske, 1994). It is the relationship between the mentor, protégé, and the organization that helps persons at all levels to *manage*, *encourage*, *nurture*, and *teach* organizational *responsibility* (Farren, Gray, & Kay, 1984). ▲

References

Alleman, E. (1982). Mentoring relationships in organizations: Behaviors, personality characteristics, and interpersonal perceptions. (Doctoral dissertation, University of Akron, 1982). *Dissertation Abstracts International, 43,* (1A), 75A.

Carden, A. D. (1990). Mentoring and adult career development: The evolution of a theory. *The Counseling Psychologist, 18*(2), 275–299.

Christie, B. A., Joyce, P. C., & Moeller, P. L. (1985). Fieldwork experience, Part I: Impact on practice preference. *American Journal of Occupational Therapy, 39,* 671–674.

Cohn, E. S. (1989). Fieldwork education: Shaping a foundation for clinical reasoning. *American Journal of Occupational Therapy, 43,* 240–244.

Farren, C., Gray, J. D., & Kay, B. (1984). Mentoring: A boon to career development. *Personnel, 61*(6), 20–24.

Gray, W. A. (1988). Developing a planned mentoring program to facilitate career development. *International Journal of Mentoring, 2*(1), 9–11.

Horgan, D. D. (1992). Multiple mentoring: All of the gain; none of the pain. *Performance and Instruction, 31*(6), 20–22.

Hunt, D. M., & Michael, C. (1983). Mentorship: A career training and development tool. *Academy of Management Review, 8*(3), 475–485.

Kram, K. E. (1985). *Mentoring at work: Developmental relationships in organizational life.* Glenview, IL: Scott, Foresman.

Kram, K. E., & Bragar, M. (1992). Development through mentoring: A strategic approach. In D. Montross & C. Skinkman (Eds.), *Career development: Theory and practice* (pp. 221–254). Springfield, IL: Charles C Thomas.

London, M., & Stumpf, S. A. (1986). Individual and organizational career development in changing times. In D. T. Hall and Associates (Eds.), *Career development in organizations* (pp. 21–49). San Francisco: Jossey–Bass.

Merriam, S. B. (1983). Mentors and proteges: A critical review of the literature. *Adult Education Quarterly, 33*(3), 161–173.

Murray, M. (1991). *Beyond the myths and magic of mentoring: How to facilitate an effective mentoring program.* San Francisco: Jossey-Bass.

Noe, R. A. (1988). An investigation of the determinants of successful assigned mentoring relationships. *Personnel Psychology, 41*(3), 457–477.

Nolinske, T. (1994). The value of the mentor–protégé relationship as perceived by the mentor, protégé, and protégé's boss. (Doctoral dissertation, Northwestern University, microfiche 943 3900).

ville, MD: American Occupational Therapy Association.

Rogers, J. C. (1986). Nationally Speaking—Mentoring for career achievement and advancement. *American Journal of Occupational Therapy, 40,* 79–82.

Schön, D. (1987). *Educating the reflective practitioner: How professionals think in action.* New York: Basic.

Progressive Student Expectations Based on AOTA's Fieldwork Evaluation

Trudy Jas-Weathers

Key Words: fieldwork education, occupational therapy • personnel management

When the Fieldwork Performance Report was first published (American Occupational Therapy Association [AOTA], Commission on Education, 1973), the occupational therapy staff at Good Samaritan Hospital in Cincinnati, Ohio, established behavioral statements for each of the 54 items. Level II fieldwork students were presented with these statements on the first day of their fieldwork and were then evaluated by their supervisor and themselves every 3 weeks thereafter, using these statements as guidelines. This schedule of evaluation had several advantages. It (a) permitted timely and comprehensive feedback, (b) provided an opportunity for the students to reflect on their own performance, (c) allowed goal setting for further student development, and (d) prevented areas from being overlooked.

In 1986, the Fieldwork Evaluation (FWE) was adopted in lieu of the Fieldwork Performance Report (AOTA, Committee for the Revision of the Fieldwork Performance Report, 1986). The addition of the domains of judgment and attitude were two of the many changes to the evaluation. The occupational therapy staff again developed behavioral statements, this time for each category of the 51 items on the FWE. These new statements totaled more than 450; reviewing them with students every 3 weeks became an overwhelming task for both supervisors and students.

Although the FWE was not designed to be used as a midterm evaluation or counseling tool (Hickerson Crist & Cooper, 1988), cost prohibited AOTA from developing a separate midterm evaluation. Therefore, AOTA's Commission on Education suggested that ratings of *satisfactory plus, satisfactory,* and *unsatisfactory* be used at the midterm evaluation for each FWE item. Our staff at Good Samaritan Hospital chose not to follow this suggestion. The FWE items were considered summative or end-performance statements, so one reason for this decision was our concern that a student might be rated *unsatisfactory* on an item that is considered a higher-level skill and is therefore not addressed until after the midterm. Receiving a large number of *unsatisfactory* or *not applicable* ratings was often interpreted negatively by students and at times may have discouraged students needlessly. This midterm problem, coupled with the time involved in reviewing our 450 behavioral statements, prompted the development of the Time Line Objectives and Counseling Tool.

Development of Time Line Objectives

Creation of the Time Line Objectives involved use of the *Taxonomy of Educational Objectives* (Bloom, 1956; Krathwohl, Bloom, & Masia, 1964) to develop learning activities and behavioral statements based on

Trudy Jas-Weathers, MHE, OTR/L, is Clinical Education Coordinator, Occupational Therapy Division, Good Samaritan Hospital, Cincinnati, Ohio 45220.

This article was accepted for publication November 13, 1989.

the FWE. The *Taxonomy* identified three domains associated with learning—cognitive, affective, and perceptual–motor. The cognitive domain involves the acquisition and manipulation of facts and is referred to in the FWE as *judgment*. The affective domain constitutes directed attention and development of values, or *attitude*. The perceptual–motor domain is characterized by growth in sensory and motor actions and is referred to in the FWE as *performance*. These domains are organized into hierarchies. Figure 1 shows the approximate relationship of the various levels to each other and illustrates the interaction between the domains at all levels.

An example of how the hierarchy relates to learning in the cognitive domain follows: A student initially learns by memorizing the muscle innervations (knowledge). The student restates this information during a case review (comprehension). The student then identifies possible return for a spinal cord–injured person based on the level of the lesion (application), predicts possible functions for the patient (analysis), and develops a treatment plan (synthesis) that can be implemented and assessed (evaluation).

Once the behavioral statements for the Time Line Objectives were completed, it was revealed that several statements were repeated in a number of the FWE items, especially in the area of attitude. For example, the expectation "Address each patient as an individual, showing consideration for age, sex, disability, and mental status" appeared often. Staff members felt that each area only needed to be addressed once. The statements were thus scrutinized for repetition, and a time frame for the achievement of each expectation was identified. For example, "Identify location of tools and supplies" should be identified during the 1st week, whereas "Explore alternate methods of achieving goals" usually is not addressed until the 9th week. The statements were then grouped according to the categories of Assessment, Treatment Planning, Reporting, Treatment, Problem Solving, and Professional Behaviors. The Reporting category was added to separate documentation procedures and interdisciplinary interaction from treatment planning in the first few weeks.

At the end of the 1st week, 22 expectations related to orientation are reviewed. At the end of the 3rd week, these 22 statements are reviewed briefly and 48 new expectations are focused on, 23 of which relate to assessment and treatment planning skills, the main tasks of the first quarter of the fieldwork experience. At the midterm evaluation (the 6th week), previous statements are reviewed to ensure that possible earlier areas for growth have been addressed, and 45 new expectations are evaluated, 22 of which relate to problem-solving skills and professional behaviors.

At this point, more than enough information is

ORIGINATION Creation of new patterns	EVALUATION Making of judgments based on comprehensive knowledge and experience	CHARACTERIZATION Performance based on a consistent and integrated set of values
ADAPTATION Modification of performance to meet special needs	SYNTHESIS Origination of new concepts based on previous knowledge and experience	
COMPLEX RESPONSE Automatic performance of complex tasks		ORGANIZATION Development and tolerance of various values; influence on others
	ANALYSIS Breakdown and reorganization of facts to clarify application	
HABITUAL RESPONSE Routine performance of tasks without supervision		VALUING Agreement with and action according to rules and previous input
GUIDED RESPONSE Performance of selected tasks with supervision	APPLICATION Use of combination of previous facts in actual situations	
SET Organization of stimuli	COMPREHENSION Translation of facts	RESPONDING Willingness to react to selected input
PERCEPTION Intake of sensory stimuli	KNOWLEDGE Intake of facts	RECEIVING Willingness to take in stimuli
PERCEPTUAL MOTOR DOMAIN[a] PERFORMANCE[b]	COGNITIVE DOMAIN[a] JUDGMENT[b]	AFFECTIVE DOMAIN[a] ATTITUDE[b]

Figure 1. Graphic description of the learning domains. *Note.* The hierarchies are shown in approximate relationship to each other. [a] (Bloom, 1956). [b] Fieldwork Evaluation terminology.

available to identify patterns in behaviors, identify strengths and weaknesses, determine general status, and predict further progress. At the 9-week evaluation, there are 18 new expectations to evaluate (see Figure 2). These cover all areas and deal with the higher levels of learning such as synthesis, evaluation, and characterization. At the 12th week, there are no

Assessment

1. Complete special evaluation (3, 5, 6).
2. Assess patient's functioning and present or modify activities/instructions accordingly (6).

Comments:

Treatment Planning

1. Consider long-term vs. short-term goals, patient status, interests, and discharge disposition in treatment plan changes (13, 20, 21).
2. Decide when patient has reached maximum benefit from treatment. Follow through with plan, as appropriate, without allowing personal biases to influence decision (22).

Comments:

Treatment

1. Recognize and adhere to modalities/approaches contraindicated in the treatment plan or patient welfare (29).
2. State awareness of precautions of patients in addition to assigned patients (28, 29).
3. Instruct patient in stress management, time management, assertive interaction, relaxation and/or work simplification techniques, as needed (34).
4. Develop and implement short-term group, which considers population needs and occupational therapy theory and is consistent with program philosophy, using novel/creative ways to meet the identified need(s) (27, 39, 40).

Comments:

Problem Solving

1. Incorporate a wide variety of activities that reflect self-care, work, and play/leisure components (37).
2. Adapt activities to maximize or minimize physical, cognitive, and/or psychological aspects of the task (37, 41).
3. Select activities that challenge the patient to function to optimum level of performance (35, 41).
4. Adapt a given activity to meet the needs of three selected diagnostic categories (35).
5. Explore alternate methods of achieving goals (35, 40).
6. Initiate problem-solving steps and modifications without reminders from supervisor (38).

Comments:

Professional Behavior

1. Report on independent reading or research related to occupational therapy during unstructured time (48).
2. Ask about and arrange attendance at in-service programs related to occupational therapy or psychiatry (48).
3. Show flexibility and efficiency in use of environment and modalities (47, 51).
4. Initiate and maintain ongoing communication with supervisor regarding case load and other activities (46).

Comments:

Figure 2. The 9-week portion of the Time Line Objectives and Counseling Tool for the psychiatric affiliation of the occupational therapy student. *Note.* The numbers in parentheses refer to the items on the Fieldwork Evaluation (FWE).

specific learning statements to be reviewed, other than general housekeeping tasks such as "Maintain caseload; function independently within constraints of the program; turn in keys"; and "Leave forwarding address." This means that all skills should be addressed, at least at the exploration level, by the 9th week, leaving the last 3 weeks for practice and mastery of the skills.

Discussion

This system of student assessment has many advantages. Students do not appear overwhelmed when the statements are presented on the first day, and they are receptive to using the statements to assess themselves every 3 weeks. The supervisor spends approximately 30 min every evaluation period reviewing the student's progress.

One specific advantage is the improved process of student assessment. Student performance is reviewed each evaluation period according to minimal competencies for that particular time period. Because the statements are grouped together, patterns of behavior are readily apparent and difficulty with particular skills is noted. Once patterns have been identified, remedial plans can be implemented to alleviate difficulties or to adapt to the learning styles of different

students. The time line structure means that supervisory meetings involve a discussion of progress, strengths, areas for growth, and overall performance, instead of a review of numerous statements. The result is a clear picture of progress; students are rarely surprised regarding the feedback received. The evaluation periods are productive for problem solving and goal setting.

The FWE form is used only at the final evaluation. At this time, all of the behavioral statements are reviewed. Any statement that was consistently not met, repeatedly met late, or met with difficulty, can easily be correlated to the items on the FWE, because the item number it relates to is noted next to the statement (see Figure 2). The final scoring of the FWE takes approximately 30 to 45 min for most supervisors.

Summary

Behavioral statements for each item of the FWE were developed according to a developmental learning hierarchy and then organized into specific categories and time frames. The performance expectations are presented to occupational therapy students in Level II fieldwork in the areas of psychiatry and physical disabilities; a similar process was used to develop performance expectations for the Level II fieldwork of those studying to be occupational therapy assistants. The advantages of this system over the system we had used previously were readily apparent: Supervisor preparation time was considerably reduced, and the content and format of the supervisory meetings changed. Meetings are now spent productively discussing strengths and patterns of behaviors, rather than reviewing endless lists of behavioral statements. ▲

References

American Occupational Therapy Association, Commission on Education. (1973). *The Fieldwork Performance Report.* Internal document.

American Occupational Therapy Association, Committee for the Revision of the Fieldwork Performance Report. (1986). *The final summary report and recommendations of the Committee for the Revision of the Fieldwork Performance Report* (resolution 584–82). Internal document.

Bloom, B. S. (Ed.). (1956). *Taxonomy of educational objectives: Handbook I: The cognitive domain.* New York: David McKay Company.

Hickerson Crist, P. A., & Cooper, R. G. (1988). Nationally Speaking—Evaluating clinical competence with the new Fieldwork Evaluation. *American Journal of Occupational Therapy, 42,* 771–773.

Krathwohl, D. R., Bloom, B. S., & Masia, B. B. (1964). *Taxonomy of educational objectives: Handbook II: The affective domain.* New York: David McKay Company.

Cooperative Education: An Alternative Level I Fieldwork

Sonia S. Zimmerman

Key Words: fieldwork education, occupational therapy

Cooperative education is an educational concept that was developed in engineering and business education during the early 1900s and was later expanded to a wide variety of fields, including the social sciences and the humanities. Grounded in John Dewey's educational philosophies of pragmatism, it connects classroom learning and paid work experience for the purpose of enhancing the educational experience of a student (Fitt & Heverly, 1990; Heinemann & De Falco, 1992; Ryder, 1987). Through cooperative education, best described as *experiential learning*, the student is able to reach understandings and make conclusions that could not be achieved through classroom instruction alone. Cooperative education puts occupational therapy students "directly in touch with the realities being studied" (Keeton & Tate, 1978, p. 2). The academic institution is responsible for building opportunities into the curriculum that make it possible for a student to leave campus and engage in productive, paid work that supports the student's career goals.

Program Description

The Cooperative Education Program at the University of North Dakota (student population: 12,000) began in 1985 and currently has 34 participating academic departments. The program served 465 students in the academic year 1991–1992 (Van Tour, 1992). Funding for the program is both institutional and federal (Title VIII of the Higher Education Act of 1965, [U.S. Department of Education, 1992]). Since 1988, the occupational therapy department has placed 10 to 12 students in the Cooperative Education Program annually—a total of 48 to date.

Cooperative education placement sites are varied and include inpatient and long-term care hospitals, nursing homes, development centers, and summer camps for special populations. Staff members from the Cooperative Education Program began the program by requesting placement site suggestions from therapists in hospitals that were already providing Level II fieldwork. This contact was advantageous because the therapists were familiar with the university's occupational therapy program and recognized the recruitment advantage that cooperative educations afforded them. As the program has grown, contacts have been made regularly through professional networks as well as through the annual Health Recruitment Fair conducted on campus. Organizations that typically hire temporary summer employees are targeted as prime candidates. Placements are made for both part-time and full-time employment. Under cooperative education, contracts with organizations differ from those used in Level II fieldwork in that they specify the salary and benefits that will be provided to the student.

The occupational therapy student who chooses to participate in cooperative education most often falls into one of two categories: (a) a preoccupational therapy stu-

Sonia S. Zimmerman, MA, OTR/L, is Assistant Professor of Occupational Therapy, University of North Dakota, School of Occupational Therapy, Box 8036, University Station, Grand Forks, North Dakota 58202.

This article was accepted for publication April 26, 1994.

dent who has completed all prerequisite courses but has not been accepted to the professional program, or (b) an occupational therapy student who is between the junior and senior year in the program and desires summer employment in an occupational therapy or related setting.

A student who has met the minimum requirements (40 hr of academic credit, including courses in introductory occupational therapy and medical terminology, and a minimum 2.7 [of a possible 4.0] grade point average) receives an orientation to cooperative education from the program's staff members. These staff members prepare the student for the interview process and direct development of an application packet, which includes a résumé, application forms, and letters of reference. The occupational therapy professor-coordinator then meets with the student to discuss available work sites and student preferences in order to match the student's needs with the employer's needs. Once the student has identified preferred sites, the application is mailed — a process that closely simulates the real-world experience of job seeking. After being approved for fieldwork at a desired site, the student enrolls in an elective course (OT 337: Cooperative Education in Occupational Therapy) for academic credit. The student then begins the work experience as a paid employee, most often as an occupational therapy aide. In this position, the student is placed under the direct supervision of an occupational therapist to eliminate licensure-related difficulties. Program participants are encouraged to consider placing students in the occupational therapy aide position to broaden the students' exposure to the occupational therapy profession.

Student objectives as well as midterm and final evaluation reports documenting student performance are completed by the on-site supervisor and provided to both the Cooperative Education Program and to the departmental professor responsible for the student.

Course Objectives

The course objectives for cooperative education in occupational therapy are similar to those of Level I fieldwork; the student is directed toward "observation and participation in selected aspects of the therapy process" (American Occupational Therapy Association, 1991, p. 7). Through this experience, the student is able to: (a) develop an appreciation for the value of the occupational therapist's role in the health care setting, (b) apply and integrate (to the best of his or her educational level) basic occupational therapy knowledge and understanding in a real-world setting, and (c) develop and apply professional behavior as a member of a treatment team.

In addition to participating in day-to-day clinical experiences, the student is asked to complete a minimum of one special project. Special projects are developed as a collaborative effort between the on-site supervisor and the student to generate products that are of mutual interest and benefit (e.g., annotated bibliographies, research papers, in-service presentations, home program packets, patient case studies).

After completing the program, the student participates in a panel presentation, sharing personal perspectives on the cooperative education experience with peers. Follow-up discussions of this sort are believed to be part of an educational process encouraging student evaluation of learning. Cooperative education students in other fields have been reported to gain "self-understanding, self-direction and the self-confidence to manage their own education and career development" (Dawson, 1989, p. 11).

Benefits

The benefits of cooperative education programs have been experienced by all parties involved, including sponsors, students, and the university. Several studies have supported the use of cooperative education placements as a way to increase productivity, principally because of the release of professional employees from clerical duties but also because of the generally high motivational level and sense of purpose on the part of the cooperative education student (Fitt & Heverly, 1992; Little, 1974; Wiseman & Page, 1983).

Another benefit involves the relationships established through cooperative education programs. Relationships between students and faculty members are strengthened. Sponsors find that their relations with colleges and universities are enhanced by the exchange of ideas among students, supervisors, and faculty members (Fitt & Heverly, 1992; Little, 1974). The benefit most often cited by participating sponsors is the opportunity to assess future graduates before hiring them for full-time employment (Fitt & Heverly, 1992; Weinstein & Wilson, 1983).

Although it may appear that the value of cooperative education is monetary, Wilson (1987) found that the most frequently cited reasons for a student's participation were related to educational gains, rather than financial or postgraduate employment. Students expressed a desire for skills, information, and insights necessary for their future careers. The issue of payment is, however, a vital part of this perception. Wilson reported that because employers are willing to pay for the work, they are more likely to have higher expectations of responsibility and performance from the student. These expectations make the work experience more realistic, challenging, and meaningful, and they encourage maturity in the student.

Fitt and Heverly (1992) described specific benefits that higher education stands to gain from cooperative education programs. These benefits included providing opportunities for students to function in the professional arena, keeping educators abreast of changing needs within the profession, and offering access to employees who may be interested in serving as adjunct faculty members. In addition, the establishment of long-term working relationships with corporate sponsors can lead to grants, scholarship monies, equipment donations, and joint research and development ventures.

Summary

The cooperative education program offered at the University of North Dakota is based on programs offered at other universities across the nation. Rewards of cooperative education programs are many, and they benefit students, universities, and sponsors alike. In addition to easing the costs of a university education, planning cooperative education experiences as part of the curriculum allows students to develop, practice, and receive feedback on the necessary professional skills vital to their success as occupational therapists. Universities and sponsors benefit from enhanced relationships and lay the foundation for joint ventures as educators and researchers.

Further research is needed to evaluate specific outcomes related to the use of cooperative education in the training of occupational therapists. This research should address issues that include evaluation tools, students' perspectives, and employers' satisfaction with the program. ▲

Acknowledgment

I thank Darlene Van Tour, PhD. and Justy A. Churchill, MA. for their assistance in developing cooperative education at the University of North Dakota's Department of Occupational Therapy and for their support in the preparation of this article.

References

American Occupational Therapy Association. (1991). *Essentials and guidelines of an accredited program for the occupational therapist*. Rockville, MD: Author.

Dawson, J. D. (1989). Educational outcomes for students in cooperative education. *Journal of Cooperative Education, 25*(2), 6–13.

Fitt, D. X., & Heverly, M. (1990). Involving the private sector with higher education. *Journal of Cooperative Education, 27*(3), 64–72.

Heinemann, H. N., & DeFalco, A. A. (1992). Dewey's pragmatism: A philosophical foundation for cooperative education. *Journal of Cooperative Education, 27*(1), 38–44.

Keeton, M. T., & Tate, P. J. (1978). The boom in experiential learning. In M. T. Keeton & P. J. Tate (Eds.), *Learning by experience—what, why, how*. New Directions in Experiential Learning, No. 1. San Francisco: Jossey-Bass.

Little, Arthur D. Inc. (1974). *Documented employer benefits from cooperative education*. Report of a study for Northeastern University. Cambridge, MA: Author.

Ryder, K. G. (1987). Social and educational roots. In J.W. Wilson & K.G. Ryder (Eds.), *Cooperative education in a new era* (pp. 1–12). San Francisco: Jossey-Bass.

U.S. Department of Education. (1992). *Fiscal Year 1992 Grant Awards*. Cooperative Education Program, Title VIII, Higher Education Act of 1965, as amended (CFDA no 84.055). Washington, DC: Author.

Van Tour, D. (1992). *Annual report of University of North Dakota cooperative education*. Grand Forks: University of North Dakota, Cooperative Education.

Weinstein, D. S., & Wilson, J. W. (1983). An employer description of a model cooperative education program. *Journal of Cooperative Education, 20*(1), 60–83.

Wilson, J. W. (1987). What students gain from cooperative education. In J.W. Wilson & K. G. Ryder (Eds.), *Cooperative education in a new era* (pp. 269–284). San Francisco: Jossey-Bass.

Wiseman, R. L., & Page, N. R. (1983). Predicting employer's benefits from cooperative education. *Journal of Cooperative Education, 20*(1), 45–59.

SECTION FIVE | Models of Fieldwork

What do we mean by *models* of fieldwork? The definition of a *model* (*American Heritage Dictionary, 2nd College Ed.,* 1983) is "a preliminary pattern," "a type or design," or "an example to be emulated." This is certainly the case with fieldwork: we have all types or designs of fieldwork programs that seem to work even though they may not follow the popular notion of fieldwork. Models can be extremely helpful when we are discussing innovative fieldwork since these types of placements are usually different from the accepted norm in clinical education. Most models reflect the changing healthcare environment and continue to offer quality clinical education to students and practitioners alike.

A traditional fieldwork model incorporates the basic essentials of an occupational therapy curriculum as stated in *The Essentials for the Accreditation of an Occupational Therapy or Occupational Therapy Assistant Program* (AOTA, 1995). Most of the models in the popular occupational therapy literature are categorized as innovative or nontraditional. This may mean that the form of supervision is different, that the student completes fieldwork at a different pace, or that the setting is new for occupational therapy service delivery. The essentials in an innovative fieldwork model are widely interpreted with continued emphasis on a quality education. These "innovative" models may actually be quite ordinary now that consumer needs and service delivery models are changing.

The American Occupational Therapy Association (AOTA) has disseminated information regarding fieldwork models to its members as an educational tool for developing quality fieldwork sites. The tra-ditional one-to-one supervision model in one setting for one extended period of time continues to be endorsed, while additional models reflecting new trends in healthcare are emerging rapidly.

The AOTA Commission on Education (COE) is made up of academic and clinical educators representative of all of our occupational therapy schools and sites nationwide who meet for guidance and to develop strategies for effective academic and clinical education. In March 1995, the COE met in Boston, Massachusetts to discuss models of innovative fieldwork. They were asked to look at the real and perceived advantages, disadvantages, barriers, resources, and strategies to implementing innovative fieldwork models as academic fieldwork coordinators and clinical fieldwork educators. The results did not necessarily reflect optimal fieldwork; however, it was the first attempt at discovering new ideas appropriate for unique fieldwork settings. Each of the models were to be considered according to the type of setting and service delivery, state licensure and reimbursement regulations, and accreditation standards. The six fieldwork models the COE identified are as follows:

1. *Community-based:* community programs for the elderly, mentally ill, and AIDS victims, sheltered workshops, and so on; education of the community about occupational therapy
2. *Remote OT Supervisor:* an OTR who is off-site or in a different building; a consultative model of student supervision
3. *Collaborative:* more than one student to one supervisor; group supervision; may also mean

more than one supervisor for one or more students

4. *Non-OT Supervisor:* a related-professions supervisor who has access to occupational therapy training and guidance; this person may be part of a large team of professionals who consult with an OTR/COTA as appropriate

5. *Consumer-based:* continuum of care with the consumer in mind; the student follows the client through the levels of service delivery and progression of independence; may mean collaboration with various facilities and therapists

6. *Part-time supervisor/student:* parttime schedule of supervisor; the student is autonomous and relies on supporting staff the other half-time; parttime student completes fieldwork in longer than traditional time but with same goals.

There is also a five-part series in quiz format on breaking down the myths of fieldwork that you will find in the *OT Week* articles included in this section. The key word in defining model is *preliminary*. We can look at these models as the beginning of greater and more rewarding developments in fieldwork.

The Student Speaks

A Field Work Experience

in Mental Retardation

Gretchen R. Beardslee
Graduate Student

A graduate student specializing in mental retardation found few pertinent electives as well as little opportunity for field work experience. A special arrangement was made for appropriate field work experiences in three types of settings—a large residential institution, school programs, and nursing care facilities. There was little time to view client changes, and rapport with patients and staff was difficult to develop. The advantages included more time with her supervisor, more exposure to organizational and administrative duties, and more exposure to a variety of settings and to the professional roles of numerous therapists. More such field work experiences should be developed to encourage new therapists to choose mental retardation as a specialty.

The education laws passed recently in many states mandate an increased need for professional services for students to 25 years of age who have mental and physical impairments. Occupational therapy clinics will need to be expanded in order to serve this population. The occupational therapists' academic education includes a good foundation for working with the physically impaired but offers the student little preparation for work in the field of mental retardation. According to a recent study, most curricula cover mental retardation only through brief introductions in psychiatric theory, pediatrics, or physical disability courses (1).

For working therapists, however, numerous workshops and conferences are available that provide specific information on the mentally impaired. Twelve percent or 20 out of 156 presentations at the 1975 American Occupational Therapy Association's fall conference pertained to mental retardation and the majority of these were about children.

As a graduate student in occupational therapy the author wished to specialize in the practice of mental retardation, but there were few electives. One psychology course provided ideological knowledge about mental retardation but no insight into the role of the occupational therapist. A unique field experience was therefore arranged—one that fulfilled the requirements of a physical dysfunction field placement. The three goals of the field work experience were: to gain exposure to settings in which the therapist works, to gain experience with evaluative procedures, and to have an opportunity to treat patients. Under the supervision of a therapist engaged in private practice who specialized in mental retardation, the student was "farmed out" to diverse settings for time periods ranging from one day to three weeks. The student toured each facility; was introduced to the clients as well as to the evaluative and treatment procedures; and discussed the role of occupational therapy in such a center with the resident therapists. Three types of settings were used: a large residential institution, school programs, and nursing care facilities. The student simultaneously participated in a University-based program to develop curriculum and inservice training for workers in mental retardation centers.

Large Residential Institution

A large residential facility is a traditional mental retardation setting in which occupational therapists practice. The student spent three days with a therapist in a 284-bed institution serving the mental and multihandicapped of all ages. In this federal- and state-funded center, the therapist was responsible for providing services to the entire population with the help of one full-time and one quarter-time aide. She concentrated on the young infirmary patient and the multihandicapped child who was severely mentally and physically disabled.

The therapist's duties included ordering and adjusting wheelchairs and adaptive equipment, as well as conducting adaptive feeding programs and a skills development group that emphasized motor and communicative growth. The last group met three times per week. The enormous case load did not allow enough time to provide direct therapy. Thus, this therapist's time was best used by giving indirect service. She provided inservice training and was a resource person to the staff in the areas of perceptual motor activity, gross-motor development, self-care, and feeding. The therapist also assisted the staff in developing creative programs for new facilities in a building addition that included a gross-motor activity room, a swimming pool, and school classrooms.

School Settings

One efficient way for therapists to disseminate knowledge is through groups. During the summer the Ingham Intermediate School District sponsored a six-week infant stimulation program designed to train mothers of handicapped children to become their children's primary therapist. A team composed of an occupational therapist, a physical therapist, a speech pathologist, and a child psychologist conducted weekly sessions with six infants, aged 6 months to two years, and their mothers. The infants' impairments included meningomyelocele, cerebral palsy, Down's syndrome, visual and auditory impairment, chromosomal abnormalities, and varying degrees of mental retardation. The infants had been evaluated prior to the course using the Denver Developmental Screening Test, the Bayley Scales of Infant Development, and developmental reflex testing.

The group met each week for a three-hour session. The format used was adapted from the *Mothers Can Help* program developed at the El Paso Rehabilitation Center (2). The session was divided into two periods. The first was a lecture and demonstration. The lectures presented general information on the infants' disabilities, techniques and positioning to influence muscle tone, range of motion exercises, speech, developmental play, feeding techniques, posture, and locomotion. The occupational and physical therapists demonstrated various procedures to use with the infants and then the mothers tried the new techniques under the therapists' supervision.

During the second half of the period the mothers met informally with the speech pathologist and psychologist to discuss feelings in common concerning their handicapped children. The mothers were also given information about resources and future special education opportunities for their children. While the mothers were meeting, the physical and occupational therapists administered therapy to the infants. Treatment consisted of positioning the children on both bolsters and therapy balls to develop head and trunk control; slow stroking, side rolling, neutral warmth, and other inhibitory techniques; and tactile, auditory, and visual stimulation. The student viewed and heard the lecture via a one-way mirror and then helped with the therapy during the second part of the session.

Preventative care programs such as infant stimulation discourage the early institutionalization of mentally retarded children. Preschool detection and therapy

contribute to their chances of becoming self-sufficient, contributing members of society. Although the emphasis is on physical management because of their age, preschool therapy can also be directed at cognitive and perceptual development. Occupational therapists' concern for the total individual makes their role a key one on the infant stimulation team.

Day Training Center

Three weeks of the field work experience were spent in the day training section of a state and federally funded school for the mentally impaired. During this period the student observed, evaluated, and planned treatment programs for two children; participated in the feeding and swimming programs for all children; and viewed a concentrated daily treatment program for one child conducted by the occupational and physical therapists. The single occupational therapist at this center was responsible for providing therapy to 35 children in the Multicap program, the section of the school that serviced children with physical as well as mental handicaps. Cerebral palsy, microcephalus, and hydrocephalus were the most common disabilities. Most of the children were wheelchair-bound and severely mentally impaired. The occupational therapist made yearly evaluations and videotapes of each child's performance and also did reflex, feeding, and manual skill evaluations.

The therapist's duties in this setting were many. She made and adapted equipment (chairs, feeding devices, splints, braces), attended cerebral palsy clinics, and trained the staff to carry out occupational therapy exercise programs. She personally administered her own treatment programs weekly with the 35 Multicap students. Other duties included writing reports, ordering, and making inventories of equipment. Formal as well as on the spot inservice sessions on the role of the occupational therapist and specific problems with the children were conducted with other staff members.

As the only therapist for 35 children, she believed her time could be best utilized by inservice with staff and parents. For example, an inservice program to train others in the construction and use of adaptive equipment and other developmental programs would give the therapist more time for direct involvement with the children most likely to benefit from her skills.

Intermediate School District

The supervisor's role as a consultant for an intermediate school system's orthopedic classroom two days per month provided the student with another exposure to occupational therapy with the mentally impaired. There were 15 children in the severely mentally impaired and trainable mentally impaired program with diagnoses of Down's syndrome, cerebral palsy, hydrocephalus, and congenital birth defects. Evaluations were conducted in the areas of primary gross motor, self-care, reasoning and problem solving, and reflexes.

Treatment techniques such as relaxation and inhibition methods, feeding, sensory stimulation, gait training, and positioning were demonstrated and taught to the classroom instructors and physical therapy aide. Specific problems that staff members were having with the students were dealt with and checked on in subsequent visits. The consultant also worked with parents and helped to familiarize the family with the treatment plan being used at school. The therapist presented formal inservice sessions on cerebral palsy and primary gross-motor development. In a setting such as this where the full-time services of an occupational therapist are not available, the consultant can provide indirect therapy through inservice training. The progress of the students and staff and the problems they encounter can be assessed during follow-up visits.

Nursing Care Homes

Many private nursing care facilities provide permanent homes for the mentally impaired. Individuals placed in such centers with full-time nursing care generally are quite physically involved, are over 25 years old, and are not in school. Four nursing care homes were visited—three had one therapist, and all had one or two aides. Each facility housed more than 100 severely mentally impaired clients from the ages of 4 to 70 years. Between 12 and 37 clients were individually treated by the therapists.

Each occupational therapy program observed in the nursing care homes emphasized different areas, but all conducted evaluations in range of motion, activities of daily living, sensation, communication, gross motor abilities, and hand function. Direct therapy was given through splinting, the use of adaptive equipment, positioning, feeding assessment and training, toileting, range of motion exercises, and developing fine motor skills. The therapists were also responsible for ordering wheelchairs. All therapists were frustrated by the enormous case loads and felt the only effective way to help the residents was by conducting inservice programs for the staff in such areas as positioning, feeding, and explaining the role of occupational therapy with multiply-handicapped individuals. The therapists in these homes felt their roles were unique because of their concern for the total psychological and physical being of the patients in contrast to other staff members whose concerns were more specialized.

University Project

Occupational therapists can extend their knowledge and skills to the mentally impaired by developing educational materials. The student's supervisor was a member of a university project that conducted inservice training programs and developed curriculum for the severely mentally impaired population. The team consisted of a speech pathologist, occupational therapist, school psychologist, and members of the special education department. The team wrote a manual for classroom instructors and aides that covered self-care, language, reasoning and problem solving, primary and fundmental gross motor, and prevocational skills training.

The project staff consulted with 25 large institutions, day care training centers of intermediate school districts, and nursing care homes throughout the state. Using the Active Response Inservice Training Method (ARITM) developed by the university, assessment and training devices were demonstrated to the aides in these different settings. The ARITM combines demonstration by the teacher and immediate practice by the students (the aides). The aides then practiced the procedures with the clients under the team's supervision. Follow-up visits to the centers helped resolve initial problems arising from the use of the assessment and training manual. During the field work experience the student attended all project committee meetings, workshops, and participated in the inservice trips to the nursing care homes.

The occupational therapist on the project, the student's supervisor, served as a consultant to the project staff, as an inservice trainer, and as a curriculum planner. Her occupational therapy skills lent themselves to self-care, provocational, and motor areas, as well as to the developmental sequence these skills follow. Because much of the population was physically impaired as well, her expertise was needed to adapt the manual to their specific needs. The therapist shared her knowledge through inservice training and consultation with professionals and paraprofessionals, thus reaching more clients than she could through direct service.

Summary and Evaluation

The traditional student field work experience is centered in one facility. Evaluation and treatment techniques are practiced with one population under the direction of a therapist working in the center. This field work experience in the field of mental retardation differed from the traditional model in numerous ways. The student received exposure and instruction in 11 treatment centers. As a traveling private practioner, the student's supervisor operated from several bases and, because the student traveled with her, she received more supervision time than most affiliates do. Through her and the many secondary

supervisors, the student received more exposure to the organizational and administrative duties of the occupational therapist than to the evaluative and treatment methods used.

The field work experience had both advantages and disadvantages. The amount of time spent at most of the centers did not permit enough opportunity to view change in the client through the evaluation, remediation, and reassessment processes of occupational therapy. Rapport was difficult to develop with the patients and staff. Not enough time was available to become proficient in all treatment techniques or to develop note-taking ability.

The advantages to a multicenter field work experience were many. The student was exposed to a variety of settings and different evaluative and treatment methods, and became familiar with the development of curriculum for severely mentally impaired clients. She met many therapists with differing styles and worked with clients of varying degrees and types of disability. It was also a unique opportunity to work with a private practitioner.

Exposure to the professional roles of numerous therapists in different settings is invaluable to the student when considering future job possibilities. This experience pinpointed areas for concentration in the remaining academic program. The supervisor acted as a resource person and role model — answered many questions and provided discussion periods. One recommendation for a similar field work experience in the future would be to allow two days per week with the same clients in one of the centers to ensure continuing treatment and observation.

The opportunities for exposure to the field of mental retardation in the occupational therapy curriculum were minimal. Through a multicenter field work experience, the student became familiar with the role of the therapist in a large institution, nursing care homes, and school settings. The therapist's role as a curriculum planner, inservice trainer, and consultant was also investigated.

The need for occupational therapists in the field of mental retardation is great. They are qualified to serve the psychological and physiological needs of the clients, and numerous positions are available in the area. It is hoped that more field work experiences like the one described above will be developed and will encourage new therapists to choose mental retardation as a specialty area.   •

Acknowledgments
The author extends appreciation to the numerous occupational therapists and to the facilities for the mentally impaired that allowed participation in their programs. The devoted concern and understanding of Virginia White, O.T.R., is also acknowledged.

This article was written when the author was a graduate student at Western Michigan University, Kalamazoo, Michigan.

REFERENCES
1. Ford LJ: Academic and clinical exposure to the field of mental retardation. *Am J Occup Ther* 27: 403, 1973
2. Cliff S, Gray J, Nymann C: *Mothers Can Help, A Therapists' Guide for Formulating a Developmental Text for Parents of Special Children*, El Paso, Texas: The El Paso Rehabilitation Center, 1974.

Gerontology

SPECIAL INTEREST SECTION NEWSLETTER

Published quarterly by The American Occupational Therapy Association   Vol. 9, No. 1, March 1986

Level II Fieldwork Education in a Home Health Care Setting

Karen Burdick, OTR
Manna Fox, OTR

The role of the occupational therapist in home health care is becoming more recognized. However educational training programs that prepare students for this setting are virtually nonexistent. Bay Valley Home Health Care is one agency changing this trend. Since January 1985, Bay Valley has accepted Level II fieldwork students from Eastern Michigan University and Western Michigan University. The occupational therapy departments at both universities and Bay Valley are pleased with the success of the home health care internship program. Students are already identified for the winter and spring semesters of 1986.

This article presents the evolution and present status of this Level II fieldwork program from the students' and fieldwork supervisors' perspectives.

Bay Valley Home Health Care is a nonprofit agency affiliated with St. Joseph Health Systems, Inc., Flint, MI. Bay Valley's catchment area includes all of Genesee County and some areas of surrounding counties. The Home Health Care Agency offers a pediatric rehabilitation program and one of the few pediatric hospice programs in the state. It also offers traditional rehabilitation and hospice programs and has a contract with a regional center for mentally retarded and developmentally disabled individuals. The occupational therapy department is aggressively active in all these areas with eight occupational therapists working either full- or part-time. Because of the diverse roles of occupational therapists at Bay Valley, the number of therapists, and their different individual areas of expertise, Bay Valley offers students a wide variety of experience and supervision.

During a 12-week internship at Bay Valley, the occupational therapy student is placed with the rehabilitation supervisor for 1 week. During that week the student is oriented to the agency, staff, documentation forms, and policies and procedures. The student also spends 1 week with a hand therapist to observe, treat, and fabricate splints. If the students' schedule permits, they may have the opportunity to observe hand surgery. The remaining 10

weeks are spent with a primary supervisor to observe other field therapists. The student accompanies the supervising therapist on each home visit, provided that prior consent is obtained from the patient. Initially, the student observes patient evaluation and treatment. At the supervising therapist's discretion, the student may progress to planning and carrying out treatment under direct supervision of the therapist. The student may also progress to evaluating, planning, and carrying out treatment independently. The supervisor is directly accessible to the student at all times. All evaluations, treatment plans, progress notes, and home programs are reviewed and co-signed by the supervising therapist.

Because of the nature of this program, the selection of students and supervisors is crucial. Bay Valley requires an interview with the rehabilitation director, the supervising therapist, and potential fieldwork students. Qualities considered important for both students and supervisors are communication and organizational skills, flexibility, self-motivation, and sensitivity.

Good communication skills are especially necessary for the home health care therapist. The lack of regular consultations with primary physicians and other therapists necessitates writing reports that are concise and accurate. Insurance coverage in home health care depends on the quality of progress notes and written evaluations. Also, phone calls are important for maintaining a good relationship between the doctor and the therapist.

Organizational skills are important for the home health care therapist. During the final portion of an internship experience, students are required to schedule their own patients. They must consider the geographic location, travel time, and time for paper work.

Flexibility is an important characteristic for therapists and students because of the treatment environment. Certain factors such as bad weather, doctor appointments, and the patient's family obligations can delay or prevent treatment. Students and therapists need to be prepared to accommodate and reschedule appointments.

Additionally, the supervisor must allow time for direct supervision and conferences with the student, for reading and co-signing documentation, and for consulting with patients and co-therapists on their impressions of the student.

Because treating patients at home is less structured than most institutional settings, students need to be relatively self-directed. Students and therapist must be willing to research an unfamiliar diagnosis and locate and contact the necessary resources. Therapists need to be holistic in their approach to patient care and able to appropriately recommend intervention by other disciplines (e.g., social work, physical therapy, etc.). Therapists must be extra sensitive to a patient's life-style, family dynamics, and privacy needs when treatment is conducted in the home.

Affiliation in a home health care setting offers special opportunities for a student. Former students of Bay Valley's program were impressed by the variety of experiences offered during their internship placement. Students felt that they had been exposed to a wide spectrum of therapy settings and clientele, and they felt confident to enter the professional world.

They particularly valued the opportunity to observe and work in the patient's environment and to identify and directly involve the patient's support system in treatment. The program offers flexibility to the student because many options for specialization are offered, and students are encouraged to emphasize their specific area of interest throughout their internship.

Many of the therapists employed by Bay Valley are in private practice and treat patients on a contract basis. Former students have appreciated the exposure to this option for occupational therapists and the experience of providing therapy on a consultant basis.

Karen Burdick, OTR, is a full-time occupational therapist and fieldwork supervisor, and Manna Fox, OTR, is a full-time occupational therapist and is completing her Level II fieldwork requirements; both are at Bay Balley Home Health Services, Flint, MI.

1

Despite the language and cultural barrier, an adventuresome OT fieldwork student discovers friendships and commonalities with OT practitioners on the Puerto Rico island

Taking the Road Less Traveled

AS I BOARDED THE PLANE bound for San Juan, Puerto Rico, I was overwhelmed by conflicting emotions of anticipatory excitement and sheer panic. Those sitting around me were fluently engaged in Spanish conversation, and everybody seemed to know one another. I was alone, knowing only a minimum of Spanish, and en route to an island where I knew nobody. I was about to begin my physical disabilities affiliation at the San Juan Veterans Administration Hospital, and I was very nervous. Nonetheless, this journey was to result in the most culturally and educationally enriching experience of a lifetime—one that I will never forget!

The idea to seek an alternative location for my affiliation began when I read an article in New York University's occupational therapy newsletter, which mentioned several educational and rehabilitation associations in Puerto Rico. As a musician and an artist, I have always been fond of Latino music and art, and I realized that an affiliation in Puerto Rico might be an opportunity to learn more about this culture. With the help of several Hispanic friends and an address list from AOTA, I sent numerous letters to various locations throughout Puerto Rico.

I received many replies, but all stated that speaking and writing Spanish would be required, a condition that I could not fulfill. My luck changed when I heard from Maria I. Rodriguez, the chief OT in physi-

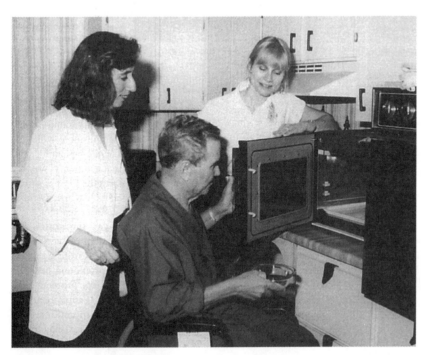

Marie Caron, *right*, observes while Zaida Garrett helps Victor Vega in a kitchen activity. During Caron's fieldwork, she was fortunate to find a mentor in Garrett.

cal disabilities at the Veterans Administration in Puerto Rico. She informed me that although Spanish was the spoken language, the staff knew English, and all documentation was in English since it was a U.S. government hospital. She also helped me locate a comfortable and inexpensive boarding house and communicated with the university on my behalf.

I was immediately impressed with the 14 OTs in the department. Without exception, they were all fluently bilingual. It was also very obvious that the therapists were abreast of the latest techniques and theories as they explained and taught me different treatment procedures. I was encouraged to research several treatment techniques in detail and had access to the hospital's extensive medical library.

While working in the department's living skills lab, I was fortunate to fulfill every student's dream, that is, to find a therapist who can be called "my mentor." Her name is Zaida Garrett, OTR/L, a therapist of 12 years. Not only did she teach me the art of helping patients relearn ADL skills, but she also demonstrated the subtle art of caring for the psychosocial well-being of her patients and that of the students under her supervision. She helped me gain confidence in my treatment skills and corrected my mistakes in a way that never made me feel inadequate or self-conscious.

She taught me the importance of being able to effectively communicate with the patient, beyond words. Often, I was only able to speak to patients in limited Spanish. I found, however, that watching and using body language can be a large part of the communication between patient and therapist. This required that I listen carefully to what the patient said, finding key words that I understood while watching the patient's facial expressions or hand motions. I, in turn, would use descriptive hand motions or actual demonstrations when talking to them.

In Puerto Rico, I was able to gain an appreciation of why occupational therapy stresses the importance of understanding a patient's culture. The Puerto Rican descends from 500 years of intermarriages between ancestors of Spanish settlers, African slaves and the indigenous Taino Indians. The mixing of these people has taken place more freely than in North America where racial barriers are more pronounced. This mixing has produced a

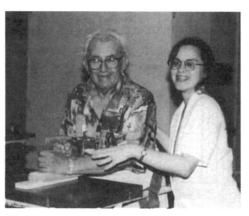

Zaira Benabe, MA, OTR/L, uses a woodworking activity to help Juan Mendez gain upper extremity strength.

culture much more tolerant of racial differences. Consequently, visitors of different backgrounds are usually received warmly, making it easy for them to mingle in Puerto Rico. By contrast, a Puerto Rican who travels to the States for the first time may experience a problem with the more conservative interracial norms and the more reserved disposition of the North American.

Also, I found the very nature of the Spanish language to be more polite than English. For example, when addressing patients, they use "Don" or "Dona," which denotes respect when talking to adults. Also, when eating, it is customary for Puerto Ricans to wish one another a pleasant dining experience with the expression "buen provecho."

Quite often, patients want to show therapists their appreciation. Accepting gifts from the patients is prohibited; however, therapists are allowed to accept food as tokens of a patient's gratitude. Often patients will bring delicious homemade or homegrown foods, such as candies, pastry, fruit, vegetables or cheese, which are then shared by all therapists in the department. Another cultural custom is touching between patient and therapist. Upon meeting or greeting a patient, it is quite customary to hold the patient's hand, and during conversation a gentle pat on the shoulder or

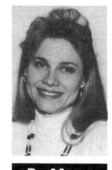

BY MARIE CARON, OTS

arm is quite appropriate. Also, saying good-bye is often done by a gentle hug or kiss on the cheek. I experienced firsthand how reassuring these touches can be. Upon my arrival, my facial expression gave away how overwhelmed I was. My supervisor noticed and reassured me with a smile and a gentle arm around my shoulder.

Although I was able to communicate to many of my patients, there were times when the language barrier made relating information or instructions to patient and family impossible. It was during these times that I realized the need for having therapists in our profession who can speak other languages. Because our profession emphasizes the whole person—psychosocial and physical—it is important that we effectively communicate with the patient. Therefore, it is our responsibility to attract and recruit minorities as students in occupational therapy. Culture is also important in understanding the norms and ways of a patient. Therefore, therapists should be recruited from all cultural and socioeconomic backgrounds. Also, the profession should support those who are interested in learning more about other cultures and backgrounds. Students who want to study a foreign language should be encouraged and perhaps financially aided by occupational therapy departments.

Organizing and arranging my affiliation in Puerto Rico was time-consuming, a bit frightening and unconventional. However, I will always remember the three months I spent on La Isla Del Encanto (the island of enchantment). Not only did I learn a great deal about occupational therapy treatment techniques and culture, but I have established professional relationships and friendships that I am sure will last a lifetime. I strongly urge other students to seek out alternative ideas for affiliations. Perhaps they may even consider the Veterans Administration of Puerto Rico as their first choice! ■

Marie M. Caron is enrolled in an entry-level master's degree program, New York University, New York City.

Level I Fieldwork
in a Daycare for Homeless Children

Margaret Drake, PhD, OTR/L, ATR

SUMMARY. The author was part of a task force that developed a mental health curriculum for a daycare for homeless children. An outgrowth of this involvement was the opportunity to use the facility as a Level I Fieldwork site. This article describes the curriculum and the student program.

INTRODUCTION

Birmingham, Alabama has a population of 800,000 people. Like most cities this size there are homeless people (LaGory, Ritchey & Mullis, 1987). More than 25% of all homeless people are single mothers with two or three preschool-aged children (Bassuk & Rubin, 1987). These mothers have often been abused by family and spouses and demonstrate greater substance abuse problems than similar domiciled women (Bassuk & Rosenberg, 1988). More than half of these mothers have had some mental health treatment before becoming homeless (Bassule, 1987).

Children in homeless shelters have also been identified as having both developmental and emotional problems (Bassuk, 1985). Approximately one half of all homeless children also have health problems (Miller & Lin, 1988) and nutritional deficiencies (Alperstein & Arnstein, 1988).

Margaret Drake is Associate Professor, Occupational Therapy Division, School of Health Related Professions at the University of Alabama at Birmingham. During part of the time she was writing this article, she was Visiting Associate Professor of Occupational Therapy at the National Taiwan University Hospital in Taipei, Taiwan.

In Birmingham there are seven shelters for homeless women and their children. While the children in these shelters do have a physical examination and the immunizations required in daycare centers licensed by the Public Health Department, they do not have a mental health evaluation. Since mental health problems are among those health problems most frequently reported (Alperstein & Arnstein, 1988; Bassuk & Rubin, 1987; Miller & Lin, 1988; Committee on Community Health Services, 1988) a role for occupational therapy assessment and intervention exists. This article describes daycare center for homeless children in Birmingham and a Fieldwork Level I program established to address the mental health needs of the children.

BACKGROUND OF THE DAYCARE PROGRAM

The Young Women's Christian Association (YWCA) has historically tried to meet the community needs of women and their families according to Suzanne Durham, director of the Birmingham YWCA. As women's needs have changed, the YWCA has adapted its programs accordingly. In the last two decades, as more and more women have been obliged to seek employment outside the home, the YWCA has responded by offering daycare for preschool-aged children. This program for 'domiciled children,' a term used to contrast those living in homes with families, with homeless children, was started 20 years ago. The Daycare for Homeless Children (DHC) was started in August 1989. It was initially funded by a grant from local financial institutions with the stipulation that the YWCA would include it in their budget the following year. The YWCA is financed by membership fees, donations and fund raisers.

In the early summer of 1989, the YWCA director was in the process of establishing a Task Force to examine the possibilities and appropriateness of development of the DHC. A social worker colleague submitted my name to her. Because of my background as a primary school teacher, an art therapist and an associate professor of occupational therapy I was the kind of resource sought for the Curriculum Committee of the Task Force. A series of meetings were held with other Curriculum Committee members in which we evaluated the existing daycare curricula and the needs of the children to be served by DHC to determine the best curriculum and services for them.

The YWCA regular daycare has approximately 80 children ages 6 weeks through 5 years in 7 different rooms. Parents pay on a sliding scale based on income. The daycare workers have limited education about normal children's needs and how to fill these needs let alone the needs of the homeless. Children are dealt with in large groups. Before the DHC was started, attempts were made to place homeless children in these classes. They were felt to be disruptive to the classes because of their different and, often greater needs. The numbers of children in these larger groups seemed to exacerbate existing behavior problems. The Committee felt that a new program needed to be developed which focussed on the specific needs of these homeless children.

THE DHC PROGRAM

In the DHC, filling the particular needs of homeless children is the central program goal. These needs relate to nutrition (Alperstein & Arnstein, 1988), emotional deprivation (Alperstein & Arnstein, 1988; Miller & Lin, 1988; Bassuk & Rubin, 1987; Committee on Community Health Services, 1988) and developmental delay (Bassuk, 1985). Further considerations in the program are: that homeless families are transient causing children to lack a sense of belonging; that frequent absences cause a lack of continuity in the school experience; that many caretakers cannot provide attachment; that they have usually lost at least one adult relative and fear further abandonment; and, that there is a severe lack of privacy living in crowded shelters.

Abraham Maslow's 'hierarchy of human needs' (1954) forms the theoretical base upon which the DHC curriculum was developed. This theory asserts that there are different levels of needs upon which human behavior is based. At the lowest level, physiological needs control how an individual responds to the environment. If the child does not have adequate, healthy air, water, and food, he or she will be unable to attempt to expend energy on higher needs. At the second level, responses to needs for safety and security dominate the child's behavior. He or she may be unable to trust any adult because previous experiences have been threatening and painful, such as abandonment or physical abuse. On the third level of feeling loved and belonging to a group such as a family, a homeless child may feel as if no place is home and no one cares. The needs of self-esteem and a feeling of being successful, Maslow's fourth level, will be difficult for a homeless child to respond to because lower-level needs have not been met. The last and highest level, 'self-actualization' which involves a child's need to be creative will be stifled because of the unmet lower needs. This theory provides an excellent framework for examining the needs and designing a curriculum for homeless children.

With this hierarchy in mind, we also incorporated elements of other curricula into our program design. A nine week program was chosen since that is the average length of stay of children in Birmingham's shelters. The program uses weekly themes related to developmental learning stages, primary relationships and the specific needs of homeless children described above. For example, one week the unit focuses on babies and their needs and provides opportunities for sibling involvement and learning lessons about babies' health needs, emotional needs, and relationships with family members are included. For another week, the topic is houses and homes. Since these children have lost their homes, they are provided opportunities through crafts, art, stories, 'the playhouse' and puppets to express their feelings of loss. Cooking and preparation of food is part of every day's activities. All of these activities address Maslow's Level 1 and 2 needs. Children have daily community outings weather permitting, in which they are taught traffic and community safety rules, a Maslow Level 2 lesson.

A typical daily schedule for 4 and 5 year olds looks like this:

7:00 - 9:00 am   Children arrive and have breakfast followed by free play.

9:00 - 10:30 am   Curriculum activities such as stories, guest speakers, art activities, pets, seasonal and holiday activities, are followed by free play.

10:30 - 11:00 am	Food preparation and snack
11:00 - 12:00 am	Physical activities such as parachute, bean-bag and ball games.
12:00 - 12:30 pm	Lunch
12:30 - 3:00 pm	Nap. Because of the noise and distraction common at night in shelters, these children often take 2-3 hour naps.
3:00 - 4:00 pm	Follow-up on morning activities related to the curriculum topic. Videos, guest speakers, sandbox, construction activities.
4:00 - 6:00 pm	Parents pick up children who have free-play while waiting.

This schedule has been successful in providing a structured and innovative curriculum at DHC. It also provides an excellent opportunity of occupational therapy involvement.

LEVEL I FIELDWORK

As I worked on establishing the DHC it became clear to me that Level I Fieldwork students could provide valuable services while having the opportunity to learn a great deal. The families and children could benefit from the newly acquired skills of our students in evaluation and treatment. Students could benefit from the opportunity to practice under supervision in this unique setting and learn about the effects of poverty and homelessness on child development. Additionally, occupational therapy's special expertise in working with 'early intervention' is well documented (Early Intervention Task Force, 1989; Schaaf and Mulrooney, 1989; Humphry, 1989; Hanft, 1988). While fieldwork is an integral part of occupational therapy curricula, it has become more difficult in the last decade to find appropriate fieldwork sites for both Level I and Level II students. Reduced funding (Leonardelli & Caruso, 1986) and staff shortages have contributed to this problem which is most acute in mental health placements. Faculty supervision of students doing fieldwork in settings where there is no occupational therapist has become more prevalent. While it is of value to faculty members to maintain clinical involvement (Brunyate, 1963; Spelbring,

1967) it can be exceedingly time consuming to establish and maintain relationships with the non-occupational therapy professionals students interact with. At DHC my involvement with curriculum development provided and easier-than-usual entré for fieldwork. This combination of factors led to the decision to place students at DHC.

Scheduling of Level I Fieldwork has been attempted in a variety of ways (Leonardelli and Caruso, 1986). At the University of Alabama Division of Occupational Therapy, it has been found that Level I Fieldwork is more satisfying for the student as well as patients and clinical staff, to have the student for 8 consecutive days, for eight hours each day. Consequently, for our seniors, the Classroom sessions end two weeks early and they spend the next eight days on their Level I Fieldwork.

In November 1989, the first placement was made for two senior students with me as their supervisor. At that time, the YWCA staff was fearful that the number of adults in the DHC as community volunteers had been overwhelming to the children. The decision was made to place each student for half the time in the DHC and half in the regular daycare where volunteers were less frequent. This reduced the number of adults to whom the homeless children were required to relate at any one time. This schedule has continued to the present (Figure 1). In the four days a student is with the homeless children, attachments are formed. The contrast between the more highly trained personnel in the DHC and the staff in the regular daycare has been instructive for students.

As clinical supervisor, I meet with the students one week before fieldwork begins to go over their schedules (Figure 1) and to explain expectations as listed below:

- To administer a mental health evaluation to one child.
- To administer a developmental evaluation to the same child.
- To discuss the results with the clinical supervisor and the daycare workers.
- To write a treatment plan based upon the evaluation results.
- To implement at least one individual activity from the treatment plan.
- To provide at least one piece of 'adaptive equipment.'
- To provide an inservice for daycare staff.
- To visit a shelter for the homeless.

FIGURE 1

Level I OT Fieldwork - YWCA
CLASS SCHEDULE

Date: March 4 - 13

PERIOD	MONDAY 4th	TUESDAY 5th	WEDNESDAY 6th	THURSDAY 7th	FRIDAY 8th
8:00 - 9:00	Meet and greet Daycare for Homeless Children enrollees. Work with them on developmental activities				
9:00 - 10:00	Orientation YWCA	Observe	Self-Esteem Activities with Regular Day Care		Self Esteem
10:00 - 11:00	Observe in Regualar Daycare	Assist in Regular Daycare	Individual Children / Cooking Session	Individual Children	and Fine Motor
11:00 - 12:00	Children's Dance Foundation			Children's Dance Foundation	Activities in DBC Children
12:00 - 1:00	Lunch	Lunch	Lunch	Lunch	Lunch
1:00 - 2:00	Start to fill out COTE Scale on Child in Regular Daycare	Decide on and familiarize self with another eval for same child using the COTE Scale	Plan and prepare activities	Plan and	Prepare
2:00 - 3:00			Score evaluation and share findings with teacher	Adaptive	Equipment To use with a child.
3:00 - 4:00	Individual Time With Regular Daycare Child				
4:00 - 5:00					

PERIOD	MONDAY 11th	TUESDAY 12th	WEDNESDAY 13th
8:00 - 9:00	Meet and greet DBC Enrollees Work with them on developmental Activities		
9:00 - 10:00	Self-Esteem and Fine Motor Activities With DBC Children		
10:00 - 11:00			Cooking Session
11:00 - 12:00	Children's Dance Foundation		
12:00 - 1:00	Lunch	Lunch	Lunch
1:00 - 2:00	Plan and Prepare Inservice Work on Regular Rx plan	Inservice with Regular Daycare teachers	Inservice Training for DBC Children
2:00 - 3:00			
3:00 - 4:00	Work with Individual DBC Children		
4:00 - 5:00			

221

Arrangements are made by me for the students to visit two of the seven shelters. On several occasions, students have pinpointed health and social problems the staff had not been aware of before. For example, the staff did not realize that the mother of one child had become involved with a men who was abusive. The student held an interview with the appropriate social worker and intervention followed.

Having two Level I students together is beneficial for the students as they give each other support. They work together to develop a plan for the 'adaptive equipment' and to execute the plan. One of the pieces of equipment was a cover made of cloth which came down over the sand-table to the floor on each side with a slit at each corner to allow it to slide on and off the table easily. The students appliqued doors and windows on the sides to make it look like a little house. Because homeless children have been found to suffer from a lack of privacy, the space under the sand-table is frequently used as a child's private place.

Each student is responsible for choosing an area to teach something to the staff and to develop an inservice training program. They then give the inservice twice, once to the regular daycare workers and once to the teachers in DHC. These have included such titles as: The Importance of Males in the Lives of Children; What is Sensory Integration?; Things to Look for in Children's Drawings; and The Importance of Games in Development.

Invariably, students have reported that it has been an invaluable experience. Several students have built such strong attachment with the children and staff that they have volunteered for weeks or months after the Level I experience was complete. The main complaint of students is that there is not an occupational therapist on site for the full eight hours. The hour I spend on a daily basis discussing the students' experience with them is felt by them to be sufficient however, since this is their first clinical experience, most would like to have an on-site supervisor.

In this day of cost containment (Shalik, 1987; Shalik & Shalik, 1988), it is important to explain that the only apparent cost to the YWCA for this entire student program is the cost of the materials for the adaptive equipment and the portion of the salary of the Director of the Daycare Programs for time spent orienting the students on the first day and, infrequently, answering their questions. The main cost is my salary which comes from the University.

CONCLUSION

The program has been in existence two years. It fills a need for finding more mental health Level I Fieldwork placements and has become a model for the development of other Level I Mental Health Fieldwork sites in the Birmingham community. Two other faculty members have also begun to supervise students in similar situations. It is a timely experience that combines the need for student placements with providing vital services to the homeless children of the community.

REFERENCES

Alperstein, G. and Arnstein, E. (1988). Homeless children--a challenge for pediatricians. *The Pediatric Clinics of North America*, 36(6), 1413-1425.

American Occupational Therapy Association, Inc. (1988). *Guide to the self-study report for an educational program for the occupational therapist*. Rockville, Maryland: Author.

Bassuk, E. L. (1985). *The feminization of homelessness; homeless families in Boston shelters*. Keynote Address for Shelter's, Inc's. yearly banquet at Harvard Science Center, Cambridge, Massachusetts.

Bassuk, E and Rosenberg, L. (1988). Why does family homelessness occur? A case-control study. *American Journal of Public Health*, 78(7), 783-788.

Bassuk, E. and Rubin, L. (1987). Homeless children--a neglected population. *American Journal of Orthopsychiatry, 57 (2), 279-286.*

Brunyate, R. W. (1963). The student in pre-clinical education. *American Journal of Occupational Therapy*, 17(4), 181-186.

Committee on Community Health Services of the American Academy of Pediatricians (1988). Health needs of homeless children, *Pediatrics*, 82 (6), 938-940.

Early Intervention Task Force (1989). Occupational therapy services in early intervention and preschool services (Position Paper), *American Journal of Occupational Therapy*, 43(11), 767-768.

Hanft, B. (1988). The changing environment of early intervention services: Implications for practice, *American Journal of Occupational Therapy* 42(11), 724-731.

Humphry, R. (1989). Early intervention and the influence of the occupational therapist on the parent-child relationship, *American Journal of Occupational Therapy*, 43(11), 738-742.

La Gory, M., Ritchey, F.J. and Mullis, J. (1987). *The Homeless of Alabama: Final Report of the Homeless Enumeration and Survey Project*, Birmingham: University of Alabama at Birmingham, Department of Sociology.

Leonardelli, C.A. and Caruso, L. A. (1986). Level I fieldwork: Issues and needs, *American Journal of Occupational Therapy*, 40(4), 258-264.

Maslow, A.H. (1954). *Motivation and Personality*, New York: Harper and Row.

Miller, D. S. and Lin, E.H.B. (1988). Children in sheltered homeless families: Reported health status and use of health services, *Pediatrics*, 81(5), 668-673.

Schaaf, R. C. and Mulrooney, L.L. (1989). Occupational therapy in early intervention: A family centered approach, *American Journal of Occupational Therapy* 43(11), 745-754.

Shalik, H. and Shalik, L.D. (1988). The occupational therapy level II fieldwork experience: Estimation of the fiscal benefit. *American Journal of Occupational Therapy*, 42(3), 164-168.

Spelbring, L.A. (1967). Upheaval in clinical education, *American Journal of Occupational Therapy*, 21(4), 205-206.

A Group Approach to Mental Health Fieldwork

Janice L. Hengel, Janice L. Romeo

Key Words: fieldwork education, occupational therapy • mental health

Fieldwork opportunities in mental health settings are limited and difficult to find. There is increased pressure for occupational therapy supervisors to accept more students although they have less time to devote to them. This article describes a group approach to training occupational therapy students that was used at one fieldwork site. The occupational therapy staff members were each responsible for specific teaching assignments that allowed them to work with a number of students simultaneously. Program development and evaluation meetings created an alternative forum for exploring ideas and practice issues and for providing guidance and supervision. This approach reduced the amount of time each therapist spent with students, provided students with several role models, and encouraged independent thinking in students.

Janice L. Hengel, MGA, MS, OTR, is Director of Rehabilitation Services, Garrett W. Hagedorn Gero-psychiatric Hospital, 200 Sanatorium Road, Glen Gardner, New Jersey 08826.

Janice L. Romeo, OTR, is Occupational Therapy Supervisor, Department of Psychiatry, Elizabeth General Medical Center, Elizabeth, New Jersey. At the time this article was written, she was student coordinator at the Garrett W. Hagedorn Gero-psychiatric Hospital.

This article was accepted for publication August 17, 1994.

As early as the mid-1970s, a critical shortage of occupational therapists practicing in mental health settings was becoming evident. The 1982 American Occupational Therapy Association (AOTA) Member Data Survey confirmed the shortage; only 9.8% of occupational therapy personnel nationwide were practicing in mental health sites (AOTA, 1984). This shortage has limited the number of fieldwork opportunities in mental health settings. One way to address the problem is "by training multiple students using alternative training models that maximize student/trainer ratios" (AOTA, 1991).

Traditional fieldwork settings pair one occupational therapist with one student (Kolodner, Weiner, & Frum, 1989); the therapist acts both as supervisor and role model to the student. This traditional approach has several disadvantages. First, it assumes that the occupational therapist with whom the student is paired has the knowledge, experience, and attitudes that make for a competent supervisor and role model; this assumption is not always accurate. Second, the one-to-one approach tends to create an experience in which the student is more likely to imitate and rely on staff members than to develop his or her own clinical reasoning skills and individual style—both of which are necessary for competent practice. Third, the approach places unnecessary demands on staff members who, under the pressures of their daily service demands, frequently view students as added work rather than as an enhancement of their own work experience. These disadvantages motivated us to develop a different approach to the traditional student fieldwork program.

This article describes a group approach to fieldwork training that has been used at Garrett W. Hagedorn Gero-psychiatric Hospital in Glen Gardner, New Jersey, for the past 3 years. In this setting, the students function as a group with a single assignment: to plan and implement an occupational therapy program. The experience was designed to engage the students in a clinical reasoning process that considers the patient's unique context in which services are delivered. It was also designed so that occupational therapy staff members could concentrate on teaching specific clinical skills in areas that have been identified as their strengths to a number of students at one time.

By analyzing and reflecting on practice issues with students, occupational therapists also enhance their own clinical reasoning skills in an ongoing process characteristic of and inherent in the development of expert practitioners (Mattingly, 1991).

The Setting

The group approach to fieldwork training was developed at Hagedorn Gero-psychiatric Hospital, a 188-bed facility that serves an exclusively psychogeriatric population. The hospital has seven units that are organized by patients' levels of functioning. Four units have 22 beds each, two units have 33 beds each, and one unit has 34 beds. Occupational therapists operate within the division of rehabilitation services, which also includes recreation, creative arts therapy, adult education, therapeutic work, physical therapy, and speech–language pathology and audiology.

An occupational therapist and a recreation staff member are assigned to each of the seven units on the basis of the conviction that all patients benefit from these services. Ongoing staffing shortages, however, have left some units without a full-time occupational therapist to provide services. All other rehabilitation disciplines are centralized and are available to the entire hospital population on the basis of need. The role of the occupational therapist on each unit is key to the provision of all rehabilitation services for that unit. The eight major components of this role in relation to the treatment team are as follows:

1. To assess the overall rehabilitation needs of the patient population
2. To define the purpose, rationale, and anticipated outcomes for all rehabilitation services
3. To develop a comprehensive rehabilitation program to meet the patients' needs
4. To negotiate with the supervisors of centralized rehabilitation staff members for needed services
5. To evaluate individual patients
6. To develop rehabilitation and occupational therapy plans for each patient
7. To develop and implement occupational therapy programs
8. To represent occupational therapy and all of the rehabilitation services on the treatment team.

In planning the students' fieldwork experience, we made several assumptions about the learning process:

1. Although students approach fieldwork with some anxiety and doubt, they have the knowledge and skills necessary for entry-level practice; however, they require the opportunity to apply their knowledge and practice their skills in order to refine them. They need supported freedom to discover and verify their abilities.
2. Each student is his or her own person. The student's task is to figure out how, within the context of that unique self, professional competence can be achieved.
3. Staff members also are students, in that they too are practicing their skills in order to refine them and are involved in a process of learning and growing.
4. Students will make mistakes and will learn from them. Without mistakes, learning is restrained.
5. Students will function competently if the environment is open and supportive.

6. What students learn in the mental health setting will transfer to other practice settings.

The Student Selection Process

The appropriateness of a fieldwork placement is based on all parties' understanding the nature of the learning program and how it relates to the needs of the students. Therefore, occupational therapy schools that have students in our program are informed about the structure of the fieldwork as well as the kind of supervision that students will receive. All prospective fieldwork students for our program are required to interview in our hospital. During this interview, the design of the program is clearly outlined and discussed. We request that each student think about the program for at least 1 week before committing to it. The final decision to participate in our fieldwork program rests with the students and the schools, not with our occupational therapy staff members. We believe that students who make the decision to participate will succeed.

There are four basic qualities that students must have to benefit from this approach: motivation, self-confidence, independence, and problem-solving skills. Furthermore, the student must be sincerely interested in mental health and in participating in a group approach to learning. Some degree of self-confidence is necessary for the student to initiate ideas and actions and to work independently. As individuals and as part of a group, students will often plan, process, and solve problems on their own before working with occupational therapy staff members. Those students who are motivated to select our hospital as a fieldwork site solely because they have been unable to locate another placement are discouraged from participating. Because we cannot completely assess students' qualities during a brief interview, we rely on the schools and the students to make this assessment. It is for these reasons that the final decision regarding fieldwork placement at our hospital rests with the students and the schools.

The Student Program

One of our 22-bed units at the hospital has been designated as the fieldwork training site. The student group, which consists of approximately four students, is assigned to plan and implement a comprehensive occupational therapy program on this unit. The unit houses low functioning patients, many of whom have organic disorders. The unit has a full-time recreation staff member assigned to it. However, due to ongoing staffing shortages, no full-time occupational therapist is assigned to this unit. Occupational therapists assigned to other units provide services to the unit as needed. The interdisciplinary team, rather than the patient population, was a factor in selecting this unit as the fieldwork site because its members tend to be receptive, supportive, and helpful to new staff members.

The students are given all of the traditional assignments that would be expected in a fieldwork experience: patient assessment, documentation, treatment planning, program development and implementation, and program evaluation. They also are asked to present both an in-depth patient treatment plan with a frame of reference of their choosing and an in-service training program to the occupational therapy or rehabilitation staff member. The students are encouraged to pursue an area of interest on another unit individually or with other students or staff members once the group has a plan for implementing its comprehensive occupational therapy program.

In order for the students to carry out their responsibilities, a process was designed that creates a structure for learning and a context for treatment planning. Learning needs are met through specific staff members' teaching assignments, and the students are guided through the patients' treatment process in a series of program development and evaluation meetings. All staff members are available as resources for feedback to analyze and reflect on practice.

Program Development and Evaluation Meetings

The occupational therapists and all other rehabilitation staff members who provide services on the fieldwork unit participate in a weekly program development and evaluation meeting. During these meetings, the students walk through the entire process of developing a program for the patients that serves to integrate all of their assignments and experiences. The format of these meetings is as follows:

1. A unit needs assessment is completed with the aggregate data from the comprehensive level of functioning rating scale for each patient. Patients' strengths and problems are identified.
2. The purpose, rationale, and anticipated outcomes of rehabilitation services and occupational therapy programs on the unit are developed on the basis of the patients' identified strengths and problems.
3. Specific programs and services to be provided by occupational therapists and other rehabilitation staff members are identified.
4. Program descriptions for the students' proposed treatment groups are written and descriptions of existing patient groups are reviewed. Once the students' treatment groups are implemented, they are observed by an occupational therapy staff member. Existing patient groups are observed by the students.
5. The program observations are processed to compare what was observed by the students with the written program descriptions and with the purpose, rationale, and anticipated outcomes for rehabilitation services on this unit. Through this process, students have the opportunity to give and receive feedback to and from each other and other rehabilitation staff members.
6. One or more patient cases are selected for review and are used to determine the effectiveness of the occupational therapy treatment. The occupational therapy assessment and treatment plan, made by the student, is reviewed and processed during the meeting to determine the relevance of the goals for the patient and the treatment groups to which the patient was referred. This determination is made by comparing the patient's goals to the anticipated outcomes of the treatment groups, as stated in the program descriptions.
7. Progress notes are reviewed and processed to determine the effects of treatment, the effectiveness of occupational therapy, and the extent to which this information was communicated to the treatment team.

Staff Member Assignments

To make the most effective use of each occupational therapist's time and to allow the students to work with as many occupational therapists as possible, each therapist accepts responsibility for one or more specific areas of instruction. Assignments are made on the basis of the therapists' individual strengths, interests, and expertise. All occupational therapists are available and willing to assist students, but specific questions and problems regarding technical skills are directed to the appropriate therapist–teacher. Although this aspect of the program may seem confusing to students at first, it quickly becomes clear. Each supervisor is responsible for guiding students in one or two of the following areas:

1. Orientation to patient charts—to orient students, during the first week, to the format and content of the patients' charts and to the hospital's approach to treatment as reflected in documentation.
2. Treatment team's role—to explain and clarify the role of the occupational therapist as rehabilitation representative within the interdisciplinary treatment team, the roles of other team members, and the treatment team process. The therapist-teacher also reviews a format for presenting evaluation findings and participating in the team process.
3. Evaluation and treatment planning—to explain how to evaluate and plan patient treatment accurately and effectively with the hospital's evaluation tool and reporting form.
4. Program descriptions—to explain and discuss the

hospital's format for writing a program description. Examples are reviewed and discussed.

5. Progress notes—to explain the hospital's format for writing progress notes and to work with students to develop their documentation skills.

6. Program development and evaluation meetings—to present an overview and chair these weekly meetings.

The occupational therapists continue in these assignments as new student groups participate in the program. This consistency affords them an opportunity to focus on refining their teaching strategies in one or two, rather than all, areas of practice.

Discussion

The reactions from students to this training approach have, for the most part, been positive. Students expressed some initial concerns about our expectations that they work independently without direct supervision at all times. Reassurance that they would be guided through the process and that they were not expected to know everything helped to reduce their anxiety. Students found the supervisory structure confusing at first but, as the program progressed, the role of each occupational therapy supervisor became clear. The students were particularly positive about the friendliness and supportiveness of the occupational therapists, other rehabilitation staff members, and the interdisciplinary treatment team. They believed that the qualities of these staff members were critical to their developing confidence and the ability to take risks. One student said, "The program is carefully structured and sets students up for success." Another student wrote

> Staff are very supportive and approachable. However, initiative on the student's part is needed to make this affiliation reach its greatest potential. Be inquisitive and willing to put your opinions in on meetings (especially with the occupational therapists). It is OK to take chances here (i.e. try something you think will work, but are unsure) and therapists don't mind talking through your questions or ideas with you. Overall, an excellent experience for the right student.

Before implementing the student program, the underlying belief of some of the hospital's occupational therapists was that there was something unsettling about this group approach; however, they could not pinpoint what it was. During discussions, discomfort was expressed about such issues as the need to be a role model for the student, to help the student, to spend time with the student, and to get to know the student well enough to judge his or her level of competence. This discomfort may have been grounded in the Accreditation Standard II.B.7.a.2 (AOTA & American Medical Association, 1991): "The ratio of fieldwork educators to students shall be such as to ensure proper supervision and frequent assessment in achieving fieldwork objectives" (p. 9). The hospi-

tal's occupational therapists interpreted this standard to mean that one student is assigned to one therapist. From discussion and dialogue it eventually became clear that discomfort was also experienced because the hospital's approach did not reflect their own fieldwork experience. This realization allowed the staff members to make a commitment to implementing the group approach on a trial basis. It then became critical for staff members to reconcile their differing personal perspectives and expectations of students, with the understanding that if consensus was not reached, conflict would arise that would create tension among staff members and confusion among students.

After approximately 3 years of experience with six groups of two to four students each and a staff of four occupational therapists, staff member feedback has, for the most part, been positive. One problem has been the formal student evaluation. Because all of the occupational therapists worked with all of the students, they contributed to each student's evaluation. As expected, there was disagreement regarding each student's performance that had to be reconciled to arrive at a rating. The process extended the time involved in completing the evaluations. Ultimately the problem was solved by having each occupational therapist complete an evaluation form on each student and each student complete a form on herself or himself. These scores then were averaged by the occupational therapy director, and all staff members' comments were incorporated into a final summary statement.

Conclusion

As the shortages in mental health practice and fieldwork training continue, occupational therapists are being challenged to create innovative fieldwork opportunities. The goal of the group approach to student learning and their supervision by staff members, as used at our hospital, was twofold: (a) to enable staff members to accommodate larger numbers of students while reducing each staff member's work load, and (b) to provide a learning experience that promotes clinical reasoning, self-confidence, and a sense of competency in mental health. Allowing each staff member to concentrate on only one or two areas of student training and to work with several students at one time has changed the nature of the staff member–student relationship. The program development and evaluation meetings have created an alternative forum for exploring ideas and practice issues and for providing guidance and supervision. Who is ultimately responsible for student learning is an issue that remains to be resolved, one that greatly affects the number of fieldwork students that can be accommodated and the amount of supervisory time required by staff members. When a student fails to assume an active role in the learning process, staff members have reverted to the more traditional and time-consuming role of directing the student through the assignments. This scenario shifts the responsibility for learning away from the student and onto the staff member and requires the staff member to spend excessive time monitoring the student's progress. The group approach requires that staff members allow students to be responsible for their own learning, regardless of whether they successfully complete their assignments.

Through the use of a group approach, students have the opportunity to learn a process for program development in addition to the specific skills needed for effective treatment. By working with several occupational therapists as well as members of other disciplines, students identify and develop their own unique and effective styles. As the student group increases its independence from staff members, the individual students develop clinical reasoning skills, self-confidence, and problem-solving skills that can be taken to any practice setting. ▲

References

American Occupational Therapy Association. (1984). *1982 Member data survey—Final report*. Rockville, MD: Author.

American Occupational Therapy Association and American Medical Association. (1991). *Essentials and guidelines for an accredited educational program for the occupational therapist*. Rockville, MD: American Occupational Therapy Association.

Kolodner, E. L., Weiner, W. J., & Frum, D. C. (Eds.). (1989). *Models for mental health fieldwork*. Rockville, MD: American Occupational Therapy Association.

Mattingly, C. (1991). What is clinical reasoning? *American Journal of Occupational Therapy, 45*, 979–986.

THE SCARCITY of occupational therapy fieldwork sites has led to an all-out search for placements in nontraditional settings. Another sort of innovative solution, however, has been adopted by Butler Hospital, an acute care private psychiatric facility in Providence, R.I. There, the setting is traditional, but the organization of fieldwork is not. OT students work in collaborative pairs, relying on each other for mutual support and for bouncing ideas back and forth. The fieldwork supervisor still provides ample guidance and feedback to each pair, but not twice the amount required for a single student, according to Mary Brinson, OTR, FAOTA, director of occupational therapy at Butler. Consequently, the overall capacity to take on fieldwork students is increased.

Brinson, AOTA's volunteer fieldwork consultant for the New England region, introduced collaborative fieldwork to Butler for the first time this quarter and has been very gratified by the results. Supervisors are able to take on more fieldwork students without feeling drained since members of student pairs problem-solve together before consulting the supervisor. Students ask fewer questions because their anxiety is reduced and confidence increased by having another student available as a "safety net." "Collaborative learning makes sense," Brinson argues. "It really comes closer to replicating practice and it also fully satisfies fieldwork requirements." She adds that AOTA has been very supportive of her efforts. Brinson is now participating in a research project designed to identify the differences between individual and collaborative fieldwork and help evaluate the latter's impact. A training video is also being made of the collaborative fieldwork experience.

The collaborative fieldwork model

ARE TWO HEADS BETTER THAN ONE?

OT staff at Butler Hospital think so. Their collaborative fieldwork model allows the facility to take on more fieldwork students with the same staff

BY BARBARA E. JOE

is not exactly new, since it has been used for some time in Canada and has been promoted in this country by Ellen Cohn, MS, OTR, FAOTA, at Tufts University in Boston. Collaborative fieldwork is, however, brand new at Butler, which previously was able to accommodate only two to four fieldwork students at a time and now has a total of nine, three working solo and six in pairs. "We decided to go ahead with this plan because we really wanted to have more fieldwork students, both to better meet educational needs and to encourage them to go into mental health," Brinson explains. "We felt this was a good way to accomplish both objectives."

Butler offers a wide range of psychiatric services, with special programs for children and adolescents, women, substance abuse, and those needing partial hospitalization. The facility has six OTs on staff, including Brinson, and four OT aides. Fieldwork students assigned there have the opportunity to observe and participate in diverse facets of psychiatric treatment. Having nine fieldwork students on board also is advantageous to the hospital, according to Brinson, because they supplement the staff, allowing the provision of more services and greater individual attention to patients, an especially important consideration in psychiatric care. PTs and other non-OT staff have enthusiastically welcomed the idea of collaborative occupational therapy fieldwork, Brinson reports.

Fieldwork students also exhibit more independence and willingness to assume responsibility when working in tandem. "They learn from each other, they observe each other," Brinson comments, adding that the pair does not necessarily take on all tasks as a twosome. They usually run groups together, but often approach a single client one-on-one, sometimes with the other partner observing. Clients do not object to the presence of so many students, Brinson says; they are accustomed to students and usually like having them around. The Butler occupational therapy department makes an effort to assure that students are well integrated into the system, and not just outsiders looking in. Brinson meets with fieldwork students as a group at least once a week and all OTs on staff function as fieldwork supervisors.

At the same time, fieldwork students are not obligated to join a pair. Butler gives them the option and also allows the students to choose their own partners instead of making assignments. Among the three current student pairs, only the members of one pair knew each other previously, Santo Russo and Scott Boris, both of Utica College of Syracuse University in N.Y. Having experienced individual fieldwork in a previous affiliation, Russo says he much prefers the collaborative system and wishes all fieldwork could follow that model. He believes it offers more variety and facilitates the transition from classroom to clinic. Russo says he has found himself to be more creative and more willing to take risks. He also finds he and his partner complement each other—"we feed off each other's strengths."

Collaborative fieldwork, Brinson feels, provides a superior learning experience. It takes away the notion that there is a single right answer known only to the experts or to the fieldwork supervisor, thereby promoting peer collaboration and practical problem solving. Butler Hospital's occupational therapy department plans to continue with collaborative fieldwork next quarter and beyond. Brinson definitely considers it "the wave of the future." ■

A 12-Month Internship Model of Level II Fieldwork

Erin Casey Phillips, Wendy Siggelkow Legaspi

Key Words: clinical competency • fieldwork education, occupational therapy • motivation

Erin Casey Phillips, MSOT, OTR/C is Staff Therapist, Milliken Hand Rehabilitation Center, Barnes Hospital, #1 Barnes Plaza Way, St. Louis, Missouri 63110. At the time of this project, she was a Clinical Instructor and Research Assistant, Washington University Program in Occupational Therapy, St. Louis, Missouri.

Wendy Siggelkow Legaspi, OTR/C, is Staff Therapist, Agana School System, Agana, Guam. At the time of this project, she was a Staff Therapist, Irene Walter Johnson Rehabilitation Institute at Barnes Hospital, St. Louis, Missouri.

This article was accepted for publication July 10, 1994.

As we approach the 21st century, our changing health care system places new and challenging demands upon service-oriented professionals. Health care providers are called upon to address these expectations with the skills necessary to respond to change. It is essential that occupational therapy continue to adapt to current changes in our health care system. A proactive approach to the development of innovative clinical training models will enable the profession to strategically plan for the future rather than react to its changes.

To meet the professional challenge for recruitment and retention and the educational demands for student supervision, many academic settings have expanded the traditional fieldwork model. As the number of fieldwork clinical sites has decreased, the interest in exploring alternatives to the traditional 6-month fieldwork experience mandated by the American Occupational Therapy Association (AOTA) (1991) has increased. Strickland and Crist (1991) evaluated the changing needs of students and practice in their workshop on fieldwork alternatives. Nontraditional fieldwork programs, such as allowing students to work part time, helps meet the needs of some students (Adelstein, Cohn, Baker, & Barnes, 1990). Other models have been created that supplement the 6-month format with programs designed to facilitate the educational process. In one model, clinical reasoning theory incorporated into the fieldwork experience acts as a foundation to enhance early skills (Cohn, 1989); in another, a stress-reducing seminar was used to help both students and supervisors turn conflict situations into part of the learning process (Yuen, 1990). The purpose of this article is to describe a 12-month internship program, to analyze the motivational operations inherent to this alternative model of the Level II fieldwork experience, and to report on what we interns saw as advantages and disadvantages of the program.

Description of Internship

A 12-month internship was created at the Irene Walter Johnson Institute of Rehabilitation in Barnes Hospital of St. Louis, in cooperation with the Washington University program in occupational therapy, to offer occupational therapy students their required Level II fieldwork experience and to simultaneously provide needed clinical services at the Institute. The internship is unlike a traditional fieldwork experience in that interns sign an employee contract, are salaried, and earn employee benefits including sick leave and vacation time, as well as medical and dental group plan benefits.

The internship is available in two tracks. In track A, the first 6 months focus on completion of Level II fieldwork experience requirements in two different occupational therapy areas within the Institute; the remaining 6 months are spent in an area in the Institute agreed upon by the intern and the Institute, according to mutual needs. Track A interns receive half the annual salary of an entry-level therapist over the 12-month internship period. In Track B, the first 3 months are completed at an outside facility and the remaining 9 months are completed in one area at the Institute. Track B interns receive three quarters the annual salary of an entry-level therapist over the 9-month period spent at the Institute.

The fieldwork opportunities offered at the Institute are in adult community programs, work performance programs, upper extremity and hand rehabilitation, acute and long-term neurology, general medicine and surgery, and community pediatrics. The Institute does not offer a fieldwork opportunity in psychiatry, at least not with patients having psychiatric disorders as the primary diagnosis. To give students more experience with psychiatric diagnoses, special emphasis is placed on investigating the psychological and emotional impact of traumatic physical injury. Where appropriate, students are encouraged to combine psychological and physical interventions into the rehabilitation treatment plan. Interns are also encouraged to take day trips to facilities within the St. Louis area that offer more specialized psychiatric services.

Selection criteria for interns include a grade point average of 2.5 or better, successful completion of occupational therapy academic requirements from an accredited education program, references from one faculty member and one Level I fieldwork supervisor, and a written essay stating the student's qualifications and what he or she hopes to accomplish during the internship. In this case, faculty members at Washington University screened and interviewed all applicants and forwarded three names to the internship committee, which was composed of Institute rehabilitation supervisors, therapists, and education coordinators. The committee then interviewed these three candidates.

An intern's progress is evaluated formally in midterm and final evaluations with the AOTA fieldwork assessment form. Progress is also monitored informally by the clinical education coordinator at Washington University, who pays attention to the intern's needs and growth areas. As Institute employees, interns also receive performance appraisals after 6 months and 1 year. Additionally, as employees, interns can take advantage of on-the-job learning opportunities such as monthly educational in-services and participation in various clinical action committees. If at any time the intern is not able to meet the requirements for Level II fieldwork or fails to pass the American Occupational Therapy Certification Board exam, employment is terminated. After completion of the 12-month internship, the student may continue employment at the Institute on the basis of his or her needs and those of the facility.

As interns, we initiated the fieldwork experience in June 1991. We both participated in Track A. The remainder of this article will discuss the intrinsic and extrinsic

motivational concepts that are enhanced by this method of clinical education, as well as the advantages and disadvantages of this type of fieldwork program.

Motivation and the Educational Process

In occupational therapy education we are taught the importance of motivation in facilitating quality performance. We teach our clients to be their own advocates and encourage internal motivation and investment as a means to overcome challenges. These issues can be applied to clinical training to determine the most effective road to clinical competency. The quality of student behavior, leading to the development of solid clinical skills, can be directly influenced by the presence of intrinsic and extrinsic motivational factors. The internship model is unique because it views the student as an employee and, through this relationship, incorporates the essential qualities of motivation into the educational process.

Application of Motivation Theory

Human behavior is influenced by both external and internal factors. Herzberg (1976) specifically delineated these factors in relation to employment and the workplace. For example, he identified hygiene (environmental and external) factors and motivator (personal and internal) factors for job satisfaction, indicating that a balance between the two was necessary for complete job satisfaction (see Table 1). Hygiene (external) factors represent the work environment (one's instinct is to avoid pain from one's surroundings), whereas the motivator (internal) factors represent the human source of happiness (one's instinct is to use personal talents and pursue psychological growth).

The internship defines students as having employee status, a well-defined place in the personnel hierarchy, with a commitment to a 40-hr work week and to the general mission of the facility. As employees, we developed a mutually rewarding investment in the Institute that resulted in personal and professional growth.

We will examine how the internal and external factors of workplace motivation are influenced by the intern-

Table 1
Profile of Motivating Factors in the Workplace

External Factors	Internal Factors
Policy/administration	Advancement
Supervision	Achievement
Interpersonal relations	Growth
Working conditions	Work itself
Security	Internal locus
Status	Responsibility
Salary	Recognition

Source: Herzberg, F. (1976). *The managerial choice: To be efficient and to be human.* Homewood, IL: Dow Jones-Irwin.

ship process. Analysis of these factors will illustrate the unique way in which employee status acts as a motivational force to enhance the fieldwork experience.

Internal Factors

Locus of control. A central idea in views of motivation is that people desire to have control over certain aspects of their lives. Rotter (1966), a social learning theorist, stated that "If the person perceives that the event is contingent upon his own behavior or his own relatively permanent characteristics, we have termed this a belief in internal control" (p. 1). As employees, we were given choice in clinical placements, a voice in program development, and the responsibility to be an active part of departmental change. We were given the resources and encouragement to exhibit power within the system, not to be controlled by it.

Self-efficacy. According to Maslow's hierarchy of needs fulfillment (1970), once basic human needs such as security and physical comfort are addressed, a person can attend to higher levels of quality performance. This theory can be applied to the internship experience as students attend to the internal factors of growth and achievement. Fieldwork students who are not on payroll struggle to deal with basic needs such as food, housing, and health care. The environmental factors inherent to the 12-month internship, such as salary and benefits, minimize the need to attend to these distractions, thus the intern is able to focus energy on a higher level of performance, such as refining clinical skills.

External Factors

Financial compensation. Money has a great influence on people (Cass, 1975), especially on students who may be encumbered with loans for their education. The salary and benefit options in the internship are attractive components reducing the need for students to finance the fieldwork experience or to request additional loans. We found this comforting and the money proved sufficient to support our basic monthly needs. Fieldwork at the Institute rewarded us for our efforts, not only educationally but financially, which created a feeling of security and an investment in the workplace. Committing to receive half salary for a full year is an obvious advantage to some students, but others rejected the idea. The important point is that this program offers an option to relieve the pressure of financial burden while allowing the individual to focus time and energy on refining clinical practice skills. Initially, money works to attract the student to the facility, acting upon the internal drive for self-preservation. Secondarily, monetary rewards relinquish this focal position, and take their place among the many environmental factors contributing to professional employee motivation. In other words, the money appears to get the students, but it is the entire package of benefits that becomes meaningful and sustains investment in the program throughout the 12-month period.

Environment. The environmental factors of interpersonal relationships, work conditions, and security were enhanced by the internship. Training in one setting decreases the amount of time spent learning procedural tasks, and the consistency of interpersonal relations afforded by the 12-month time span provides for greater teamwork than is found in a 6-month experience. For example, time required to orient new students at 3 months and new employees at 6 months was used to sharpen clinical skills and open opportunities for ongoing collaborative research and program developments. By contracting to remain at a single facility, we felt secure about the immediate future. There was no stress triggered by an upcoming job search. The relationships developed with our supervisor, occupational therapy staff members, and interdisciplinary team members were enhanced by the consistency of the workplace environment. We were able to observe various management and treatment styles and develop personal attributes that were recognized and respected as they supplemented those of existing colleagues. Our familiarity with physician referral sources enhanced communication and treatment effectiveness. As noted here, the benefits of the 12-month consistent environment lead to both personal and professional growth.

As Herzberg (1976) stated, a balance of internal and external factors leads to job satisfaction and subsequently to a higher quality of work performance. A 12-month internship model of clinical training promotes this balance by providing the student with employee status and the benefits inherent to this position. The internal and external motivators unique to the workplace are incorporated into this model of Level II fieldwork and lead to greater professional development and clinical competency.

Advantages and Disadvantages of the Program

The program can be evaluated from the perspective of both the facility and the student. Advantages to the student include all the environmental motivators previously discussed: salary, benefits, and employee status. The student intern is also able to explore a variety of clinical settings throughout the 12-month period. Although variety may be offered, training at a single facility is seen by some students as a limitation of resources and a definite disadvantage of this type of program.

The facility, by providing the internship, is receiving an intern who is committed to its system and will have training in many different service areas. Facilities are able to interview the internship candidates and choose a good fit, which will enhance retention and job satisfaction.

One drawback to this model is that it requires cooperation from facilities that are large enough to offer the student a variety of experiences. Without this element, the intern may not develop the range of competencies necessary for future function in a diverse health care profession.

The rewards and sacrifices of this type of fieldwork model must be weighed on an individual basis. The program establishes a solid alternative to the traditional approach. As more nontraditional students enter the field, occupational therapy clinical training models must also consider nontraditional options to meet changing needs.

Conclusion

The intended outcome of the Level II fieldwork experience is growth in clinical and professional skills. Certainly a 12-month fieldwork experience provides more opportunities than a 6-month experience for this growth. This article has provided educators with information on an alternative clinical education fieldwork model based on motivation theory that facilitates desired professional development and clinical competency. By examining aspects of motivation, we can more effectively promote goal-directed behavior in the development of occupational therapy practice skills, and subsequently use this information in the initiation and evaluation of new clinical education models. ▲

Acknowledgments

We thank Carolyn Baum, PhD, OTR, FAOTA, for her continued support of our professional growth, and Karen Barney, MS, OTR/C, and Monica Perlmutter, MA, OTR/C, for their persistence in developing the internship program at Washington University Medical Center.

This article is based in part on a presentation made at the Commission on Education Annual Meeting (short papers forum) at the 73rd Annual Conference of the American Occupational Therapy Association, June, 1993, Seattle, Washington.

References

Adelstein, L. A., Cohn, E. S., Baker, R. C. & Barnes, M. A. (1990). A part-time level II fieldwork program. *American Journal of Occupational Therapy, 44,* 60–65.

American Occupational Therapy Association. (1991). *Essentials and guidelines for an accredited educational program for the occupational therapist.* Rockville, MD: Author.

Cass, E. L., Zimmer, F. G. (1975). Monetary rewards—People do not work for bread alone, or do they? In E. L. Cass & F. G. Zimmer (Eds.), *Man and work in society* (pp. 135–150). Nutley, NJ: Sax Lewis Faulken.

Cohn, E. S. (1989). Fieldwork education: Shaping a foundation for clinical reasoning. *American Journal of Occupational Therapy, 43,* 240–244.

Herzberg, F. (1976). *The managerial choice: To be efficient and to be human.* Homewood, IL: Dow Jones-Irwin.

Maslow, A. H. (1970). *Motivation and personality.* (2nd ed.). New York: Harper & Row.

Rotter, J. B. (1966). Generalized expectancies for internal versus external locus of reinforcement. *Psychological Monographs, 80*(1, No. 609), 1.

Strickland, L. R., & Crist, P. (1991, June). *New alternatives for fieldwork education: Opportunities unlimited.* Workshop presented at the 71st Annual Conference of the American Occupational Therapy Association, Cincinnati.

Yuen, H. K. (1990). Fieldwork students under stress. *American Journal of Occupational Therapy, 44,* 80–81.

Level I
Field Placement
at a Federal
Correctional Institution

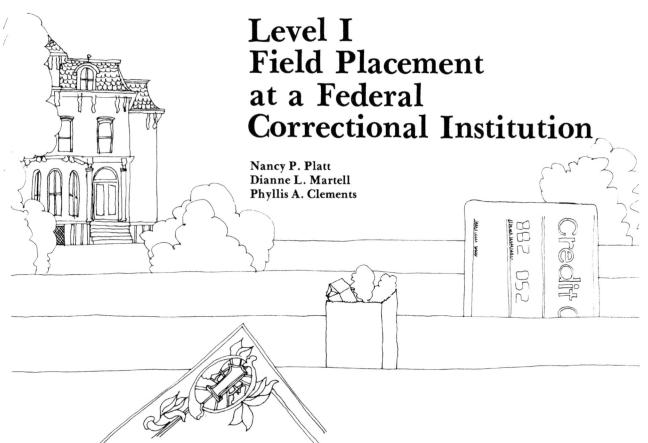

Nancy P. Platt
Dianne L. Martell
Phyllis A. Clements

*Two senior occupational therapy
students at Eastern Michigan
University were assigned during
consecutive semesters to a Level I
field placement at a Federal correctional institution and were supervised by a faculty member. Each student led a group of men in a life
planning and work readjustment
program. The program development, implementation, and evaluation of the experience are discussed
here.*

Nancy P. Platt, *OTR, is a visiting
lecturer at Eastern Michigan University, and has completed the requirements for a master's degree
from The University of Michigan.*

Dianne L. Martell and **Phyllis A.
Clements** *are graduates of the oc-
cupational therapy program at
Eastern Michigan University.*

S tudents in the occupational therapy program at Eastern Michigan University (EMU) are required
to complete both a mental health
and a physical function field work
experience during the final two semesters of their senior year. As basic
initial learning experiences that include directed observation and participation, these fall in the Level I
category of field work experience (1).

Halfway houses, community
centers, and other community programs have served as placement sites
for the EMU students for several
years, giving them an understanding
of how occupational therapy can
function in a nonmedical setting as
well as the therapist's relationships
with nonmedical personnel. Students
have had the opportunity to observe
and evaluate people from a social
health perspective, as well as to set
goals in "prevention and health

maintenance, remediation, daily life
tasks, and vocational adjustment."
(1) Concurrently, the personnel at
those facilities have increased their
understanding of occupational
therapy.

Program Development

Milan Federal Correctional Institution (FCI), located 15 miles from
EMU's campus, is a maximum
security prison housing 700 men
from 18 to 28 years of age. The institution's chief psychologist assisted
in organizing the occupational
therapy group. An EMU faculty
member and a selected student led
the weekly meetings. As the semester
progressed, the student accepted increased responsibility for the leadership of the group, and the faculty
member attended the meetings less
frequently. The student and faculty

supervisor met weekly on campus to consult regarding the group meetings and the student's work.

Description of Placement

First Semester. Six men who resisted participation in other prison groups were selected for the occupational therapy group. Dealing in narcotics, car theft, and armed robbery were among the offenses represented by those selected.

Initial meetings consisted of introductions of the group members and descriptions of prison life by the inmates. The student explained to the men that the therapists were to assist them in exploring their individual skills and interests in relation to work, leisure, and self-care activities. The men expressed an interest in gaining experience in preparing job applications and improving job interview skills.

The student and supervisor identified in the meetings the behavioral objectives for the occupational therapy group members: 1. to explore interests and needs in work, leisure, and self-care; 2. to develop the program agenda around these areas; 3. to regularly assess their own participation and value derived from the meetings.

Outside speakers were invited to discuss various aspects of job seeking; the men practiced completing job applications; and role playing in job interviews was recorded and critiqued by the group members. A booklet by R. Bolles (2) helped the men to assess their work skills. With practice and discussion the men showed improvement in the basic skills used in job seeking, and one inmate, who had never previously filled out a job application, was able to set more positive goals and to clarify his career interests with the support of other group members. He subsequently applied for and received a basic education grant enabling him to pursue a college education upon release from the prison.

Initial sessions were marked by resistance from the men in expressing themselves and in working with the others. Group discussions centered around issues such as societal prejudice toward exconvicts and prison politics. They also expressed negative attitudes toward society. In time, the men exchanged ideas and opinions more freely. They began to talk about themselves, their frustrations and needs, and their ambitions. Ultimately, they accepted increased responsibility for planning and carrying out group activities. They worked with each other to minimize disruptive behaviors.

The group activities were generally of an unstructured nature, and discussions were a principal part of every meeting. The student gained leadership skills and effectively handled her own and the group members' frustrations and disappointments as well as difficult staff relationships. At the semester's conclusion the student came to believe that the occupational therapist could make a significant contribution in a prison setting.

Second Semester. Consumer education was the basis for programming during the second semester. The two objectives were: to promote knowledge of consumer skills; and to facilitate adjustment to the community upon release through knowledge of community resources.

The program included presentations on money management, the proper use of credit, purchasing food and clothing, and locating appropriate housing. The presentations were supported by audiovisual materials, pamphlets, articles, and books obtained from the Michigan Consumer Education Library. The topics were discussed and newly learned skills such as money management were practiced.

During the practice sessions, the men were able to analyze their consumer skills and specific planned living situations. One session provided the opportunity for reality oriented problem-solving. One inmate, working with the student therapist individually, was asked to construct a budget that he might use when released. He prepared a list of estimated yearly expenses and projected an income from his first job after release from prison. A comparison of the estimated expenses and projected income revealed that his expenses were twice that of his earnings. With guidance he was able to eliminate unnecessary items and to reach a more practical budget, one within his means.

Local businesses and agencies were invited to make presentations to the group. The topics were banking and credit union services, employment, housing, consumer rights, insurance needs, and credit and contract rights. The presenters included a banker, a credit union representative, a tenants' union representative, a college professor, an insurance agent, and a consumer advocate.

Attendance diminished from six to two group members during this semester, and there are several possible reasons for this: The men's priority needs were not being met; they may have felt uncomfortable with the degree of structure or the methods of the program; they may have lacked interest in the activities or subjects.

A pre-release group of 15 men was then added to the group for the guest presentations. The pre-release group was responsive to the community resource programming, and many of the men said they had been unaware of the services and agencies presented. At the conclusion of the second semester the men had gained a more favorable perception of the community's interest in assisting the ex-offender. The community participants were enthusiastic about the program and expressed willingness to participate again in pre-release groups. The student gained experience in exploring community resources and an awareness of employment opportunities for the occupational therapist in the correctional setting.

At the conclusion of each semester the student and supervisor prepared summary letters for inclusion in the inmates' case files. A memorandum describing the occupational therapy program was distributed to the warden, case managers, and other prison staff.

Conclusion

The fieldwork experience at a Federal correctional institution was believed to be helpful to the students, the inmates, the institution, and the community. The students gained experience in group leadership, identification of clients' needs, and resourcefulness. They identified the role of occupational therapy and experienced some of the satisfactions and challenges of working in a non-medical setting.

The inmates in the group were provided with opportunities to identify and discuss their needs, to assess their personal skills, and to re-evaluate their views of community concern for the ex-offender. It is believed the men increased their knowledge of practical skills for a lawful future life.

The staff and inmates became more aware of occupational therapy and its potential for contributing to programs in a correctional setting; the dozen guest speakers from the community became more involved in the institution, and the staff gained information and resources for use in future pre-release groups.

Acknowledgment

Gratitude is extended to Dr. Tom Rosenbaum, Father Mark Santo, Mr. Henry Lams, and Ms. Ardeth Alderdyce for their contributions to the program.

REFERENCES

1. *Essentials of an Accredited Educational Program for the Occupational Therapist,* Rockville, Maryland: The American Occupational Therapy Association, Inc., 1973
2. Bolles R: *The Quick Job-Hunting Map,* Berkeley, California: Ten Speed Press, 1975

The American Journal of Occupational Therapy **387**

NEWS FROM THE FIELDWORK CORNER

As we enter a new year, fieldwork continues to be an integral component in occupational therapy education and in AOTA's strategic plan to maintain the viability of the profession. This year, fieldwork issues will revolve around a changing health care environment and increased numbers of students enrolling in occupational therapy education programs. With this first fieldwork column of the new year, we hope to communicate with OT practitioners, educators, and students regarding issues of concern in fieldwork and provide information on fieldwork resources available from the national office and nationwide.

A good place to start is to remind you about the network of regional fieldwork consultants available nationwide to use as a resource on fieldwork issues. For our purposes, the country has been divided into nine regions, with consultants available in each region. The individuals selected for these positions are recognized in their communities and regions for a certain level of fieldwork expertise.

The consultants participate in local and regional fieldwork councils and workshops, as requested by the schools or fieldwork clinical sites. Clinical fieldwork educators often seek out the consultants in their respective regions for advice or knowledge about particular fieldwork issues and concerns. Academic faculty will often present workshops in tandem with the regional fieldwork consultants for the clinical educators in their regions.

The regional fieldwork consultants meet once a year for information exchange and strategic planning in fieldwork; they may also present a small workshop to local constituents. Popular topics for workshops and fieldwork council meetings that the consultants have been involved in are supervision, identifying the developmental needs of students, OTR/OTA supervision collaboration, and innovative fieldwork models.

If you wish to access this network, use the roster on page 9 to determine who your regional fieldwork consultant is according to where you live and then call him or her directly. You may also contact me at the national office.

The consultants' role is to facilitate communication between clinical educators in fieldwork; therefore, they are ready and willing to answer questions on behalf of AOTA and according to their own experiences. Please feel free to utilize the network as often as you desire.

OT practitioners will be experiencing new and different service delivery models in the next few years; fieldwork will need to reflect the changes that are occurring in the health care environment. The regional fieldwork consultants can ease this transition while also helping to provide quality education. The consultants would appreciate hearing from you. —*Christine Rogers, MA, OTR/L, AOTA's fieldwork education program manager; 1383 Piccard Drive, P.O. Box 1725, Rockville, MD 20849-1725; (301) 948-9626, ext. 376*

NEWS FROM THE FIELDWORK CORNER

In the last five years, AOTA has advocated for innovative fieldwork experiences for Level II students. Due to a changing health care environment and increased competition for clinical placement, the need for innovative clinical placements has emerged in all areas of the country. As fieldwork constituents, we often conjure up various notions of what innovative fieldwork means. AOTA's fieldwork issues committee (FWIC) has selected models of innovative fieldwork from across the country. We hope to highlight one of these models each month. We will begin with a residential center for children and adults with developmental disabilities in Madison, Wis.

The Central Wisconsin Center is a residential setting for children and adults with developmental disabilities such as developmental delay and learning disabilities. The OT practitioners serve these individuals who currently live in the community or at the center.

The clinical education coordinator is Karen Kinnamon, OTR. Kinnamon meets with the staff initially to determine which of the 10 OTRs on staff would best suit the OT students' needs for fieldwork learning experiences. During the course of the students' affiliation, they may have two to three clinical supervisors in addition to Kinnamon. These OTR supervisors work in various settings within the 500-bed center, such as pediatrics, severely profound mental retardation, behavioral problems, and learning disabilities. The students, therefore, are exposed to a variety of populations and diagnoses.

The OTRs supervise the students' treatment and documentation, and Kinnamon confers in team meetings with the supervisors for the students' midterm, final, and weekly supervision meetings on a regular basis. The center has two part-time COTAs, who also participate and contribute to the students' program.

Kinnamon will coordinate fieldwork for up to five students at one time, from both levels of occupational therapy education. The OTRs have the primary responsibility for supervision of the OTA and OT students, with input from the COTAs. Joint treatment sessions with physical therapy interns and staff are encouraged.

At the Central Wisconsin Center, having multiple students affiliating at one time has been a positive experience. The program is structured to encourage teamwork and the participation by a majority of the OTRs on staff. Kinnamon does note a few problems with this structure; for example, some students find it difficult to match—and feel comfortable with—their different supervisors' writing styles for documentation purposes.

The FWIC selected this clinical site as innovative because of the unique supervision style, with multiple students affiliating at one time, and more than one supervisor for each student. In addition, the setting is appealing for the range of clients the center serves.

The Central Wisconsin Center, of Madison, Wis., is an example of the opportunities we have to expand and improve fieldwork education. Please contact me with questions regarding innovative fieldwork or this clinical site in particular. I can be reached Monday through Friday, 9 a.m. to 5 p.m. EST, at 1-800-877-1383, ext. 376. —*Christine Rogers, MA, OTR/L, AOTA's fieldwork education program manager*

OT WEEK / MARCH 17, 1994 **11**

NEWS FROM THE FIELDWORK CORNER

As an active fieldwork task group, the Fieldwork Issues Committee (FWIC) intends to fulfill AOTA's strategic plan of promoting innovative models of mental health and other types of fieldwork in light of changing service delivery models in health care. This is the second column to highlight such programs. This second model is a community-based psychosocial, drop-in program in St. Paul, Minn.

The Apollo Center of People Inc. is a drop-in program for adults with chronic mental health problems. Diagnoses include hearing and visual impairments, chemical dependency and dual disabilities. Shelly Linda, COTA, is the primary occupational therapy supervisor for four to six week COTA Level II student placements. Therapeutic recreation specialists and counselors also participate in the supervision process, as the whole team is responsible for the service delivery to the clients.

There are usually two to three COTA students affiliating at one time at the Apollo Center. They work very closely with the COTA initially, and then they are expected to gain more independence as they progress in their fieldwork experience. They may colead in-house activities and outings with the COTA and the other professional staff. Formal meetings with the students and the supervising COTA are held weekly and informal meetings are held as necessary.

Linda draws from three occupational therapy assistant programs in the region for Level II fieldwork placements, and good communication and collaboration with the academic fieldwork coordinators has been essential.

The FWIC selected this clinical site as innovative because of the unique supervision style at this setting (the COTA is the primary supervisor with an OTR reg-ularly available for consultation and supervision), and the appeal of the community-based program for people with chronic mental illness. As a COTA, Linda also relies on the strong relationship with the occupational therapy assistant programs and her teamwork with the other professionals at the center.

The Apollo Center of People Inc. is an example of the opportunities we have to expand and improve fieldwork education in mental health. If you have questions regarding innovative fieldwork or this clinical site in particular, please call me. If you are a fieldwork supervisor, student, or coordinator and feel that you may have a unique or creative fieldwork program, please contact me by phone or letter with your name, address, phone number, and facility. You can reach me Monday through Friday from 9 a.m. to 5 p.m. at 1-800-SAY-AOTA, ext. 376 (members) or (301) 948-9633, ext. 376 (nonmembers). Address your correspondence to AOTA, Fieldwork Education Program Manager, Education Department, 1383 Piccard Drive, P.O. Box 1725, Rockville, MD 20849-1725.

—Christine Rogers, MA, OTR/L,
AOTA's fieldwork education program manager

NEWS FROM THE FIELDWORK CORNER

Wendy Presecan, OTS, from Towson State University, Md., shares a personal account of her innovative fieldwork experience at Way Station Inc., in Frederick, Md.

I am shocked! I never thought I would choose mental health as my career focus in occupational therapy. Don't get me wrong, I thought mental illness was interesting but I had difficulty seeing any concrete benefits of treatment. My Level II fieldwork in psychiatry at Way Station Inc. in Frederick, Md., changed my attitude and my career goals.

Way Station is a community rehabilitation facility that focuses on re-entry of individuals with severe mental illness into the community. It does not have a traditional occupational therapy department and the Level II occupational therapy program was just beginning. A COTA student and I would be the first to participate and would be instrumental in the program's development.

Accepting the challenges this fieldwork offered was one of the best choices of my life. I became involved in a program that was concerned with facilitating "normalcy" in the lives of people with mental illness. This approach sounds like common sense, but I found this concept lacking in some of my other psychiatric experiences. My responsibilities at Way Station were varied, and at first I found it difficult to determine the function of occupational therapy in some of my assignments. I eventually realized that as an OT student I had special training and a way of looking at situations that was different from anyone else.

I used my training to help the direct service providers at Way Station do their job more effectively. I was responsible for a small caseload, so I had exposure to traditional methods of direct service. The nontraditional aspect of this fieldwork placement required that I act as a program consultant. I worked closely with my supervisor, Diana Ramsay, OTR/L, to understand my place in this framework, and to understand the principles of consultation. I worked collaboratively with direct service providers, who were primarily paraprofessionals. Together we developed a number of programmatic systems for training consumers in goal-related tasks at Way Station. For example, I worked collaboratively with my supervisor in the development of a job matrix system that would match a consumer's skills and rehabilitation goals with appropriate Way Station activities. I also assisted senior management staff in developing a quality assurance framework.

Working on several of these projects with a COTA student, Michael LaPole, gave me the opportunity to explore OTR-COTA collaboration and role delineation. I gained an appreciation for the COTA's skills in task analysis. I often had a broad focus on our projects, and it was useful to have Michael to keep me focused on specifics!

An important result of this experience is that I learned that all the course work I suffered through really did have a purpose and a practical application. Occupational therapy's philosophical concepts and their uses were vague to me at the beginning of my fieldwork. The theories became clear as I found myself using this knowledge base to explain the purpose and the role of occupational therapy to consumers and staff at Way Station. I realized that people with severe mental illness are just like anyone else, and they are not to be feared. In fact, these people are incredibly brave.

I was lucky enough to find a fieldwork setting in which all my course work fit. I was able to use all of my specialized skills to facilitate Way Station consumers' independence and quality of life.

I have been hired by Way Station to begin work as soon as my last fieldwork experience is completed. I have never been more excited about the contributions I can make to my consumers, occupational therapy and mental health!

Want to learn all about other innovations in fieldwork? Then come to Boston and attend the regional fieldwork consultants workshop on Sunday, July 10, 2:30-5:30 p.m., workshop A15 at conference.

We are now in the seventh month of our continuing series on innovation in fieldwork. For the past six months, I have been highlighting innovative models of fieldwork. I thought I would take a break from our series and review and define innovation in fieldwork. The Fieldwork Issues Committee (FWIC), in 1992, developed the Recommendations for Expanding Fieldwork document, which serves as a good reference point for innovative fieldwork models and is reprinted below. I would encourage you to follow up with the resources listed for further clarification of AOTA's viewpoints on innovative fieldwork.

Recommendations for Expanding Fieldwork

Rationale

Traditionally, fieldwork has been an experience where a student spends six weeks to three months at one facility with a single supervisor, often at a hospital or primary health care setting. Many factors are influencing the way occupational therapy practice and clinical education are provided. These factors include an increasing demand for OT services in expanding practice arenas, humanpower shortages, increasing numbers of students needing fieldwork placements, students with special needs, and a shrinking number of fieldwork placements. Occupational therapy's growth into broader practice arenas provides us with an opportunity to expand and improve the fieldwork education component to reflect current practice. This is an essential consideration in preparing students for entry-level practice.

Examples

Alternate fieldwork options that reflect current practice might include: part-time scheduling, e.g., half days for six months; flexible fieldwork schedule, e.g., longer than three months at one setting; part-time OT supervisor, e.g., placement with consulting OT; rotating through several programs at one setting; multiple sites, either with similar or different caseloads/focus, and with one or more supervisors; combined experiences, e.g., psychiatric and physical dysfunction, adult and pediatrics; one supervisor supervising more than one student simultaneously; newer practice or setting areas, e.g., chronic pain program; Alzheimer's program; head trauma; head start center; senior citizen center; special education center; work hardening/industrial injury center; rural home health; geropsychiatry; wellness program; department of corrections; substance abuse center; school affirmative action programs; retirement home; private practice; forensic mental health unit; adaptive living skills program; prevocational or vocational; cognitive retraining; health education center; administration/supervision; hospice programs; adaptive sports; family crisis centers; AIDS clinics and programs; camps; homeless shelter or soup kitchen; community-based programs.

Criteria

Fieldwork is a collaborative effort between students, clinicians and educators. Ideas for placement may originate with an academic program or with a practitioner. The following criteria may help indicate whether your practice would be appropriate as a fieldwork placement.

● Your practice provides opportunities for a student to:
   —learn OT skills and concepts, either general or specialized
   —apply OT skills and concepts, learned in the academic setting
   —experience success as a result of their OT intervention
   —communicate with other individuals in a professional manner
● You are interested in supervising students
   ● You are willing to collaborate with an academic fieldwork coordinator to plan and implement a student placement

Resources

Any of the following resources would be able to offer further assistance: Christine Rogers, MA. OTR/L, fieldwork education program manager, (301) 948-9626, ext. 376: regional fieldwork consultants' network; academic fieldwork coordinators (at all OT or OTA educational programs; COE fieldwork representatives—check with the educational programs.
—*Christine Rogers*

NEWS FROM THE FIELDWORK CORNER

An Innovative Program in South Dakota

In our continuing series on innovative fieldwork models, I am pleased to highlight the South Dakota Developmental Center at Custer (SDDC-C).

The SDDC at Custer is located in a rural setting with the nearest town having approximately 3,000 to 4,000 people. The institution is in the country and the school systems are small. Laura Burden, OTR, is an employee at the SDDC-C and a co-op that providers services to two school districts.

The SDDC at Custer serves individuals with severe, profound, multiple disabilities, and the school system provides occupational therapy services to children with sensory integration and fine motor deficits, in addition to other typical school interventions.

Burden has coordinated a small student program where the students practice occupational therapy at SDDC-C, the two school districts, and occasionally home health. The student is supervised directly by an OTR part-time or full-time per week at SDDC (with COTA input) and part-time in the school systems. Primarily, OT students have affiliated with Burden; however, the possibilities exist to begin OTA student supervision. The potential for growth, in terms of OT/OTA student programming and serving additional settings within the rural area, is apparent.

The student travels with Burden to the school settings to provide direct OT service and receive direct supervision. According to feedback from the students, this seems to be an ideal way to facilitate the mentoring process, especially with time during the drives up and back to discuss the cases and the supervisory process.

We have chosen this fieldwork setting as innovative due to its rural service delivery in multiple settings. The positive student feedback is testimony to the success of multiple settings with adequate supervision and the vast amounts of learning that a student experiences in a rural area.

If you are a fieldwork supervisor, student, or coordinator and feel that you have a unique or creative fieldwork program, please contact me by phone or letter with your name, address, phone number, and facility. You may contact me at AOTA, Education Department, 1383 Piccard Drive, P.O. Box 1725, Rockville, MD 20849; 1-800-SAY-AOTA, ext. 376. —*Christine Rogers, MA, OTR/L, AOTA's fieldwork education program manager*

NEWS FROM THE FIELDWORK CORNER

This month's innovative fieldwork setting is the ALS Regional Center, St. Peter's Hospital in Albany, N.Y. We chose this program for its unique learning opportunities with patients diagnosed with progressive degenerative neurological disease.

The ALS Regional Center provides services to 17 upstate New York counties. Primary intervention is for those diagnosed with ALS, and approximately 10 percent of the clients have other motor neuron diseases.

Dennie Whalen, OTR, one of two OTRs on staff, speaks fondly of the fieldwork students and their growth experiences at the ALS Regional Center. In addition to Whalen, who is also the fieldwork coordinator, the ALS Center is staffed by Barbara Thompson, OTR, and Karen Spinelli, RN. Students regularly follow patients and families in a variety of settings, including hand, outpatient, short-term inpatient and long-term care facility. They work collaboratively with the interdisciplinary team and with the community. The OT and OTA students' participation in groups such as the support group for the caregivers of children, a hospice training program, and attendance at one evening memorial service as part of bereavement follow-up are an important aspect to their experience at the ALS Center. According to Whalen, these are life experiences that contribute to the personal and professional development and maturity level of each student and staff member. The hospice training program and ex-

posure to St. Peter's Hospital also prepare a student for possible entry into a hospice model of occupational therapy service delivery.

In addition to typical documentation requirements, a student is required to complete an independent project. This has taken innovative forms such as guided imagery tape for an ALS spirituality group, the development of a children's support group, and the use of a life review project for the client who wishes to leave a legacy for family or friends.

Because of the challenging nature of this type of fieldwork, Whalen stresses that this opportunity is for the relatively autonomous, self-starting, and flexible student. The OTs at the ALS Center believe that they can provide a tremendous opportunity for creative approaches to treatment planning and practice of more nontraditional approaches in occupational therapy, along with personal growth.

Students have been a part of the ALS Regional Center because of the staff insights into innovative learning opportunities at their challenging setting and because of the teamwork of other disciplines in training the OT students. OT students have been affiliating with the ALS Regional Center since 1990; currently the center has arrangements with five colleges and universities.

The ALS Regional Center is an excellent example of a unique fieldwork setting for both levels of OT students, and one that we will continue to support.

Please contact me if you have questions or concerns about innovative fieldwork at 4720 Montgomery Lane, P.O. Box 31220, Bethesda, MD 20824-1220; 1-800-SAY-AOTA (members), (301) 652-AOTA (nonmembers), Monday-Friday, 7:30 a.m. to 3:30 p.m. —*Christine Rogers, MA, OTR/L, AOTA's fieldwork education program manager*

NEWS FROM THE FIELDWORK CORNER

I received the following letter from Deborah Waltermire, OTR/L, fieldwork education coordinator at the Sheppard and Enoch Pratt Hospital in Baltimore, Md. This is a wonderful example of an innovative fieldwork setting in mental health, and one that I am pleased to highlight this month as part of our continuing series.

"I am writing to tell you about a new fieldwork placement that we have developed at the Sheppard Pratt Health System. Although we continue to provide traditional inpatient and day hospital fieldwork experiences, we have recently started using a community psychosocial rehabilitation program for fieldwork.

New Ventures is a community psychosocial rehabilitation program located in Cockeysville, Md.—about six miles from our main hospital campus. They provide a clubhouse model of social support and recreational activities as well as prevocational skills training and other vocational programs.

In January 1994, we began a Level II fieldwork program with New Ventures. Because New Ventures does not have an OT on staff, OT interns spend two days a week there and three days a week at the main hospital. This combination provides interns with necessary occupational therapy supervision and role-modeling at the main hospital.

Direct supervision at New Ventures is provided by a licensed social worker. The social worker and the primary OT supervisor discuss the intern's issues and needs via telephone usually every other week. Part of the primary OT supervision time is allocated for discussion of New Ventures and the intern's roles and expectations, etc. A basic list of fieldwork objectives and guidelines for occupational therapy interns at New Ventures was also developed.

So far, the interns have really enjoyed this combination of inpatient and community fieldwork. They are experiencing a continuum of care in mental health, and have been able to work with clients on independent living skills since many of the clients are living in supervised apartments. The interns at New Ventures usually work on an administrative project such as member satisfaction surveys and program development. Such projects provide them with opportunities to use their occupational therapy training in an almost consultative role (with supervision from their primary OT supervisor) and help the interns learn about the potential role of OTs as consultants in mental health—especially community-based programs.

This has been an exciting program for us. The program director at New Ventures has also been pleased with the contributions that OT students have made to the program."

Please contact me if you have questions or comments about innovative fieldwork at 4720 Montgomery Lane, P.O. Box 31220, Bethesda, MD 20824-1220; 1-800-SAY-AOTA (members); (301) 652-AOTA (nonmembers), Monday-Friday, 7:30 a.m. to 3:30 p.m.

—*Christine Rogers, MA, OTR/L,*
AOTA's fieldwork education program manager

NEWS FROM THE FIELDWORK CORNER

It is now April, and we are in our second year of highlighting innovative models of fieldwork from around the country. We have also just wrapped up this year's AOTA Annual Conference and Exposition in Denver, where there were many opportunities to learn more about fieldwork. This is a good time to stop, take a breather and keep you posted on some of the national level fieldwork activities that you will need to be aware of.

One of the most often asked questions centers around the proposed revision of the fieldwork evaluation forms. This will be a two-phase project, which commenced in January. Phase I, which will take approximately one year, involves the identification of student learning outcomes (behavioral objectives that reflect a student's academic readiness prior to fieldwork). Phase II will be the development of the fieldwork evaluation tool for both levels (OT and OTA) using the student learning outcomes to guide this process, and with consultation from a research firm. We anticipate that this will be a three- to five-year project, including the field testing, so stay tuned.

Two documents, the fieldwork data form and the student evaluation of fieldwork experience, have also been revised and they will be available from the educational programs this year.

The fieldwork for the future (FWFF) task force also presented their recommendations to the Representative Assembly in Denver. This is the group that was charged to look at the future direction of fieldwork and to make recommendations for change. Stay alert to *OT Week*, contact the schools you have relationships with, and participate in your local or regional fieldwork councils for more information about the implementation of these recommendations.

One of the most rewarding fieldwork activities occurred in February at the national office. Focus groups were held to explore the thoughts and feelings of current fieldwork supervisors as well as practitioners who have not participated in student supervision or supervised students for a long period of time. The purpose of the focus groups was to gain valuable insight about the realistic and perceived benefits and restraints to student supervision. We will value and use this information as we evaluate the current fieldwork system.

Many of you are familiar with the AOTA *Fieldwork Centers Book*, which is updated and published annually. We have solicited the interest of a core group of schools to help us pilot a project where the academic fieldwork coordinators from these schools would help AOTA keep a more accurate and useful listing of fieldwork sites through Reliable Source. We hope to evaluate the feasibility of this project by mid-summer.

Let's talk innovation! The February issue of the *American Journal of Occupational Therapy* is devoted to new approaches to fieldwork education. A must-read for administrators, fieldwork coordinators, clinical supervisors, and practitioners and students.

The regional fieldwork consultants will be visible this year in their regions spreading the word on the FWFF recommendations and continuing to help members implement some of the innovative fieldwork models that we have been discussing this year. I must take the time to do a bit of recruiting for the three vacant regional fieldwork consultant positions. These would be OTs like yourself who live and work in either the Pacific Southwest, the South/Southwest, or the Central Midwest regions. If you have been supervising students for a minimum of five years, call me. This could be an exciting way to become involved.

The national activities surrounding fieldwork are exciting, challenging, and a little scary. I hope I have been able to provide you with some insight as to the extent of change that our profession is facing regarding our fieldwork system. As members of AOTA, it is certainly time for you to keep abreast and aware of these changes, and to share this information with your peers.

Please call me if you would like to know who your regional fieldwork consultant is (or if you think you may be interested in a position), and for any questions surrounding fieldwork and innovation. You can reach me Monday through Friday, 7:30 a.m. to 3:30 p.m. EST, 1-800-SAY-AOTA, ext. 2936 (AOTA members); (301) 652-2682, ext. 2936 (nonmembers); or 1-800-377-8555 (TDD users).

A special thank-you to the Baltimore-Washington Metropolitan area clinicians who participated in our first-ever fieldwork focus groups, and to all of you who responded to my initial questionnaire—it is wonderful to see such interest.

—Christine Rogers, MA, OTR/L,
AOTA's fieldwork education program manager

Go for the

The following article appeared in OT Week's Today's Student. *Put yourself in the place of the student as you read it. I think you will find a unique perspective that will help you supervise students more effectively or entertain the idea of supervising a student*

By
Christine
Rodgers,
MA,
OTR/L

SO YOU WANT TO GO ON FIELD-WORK? And you want to successfully pass fieldwork! What is all this talk about innovation in fieldwork? Does this mean you'll be inventing a new system of fieldwork? Is there such a thing as Newton's (or even Murphy's) law in fieldwork?

Murphy's law, gratefully, does not seem to be a factor in grappling with fieldwork, and Newton's laws are much too rigid, to say the least! What we do have are the "Essentials" of fieldwork. The "Essentials and guidelines for an accredited educational program for the occupational therapist/occupational therapy assistant" is occupational therapy's answer to a universal guide to OT education and fieldwork. With additional official guidelines to help interpret the "Essentials," we can go for the gusto and create innovative clinical learning experiences.

Before we go any further with this notion, a brief definition of the "Essentials" is in order. This is the document to which all OT education programs must adhere in order to achieve and maintain accreditation. Since fieldwork is a vital link between education and practice, it has its own section in the "Essentials." Educators, clinical practitioners, and students must follow the "Essentials" as part of our standards of practice. As a profession, we of course recognize the need to interpret this document,

and that leads us to our official guidelines for fieldwork experience. As a student, your role is to grasp some of the main concepts of the "Essentials," so that you can better discuss fieldwork opportunities with your school coordinator, and be better prepared as a professional in a changing workplace environment.

So *what, where,* and *how* does innovative fieldwork fit in all of this and should students be excited about these opportunities? The answer, without reservation, is yes. Students will be meeting the future needs of our profession. These needs are ever-changing, so what better way than for students to position themselves in settings such as community centers, home health, senior day care centers, and school systems. Have you thought about part-time fieldwork in two different settings, pairing up with another OT student during fieldwork, or affiliating for six months in one setting? There are a myriad of creative and worthwhile fieldwork opportunities for students of today as we approach the 21st century.

My instincts now lead me to guide you through the "Essentials" of fieldwork, so that you will be prepared for your fieldwork journey.

First and foremost, you must subscribe to the standards of the profession, including the code of ethics. These beliefs and behaviors are fundamental to any fieldwork experience, and they are

the foundation upon which your OT career is built. You will find the code of ethics and standards of practice in the OT literature and from AOTA.

Fieldwork objectives should be collaboratively developed between the school, clinical site, and the student. This is especially important in innovative fieldwork settings; the effort to develop objectives for a traditional or innovative type of fieldwork setting is paramount to a successful experience. Regular communication with your fieldwork coordinator and clinical supervisor is tantamount to a fieldwork experience that meets your expectations. Routine feedback about the objectives before and during fieldwork can help to ensure a positive experience.

Level II fieldwork is designed to promote clinical reasoning, reflect practice, communicate and model professionalism, apply ethics as it relates to the profession, and expand OT clinical competencies related to human performance intervention. This is attainable in all settings where there are OTRs. You will want to discuss with your fieldwork coordinator the possibilities that could exist where there may not be full-time, one-on-one supervision.

GUSTO!

Supervision must always be provided by an OTR with a minimum of one year of clinical experience. Your school, in collaboration with you, can consider and explore the legal, ethical, and professional ramifications of an innovative setting.

The ratio of fieldwork educators to students shall be appropriate for proper supervision and frequent assessments in achieving the fieldwork objectives. The quantity and quality of supervision are subject to interpretation of individual clinical programs, state regulations, standards of practice, ethical responsivilities, and the student's learning needs. There can be very positive fieldwork supervision in certain nontraditional settings, provided these factors are taken into account. Keep in mind that it takes effort to develop a model of fieldwork where the model of supervision may differ from the norm.

Fieldwork can be provided with various groups across the life span, people with psychosocial and physical performance deficits, and various service delivery models. For example, innovative models that we know about include an all-male, 3,000-bed medium security prison that offers rehabilitation and psychiatric services to its population and an ALS center that runs extensive patient and caregiver education programs as their primary OT focus. Some students affiliate in one place for their entire fieldwork experience; they may rotate among different units within the facility or work with pediatrics and geriatrics in a home health environment. The primary concern is that the fieldwork remains reflective of current practice in the profession.

If problems should arise at any time during your fieldwork, the communication channels with your school and your supervisor need to be in place. Your school is responsible for passing you on fieldwork; and your school has established a relationship with the clinical site and relies on your supervisor(s) for feedback and input. It is of critical importance that you establish regular and routine communication, especially in nontraditional clinical settings.

Take responsibility for your own learning; in innovative settings you may not always be privy to traditional learning experiences or OT peers other than your supervisor. Augment your learning with trips to other facilities, extra reading assignments, brainstorming with your faculty, or tackling new program development.

Be aware of fieldwork myths. What may seem "wrong" in one setting may be quite appropriate in another. What doesn't work in one setting may work in your placement. Be leery of comparisons among classmates of the "ideal" fieldwork placement; each and every fieldwork setting has the potential to make you a competent entry-level therapist.

Finally, use your national association! We are here as a resource and for guidance. The education department has devoted the past years to developing, encouraging, and fostering the implementation of innovative fieldwork models. You will be the future for occupational therapy; it is you who we encourage to participate in the world of innovation.

In closing, I would like to note that the "rules" of fieldwork are not so set in stone. We, as a profession, have guidelines to help you interpret the fundamental legal and ethical aspects of fieldwork. Beyond this lies a genuinely exciting and rewarding career in occupational therapy.

Christine Rogers is AOTA's fieldwork education program manager.

NEWS FROM THE FIELDWORK CORNER

As part of the continuing series on innovative fieldwork, I talked with Heidi Furth, OTR, who practices at the Good Samaritan Hospital, Center for Continuing Rehabilitation (CCR), in Puyallup, Wash. I was immediately attracted to the variety of services the CCR offers to both consumers and OT students in the community. The

CR is a postacute community-reintegration program for adults with head injuries. The program's desired outcomes target the improved skill and increased independence within the client's home, community and work. The OTs, as part of the interdisciplinary team, facilitate the clients' life-care planning, including accessing mental health services, referrals to hand clinics, ADL training, and other hospital services.

What makes the fieldwork program at CCR so innovative? The CCR therapists provide occupational therapy in the home and in supervised-living apartments in the community. They also receive direct admissions from acute care and treat between 12 and 14 clients in the clinic, with some clients commuting as outpatients. OT fieldwork students have a unique chance to become involved in all of these services as part of their learning continuum.

The CCR inpatient and outpatient clinics offer fieldwork Level I and II experiences with direct one-on-one supervision. The OT practitioners also hope to have Level II fieldwork students participating in the home health program and/or float between the center-based and home health service-delivery models. Another opportunity for fieldwork students at CCR is to provide supervision for OT students from the University of Puget Sound who are working in the community living program. This program provides apartments for patients and families who are receiving services from Good Samaritan/CCR and who require continued 24-hour care. Fieldwork students are often hired to provide caretaking services as aides to the clients living in these apartments. Excellent related learning experiences are provided and professional development for both the fieldwork II students and the university students is promoted. This collaboration between students also provides program-planning experience in the community and home environment.

The OTs at Good Samaritan/CCR work with both Level I and II fieldwork students from the professional level and are preparing for a fieldwork program with OTA students as well. Further, the OT staff and other team members are able to provide unique learning experiences in a variety of ways, including center-based, home care, and community living services for clients age 17 and over with head injuries. It is exciting to think that a fieldwork student can tap into all these services as part of the personal learning and development opportunities offered at CCR.

If you would like more information about Good Samaritan/CCR, please contact me at 1-800-SAY-AOTA (members) or (301) 652-2682, ext. 2936.

—Christine Rogers, MA, OTR/L, is AOTA's fieldwork education program manager

FIELDWORK CORNER

The last 18 months of this column have been devoted to describing innovative fieldwork models in a variety of practice settings. These have been based on real OTs in real settings who have succeeded in employing new ideas and supervision styles in Level II fieldwork.

As OT fieldwork supervisors and students, we should function with a degree of comfort when it comes to trying new things in fieldwork. The innovative models that I have presented thus far may still cause some disconcertion on the part of OT educators, students and practitioners, so perhaps we should look at what AOTA says about fieldwork (Levels I and II) to provide this comfort level for therapists supervising students.

The 10 quiz items below are the first in a five-part quiz series on all aspects of fieldwork. The fieldwork statements represent the AOTA essentials for accreditation; AOTA guidelines for fieldwork Levels I and II; innovative fieldwork models; the rights and responsibilities of students, sites and schools; and fieldwork myths. Your goal is to distinguish fact from fiction in the 10 statements.

So, pick up your pencil and get started. Each fieldwork statement below corresponds to one of the fieldwork categories listed below: A, B, C, D, or E. Place the appropriate letter (only one) in the column to the left of each of the statements.

Remember, this is the first part of a five-part quiz series on AOTA and fieldwork. Stay tuned to the monthly "Fieldwork Corner" column in *OT Week* for the entire series. Collect the entire series and share the information with your clinical site and school. Future articles will address each statement in more depth to help you interpret the correct answers. I can be reached Monday through Friday, 9 a.m. to 5 p.m. eastern time at 1-800-SAY-AOTA, ext. 2936. —*Christine Rogers, MA, OTR/L, is AOTA's fieldwork education program manager*

Categories

A = The Essentials for an Accredited Educational Program for the Occupational Therapist/Occupational Therapy Assistant. This is the document to which all OT educational programs must adhere to achieve and maintain accreditation. Schools must demonstrate substantial compliance with the "Essentials" and report to the Accreditation Council for Occupational Therapy Education.

B = Guidelines for Fieldwork Levels I and II. These are Commission on Education (COE) documents and are guidelines only. They are not regulations, but what the COE says if you ask AOTA to interpret the "Essentials."

C = Innovative Fieldwork Models. This is information that is disseminated from AOTA about innovative fieldwork models. They are suggestions and recommendations about innovative fieldwork.

D = Rights and Responsibilities of Students, Schools and Sites. This material interprets the fundamental rights and responsibilities (including legal, ethical, and professional) of students, schools, and sites.

E = Fieldwork Myths. This is information about fieldwork that circulated in the OT community that may or may not be true.

Statements

_____ 1. The fieldwork site should have a stated philosophy regarding service delivery.

_____ 2. Supervision must be provided by an OTR on Level II fieldwork.

_____ 3. Supervision must be provided by an OTR with a minimum of one year of experience.

_____ 4. A school or a site can develop its own Level I fieldwork evaluation form.

_____ 5. Fieldwork should be completed within 24 months of the OT academic program.

_____ 6. The student should not miss more than three days of fieldwork.

_____ 7. A fieldwork consultant can be used to supervise students part-time or full-time in fieldwork.

_____ 8. The fieldwork evaluation form is a required performance evaluation.

_____ 9. A supervisor should have no more than three students at a time.

_____ 10. A student must file a formal grievance with the school first if problems with fieldwork grade arise.

(*Answers: 1.B 2.A 3.A 4.D 5.A 6.E 7.C 8.E 9.E 10.D*)

This is the second installment of a five-part series of fieldwork quiz questions (see the July 13 issue for Part 1). Remember, the questions and answers that you find here are meant to increase your comfort level with trying new things in fieldwork. Collect the entire series and share the information with your clinical site and school. Future articles will address each statement in more depth to help you interpret the correct answers. I can be reached Monday through Friday from 7 a.m. to 3:30 p.m. eastern time at 1 (800) SAY-AOTA, ext. 2936, if you have questions or comments.

Each fieldwork statement below corresponds to one of the fieldwork categories listed below: A, B, C, D, or E. Place the appropriate letter (only one) in the column to the left of each of the statements. —*Christine Rogers is AOTA's fieldwork education program manager*

Categories

A = The Essentials for an Accredited Educational Program for the Occupational Therapist/Occupational Therapy Assistant. This is the document to which all OT educational programs must adhere to achieve and maintain accreditation. Schools must demonstrate substantial compliance with the Essentials and report to the Accreditation Council for Occupational Therapy Education.

B = Guidelines for Fieldwork Level I and II. These are Commission on Education (COE) documents and are guidelines only. They are not regulations, but what the COE says if you ask AOTA to interpret the Essentials.

C = Innovative Fieldwork Models. This is information that is disseminated from AOTA about innovative fieldwork models. They are suggestions and recommendations about innovative fieldwork.

D = Rights and Responsibilities of Students, Schools and Sites. This material interprets the fundamental rights and responsibilities (including legal, ethical, and professional) of the student, school, and/or site.

E = Fieldwork Myth. This is information about fieldwork that circulated in the OT community that may or may not be true.

Statements

_____ 11. Entry-level OTR must have routine supervision.

_____ 12. A supervisor must be present at least half of the time.

_____ 13. Fieldwork must be a minimum of two three-month affiliations.

_____ 14. Fieldwork experience must be three months in mental health and three months in physical disabilities.

_____ 15. Schools can require more than the minimum of three months (OTA) or six months (OT) of fieldwork.

_____ 16. The fieldwork experience shall be evaluated by the student using the AOTA "Student Evaluation of Fieldwork Experience" form.

_____ 17. The school submits names of eligible candidates to sit for the national registration exam.

_____ 18. International fieldwork is for OT programs only.

_____ 19. National Office internships are for OT students only.

_____ 20. Fieldwork can be in any setting where there is OTR supervision.

Answers (11. B, 12. E, 13. E, 14. E, 15. D, 16. D, 17. D, 18. E, 19. E, 20. C)

This is the third installment of a five-part series of fieldwork quiz questions. Remember the questions and answers that you find here are meant to increase your comfort level with trying new things in fieldwork. Collect the entire series and share the information with your peers. Future articles will address each statement in more depth to help you interpret the correct answers. I can be reached Monday-Friday from 7:30 a.m. to 3:30 p.m. eastern time at 1 (800) SAY-AOTA, ext. 2936, if you have comments or questions.

Each fieldwork statement below corresponds to one of the fieldwork categories listed: A, B, C, D, or E. Place the appropriate letter (only one) in the column to the left of each of the statements. —*Christine Rogers is AOTA's fieldwork education program manager*

Categories

A = The Essentials for an Accredited Educational Program for the Occupational Therapist/Occupational Therapy Assistant. This is the document to which all OT educational programs must adhere to achieve and maintain accreditation. Schools must demonstrate substantial compliance with the Essentials and report to the Accreditation Council for Occupational Therapy Education.

B = Guidelines for Fieldwork Level I and II. These are Commission on Education (COE) documents and are guidelines only. They are not regulations, but what the COE says if you ask AOTA to interpret the Essentials.

C = Innovative Fieldwork Models. This is information that is disseminated from AOTA about innovative fieldwork models. They are suggestions and recommendations about innovative fieldwork.

D = Rights and Responsibilities of Students, Schools and Sites. This material interprets the fundamental rights and responsibilities (including legal, ethical, and professional) of the student, school, and/or site.

E = Fieldwork Myth. This is information about fieldwork that circulated in the OT community that may or may not be true.

Statements

_____ 21. Must have a written contract between clinical site and school for fieldwork.

_____ 22. Must use fieldwork evaluation form at midterm.

_____ 23. There is an AOTA-required passing score (criteria score) on the fieldwork evaluation form.

_____ 24. Can pair OT with OTA students on fieldwork.

_____ 25. AOTA advocates for two students to one supervisor in certain settings.

_____ 26. There can be non-OT supervisors for Level I fieldwork.

_____ 27. A student can spend six months in one setting for fieldwork.

_____ 28. A student can complete fieldwork part-time.

_____ 29. A student can meet psychosocial objectives in a physical disability setting to fulfill mental health requirement.

_____ 30. Fieldwork can occur in the home health setting

Answers: 21. A 22. E 23. E 24. C 25. C 26. A 27. C 28. C 29. C 30. C

This is the fourth installment of a five-part series of fieldwork quiz questions. Remember the questions and answers that you find here are meant to increase your comfort level with trying new things in fieldwork. Collect the entire series and share the information with your peers. Future articles will address each statement in more depth to help you interpret the correct answers. I can be reached Monday-Friday from 7:30 a.m. to 3:30 p.m. Eastern time at 1(800) SAY-AOTA, ext. 2936, if you have comments or questions.

Each fieldwork statement corresponds to one of the fieldwork categories listed below: A, B, C, D, or E. Place the appropriate letter (only one) in the column to the left of each of the statements. —*Christine Rogers is AOTA's fieldwork education program manager*

Catagories

A = The Essentials for an Accredited Educational Program for the Occupational Therapist/Occupational Therapy Assistant. This is the document to which all OT educational programs must adhere to achieve and maintain accreditation. Schools must demonstrate substantial compliance with the Essentials and report to the Accreditation Council for Occupational Therapy Education.

B = Guidelines for Fieldwork Level I and II. These are Commission on Education (COE) documents and are guidelines only. They are not regulations, but what the COE says if you ask AOTA to interpret the Essentials.

C = Innovative Fieldwork Models. This is information that is disseminated from AOTA about innovative fieldwork models. They are suggestions and recommendations about innovative fieldwork.

D = Rights and Responsibilities of Students, Schools and Sites. This material interprets the fundamental rights and responsibilities (including legal, ethical, and professional) of the student, school, and/or site.

E = Fieldwork Myth. This is information about fieldwork that circulated in the OT community that may or may not be true.

Statements

_____ 31. School faculty can be fieldwork supervisors in certain settings.

_____ 32. The clinical site is responsible for the grading of fieldwork.

_____ 33. Fieldwork objectives should be collaboratively developed.

_____ 34. There is a minimum of 940 hours of fieldwork for OT students.

_____ 35. The school determines a student's fieldwork grade.

_____ 36. International fieldwork must be provided where there is no language barrier.

_____ 37. Fieldwork should promote clinical reasoning.

_____ 38. Fieldwork objectives must be documented.

_____ 39. Fieldwork objectives should reflect role delineation between professional and assistant level students.

_____ 40. The ratio of fieldwork educators to students must ensure adequate supervision.

Answers: 31. C, 32. E, 33. A, 34. A, 35. A, 36. D, 37. A, 38. A, 39. B, 40. A.

OT WEEK / NOVEMBER 2, 1995 **7**

Advice on Fieldwork

What should be done if a supervisor is unable to be on-site while a student is working in the clinic? Is this OK? Many fieldwork educators become ill for a few days or wish to take vacations or attend continuing education workshops off site; what would AOTA say?

In fieldwork, there may not always be concrete answers, and this is a fairly complex question. First, you should designate a person as the party who is responsible for the student in your absence (this must be done for liability). The responsible party could be an occupational therapist or a certified occupational therapy assistant who is on staff or another member of the health care team. When you have selected this person, make sure that this change in authority is clear to both the student and the practitioner in charge. You should then contact the academic fieldwork coordinator at the student's school and apprise him or her of the situation. Remember, communication is key in this temporary situation so that all of the professionals are aware of and in agreement with your plan. Additionally, you can modify the student's fieldwork objectives for the time you are away (e.g., less caseload and more program planning).

Second, all of our AOTA documents refer to the professional and ethical judgments of the occupational therapy practitioner when it comes to supervision of the student. *Occupational Therapy Roles* states that supervision is provided "by an administrator or specifically designated individual. The level of supervision varies with the skills of the educator, complexity of setting, and nature of student's learning needs." The *Essentials and Guidelines for an Accredited Program for the Occupational Therapist/Occupational Therapy Assistant* states, "The ratio of fieldwork educators to students shall be such as to ensure proper supervision and frequent assessment in achieving fieldwork objectives." And finally, the *Guidelines for an Occupational Therapy Fieldwork Experience—Level II* state, "The ratio of fieldwork educators considered adequate to carry out a fieldwork experience is dependent upon the complexity of the service and the ability to ensure proper supervision and frequent assessment in achieving fieldwork objectives."

AOTA encourages occupational therapists to consider the context of their work environment and their students' learning needs. Often clinicians are also bound by their employers and staff philosophies on clinical education and supervision (in terms of the amount and structure of supervisory sessions). Please remember that good communication with the student, your peers at your clinical site, and the faculty at the student's school will help ensure a smooth experience for your student while you are away.

If you have any questions or comments, contact Christine Rogers, Fieldwork Education Program Manager, AOTA, 4720 Montgomery Lane, PO Box 31220, Bethesda, MD 20824-1220, 1-800-SAY-AOTA, ext. 2936 (members), or 301-652-2682, ext. 2936 (nonmembers). All of the documents mentioned in the article above are available from AOTA's Products department.

Congratulations! You have made it to the final segment of this five-part quiz series. Once you complete this last section, you will be ready to tackle new fieldwork models and expand your current student program.

Remember, this quiz is designed to increase your comfort level with our current fieldwork system and to provide information from AOTA to help you design your programs. The key is to collaborate in an ongoing manner with the education program, the student, and your fellow OT peers to provide a quality fieldwork experience.

Stay tuned for future fieldwork corner articles. I can be reached Monday through Friday from 7:30 a.m. to 3:30 p.m. eastern time at 1-800-SAY-AOTA, ext. 2936, if you have comments or questions.

Each fieldwork statement corresponds to one of the fieldwork categories listed below: A, B, C, D, or E. Place the appropriate letter (only one) in the column to the left of each of the statements.

—Christine Rogers, MA, OTR/L, AOTA's fieldwork education program manager

Categories

A = The Essentials for an Accredited Educational Program for the Occupational Therapist/Occupational Therapy Assistant. The document to which all OT educational programs must adhere to achieve and maintain accreditation. Schools must demonstrate substantial compliance with the Essentials and report to the Accreditation Council for Occupational Therapy Education.

B = Guidelines for Fieldwork Level I and II. These are Commission on Education (COE) documents and are guidelines only. They are the COE's interpretation of the Essentials.

C = Innovative Fieldwork Models. This information is disseminated from AOTA about innovative fieldwork models. They are suggestions and recommendations about innovative fieldwork.

D = Rights and Responsibilities of Students, Schools and Sites. This interprets the fundamental rights and responsibilities (including legal, ethical, and professional) of the student, school, and/or site.

E = Fieldwork Myth. This information is circulated in the OT community and may or may not be true.

Statements

_____ 41. There should be regular communication between the school and the clinical site.

_____ 42. Schedule design of Level I will depend on the type of setting and the curriculum of the school.

_____ 43. Level I fieldwork can be supervised by any qualified personnel.

_____ 44. Level I fieldwork can substitute for any part of Level II fieldwork.

_____ 45. OTA fieldwork must be completed in 18 months from academic program.

_____ 46. The school collaborates with the clinical site and student only in arranging fieldwork placement.

_____ 47. AOTA approves fieldwork sites.

_____ 48. Students have a choice whether to sign release of information.

_____ 49. Supervision should be provided daily and/or weekly as an essential part of the program.

_____ 50. Fieldwork must follow AOTA's standards of practice and code of ethics.

Answers: 41. B, 42. B, 43. A, 44. E, 45. A, 46. D, 47. E, 48. D, 49. B, 50. A

Corner by Christine Rogers Privott

Home Health

It is the start of another calendar year for fieldwork and another year for OT practitioners to consider innovations in fieldwork. The home health setting is an emerging practice arena for OT students that exhibits some uncertainty in terms of supervision guidelines.

The following profile of Willowbrook Home Health Care Inc. is a result of talking with Ted Krackowiak, OTR/L, who has been an OTR for eight years and has incorporated student programming into his daily role as a home health OTR.

Willowbrook is a full service home health agency based in Tennessee that provides OTs, PTs, speech therapists, nursing staff, home health aides, social workers, and various specialists. It provides services in 18 counties in middle Tennessee to clients who are primarily diagnosed with orthopedic and neurologic conditions. Most of its clients are insured by Medicare/Medicaid and private plans.

Krackowiak has been working primarily with Level II fieldwork students, who are paired up for home visits and supervised by him on a daily basis. The students see clients in the inner city as well as small rural communities, which provide for an eclectic mix of treatment opportunities requiring flexibility and good organizational skills. The daily schedule can be quite unpredictable. As with most student fieldwork, the experience is progressive, so that the student is able to treat clients independently with minimal supervision near the end of the program. Currently, one other OTR and two COTAs are participating in student supervision.

The fieldwork student also has the opportunity to travel with members of the other disciplines at Willowbrook to learn professional role interaction. Most of the one-on-one supervision occurs during the course of the day as the pair drives to and from clients' homes. This seems to be an excellent method for ongoing supervision. The Willowbrook administration has pledged full support for the student fieldwork program and has a good relationship with the student OT education program. Willowbrook is also currently developing a new student manual with hopes for expanding their student program.

The AOTA supervision guidelines remain basic to allow for professional interpretation of what is appropriate for each particular setting. The AOTA *Guidelines for Occupational Therapy Practice in Home Health* (1995) states that "all levels of practitioners should recognize that ongoing supervision is a necessary component of the practice setting . . . specific supervision requirements vary according to public health, state, and agency rules and regulations." The AOTA Commission on Education *Guidelines for Level II Fieldwork* (1993) recommends that a supervisor be present at least half of the time. These are, however, only guidelines and subject to further interpretation in the home health setting. It is important to remember that supervision is an interactive process that requires both the OTR/COTA and the student to share responsibility—the OTR/COTA should provide supervision and the student should seek it (*Guidelines for Occupational Therapy Practice in Home Health*).

Willowbrook is a good example of an agency that is able to offer student fieldwork with regular supervision in a community setting. Of importance to any home health fieldwork experience is the student's preparedness to practice in a less structured environment with different supervision expectations. The fieldwork educator can also consider new models of supervision while demonstrating good professional judgment in supervising the student. It is apparent in today's health care environment that we should be moving our services toward the community, and it begins with fieldwork. The supervision guidelines for students in home health allow practitioners to interpret their student program individually.

Resource List

In collaboration with the home health and community SIS, I would like to start a resource list of OTR/COTA practitioners who are involved with student fieldwork in home health. This list would contain individuals involved in home health fieldwork and who could serve as a resource for inquiries about different supervision styles and learning needs for students in home health. If you are interested, please call me, Christine Rogers Privott, MA, OTR/L, AOTA fieldwork education program manager, at 1-800-SAY-AOTA, ext. 2936 (members) or (301) 652-2682, ext. 2936 (nonmembers).

— Christine Rogers Privott is AOTA's fieldwork education program manager.

Call 1-800-SAY-AOTA for membership information and benefits.

January 25, 1996 / OT WEEK **9**

Corner by Christine R. Privott, MA, OTR/L

Last month's column discussed home health fieldwork as an emerging innovative fieldwork model. This month, I will discuss one of the more apparent innovative fieldwork models, which is the collaborative supervision model, or more than one student to a supervisor. For some of you this model may no longer seem different or innovative, but for others, collaborative fieldwork connotes double the amount of work!

In its simplest form, this model places more than one student (typically a pair) with one primary supervisor. The pair of students may be predetermined by the school, or the clinical site may assign the pairs, depending on the number of fieldwork students scheduled at the clinical site. The OT supervisor meets with the group initially for orientation and to discuss strategies for client treatment in a group supervision model. The supervisory feedback sessions typically evolve to once a week, since the students quickly learn the benefits of peer feedback and mentoring; other members of the health care team are also involved in the day-to-day supervision. Client treatment can be provided by both students together and often both students run groups together as well. While sharing a full staff caseload, students also work with a client one-on-one as the student partner observes, periodically switching roles. The students

must be evaluated for competency at midterm and near completion of the fieldwork experience, and this is achieved by meeting with both students and allowing some time for individual consultation.

Students' perspectives of this collaborative approach to fieldwork have been positive and have resulted in worthwhile outcomes. They see themselves as better prepared for actual practice and comfortable that they have fully achieved fieldwork requirements. They also report increased creativity in the practice environment. Fieldwork supervisors extol the benefits of collaborative fieldwork because the students tend to problem solve together and they exhibit increased independence and confidence overall. In this day of managed care, the collaborative approach to fieldwork also gives us some tangible benefits in terms of a cost-benefit analysis; more than one student at a site can contribute to more provision of services while providing more individual attention to the clients.

To sum up, I would be remiss if I did not mention a few possible drawbacks to the collaborative learning process. The paired students may progress at a different pace and develop their own group dynamics separate from the larger group dynamics of the OT department. Supervisors should always allow for the option of disbanding the pair and facilitating one-on-one supervision during the fieldwork. The collaborative model can allow for ample supervision and feedback to the students, but not twice the amount of time and effort.

If you have questions or concerns, please contact Christine R. Privott at 1-800-SAY-AOTA, ext. 2936 (members) or (301) 652-2682, ext. 2936 (non-members).

1+1=2?

Call 1-800-SAY-AOTA for membership information and benefits.

February 29, 1996 / OT WEEK 7

Models of Fieldwork | 347

Corner by Christine R. Privott, MA, OTR/L

What Does It Take to Become a Fieldwork Supervisor? Do You Know How to Get Started?

Well, look no further! I am here to tell you that becoming a fieldwork supervisor is achievable and believable. There are basically two questions integral to the recruitment of the new fieldwork supervisor—What are the AOTA guidelines for student supervision? What are the intrinsic values associated with mentoring a student?

First, what are AOTA's minimum requirements for supervising students? The AOTA "Essentials for an Accredited Educational Program for the Occupational Therapist and Occupational Therapy Assistant" states:

• **Level II: OT/OTA student supervision shall be provided by qualified personnel including, but not limited to, certified occupational therapists, certified occupational therapy assistants, teachers, social workers, nurses, and physical therapists.**

• **Level II: OT student supervision shall be provided by a certified occupational therapist with a minimum of one year experience in a practice setting.**

OTA student supervision shall be provided by a certified occupational therapist or a certified occupational therapy assistant with a minimum of one year experience in a practice setting.

The AOTA and OT and OTA education programs have additional fieldwork supervision training resources available for the critical development of your role as a student supervisor. Keep in mind that the one year experience "rule" should apply to those OT practitioners who have passed the national certification exam and have started work as an OTR or a COTA.

Now let's take a look at the extrinsic and intrinsic rewards of becoming a fieldwork supervisor. Supervising students can:

* **Provide a sense of personal pride**
* **Enhance personal and professional development**
* **Offer an opportunity to give back to the profession**
* **Bring new ideas to the clinic**
* **Provide an opportunity to be part of a mentoring facility**
* **Expose clients and staff to the latest techniques and theories in the field**
* **Foster a beneficial relationship with academia**
* **Offer an opportunity to see that clients respond well to students**

Becoming a fieldwork supervisor can be reminiscent of all of those characteristics that led you to the profession in the first place; patience, creativity, tolerance, and open-mindedness.

Hopefully you are now aware that: AOTA wants you to be a fieldwork supervisor. You meet the minimum eligibility requirements for student supervision. You know that AOTA and the education programs have resource materials available to you. You can truly make an impact on the profession. You see intrinsic value in mentoring a student.

You are ready to garner administrative support and present your proposal to your manager. You may need to ask yourself, why does an organization participate in OT fieldwork?

✓ **Occupational therapists have a responsibility to share skills and knowledge just as an organization must provide quality health care**

✓ **Participation in fieldwork is an excellent recruitment technique and good public relations with universities and communities**

✓ **Teaching students creates new projects and activities that are appreciated by all**

✓ **Student teaching contributes to the education of all health care providers**

Overall, supervising students is an enriching experience that truly benefits everyone involved. There can be obstacles in setting up a fieldwork program yet AOTA and the education programs can be instrumental in guiding you and tapping into resources.

We also have a fieldwork brochure, "Say Yes to Fieldwork! Occupational Therapy Clinical Education Is for You!" that includes the above information and additional helpful tips from colleagues on how you can become a fieldwork supervisor. I would encourage you to request a sample brochure from the AOTA education department, to entice your peers to supervise students!

Please call AOTA's education department, (301) 652-2682, ext. 2930, for further information.

Remember, becoming a fieldwork supervisor is achievable and believable! —*Christine Privott is AOTA's fieldwork education program manager.*

The American Occupational Therapy Association, Inc.

Advice on Fieldwork

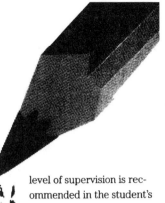

How should Level II fieldwork supervisors use the fieldwork evaluation forms with their students? How are the scores converted to grades? The use of the fieldwork evaluation forms varies from placement to placement and often even within the same placement among fieldwork educators. All clinical performance evaluations may be interpreted differently and are therefore subjective to some extent. In order to minimize the subjectivity and evaluate each student more objectively, AOTA encourages the fieldwork site supervisor to write behavioral objectives for each of the items on the fieldwork evaluation forms; however, writing and implementing fieldwork objectives does not necessarily eliminate the confusion over scoring and interpretation.

The final responsibility for grading the student on fieldwork rests with the student's education program representative (e.g., program director, academic fieldwork coordinator). This person will have a scale set up for either pass/fail or a numerical grade. The education program representative usually develops these grading scales after consulting with the fieldwork educators from various sites and other educators in the region. AOTA recommends that fieldwork evaluation scores be used as a guidance tool to determine the student's overall level

of competency. Ideally, the fieldwork supervisor, in consultation with other staff when appropriate, evaluates and determines the student's readiness for entry-level practice, and the fieldwork evaluation score supports this opinion. This should be a comprehensive assessment of the student, including not only the AOTA fieldwork evaluation score but the clinical, ethical, and professional judgment of the supervisor. After a thorough review and discussion with the student, followed by recommendations, the fieldwork evaluation form is sent to the education program representative for review and scoring according to the program's grading system.

What would be appropriate in a situation where the fieldwork supervisor rates the student using the AOTA fieldwork evaluation form, and the student's score, according to AOTA guidelines, is borderline passing? The supervisor should ask for input from other staff members and the academic fieldwork coordinator regarding the student's competency to practice. The supervisor should further demonstrate professional reasoning and judgment in recommending this student for entry-level practice, without focusing on the AOTA score. Would this student do well in a different setting? What

level of supervision is recommended in the student's first practice setting? Would this student succeed under different circumstances? Are the items on the fieldwork evaluation form truly reflective of the student's potential? What are the questionable items, and would the student respond well to suggested remediation activities? Remember, the strategies and recommendations should still be indicative of what any entry-level therapist typically would learn on his or her first job. The supervisor should also request a copy of the education program's grade policy from the academic fieldwork coordinator before forming a final opinion.

It is critical that there be a certain level of trust between the education program representatives and the fieldwork site supervisors to ensure proper interpretation of fieldwork scores. The education program faculty select the fieldwork sites and clinical educators to train and prepare their students for entry-level practice. Fieldwork site supervisors are obliged to provide their professional interpretation of a student's performance and to use the fieldwork evaluation tool and subsequent scores for guidance.

Remember that the first page of the evaluation forms contains a comment section in which the fieldwork educator can summarize or include areas not covered in the evaluation. A separate letter can be written and used to elaborate on matters of student competency or to serve as a reference. Continuous communication is vital during any aspect of fieldwork; there should be no surprises at the end!

If you have any questions or comments, contact Christine R. Privott, Fieldwork Education Program Manager, AOTA, 4720 Montgomery Lane, PO Box 31220, Bethesda, MD 20824-1220, 1-800-SAY-AOTA, ext. 2936 (members), or 301-652-2682, ext. 2936 (nonmembers).

Three Faculty-Facilitated, Community-Based Level I Fieldwork Programs

Kay Rydeen, Lisette Kautzmann, Mary K. Cowan, Penny Benzing

Key Words: education, occupational therapy • fieldwork, occupational therapy, Level I • teaching methods

Finding sufficient placements for students' Level I fieldwork experiences has become a major challenge in occupational therapy education and has led to the increased involvement of faculty members in facilitating these experiences. The conceptualization, site selection, program implementation, and outcome of three faculty-facilitated Level I fieldwork programs, designed for occupational therapy fieldwork students at Eastern Kentucky University, are presented here. The first program involved moving a faculty member and students to a small town in the mountains of Eastern Kentucky for 4 weeks and assigning the students to pediatric fieldwork at local agencies. The second, organized and developed by a faculty member and implemented by faculty members and students, provided an enrichment opportunity to adult consumers of psychosocial services. The third, also organized and developed by one faculty member and implemented by faculty members and students, provided day-care services to persons with Alzheimer's disease. In all three programs, persons receiving services as well as the agencies, students, and faculty members benefited from the experience. The use of faculty role models is recommended to demonstrate and reinforce the application of theory to practice.

Kay Rydeen, MOT, OTR/L, is Assistant Professor and Level I Fieldwork Coordinator, Eastern Kentucky University, College of Allied Health and Nursing, Department of Occupational Therapy, 103 Dizney Building, Richmond, Kentucky 40475-3135.

Lisette Kautzmann, EdD, OTR/L, FAOTA, is Associate Professor, Eastern Kentucky University, College of Allied Health and Nursing, Department of Occupational Therapy, Richmond, Kentucky.

Mary K. Cowan, MA, OTR/L, FAOTA, is Professor and Level I Fieldwork Coordinator, Eastern Kentucky University, College of Allied Health and Nursing, Department of Occupational Therapy, Richmond, Kentucky.

Penny Benzing, MA, OTR/L, FAOTA, is Associate Professor, Eastern Kentucky University, College of Allied Health and Nursing, Department of Occupational Therapy, Richmond, Kentucky.

This article was accepted for publication February 14, 1994.

The purpose of Level I fieldwork is to provide students with experiences that enrich didactic course work through directed observation and participation with varied populations in selected aspects of the occupational therapy process (American Occupational Therapy Association, 1991). The conceptualization and delivery of Level I fieldwork stem from each academic program's priorities, philosophical base, conceptual model, and internal and external resources and constraints. Therefore, it is important to describe the academic setting that propelled and nurtured the development of each program described in this article.

Eastern Kentucky University is a regional, public university with an enrollment of 15,000 students. It is located in Richmond, Kentucky, a rural town 26 miles south of Lexington, one of the state's two major urban centers. The university's service region covers the Appalachian mountain area of southeastern Kentucky. The Department of Occupational Therapy is located in the largest college on campus: the College of Allied Health and Nursing. The university is not affiliated with a medical school or clinical facility.

Since the occupational therapy program began in 1976, the number of students and faculty members has increased rapidly. In addition to the graduate program, 50 students are admitted each semester as second-semester sophomores in the undergraduate program. Sixteen students are admitted once per year to the post-baccalaureate program. There are 24 full-time, tenure-track faculty members. The curriculum is based on concepts of human adaptation across the life span. Students are required to complete three Level I fieldwork experiences that provide opportunities for them to apply these concepts to each of the following life span divisions: children and adolescents, adults, and elderly persons. Approximately 170 students are enrolled in Level I fieldwork each semester.

History of the Level I Fieldwork Program

Early in the development of the university's occupational therapy program, it was recognized that because of the rural character of the region and the small number of occupational therapists in the state, there would be a need to use nontraditional sites for Level I fieldwork placements. Several strategies were developed to support this effort, including the designation of three faculty members as Level I fieldwork coordinators, the organization of fieldwork into small class sections supervised by academic faculty members, and the use of university vehicles for transporting students to fieldwork sites.

The three faculty members designated as Level I fieldwork coordinators hold the primary responsibility for site development. They also determine student placement, learning objectives, academic requirements, and evaluation methods. One coordinator is responsible for fieldwork experiences with children, one for experiences with adults, and one for experiences with elderly persons. Each coordinator strives to develop Level I fieldwork sites within the university's service region.

Level I fieldwork was designed to be provided in small class sections of six students each to ensure adequate faculty supervision of students assigned to fieldwork in widespread locations. Each class section is supervised by a faculty member. These faculty members are responsible for all course-related activities, including the observation of students at their fieldwork sites and the grading of fieldwork assignments. Student evaluations are based on specific learning objectives. These objectives are organized under three domains: attitudes, knowledge, and performance (Gronlund, 1991). As students progress through Level I fieldwork experiences, general instructional objectives and specific learning outcomes reflect higher levels of performance (Gronlund, 1991).

Students begin Level I fieldwork during their junior year in the occupational therapy program. In accordance with the program's curriculum design, students are first assigned to sites in which services are provided to children. During their senior year in the program, students complete two additional fieldwork assignments: one with adult populations and one with elderly persons. Students' fieldwork experiences occur concurrently with or after completion of didactic course work specific to the respective life span division.

Typically, students spend approximately 6 hr per week throughout a semester at an assigned site. These sites are within a 1-hr driving radius of the university. This proximity allows students to complete their fieldwork commute either immediately before or after attending classes on campus. Over the years, a variety of scheduling options have developed. Students may choose to complete their fieldwork assignments by attending sites once per week (full day) or twice per week (half day) throughout the semester, or they may complete their assignments during the week of spring break or during the 4-week intersession that follows the spring semester and precedes summer school.

Since its inception, the university's occupational therapy program has developed a variety of nontraditional fieldwork experiences. Students have had Level I fieldwork experiences in Head Start programs, senior citizens' centers, adult day-care centers, and outpatient mental health programs. Faculty members have become used to working with these nontraditional fieldwork sites.

This history, coupled with administrative support from all levels of the university, prepared occupational therapy faculty members to take the next step in developing and implementing Level I fieldwork programs. This article describes three unusual approaches to Level I fieldwork. These approaches were created and directly facilitated by faculty members, and they reflect the most recent national trends in the evolution of Level I fieldwork.

Literature Review

A number of innovative models of fieldwork have been reported in the literature. Articles published in the 1970s have described fieldwork in nontraditional sites, including a parent education program (Grossman, 1974), human services agencies (Cromwell & Kielhofner, 1976), and a camp for diabetic children (Gill, Clark, Hendrickson, & Mason, 1974).

A more recent trend in fieldwork is for students to serve as program staff members and academic faculty members to serve as supervisors. Implementation of this type of Level I fieldwork has been reported in the following settings: a federal correctional facility (Platt, Martell, & Clements, 1977), a college-based community clinic (Kimball, 1983), a program for long-term psychiatric patients in a Veteran's Administration hospital (Cole, 1985), classes demonstrating communication techniques for children with handicaps (Kramer, 1985), and a service learning model in pediatrics and physical disabilities (Germain, Miller, & Pang, 1986). In a program described by Neistadt and O'Reilly (1988), students, who were supported by off-site faculty members, served as volunteers in a variety of settings and led groups in the development of independent living skills. Subsequent findings revealed that this program was successful in facilitating student learning and service provision in clinical sites that served young adults and populations that routinely used group treatment (Niestadt & Cohn, 1990b).

Initiating a Residential Fieldwork Experience

Conceptualization

With the financial assistance of a rural health grant and Kentucky's Area Health Education System, which supports rural fieldwork experiences for students in health care professions, a residential fieldwork option was first developed for the 1991 intersession. Under this option, six junior-year occupational therapy students and their faculty supervisor worked and lived in a rural Kentucky community for 1 month while completing a Level I fieldwork experience in pediatrics. The students were placed in various nontraditional sites that served children. The faculty supervisor traveled between these sites and provided supervision to the students and consultation services to the agencies.

Site Selection

Hazard, Kentucky, was chosen for this residential experience for several reasons. It is a community of approximately 15,000—a population large enough to offer many local services that would benefit from occupational therapy. Although occupational therapy services in Hazard and in its surrounding counties are very limited, Hazard was able to offer the program multiple support services through its local Area Health Education Center (AHEC). In addition, because Hazard is located in a mountainous area of southeastern Kentucky, it offered students a unique opportunity to live in and provide services to a new and different culture.

Personnel from the AHEC office in Hazard assisted considerably in the development of this fieldwork experience. They obtained housing in a local hotel for the students and the faculty supervisor at a reduced rate. An AHEC administrator contacted and compiled a list of programs that served children and adolescents. The university's pediatric fieldwork coordinator and the faculty supervisor assigned to Hazard then selected the final fieldwork sites. Four programs in or near Hazard were selected. They included: (a) a day-care program for preschool children, (b) a Head Start program for at-risk children, (c) a residential school for children with behavioral disorders, and (d) an early intervention home-based program for children with handicaps. In addition, AHEC personnel assisted the faculty supervisor in planning regional field trips for the students to enhance their community awareness and cultural experience. These field trips included a visit to Appalshop (an organization that supports Appalachian culture), a tour of a coal mine, and a hike in the Appalachian mountains.

Program

The faculty supervisor contacted each agency that had been selected and consulted with the on-site supervisor to determine areas for student placement and to organize the student role (from observer to implementor) within the agency. The faculty supervisor was available to orient staff members at each site to Level I fieldwork. This orientation included explaining the purpose and function of the pediatric fieldwork experience, explaining the role of occupational therapy within the context of the site, and coaching staff members as needed in regard to faculty members, students, and fieldwork responsibilities.

Each student was assigned to one of the four sites and introduced to the on-site supervisor at the respective agency. These supervisors represented the professions of education, recreational therapy, and social work. Each on-site supervisor was responsible for providing students with an orientation to the agency, an assignment of responsibilities, and an evaluation of performance.

At each agency, students provided the children with individual and group activities that would facilitate their sensorimotor development and play skills. With the assistance of the faculty supervisor, students screened children for developmental and sensorimotor problems. The faculty supervisor was available to demonstrate specific testing procedures and to coach students on how to acknowledge and appreciate the developmental abilities of these children. During weekly discussions, the faculty supervisor emphasized therapeutic communication and cultural understanding.

Outcomes

At the end of the 4 weeks, the students were given the opportunity to reflect on the value of their experiences. Some of their comments follow:

> I think the most important thing that I have gained from this experience is a more open mind. All the classes in the world cannot accurately show you how important it is to take a person's culture seriously, to always take into account what is important to each person, what they value, how they deal with things, and who is important in their life. These issues are highly controlled by a person's culture. If you don't have an open, inquisitive, and caring attitude about these issues, very little will happen in a client–therapist relationship—successful treatment will not exist.

> The benefits are numerous, but being around the culture is a learning experience . . . as well as the closeness of the students. They worked well together and seemed to help each other when needed. It's also a chance to get individualized attention from instructors.

Students not only reflected on Appalachian culture and the support of the other students and faculty member, they also recognized the need for occupational therapy services in the region. One student stated, "It is rewarding to know you've made a difference in these people's lives." Another student said, "There is a great need for occupational therapists in this area." Twelve of the 18 students who have participated in this fieldwork experience since 1991 have stated that they would return to work in this area of Kentucky if the opportunity arose.

This experience has proved to be meaningful not only to the students, but also to the agencies. Agency personnel and community members of Hazard have continually demonstrated how much they appreciate the visiting faculty members and students. Each agency has requested continued participation in this fieldwork program.

Initiating a Program in a Community Mental Health Agency

Conceptualization

Community-based psychosocial rehabilitation programs that are part of comprehensive care centers were among the first nontraditional sites chosen for the university students' Level I fieldwork experiences. Because there are no occupational therapists employed in these outpatient mental health programs, Level I fieldwork students were integrated into the existing programs and received on-site supervision from staff members who represented the disciplines of social work, psychology, and nursing. Faculty supervisors were responsible for reviewing students' documentation, visiting the sites as needed, and helping students apply their occupational therapy knowledge and skills to the clinical setting. Although these were appropriate settings for Level I fieldwork students, faculty members recognized that at many of these programs, on-site staff members were inexperienced in planning and implementing purposeful activities. Therefore, a decision was made to develop a new fieldwork program that could serve as a model for Level I fieldwork experiences in community-based mental health settings.

Site Selection

In choosing a fieldwork site, the following criteria were observed: (a) the site had not been used previously for occupational therapy fieldwork, (b) the site was within a 1-hr driving radius of the university and within its designated service region, and (c) the agency was committed to student education.

With assistance from the Central Administration Office of the Kentucky Department of Mental Health, the psychosocial rehabilitation program of the Cumberland River Comprehensive Care Center was selected. This site, located in Corbin, Kentucky, met all of the preestablished criteria. Although a variety of activities and work assignments were included in the psychosocial rehabilitation program, these activities did not include a wide range of functional tasks or offer as much consistency and structure as the proposed program.

The staff members and the consumers of the center were enthusiastic about the program. Staff members were pleased because the proposed fieldwork activities provided an additional dimension to the existing program without an additional cost to them. Staff members were not required to plan educational experiences for the fieldwork students or supervise them directly; however, the staff members willingly extended themselves by offering personal and administrative support to the program. Consumers were asked whether they would be willing to help the students practice the skills that they had been learning in their classes. They readily agreed.

Program

The students and faculty supervisor provided an enrichment program that was open to anyone who attended the existing psychosocial rehabilitation program. The enrichment program was offered once per week and was held in a house that served as a group home and halfway house for the consumers. The living room, dining area, and large back yard were used for activities. These activities were scheduled from 9:00 a.m.–10:45 a.m. and from 11:45 a.m.–2:00 p.m. Between these two periods, the students and faculty supervisor joined the consumers and staff members for lunch. The students and the faculty supervisor used the time spent traveling to and from the site to discuss students' observations and performance and to plan activities for the following week.

With guidance from the faculty supervisor, the students assumed responsibility for planning and structuring the activities and the environment for consumers. Like the psychosocial rehabilitation program, the enrichment program was based on the concept of consumer empowerment. Allen's work (Allen, Earhart, & Blue, 1992) on cognitive levels, including structuring the environment to match each person's ability to process sensorimotor information, provided the basis for program planning. King's (1990) work on the use of movement and Kielhofner's (1992) Model of Human Occupation also guided program development. Activities were selected that would provide consumers with opportunities to learn functional performance skills, practice coping and interpersonal skills, increase self-esteem and self-confidence, and promote a sense of mastery.

Students had the opportunity to administer selected evaluations to consumers and use the results to aid in planning appropriate activities. The Allen Cognitive Level Test–90 (Allen et al., 1992) was used to assess consumers' abilities to process new sensorimotor information. Students used functional performance evaluations of consumers' daily living skills and assessments of their role performance to guide the selection of psychoeducational topics and activities.

Although the assessments were administered individually, all of the other activities were completed in groups. The high ratio of students to consumers allowed individual support and attention to consumers during group activities. This individual support and attention, coupled with faculty expertise, made it possible for severely disorganized consumers to participate appropriately in the program. Students used a psychoeducational approach to provide consumers with information and engage them in grooming and hygiene, money management, and stress reduction activities. The students found the Independent Living Skills group protocols for adults (Neistadt & Cohn, 1990a) to be very helpful in planning and implementing activities.

Because opportunities to engage in physical activity were lacking in the consumers' lives, gross motor activities (e.g., new games, relays, balloon volleyball) became a vital component of the program. These activities generated a considerable amount of laughter and interaction. They catalytically drew consumers to the program and solidified their interest in attending.

Outcomes

The program proved to be extremely beneficial both for students and for consumers. The students learned to feel comfortable while interacting with consumers. They gained confidence in their abilities to plan and structure activities and environments. They became more adept in administering several evaluation instruments. They were able to move from a focus on their own behavior and performance to a focus on consumers' needs and on facilitation of adaptive responses. They learned to look beyond diagnosis and symptomatology to recognize the individual person struggling to live with the effects of severe and persistent mental illness.

Students also recognized their growth in these areas. Their written responses indicated that they were surprised by their enjoyment of the experience. Many reordered their list of practice preferences, placing mental health higher on their priority scale of practice settings. Students also realized how they could apply what they had learned in this fieldwork experience to Level II fieldwork and to future work situations.

Students indicated that the presence of a faculty member role model was critical to their growth and confidence in interacting with consumers and in implementing group activities. In addition, their prolonged exposure to the same consumers helped give them the insight and information that they needed to document the consumers' behavior and performance in progress notes and treatment plans. An added benefit was the opportunity for students to work as a fieldwork team in planning and implementing the program.

The agency has been pleased with the outcomes of the program. Staff members were impressed with the students' abilities to engage the consumers in purposeful activity. In addition, staff members have reported observable changes in the consumers since the fieldwork program was initiated. The consumers are more animated,

more spontaneous, and less socially isolated during group activities. They have learned new skills and are able to use them in their everyday lives. Although the program's structure and activities have had positive effects on all of the participants, the program has been particularly valuable for those persons who had been too disorganized to participate regularly in the existing psychosocial rehabilitation program. The structure and specificity of the activities, combined with the high student-to-consumer ratio, allowed these persons to engage in the activities appropriately and successfully.

This program has been offered for five semesters. When each semester has ended, the consumers, staff members, and students have expressed enthusiasm for the program's continuation.

Initiating an Alzheimer's Day-Care and Respite Program

Conceptualization

This fieldwork opportunity differs from the two preceding experiences in that it was not built on an existing program; instead, it was planned, developed, and implemented by one of the faculty members in the university's occupational therapy department. It continues to be coordinated by departmental faculty members; the only on-site staff member involved in this day-care and respite program is the one faculty member who serves as both the academic supervisor of the students and as the director and site supervisor of the day-care and respite program.

Because there were no day-care programs within a 30-mile radius of Richmond for persons with Alzheimer's disease, the development of an Alzheimer's day-care and respite program that would meet the needs of these persons, their caregivers, the community, and the university's fieldwork students seemed appropriate and timely. The process of gathering information for adult day care and dementia-specific day care began with a literature review (American Occupational Therapy Association, 1986a, 1986b, 1986c; Gitlin & McCracken, 1991; Goldston, 1989; Hasselkus, 1992; Panella, 1987; Smith, 1986; Webb, 1989). Additional information was gathered through one faculty person's attendance and participation in workshops and conferences on Alzheimer's disease. This person also visited model programs and consulted with their staff members. The program was heavily publicized during the summer before it was implemented. News releases were sent to all area physicians, local hospitals, nursing homes, the local home health agency, area churches, the regional Alzheimer's Association, and the Alzheimer's Disease Research Center. Area newspapers and radio stations carried information and updates about the program.

Site Selection

The Baptist Student Center, located on the university's campus, donated its facility at no charge to the day-care and respite program for one day per week. The center has a very large all-purpose room with an adjoining kitchen and bathrooms, as well as ample, convenient parking. These features were well-suited for the program and for its participants.

Program

The program was held one afternoon per week from 12:30 p.m.–4:00 p.m. Students met the faculty supervisor–program director from 11:00 a.m.–12:15 p.m. to discuss the day's program and review the participants' cases. Each student was assigned to one participant per day. The primary emphasis of the program was on the appropriate use of goal-directed activities for persons with Alzheimer's disease.

At the beginning of the semester, each student completed an assessment of one of the program participants. This information was used to help determine the functional abilities of individual participants and of the group. Examples of assessment tools used included the interview of a family member, which provided information on a patient's life history, the Parachek Geriatric Rating Scale (Parachek & King, 1986), the Mini-Mental State Exam (Folstein, Folstein, & McHugh, 1975), and the Allen Cognitive Level Test 90 for cognitive disabilities (Allen et al., 1992).

On the basis of students' assessments, appropriate goals were developed for the program participants, and activities that best met these goals were selected. Activities focused on physical and gross motor and psychosocial skills, including exercise, movement, and games. In addition, arts and crafts, baking and cooking, and mental and memory activities appropriate for each program participant's level of cognitive functioning were used. Each student was responsible for planning and implementing the day's activities for two afternoons during the semester.

Outcomes

The day-care and respite program has now been used as a fieldwork site for five semesters. During this period, the university's occupational therapy department and the community of Richmond have gained a valued resource. The vitality of the program has been maintained through the commitment of the faculty coordinator and students and through the continued interest of the families who use and commend its services.

The persons with Alzheimer's disease who have taken part in the program have also benefited from the activities. Many of the participants have been able to remain in their home settings because respite services provided family members with time for self-renewal. One family member stated, "I know that once a week for 3½ hours I can leave Mom with you and know that she's safe and loved, and I can do something for me and not feel guilty."

Students have described this fieldwork experience as extremely "educational, worthwhile, and meaningful." The students involved have developed an awareness of the personal, familial, and social ramifications of Alzheimer's disease. Through ongoing interactions with these persons, students have also developed an appreciation for the individuality of each program participant. Students have come to recognize the significance of the moment for these program participants, and they have based structured activities on the participants' habitual behaviors. Students have completed this fieldwork experience with the requisite skills needed to work with persons with Alzheimer's disease and with their families.

Discussion and Conclusions

The use of academic faculty members to plan and implement Level I fieldwork has been an effective means to increasing the number of sites available for fieldwork placements. At Eastern Kentucky University, administrative support and faculty member familiarity with student supervision in nontraditional fieldwork sites have resulted in the development of three highly innovative programs previously unserved by occupational therapists. Developing and implementing these three programs accomplished the initial objective of providing additional placements for Level I fieldwork students. The programs provided services to persons who did not have access to occupational therapy. The recipient communities and agencies have reported continued interest and support for the programs.

Both students and faculty members perceived the fieldwork experiences as beneficial. Students felt supported by their close working relationships with faculty supervisors and, as a result, were willing to take on new responsibilities and challenges. Faculty members valued the opportunity to model professional behavior, skills, and clinical reasoning to their students. In addition, faculty member role models within practice settings help students bridge the gap between theory and practice. This close working relationship between students and faculty members has additional benefits. As reported by Wittman (1990); Barris, Kielhofner, and Bauer (1985); and Depoy and Merrill (1988), the use of faculty member role models to demonstrate the application of theory to practice and to describe the clinical reasoning process is one way of reducing the disparity between occupational therapy education and clinical practice. ▲

Acknowledgments

We thank all of the community agencies who have assisted in the development of these Level I fieldwork opportunities. These experiences would not have come to fruition without their support.

References

Allen, C. K., Earhart, C. A., & Blue, T. (1992). *Occupational therapy treatment goals for the physically and cognitively disabled*. Rockville, MD: American Occupational Therapy Association.

American Occupational Therapy Association. (1986a). Occupational therapy in adult day-care. *American Journal of Occupational Therapy, 40,* 814–816.

American Occupational Therapy Association. (1986b). Occupational therapy services for Alzheimer's disease and related disorders. *American Journal of Occupational Therapy, 40,* 822–824.

American Occupational Therapy Association. (1986c). Roles and functions of occupational therapy in adult day-care. *American Journal of Occupational Therapy, 40,* 817–821.

American Occupational Therapy Association. (1991). *Essentials and guidelines for an accredited educational program for the occupational therapist.* Rockville, MD: Author.

Barris, R., Kielhofner, G., & Bauer, D. (1985). Educational experience and changes in learning and value preferences. *Occupational Therapy Journal of Research, 5,* 243–256.

Cole, M. B. (1985). Starting a Level I fieldwork program. *American Journal of Occupational Therapy, 39,* 584–588.

Cromwell, F. S., & Kielhofner, G. W. (1976). An educational strategy for occupational therapy community service. *American Journal of Occupational Therapy 30,* 629–633.

Depoy, E., & Merrill, S. C. (1988). Value acquisition in an occupational therapy curriculum. *Occupational Therapy Journal of Research, 8,* 259–274.

Folstein, M. F., Folstein, S., & McHugh, P. R. (1975). "Minimental state": A practical method for grading the cognitive state of patients for the clinician. *Journal of Physical Therapy Research, 12,* 189–198.

Germain, A. C., Miller, P. A., & Pang, S. (1986). From theory to practices: Service learning in occupational therapy. In *Proceedings of occupational therapy education: Target 2000* (pp. 145–149). Rockville, MD: American Occupational Therapy Association.

Gill, A. A., Clark, J. A., Hendrickson, F. R., & Mason, C. L. (1974). A student practicum experience. *American Journal of Occupational Therapy, 28,* 284–287.

Gitlin, S. D., & McCracken, A. L. (1991). A unique teaching opportunity: A specialized facility for persons with Alzheimer's disease. *Educational Gerontology, 17*(6), 621–629.

Goldston, S. M. (1989). *Adult day care. A basic guide.* Owings Mills, MD: National Health.

Gronlund, N. E. (1991). *How to write and use instructional objectives* (4th ed.). New York: Macmillan.

Grossman, J. (1974). Parent education–community experience for students. *American Journal of Occupational Therapy, 28,* 589–591.

Hasselkus, B. R. (1992). Meaning of activity: Day care for persons with Alzheimer disease. *American Journal of Occupational Therapy, 46,* 199–206.

Kielhofner, G. W. (1992). *Conceptual foundations of occupational therapy practices.* Philadelphia: F. A. Davis.

Kimball, J. G. (1983, Spring). The community occupational therapy clinic: one answer to providing fieldwork I experiences at a rural college. *O.T. Education Bulletin,* 13–16.

King, L. J. (1990). Moving the body to change the mind: Sensory integration therapy in psychiatry. *Occupational Therapy Practice, 1,* 12–22.

Kramer, P. (1985, Fall). A unique Level I fieldwork experience: The student as therapist. *O.T. Education Bulletin,* 11–12.

Neistadt, M. E., & Cohn, E. S. (1990a). *An independent living skills model for Level I fieldwork.* Rockville, MD: American Occupational Therapy Association.

Neistadt, M. E., & Cohn, E. S. (1990b). Evaluating a Level I fieldwork model for independent living skills. *American Journal of Occupational Therapy, 44,* 692–699.

Neistadt, M. E., & O'Reilly, M. (1988). Independent living skills groups in a Level I fieldwork experience. *American Journal of Occupational Therapy, 42,* 782–786.

Panella, J. (1987). *Day care programs for Alzheimer's disease and related disorders.* New York: Demos.

Parachek, J. F., & King, L. J. (1986). *Parachek geriatric rating scale* (3rd ed.). Phoenix: Center for Neurodevelopmental Studies.

Platt, N. P., Martell, D. L., & Clements, P. A. (1977). Level I field placement at a federal correctional institution. *American Journal of Occupational Therapy, 31,* 385–387.

Smith, D. A. (1986). Theory guided intervention with Alzheimer's disease clients in a Level I practicum. In *Proceedings of occupational therapy education: Target 2000* (pp. 170–174). Rockville, MD: American Occupational Therapy Association.

Webb, L. C. (Ed.). (1989). *Planning and managing adult daycare: Pathways to success.* Owings Mills, MD: National Health.

Wittman, P. P. (1990). The Issue Is — The disparity between educational preparation and the expectations of practice. *American Journal of Occupational Therapy, 44,* 1130–1131.

The Student Speaks

Aquatics in Occupational Therapy

Christine Tank, *Student*
University of Wisconsin

As a former swimming instructor and presently an occupational therapy student, a special issue on aquatics for the handicapped in *The Therapeutic Recreation Journal* (vol 10, no 2, 1976) suggested some possibilities for using the knowledge and resources of occupational therapy in conjunction with swimming activities for the disabled population.

One article, "Academic remediation in aquatics," by Louise Priest, discussed water activities that could be used to encourage transfer of learning in such areas as visual and auditory discrimination, eye-hand coordination, spatial and kinesthetic awareness, task completion, and sequential thinking. Several games and activities were suggested to achieve these areas of learning. The article, "Aquatics games, a multidisciplinary teaching method for the handicapped," by Linda Melvin, also discussed transfer of learning but included the therapeutic value of movement skills, perceptual motor development, pre-academic and academic skills achieved through swimming. A third article, "Movement exploration in aquatics," by Louise Priest, stressed the importance of movement capabilities and perceptual awareness of space in disabled persons prior to teaching specific swimming skills.

On reading about these concepts within the context of swimming activities, it seemed that here were areas in which therapists had the background and ability to define the prerequisite developmental skills. A therapist could use swimming as a specific therapeutic medium, a goal-directed activity for psychological support in which secondary goals can be achieved, or as activity to develop the prerequisite skills needed for actual swimming techniques. A team approach in a total swim program could involve occupational therapists, water safety-trained instructors, physical therapists, recreation therapists, and education directors.

A fourth article, "Integrating families of handicapped individuals in the public swimming facility," by Robert Lyttle, which discussed a program where the nonhandicapped and the handicapped were successfully integrated for instruction purposes, suggested another possible role for the therapists, namely that of the consultant. The therapist has a background in identifying special problems of the handicapped (i.e., architectural barriers, integration into the social system, evaluation, and treatment planning). Occupational therapy could also play a role in family involvement, public education, and awareness in community organizations. Involvement

in new programming, as described in the article, "Swimming for senior citizens," by Carol Cooper, suggested yet another possibility for the therapists—that of program coordinators.

I think this could be an exciting area for occupational therapy involvement—with possibilities of developing a dynamic team approach. For any therapist using swimming in the treatment area, presenting such information in *AJOT* would be of professional interest.

Nontraditional Field Work Experiences

Roseanne Pascoe
Student
Eastern Michigan
University

Cromwell and Kielhofner's "An Educational Strategy for Occupational Therapy Community Service" (November/December 1976 AJOT) deserves recognition by all occupational therapy educators and curricula advisors. It clearly describes efforts at the University of Southern California to balance training of both traditional hospital practice and community health roles. As an expression of approval of this increased emphasis on community experience, I would like to tell about my preclinical experiences in nontraditional settings.

These experiences consisted of defining and establishing my role as an occupational therapist in two settings: a psychiatric half-way house and an intermediate school district. The emphasis of supervision was to foster my independence in developing and implementing therapy programs. With few role models and precedents available, I had to acquire the ability to solve problems— to assess, formulate, and implement strategies of intervention. Treatment programs were formulated through research, trial and error, discussion with other health professionals, and lengthy problem-solving periods. In treatment implementation, I established the professionalism of occupational therapy for other health professionals and for myself. My self-confidence and autonomy increased because I began to design and actualize my professional potential.

The use of nontraditional settings can be a benefit to educators. Seeking out and establishing community placements helps to fill student quotas and increases the profession's visibility in the surrounding community.

I found only two disadvantages in these *nontraditional* preclinicals. As Cromwell and Kielhofner mentioned, at the outset I remember feeling totally overwhelmed. This initial feeling made later treatment accomplishments seem even greater. Subsequently, in traditional field work experiences, I lacked knowledge and practice of concrete clinical treatment modalities—for example, I had no experience in prescribing craft activities or adaptive devices. To make up for this lack of clinical knowledge I relied on my developed problem-solving ability and ability to research for the knowledge.

In retrospect, for me this background in nontraditional community settings created a professional strength, the ability to assess an unfamiliar setting, and to formulate and implement its treatment program. I urge all educators and curricula advisors to offer students the opportunity for such preclinical experiences.

SECTION SIX

International Occupational Therapy Articles

This section is a small collection of international articles discovered during the literature search for this anthology. The articles are primarily from Canada and Britain, and they are by no means representative of research on fieldwork worldwide. They are included as a supplemental source of ideas and strategies for fieldwork.

Contracting in Fieldwork Education: The Model of Self-Directed Learning

Barbara Gaiptman, Arlene Anthony

Key Words:

- Fieldwork Education
- Learning

Abstract

The educational role of fieldwork supervisors has become an increasingly salient one in Occupational Therapy programs. This paper discusses the model of self-directed learning and the use of this model as a framework for the fieldwork education of occupational therapy students. The assumptions underlying the model of self-directed learning are presented and contrasted with the assumptions underlying the traditional model of learning in fieldwork education. The learning contract as a tool in the implementation of the model of self-directed learning is described and the four components of the learning contract are discussed. Areas for further investigation are identified.

Barbara Gaiptman, M.Ed., O.T.(C), is an Assistant Professor and Fieldwork Coordinator within the Division of Occupational Therapy, Department of Rehabilitation Medicine, University of Toronto, 256 McCaul Street, Toronto, Ontario, M5T 1W5.

Arlene Anthony, M.Ed., O.T.(C), is an Assistant Professor and Fieldwork Coordinator within the Division of Occupational Therapy, Department of Rehabilitation Medicine, University of Toronto.

This paper is based on a presentation made at the Annual C.A.O.T. Conference in St. John, New Brunswick, in June, 1987.

The value of an effective fieldwork program in the development of professional occupational therapists cannot be underestimated (Presseller, 1983; Stan, 1987). The subject of fieldwork education has begun to receive increased attention in Canadian occupational therapy literature. Recently, much that has been written on the subject of fieldwork education in Occupational Therapy has focused on specific issues such as fieldwork education standards, evaluation, etc. (Polatajko, Ernest, & MacKinnon, 1987, Tompson & Tompson, 1987). Krefting (1985) notes that the use of conceptual models is critical to the provision of effective occupational therapy service. It is equally important to examine the educational theories underlying the fieldwork experience and to analyze the implications of these theories for both the student and the supervising therapist involved in the fieldwork process.

Fieldwork education in Occupational Therapy has been viewed as a collaborative process between academic and clinical facilities with the clinic identified as the environment in which the student is expected to integrate academic theory with clinical practice (Christ, 1986). Little has been written, however, about how this integration actually occurs.

As in many other professional education programs, fieldwork education in Occupational Therapy was historically based upon an apprenticeship model of learning. The primary focus was placed upon the student's learning through doing. It was expected that the knowledge, values, and clinical skills of the supervising therapist would be acquired, primarily by the student observing an experienced clinician, and then modelling his/her own behaviour upon that of the clinician. This approach to learning appeared to focus primarily on the development of clinical skills and to omit reflective and conceptual activities, key components in the integration of knowledge and development of professional practice (Bogo & Vayda, 1986; Tompson & Tompson, 1987).

At one Canadian university it was felt that this approach to fieldwork education did not accurately reflect the values and philosophy of the occupational therapy program, that is, to graduate occupational therapists who were effective, innovative clinicians, committed to critical thinking, continuing learning, and self-appraisal (University of Toronto, 1983). In addition to the concern about the underlying philosophy of the fieldwork education program, other problems had been identified that intensified the need for the implementation of a new approach to learning in fieldwork education. These same concerns were recognized and effectively summarized by Leonardelli and Gratz (1985).

1. Inconsistency between the students and the fieldwork supervisors regarding expectations of student performance;
2. Incompatibility between student expectations and the realities of the fieldwork facility;
3. Inconsistency between the educational institution and fieldwork facilities regarding expectation of student performance during the fieldwork placement.

If one examines the purposes of both university programs and clinical facilities, the occurrence of these problems is not surprising. Both of these institutions are philosophically very different. The purpose of a university based program in Occupational Therapy is to graduate occupational therapists for practice and to critically evaluate and expand upon the body of knowledge upon which occupational therapy practice is based. The purpose of the majority of clinical facilities is to provide occupational therapy services to people in need. Whereas the valued activities of a university based program are research, scholarship, and teaching, the valued activities of clinical facilities is primarily the delivery of effective services (Bogo & Vayda, 1986). Although the differences between the two systems can create a dynamic tension that is productive, the differences can, as well, create difficulties for the student who is attempting to reconcile the requirements of the academic program with the expec-

tations of the clinical facility.

The purpose of this paper is therefore: 1) to describe a model of learning in fieldwork education which encourages communication and collaboration between students, university, and fieldwork facilities, and is derived from adult education theory; 2) to analyze specific key educational issues from the perspective of adult education theory; and 3) to describe the practical implementation of this model through the use of learning contracts.

Self-Directed Learning

The model of self-directed learning was selected to provide the framework for the development of the fieldwork education program. In its broadest meaning, self-directed learning describes "a process in which individuals take the initiative with or without the help of others in diagnosing their learning needs, formulating learning goals, identifying human and material resources for learning, choosing and implementing appropriate learning strategies, and evaluating learning outcomes" (Knowles, 1975, p. 18).

This model is based on the work of Malcolm Knowles who has practised extensively in the field of adult learning. Knowles (1975) refers to adult education as "andragogy" and differentiates it from pedagogy which refers to the teaching of children. There are major differences in the underlying assumptions of andragogy and pedagogy which Knowles (1975) identifies:

1. The Concept of the Learner: The pedagogical model attributes to the instructor the responsibility for making decisions regarding the content and pacing of the learned material. The andragogical model assumes that as a person grows and matures his/her self-concept changes from total dependency to increasing independence and self-directedness. Adult learners experience the need to be perceived as self-directing. A learning situation that puts the learner in a role of dependency can create conflict and resistance.
2. The Role of Experience: The learner's previous experiences are not viewed as an important resource in a pedagogical model — it is the experience and knowledge of the instructor that is of prime importance. Emphasis is on the methodology by which information is transmitted from instructor to student. The andragogical model acknowledges

the differences in student's previous experiences and emphasizes the need for individualized learning plans and experiential learning techniques.
3. Readiness to Learn: The pedagogical model assumes that the student is ready to learn required material because of his/her age or the completion of prerequisite academic courses. The andragogical model, however, assumes that an adult's readiness to learn is related to the need to know or do something in order to perform more effectively in some aspect of his/her life.
4. Orientation to Learning: The pedagogical model assumes that students are subject- oriented in their learning. Material is organized and presented by the instructor according to the logic of the subject matter. The andragogical model recognizes that adults have a problem-centered orientation to learning. Learning experiences are considered to be most significant if they focus on relevant meaningful situations.
5. Motivation to Learn: The pedagogical model emphasizes external pressures such as grades, consequences of failure, competition, etc., whereas the andragogical model acknowledges that adults respond most effectively to internal rewards such as a sense of accomplishment and increased self-esteem.

The differences between the two models result in very different approaches to the educational process (Knowles, 1985). The pedagogical model is primarily a "content plan" with emphasis on the organization, sequencing and methodologies of both the transmittal of information and the evaluation of learning. The andragogical model is a "process design", the primary focus is on the facilitation of learning. The implication of these differences for fieldwork education is that the supervisor is not viewed primarily as an instructor of specific content but as a collaborator in the design of effective processes by which the student can acquire required content.

There are two main elements to consider in the application of the model of self- directed learning. The first is the establishment of a climate that is conducive to learning. The characteristics which promote an optimal learning climate are collaboration, mutual respect, openness, trust, flexibility and supportiveness. Christie, Joyce and Moeller (1985), in a study designed to identify the distinguishing characteristics of effective and ineffective supervisors found that students described effective supervisors as possessing very similar characteristics as those described by Knowles. The second element to consider is involvement of the student in all stages of the learning process. This is facilitated through the use of learning contracts.

The andragogical process stresses the importance of a shift in role for both the student and the supervisor. The student must perceive him/herself as being an active participant in the learning process rather than a passive recipient of information. This implies that the student must develop skill in diagnosing learning needs and formulating specific learning objectives. In order to do this the student must develop the ability to honestly evaluate his/her strengths and weaknesses and identify learning needs. The student must be involved in developing strategies for meeting his/her objectives and therefore must become aware of the specific techniques by which he/she learns most effectively. Because the student has to take responsibility for learning outcomes, he/she must also develop the ability to identify which objectives were met and to critically evaluate his/her own behaviour. The model emphasizes the collaborative nature of the supervisory relationship and thus the student must develop skill to work effectively with a supervisor and to be able to give and receive feedback without allowing it to interfere with the learning process.

Implementation of this model requires that the supervisor's perception of his/her role shift from that of instructor and supplier of information to facilitator of the student's learning. In order to do this effectively, there are skills that are required of the supervising therapist. The supervisor must learn to feel comfortable in an educational situation in which he/she does not have total control over the student's learning experience. The therapist must establish a balance between encouraging the student's self-directedness and requiring an acceptable standard of performance (Price, 1976). The supervisor in the clinical setting must encourage the student to share previous learning experiences and to use this information in the diagnosis of learning needs and development of objectives. To aid the student in meeting learning objectives the supervising therapist must encourage the student to use a variety of resources and strategies. The therapist must discuss the resources he/she possesses which may be useful to the student and encourage the student to seek out other resources in the facility as well. The student's self-evaluation of his/her learning is integral to the model, thus it is crucial that the therapist and student work collaboratively to encourage the student to feel comfortable to discuss difficulties and to identify areas of concern.

Learning Contract

Although not essential to the model of self-directed learning, the learning contract is an effective tool by which to implement the model, particularly in a professional education program, because of the flexibility that the contract provides to blend the imposed requirements of a professional education program with the student's personal goals and need to be self-directing (Knowles, 1975). The contract is a written document that is developed by the student in conjunction with his/her supervising therapist. Though based on the performance objectives developed by the university program and clinical facilities, the contract individualizes the student's learning program and makes explicit the responsibilities of both the student and the supervising therapist.

Formulating the contract is a dynamic process. Through the contracting process

Table 1

UNIVERSITY OF TORONTO Occupational Therapy Learning Contract

Learning Objective	Learning Resource	Evidence	Validation
What do you want to learn or develop? Consider your own competency levels and the opportunities available within this facility.	What will you utilize to achieve your learning objectives? Where can you find information? Be specific, consider how you learn best.	How can you show to yourself and your therapist that you have met your learning objectives? What proof will you offer and when?	How do you want your evidence to be evaluated? By whom? When? What are the criteria for evaluation?
To perform safe and efficient transfers under minimal supervision by the end of the three-week placement. (C.V.A. pt.) (chair—chair)	- observe supervising therapist - observe other therapists within the department - practice on other students - class notes - readings - perform several transfers (practice) under maximum supervision	Perform transfers in competent fashion by the end of week three.	Verbal feedback from supervising therapist: 1. appropriate positioning and stabilization 2. safety precautions, e.g. wheelchair brakes 3. appropriate transfer method selected and demonstrated 4. feedback from patient (pt. felt safe, yes/no with student) 5. student's personal feelings after transfer
To develop rapport with adult day patients in a Psychiatric Day Hospital.	- observe therapist and team members - talk to other students about their experiences - refer to class notes - read patient charts	Demonstrate rapport by midterm 1. good eye contact 2. tone of voice 3. posture 4. spontaneous 5. calm appearance 6. sense of humour	Therapist collects feedback from other members of the team - comments on the strengths and weaknesses on evidence identified at midterm and weekly afterwards

DATE NEGOTIATED: _____ STUDENT: _____

COMPLETED: _____ THERAPIST: _____

the supervising therapist and student assess the student's levels of competency in different areas and identify the student's expectations. The supervising therapist and student discuss the supervisor's resources, plan learning experiences that will facilitate growth within the student, and negotiate how the student will identify the effectiveness of his/her learning (Flanigan 1974; Fox 1983). Significant learning should take place as a result of the contracting process. Flanigan (1974, p 35) states that the "suggestion of a learning contract in itself requires the student to consider 'perceived discrepancies' between his level of functioning and his potential level." Clancy (1985) has observed that participation in goal setting may develop within students more commitment to the learning process. The contract, once written, should not be viewed as static or binding but used flexibly to allow for changes as objectives are met and new objectives are developed (Fox 1983; Knowles 1975).

A discussion of each section of the learning contract will help to illustrate the manner in which the contract is used in fieldwork education in Occupational Therapy (see Table 1).

Objectives

In the Objectives section of the contract the student identifies what he or she wishes to learn or develop (see Table 1) and then translates these needs and interests into learning objectives (Clancy, 1985). The objectives are derived from information that is retrieved from a variety of sources including university and clinic performance objectives, student's learning needs and the orientation to the resources of the clinical facility. The objectives that the student writes fall into one of the following three groupings: cognitive, affective and psycho-motor (Bloom, 1956). The cognitive or conceptual domain includes those objectives which deal with recall or recognition of knowledge and the development of problem-solving skills. The affective or emotional domain includes those objectives which emphasize a feeling tone, attitudes, or values. The third domain is the psycho-motor or motor skill area and refers to those objectives which emphasize the development of clinical skills. As stated previously, in order for the objectives to be relevant, the supervising therapist and student must obtain a baseline understanding of the student's performance. This can be done in a variety of

ways including observation by the student of the supervising therapist and discussion of the student's observations, or observation of the student's interaction with clients. The objectives are stated in terms that clearly identify the behaviour or skills to be developed and define the clinical areas in which the behaviours are to operate. Verbs such as define, identify, and interpret are examples of verbs that specify behaviour.

The therapist's major responsibilities during this stage include the establishment of an effective climate for learning, providing the student with a clear orientation to the facility, and helping the student to explore the skills that each individual brings to the clinical setting. Clearly stated objectives provide both the student and supervisor with consistent measurable expectations for the placement.

Learning Resources and Strategies

In the second section the student describes how he/she proposes to go about accomplishing each objective (see Table 1). The student identifies the resources, both material and human, to be used and the learning strategies that will be employed. The more specific the student is in describing learning resources and strategies, the more helpful the supervising therapist can be in facilitating the learning process (Knowles, 1975).

There are a variety of learning strategies or resources that can be utilized. These vary according to the student's learning style and the supervisor's facilitating style. Individual teaching and learning styles of both the supervisor and student are important factors which can influence the learning process and should be clarified during the contracting. Examples of some learning strategies include: observation of supervising therapist, assisting the therapist, practice sessions with other students, discussion, role play, use of video playback monitors, literature, class notes, etc.

Although it is acknowledged that the relationship that the student establishes with the supervising therapist is an important learning resource, the student is also encouraged to consider other students and therapists within the clinical facility as resources. Efficient use of a variety of resources decreases the likelihood of dependency on the supervising therapist and enables the student to work more independently.

Evidence

In the evidence section the student specifies the behaviours that will demonstrate that the learning objectives have been met. The student defines what is to be measured or evaluated. As an example, if the student's objective has been to perform a specific assessment under minimal supervision, the evidence will be that the assessment has been performed under minimal supervision on a certain date. However, if the learning objective focused on the student's learning to feel comfortable with patients, the evidence would be a list of the observable behaviours that the student will demonstrate to show that he/she is comfortable with patients. The evidence should have a date assigned to it so that both the student and the supervising therapist are in agreement as to when the student will have met the objective. In order to avoid student anxiety close to the end of the placement, it is important to ensure that targeted dates to meet objectives are scheduled throughout the placement.

Validation

In the validation section (see Table 1) the student, in conjunction with his/her supervising therapist, specifies the criteria by which the evidence will be evaluated. This process occurs at the time when the contract is formulated, long before the evaluation actually takes place. The criteria stated vary according to the type of objective that has been developed, i.e. knowledge, skill, and/or attitude. Congruent with the androgogical model, the student participates in this component through a process of self-evaluation. The supervising therapist does carry primary responsibility for evaluation and validation, however, other professional staff within the facility are frequently asked to be involved as well. Feedback on the identified criteria should provide the student with knowledge of strengths and weaknesses, as well as strategies to improve performance. The evaluation process should lead to a redefining of learning needs (Bogo, 1986). Table 1 presents examples of learning objectives that were developed by two level one students during their first clinical placement.

As this is a professional education program, it is not feasible that the student receive feedback only on the areas identified in the contract. The areas identified by the student and agreed upon by the supervising therapist do, however, become the focus for learning in the placement.

Conclusion

The assumptions underlying the model of self-directed learning and the related methodological implications provide a framework which offers the opportunity to design an occupational therapy fieldwork education program that addresses the needs of individual students, university programs, and clinical facilities. In situations where students encounter difficulties, the use of the learning contract can be very valuable. As Bogo (1986, p. 78) states: "Focusing on the process of learning and the changed behaviour expected may help the student partialize the task and reduce anxiety." The learning contract can be an important tool in clearly identifying the areas of difficulty and making explicit the expectations of both supervising therapist and student.

Occupational therapy students are involved in fieldwork placements which can be as brief as four weeks and generally no longer than three months. This requires the student and supervising therapist to plan the stages of the learning experience as early as possible so that the student can maximize his/her learning experience.

Discussion regarding previous personal and professional learning experiences and the process of negotiating the learning contract are helpful in facilitating the development of the supervisory relationship early in the placement.

The realities of the current manpower shortage in Occupational Therapy may necessitate utilization of a variety of supervisor:student ratios in fieldwork education (Tiberius & Gaiptman, 1985). The application of the model of self-directed learning makes possible individualized student learning and provides direction to the learning experience.

There are many aspects of the implementation of this model that require investigation but any investigation of learning outcomes is predicated on the assumption that supervising therapists and students are, in fact, implementing the strategies of self- directed learning. It is recommended that research into the evaluation of the application of the principles of self-directed learning to fieldwork education be conducted. Some of the questions to be investigated include:

1. Are students and therapists utilizing the strategies of self-directed learning?
2. What are the barriers that prevent utili-

zation of the strategies of self-directed learning?
3. Can certain students be identified who respond most favourably to the self-Directed learning approach and should this potential be considered in the selection of candidates for professional programs adopting this model?
4. Are there distinguishable types of supervisors who function best within this model?
5. Is there a specific type of educational experience that would best prepare students and clinicians for their involvement in the self-directed learning process?
6. Does the model, if implemented, help students develop skills that prepare them for their ongoing need for education as professionals?

Occupational Therapy is a profession which requires as a fundamental skill the ability to deal with complex and often unique clinical problems. It is not feasible to believe that students will learn all they need to know in an undergraduate program. University programs must recognize that professional education must include not only the transmission of specific knowledge, attitudes, and skills, but should focus on the process of learning and on the development of the skills of inquiry. The implementation of the model of self-directed learning in fieldwork education prepares students for the continuing need for education that will be critical for them as professional occupational therapists.

REFERENCES

Bloom, B. (Ed) (1956). *Taxonomy of educational objectives: The classification of Educational Goals*. New York: David McKay.

Bogo, M. & Vayda, E. (1986). *The practice of field instruction in social work theory and process*. Toronto: University of Toronto Press.

Christ, P. (1986). *Contemporary issues in clinical education*. Thorofare, N.J.: Slack.

Christie, B.A., Joyce, P.C., & Moeller, P.L. (1985). Fieldwork experience, part II: The supervisor's dilemma. *American Journal of Occupational Therapy, 39*, 675-681.

Clancy, C.A. (1985). The use of the andragogical approach in the educational function of supervision in social work. *The Clinical Supervisor, 3*(1), 75-86.

Flanigan, B. (1974). Planned change and contract negotiation as an instructional model. *Journal of Education for Social Work, 10*(2), 34-39.

Fox, R. (1983). Contracting in supervision: A goal oriented process. *The Clinical Supervisor, 1*(1), 137-149.

Knowles, M. (1975). *Self-directed learning: A guide*

for learners and teachers. New York: Association Press.

Knowles, M. & Associates (1985). *Andragogy in action*. San Francisco: Jossey-Bass.

Krefting, L.H. (1985). The use of conceptual models in clinical practice. *Canadian Journal of Occupational Therapy, 52*, 173-178.

Leonardelli, C.A., & Gratz, R.R. (1985). Roles and responsibilities in fieldwork experience: A Social systems approach. *The Clinical Supervisor, 3*(3), 15-24.

Polatajko, H., Ernest, M. & MacKinnon, J. (1987). Computerized fieldwork data base: Applications and implications. *Canadian Journal of Occupational Therapy, 54*, 263-267.

Presseller, S. (1983). Fieldwork education: The proving ground of the profession. *American Journal of Occupational Therapy, 37*, 163-165.

Price, H.G. (1976). Achieving a balance between self-directed and required learning. *Journal of Education for Social Work, 12*(1), 105-112.

Stan, J. (1987). National perspective: Fieldwork—whose job is it anyway? *Canadian Journal of Occupational Therapy, 54*, 233-234.

Tiberius, R., & Gaiptman, B. (1985). The supervisor-student ratio: 1:1 versus 1:2. *The Canadian Journal of Occupational Therapy, 52*, 179-183.

Tompson, M.A. & Tompson, C. (1987). The evolution of standards for the fieldwork component of the curriculum. *Canadian Journal of Occupational Therapy, 54*, 237-241.

University of Toronto (1983). Division of Occupational Therapy, *Mission Statement*, unpublished document.

Acknowledgements

The authors wish to acknowledge the contribution of the many occupational therapists who have worked towards the implementation of the model of self-directed learning in the fieldwork education program at University of Toronto. The learning contract form was introduced by Mona Callin, B.N., M.Ed., McMaster University, School of Nursing, at a workshop on self-directed learning at University of Toronto, April, 1981.

Résumé

Le rôle pédagogique des superviseurs de stages devient de plus en plus marquant dans les programmes d'ergothérapie. Cet article illustre le modèle d'apprentissage auto-dirigé et l'utilisation de ce modèle en tant que guide pour la formation pratique des étudiants en ergothérapie. Les hypothèses sous-jacentes au modèle d'apprentissage auto-dirigé sont élaborées et mises en parallèle avec celles de l'apprentissage traditionnel pour la formation pratique. Le contrat d'apprentissage en tant qu'outil dans la mise sur pied du modèle d'apprentissage auto-dirigé est décrit ici et les quatre composantes du contrat d'apprentissage y sont présentées. Les domaines susceptibles de faire l'objet d'investigations futures, sont identifiés.

The Application of Cognitive Style Research to Fieldwork Education

by Barbara Gaiptman

Abstract

Each individual demonstrates a distinct style of gathering and organizing information or accumulating knowledge. This paper describes the cognitive style of field dependence versus field independence. The literature on cognitive style research is discussed and applied to the supervision process that occurs in fieldwork practice. Implications for the future development of fieldwork education programmes are presented.

Introduction

For some time now, psychologists have been aware of the influence of cognitive style, or the learning style, of students and the instructional style of teachers on learning performance or learning outcome (Messick, 1976). According to Cross (1976), however "not one teacher or counsellor in a hundred knows anything at all about cognitive styles despite the fact that the research on cognitive styles has been going on for some twenty-five years in psychology laboratories" (p. 112). The issue of cognitive or learning style, particularly as it impacts on student performance in fieldwork education, has not been addressed by occupational therapists. Since performance in clinical practice may be influenced by both the student's learning style and the supervising therapist's instructional style, it would seem necessary for occupational therapists who supervise students to become aware of this interaction.

Barbara Gaiptman, B.O.T., O.T.(C) is Assistant Professor and Clinical Coordinator at the University of Toronto, Division of Occupational Therapy, Department of Rehabilitation Medicine, Toronto, Ontario, M5T 1W5.

The premise on which this paper is based is that the role of an effective clinical supervisor encompasses three major functions: a) clinical teaching, b) counselling, and c) administrative instruction (Schwartz, 1984). If a clinical supervisor's cognitive style influences his/her way of teaching and a student's cognitive style influences his/her way of learning, a match or mismatch in cognitive style between supervising therapist and student has important consequences for the learning process (Wilkin, p. 57).

> *A match or mismatch in cognitive style between supervising therapist and student has important consequences for the learning process.*

The purpose of this paper is, therefore, to 1) explore the literature on cognitive style, in particular, the cognitive style of field dependence versus field independence; 2) apply the research on cognitive style to the area of supervision in clinical practice; and 3) make recommendations for the development of the fieldwork education

program in an undergraduate occupational therapy program at a Canadian University.

The primary responsibilities of a university programme clinical coordinator are the planning, development, and monitoring of the fieldwork education component. Through experience it has become clear to this author that there are major problems associated with the programme of clinical practice. These issues are: 1) the lack of attention that has been paid to the supervisory skills of fieldwork instructors who are inevitably responsible for the quality of fieldwork instruction; 2) the difficulties that occur in clinical practice as a result of what appears to be interpersonal difficulties between supervising therapist and student; and 3) the lack of consistency in therapists' perceptions of student performance from one clinical setting to another, evident in the dramatically different clinical evaluations a student receives from different therapists. This author has begun to hypothesize that perhaps some of the problems associated with the varying evaluations of student performance — those that have traditionally been referred to as a "personality conflict between student and fieldwork instructor" — may be influenced by two primary factors: 1) the differences in learning style of the occupational therapy student and teaching style on the part of the fieldwork supervisor; and 2) the varying aptitudes of students either for the scientific and analytical approach to treatment as compared to the more humanistic orientation to treatment, e.g., neurosciences versus psychosocial dysfunction (Messick, 1976). Witkin (cited in Cross, 1976) stated "Cognitive style is a potent variable in students' academic choices and vocational preferences: in students' academic development throughout their school career; in how students learn and teachers teach; and in how students and teachers interact in the classroom" (p. 112).

The cognitive style selected for discussion in this paper is that of field dependence versus field independence primarily because of its discussion of interpersonal competencies, an essential skill in the development of student occupational therapists.

Programme description

It is important to the development of this paper to briefly describe the model of clinical practice at one Canadian university. Students are assigned to hospitals or community agencies by the university coordinator for a physical medicine or psychosocial placement. It then becomes the responsibility of the agency or hospital student coordinator to assign the student to his/her supervising therapist. The assignment is based on the identified learning needs of the student, e.g., for neurological experience. The supervising style of the therapist and the learning style of the student are not taken into account.

The philosophy of self-directed learning serves as a theoretical framework for clinical practice. Each student is expected to negotiate the development of a mutually agreed upon learning contract with his/her fieldwork instructor. The purpose of this contract is to ensure that the planning of the fieldwork experience becomes a shared responsibility between student and supervising therapist. By participating in the process of identifying learning needs, setting objectives, identifying resources and strategies, and evaluating learning outcomes each student should develop a committment to the learning experience (Knowles, 1975). It is expected that the learning contract serves to facilitate the communication process between therapist and student.

Cognitive style

"Cognitive Style refers to the information processing habits that typify an individual's mode of perceiving, thinking, problem-solving and remembering" (Macneil, 1980 p. 354). Each one of us possesses a distinct style for gathering and organizing information or accumulating knowledge. Certain individuals concentrate on a methodical and orderly approach to problem solving while others typically utilize an intuitive approach. Some people do their best learning in collaboration while others prefer independent study (Cross, 1976). Messick conceptualized these cognitive styles as "stable attitudes, preferences or habitual strategies" (Messick, 1976 p. 5).

It is important to distinguish cognitive styles from abilities. Cognitive style refers to the consistent manner by which an individual organizes and processes information. Cognitive styles develop slowly, remain stable over the years, and influence all human activities. Cognitive styles differ from abilities in a number of ways. Abilities refer to intellectual abilities and imply the measurement of an individual's capabilities. Abilities are value directional, that is, having more is better than having less. A particular cognitive style, however, is valued according to the circumstances. Messick (1976) uses the example of spatial ability to illustrate the concept. High spatial ability predisposes an individual to achieve in certain tasks; its absence implies that the individual will more likely not succeed in those areas. Cognitive styles on the other hand range from one extreme to another with each end having different implications for performance and aptitude.

Various dimensions of cognitive style have been identified over the years. The concept of field dependence/field independence was first introduced by Witkin and associates in 1954. Their interest at that time was in the area of perception, particularly in the difference between global and analytical ways of perceiving the environment (Cross, 1976).

A variety of tests have been developed to illustrate the difference between field dependence/field independence. In early experiments, subjects, seated on tilted chairs in tilted rooms, were asked to adjust both the chairs and their bodies to the upright. Witkin demonstrated that certain groups of individuals consistently aligned themselves with the tilt of the room whereas others were able to ignore their surroundings and through internal cues adjust their bodies to an upright position. In another exercise, subjects seated in a dark room, presented with a bright rod in a bright picture frame which was tilted, were asked to place the rod in an upright position. Again, results indicated that some individuals aligned the rod to the slant of the frame, whereas other were able to set the rod upright. Later, experiments were carried out with figure drawings; in these, some individuals were unable to locate line figures embedded in complex designs, whereas other individuals were able to distinguish the figures as separate from the background (Cross,, 1976). Witkin designated those individuals who relied on their environment for their orientation (i.e., they demonstrated less ability to deal with parts of the field separately) as being field dependent. Field dependent individuals are generally noted to be more attentive to an entire situation; they seem to be more adept and sensitive to social situations where they demonstrate effective interpersonal skills. They are described as being more susceptible to external influences and appear to have more difficulty with tasks that require analytical abilities (Cross, 1976, Mcleod, 1979-80, Messick 1976).

Field independent individuals, on the other hand, consistently utilized internal cues to orient themselves during the experiments. Field independent individuals are described as being able to deal with situations in an analytical manner; they tend to process information with greater isolation from the environment, and perform well at tasks that require differentiation and analysis. They are depicted as having less well-developed interpersonal skills (Cross, 1976, Jacob, 1982, Mcleod 1979-1980).

Review of the literature

Many researchers have studied the interaction between students' learning styles, teachers' instructional styles and learning outcome. A brief review of studies which may have implications for the supervisor-student relationship follows.

Andrews (1981) investigated how teaching methods and students learning style affect learning outcome. Although he presented several hypotheses, the one that is of particular interest here is the hypothesis that students will be able to learn more in settings which allow them to interact more effectively with their instructor. He suggested that effective interaction arises when interpersonal patterns between course instructors and students mesh; the students are comfortable in the relationship with the instructor, and are then able to focus their energy on academic learning. He explored two distinct instructional strategies (Instructor Centered versus Peer Centered) in chemistry classes which were led by teaching assistants. The student's learning style was evaluated on the Grasha Reichmann Student Learning Style Scale and measured along collaborative/competitive dimensions. His results indicated that the dynamics of compatibility between student learning style and section format were stronger than the differences. The Peer Centered approach was most beneficial for collaboratively oriented students

whereas competitive students learned best in an Instructor Centered approach. He suggested that course instructors should capitalize on the fact that students, consciously or unconsciously, select learning resources to match their learning style. He recommended that instructors should provide students with information about their learning style to help them to become more effective learners (Andrew, 1981).

The philosophy of self directed learning serves as a theoretical framework for clinical practice.

Packer & Bain (1978) investigated the effects of teacher-student cognitive style matching and mismatching on both interpersonal ratings and objective measures of student learning. They compared two cognitive styles, namely, field dependent/field independent and serialist/holist. Serialist/holist refers to an alternate dimension of learning style. Persons described as serialist generally concentrate on a step-by-step approach to learning. A holist learning style generally indicates a more global approach to learning. (Entwistle, 1981). Packer and Bain tried to determine if the effects of matching and mismatching were mediated by differences in instructional strategies. They hypothesized that teachers' cognitive styles may influence their skill with different instructional methodologies. The task was to teach the mathematical concept of network tracing.

The results indicated that students' learning outcome and subjective evaluation of the ease of learning, as well as teachers' ability to interact with students, may benefit from matching, but only at the extremes of field dependence/field independence. No significant results were achieved when serialism/holism was used as the measure of

cognitive style. The results suggested that: 1) the disadvantages of field dependent students in the area of math may be minimized by assigning them to teachers who are also field dependent and 2) teachers' cognitive style did not seem to be as important in the learning outcome of field independent students. However, this result may be influenced by the aptitude of field independent students for math.

Jacobs (1982) investigated the relationship between cognitive style (field dependent/field independent), proctor-student interactions and the achievement of students in a Personalized System of Instruction course on Cybernetics. Three styles of proctor-student interaction were measured: 1) specific to course objectives, 2) related to content in some manner, and 3) unrelated to course, concerned with non-academic matters. The results indicated that there were significant differences in the social behaviour of the two groups but not in their achievement in the course. There was a greater tendency for field dependent students to obtain specific course information through social contacts with proctors whereas there was no significant difference between the two groups in the frequency of their interactions with their proctors.

Macneil (1980) investigated the relationship between instructional style, cognitive style and learning performance. Three levels of instructional style were utilized: 1) discovery 2) expository and 3) no treatment. Cognitive style (field dependence/field independence) was identified through performance on the Group Embedded Figures Test. The task was to provide students with an introduction to behaviour modification. The results of the study indicated that the learning performance of students was not affected by a particular style of instruction irrespective of cognitive style. Macneil suggested several interesting explanations for the results. It may have been that: 1) although the reliability of the evaluation test designed to test knowledge was high the difficulty index was not as high as it might have been, 2) the nature of the subject matter did not require either a high degree of analytic ability or social skills, and 3) the results were affected by the fact that all of the instructors were categorized as field dependent (Macneil, 1980).

Di Stefano (1969, cited in Witkin, 1976) noted that teachers and students matched for cognitive style described each other in highly positive terms whereas teachers and students who were not matched, tended to describe each other more negatively. Teachers tended to place a higher value on the intelligence of students who were similar to themselves in cognitive style. Witkin (1976) noted that persons matched for cognitive style appear to get along better. He suggested that this is a result of: 1) shared foci of interest, 2) shared personal characteristics, and 3) similarity in communication modes which encourages easier and more effective communication.

Another important issue which is a function of cognitive style is that of aptitude. Witkin (1976) stated that cognitive style is a dynamic variable that affects a number of areas, one of these being vocational preference. Quinlan & Blatt (1973, cited in Witkin, 1976) found that high achieving students in psychiatric nursing tended to be significantly more field dependent than high achieving students in surgical nursing. Nagle (1968, cited in Witkin) indicated that first year graduate students in clinical psychology were more field dependent than students entering a programme in experimental psychology.

Differences have, as well, been noted in the behaviour of psychiatric therapists. Pollack & Kiev (1963, cited in Witkin, 1976) and Witkin, Lewis & Weil (1968, cited in Witkin, 1976) noted that field dependent therapists tended to favour styles of therapy that focus on interpersonal relationships with the patients whereas field independent therapists tended to favour directive, noninvolving approaches to treatment. Greene (1972, cited in Witkin, 1976) noted that therapists selected more supportive therapy for field dependent patients than they did for field independent patients.

Chickering (1976) pointed out that contract learning, an approach designed to increase the opportunity for individual learning, may create problems for both the field dependent and field independent student. The development of the contract provides a rich opportunity for human interaction which may be particularly difficult for field independent students whereas the field dependent student may have more difficulty in analysing and identifying his/her learning needs.

Little attention has been paid to the role of fieldwork supervisors, who are inevitably responsible for the quality of the fieldwork programme.

Application of the literature to the supervision process

Although the educational process that occurs in the academic setting is not the same as that happening in the clinic there is probably sufficient similarity between the two situations that factors which affect students' learning in the classroom may also influence students' learning in the clinic. Indeed if one conceptualizes the clinical supervisor's role as including clinical teaching then it does appear that clinical performance or learning outcome may be influenced both by supervising therapist's teaching style and student's learning style. In this section an attempt will be made to integrate the literature previously described with issues relating to fieldwork education.

As previously discussed, Witkin (1976) noted that cognitive style is an important reason for the student's academic choice and vocational development. Although it has been recognized by the faculty of the Division of Occupational Therapy that there are certain students who consistently experience more difficulty with the biomedical sciences than with the social and behavioural sciences, and visa versa, the achievement of these students has never been closely monitored, particularly as it relates to performance in clinical practice. The work of Quinlan & Blatt (1973, cited in Witkin, 1976) and Nagle (1968, cited in Witkin, 1976) reinforce the idea that occupational therapy students should be provided with feedback about their aptitude and learning style in order to help them to identify their strengths and weaknesses and to allow them to anticipate problems that they may encounter in clinic.

The results of the studies on cognitive style are variable. Packer & Bain (1978) reported that only students who scored at the extremes of the Group Embedded Figures Test may benefit from a matching process, particularly in a subject area that has been identified as difficult for each cognitive style. Di Stefano (1969, cited in Witkin, 1976) noted that students and instructors matched for cognitive style described each other in positive terms. Andrews (1981) pointed out that when interpersonal communication between instructor and students mesh, the student is then able to direct his energies into learning.

What implications do these studies have for the supervision process? If we were to hypothetically assign a student, who had scored at the low end on the Group Embedded Figures Test, (i.e. who was field dependent) to a placement in a neurological setting to be supervised by a therapist who has been classified as field independent, the potential problems that we could create for student learning are obvious, e.g., little aptitude for a subject area, communication difficulties between student and therapist that may interfere with learning, and student and therapist potentially viewing each other in negative terms. The disadvantages for this student could perhaps be minimized by assigning the student to a field dependent therapist (Packer & Bain, 1978).

Jacobs (1982) reported that field dependent students are more likely to approach their proctors for course related information than are field independent students. In my experience, I have frequently encountered supervising therapists who have expressed serious concerns that certain students present as very "dependent", frequently asking questions of clinicians that could easily be answered by consulting charts or textbooks. Although one cannot assume that this trait is common to all individuals whose cognitive style is classified as field dependent, it is certainly a subject that would benefit from further study.

Macneil's (1980) results may explain why many students perform well in the area of chronic care. The staff in chronic care settings, because of their holistic approach to treatment, generally value both the interpersonal and analytical skills of therapists. Each student, therefore, has the opportunity to be recognized for his/her strengths.

Another major problem that has been noted with the fieldwork programme is that of the inconsistent evaluations that are received by students in the same area of practice. Students currently are assigned to approximately four psychiatric placements, with a different supervising therapist in each placement. Referring back to the studies of Witkin, Lewis & Weil (1968, cited in Witkin, 1976) and Pollard & Kiev (1963 cited in Witkin, 1976) the fact that students may not receive consistent feedback from supervising therapists about their performance in clinic presents as no surprise.

It is becoming clear that cognitive styles and, in particular, the supervisor's teaching style and the student's learning style likely have a major impact on learning outcomes, or student performance, in clinic.

Implications for the fieldwork education programme

The literature on cognitive style must be considered in the future planning and development of the fieldwork education programme. The first point to be discussed is that of "matching the cognitive style of the learners to the teaching resources of the institution" (Cross, 1976, p. 126). Should therapists and students be matched for clinical practice? To what extent is the matching of cognitive styles beneficial? Cross discuses four options for matching: 1) a challenge match, i.e., placing the student in an uncomfortable situation so that he is forced to develop; 2) a remedial match, i.e., placing the student in a situation to try to correct his weakness; 3) a compensatory match;

Through experiential activities therapists would be provided with the opportunity to identify their own learning style.

---

i.e., the student learns to compensate for deficiencies by utilizing skills that are more developed; and 4) a capitalization match, i.e., the student is placed in a match to capitalize on his unique strengths (Cross, 1976). Although there are four matching strategies to select from, there are, for this writer, conceptual and logistical problems that interfere with the implementation of any of the above strategies. In planning the fieldwork programme is is essential to consider both the optimal setting for clinical learning as well as the working environment that will confront the student upon graduation. It is fundamental to the practice of occupational therapy that students graduate with the ability to work with both clients and other professionals whose cognitive style may be very different from their own. In addition to the conceptual problems associated with any matching scheme, the logistical problems are overwhelming. There are currently 130 students in this oc-

cupational therapy programme, 88 of whom are in clinical practice in approximately 35 facilities at any one time. The problems associated with attempting to match the learning style of 88 students with the teaching style of 88 therapists leaves the writer (whose responsibility it would ultimately be) quivering. It would appear that there are alternate solutions to be considered prior to subscribing to a proposal for matching student and therapist.

It might be suggested that, rather than have the university coordinator assume the responsibility for the matching process, an interview system be set up in which students would be responsible to apply for, and negotiate, their own placements. Referring to the results of Oltman, Goodenough, Witkin, Friedman & Friedman (1975, cited in Witkin, 1976) therapists and students would identify in a very short time if they felt comfortable with each other. This strategy, however, seems more appropriate for a graduate programme where smaller numbers of students are in fewer placements for a longer period of time. The most feasible and exciting strategy appears to be the development of an education programme in which occupational therapy fieldwork supervisors would be provided with an opportunity to learn about educational philosophy as well as to develop the skills necessary to become effective supervisors. As previously stated, little attention has been paid to the role of fieldwork supervisors in occupational therapy, who, in reality, are inevitably responsible for the quality of the fieldwork programme. It is the writer's goal to develop an educational programme for supervisors utilizing a small group format. A major component of this programme would include discussion of cognitive styles, specifically the interaction between learning style and teaching style and its effect on learning outcome. Through experiential activities therapists would be provided with the opportunity to identify their own learning style. The goal of this exercise would not be to label either therapists or students, but to help therapists to become aware of the differences in learning style, and to bring to their awareness the fact that, they too, because of their cognitive style, supervise and teach by the methods which are most comfortable for them (Cross, 1976). The facilitator's goal would be to structure and plan the learning experience so that participants would be provided with the opportunity to discuss issues such as: 1) the impact of their cognitive styles on the way they prefer to supervise students, and 2) the ways in which they could adapt their teaching styles and supervisory approach to different students to facilitate learning. Similarly, as part of their orientation to clinical practice, students would be exposed to a similar process in order to help them to know themselves better and to enable them to become more effective learners (Andrew, 1981).

It does not seem feasible, or perhaps even a beneficial strategy, to match learning styles of therapists and students. Perhaps what may turn out to be as effective is to provide both therapists and students with some awareness of their cognitive styles to help both groups to facilitate the supervision process in the clinical setting.

Conclusion

This review of cognitive styles has helped the writer to develop a frame of reference by which to better understand what happens between supervisor and student in the clinical setting. Traditionally the majority of student/therapist problems in clinical placements have been classified as interpersonal difficulties. There is a great deal of value in beginning to utilize cognitive style as a conceptual approach to better understand both problems and process in fieldwork education. In order to more effectively apply cognitive style research to field work education it will be important to investigate alternate learning and cognitive processes as well as to evaluate the validity of such an approach to clinical education.

REFERENCES

Andrews, J.D.W. (1981). Teaching Format and Student Style: Their Interactive Effects on Learning, *Research in Higher Education*, *14*, 161-178.

Canadian Association of Occupational Therapists, Standards for the Education of Occupational Therapists in Canada, *The Association*, June 1980.

Chickering, Arthur. W. (1976). Commentary: The Double Bind of Field Dependence/Independence in Program Alternatives for Educational Development in Messick, S. and Associates (1976). *Individuality in Learning*: San Francisco: Jossey-Bass.

Cross, K.P. (1976). *Accent on Learning*, San Francisco: Jossey-Bass.

Entwistle, Noel (1981). *Styles of Learning and Teaching*, Chichester: John Wiley & Sons.

Jacobs R.L. (1982). The Relationships of Cognitive Style to the Frequency of Proctor/Student Interactions and Achievement in a PSI Course, *Journal of Industrial Teacher Education*, *19*, 18-26.

Knowles, M. (1975). *Self-Directed Learning* Chicago: Associated Press.

Macneil, R.D. (1980). The Relationship of Cognitive Style and Instructional Style to the Learning Performance of Undergraduate Students. *Journal of Educational Research*, *73*, 354-359.

Mcleod, D.B., Adams, U.M. (1979-1980). The Interaction of Field Independence with Small Group Instruction in Mathematics. *Journal of Experimental Education*, *48*, 118-124.

Messick, S. And Associates (1976). *Individuality in Learning*: San Francisco: Jossey-Bass.

Packer, J., Bain, J.D. (1978). Cognitive Style and Teacher Student Compatibility. *Journal of Educational Psychology*, *70*, 864-871.

Schwartz, K.B. (1984). An Approach to Supervision of Students on Fieldwork. *The American Journal of Occupational Therapy*, *38*, 393-397.

Witkin, H.A. (1976). Cognitive Style in Academic Performance and in Teacher-Student Relations in Messick, S. and Associates (1976), *Individuality in Learning*: San Francisco: Jossey-Bass.

Résumé

Chaque individu a sa manière propre de recueillir et d'organiser les informations ou d'accumuler les connaissances. Cet article décrit le style cognitif dépendant du milieu clinique versus un style cognitif indépendant de ce milieu. Les articles traitant de recherches sur les styles cognitifs sont examinés et leurs données sont appliquées au processus de supervision courants lors des stages cliniques. On y discute également des répercussions possibles, à l'avenir, sur le développement de programmes éducatifs basés sur les stages cliniques.

Evaluation of the Usefulness of Objectives in Fieldwork Experiences

Bonnie Hawkes and Sue Ryan

Abstract

This paper presents a pilot study which investigated students' and therapists' perceptions of the value of objectives in structuring fieldwork experiences. The method in which the objectives were presented and their content is described. The model used to guide the therapists in the development of the objectives is outlined together with the study procedures. Results of this study and their implications for educators and therapists who plan and organize fieldword experiences are also discussed.

The pilot study on which this paper focuses investigated three areas related to fieldwork objectives; (1) students' and therapists' perception of the value of objectives in structuring fieldwork experiences, (2) the format in which the objectives were presented to students and therapists (particularly with regard to their clarity), and (3) the degree to which the broad content of the objectives was applicable to all clinical areas within one occupational therapy department.

This paper will be divided into five major sections: the literature review, the development of objectives in the participating facility, an outline of the study methods (which will include questionnaire development, subject selection and study procedures), data analysis and results, and implications of the study.

Literature Review

Within the field of education and health sciences numerous authors for example, Boyle (1981), Mager (1962), Gronlund (1978) and Caput (1976) have expounded the use of objectives as a necessary ingredient of all instructional programs. Research into the use of objectives (whether or not they improve, clarify or enhance learning experiences) has been largely limited to studies on their use in the school system. Empirical evidence on objectives which has relevance to this study suggests that (1) generally stated objectives are as useful as specifically stated objectives, and (2) objectives have a role to play in criterion-referenced evaluation (Davies, 1976). Further observations from some of these authors, for example Perry (1981), Windom (1981) and Reilly (1980) which have not been substantiated by research, suggest additional uses for objectives in occupational therapy fieldwork. These are — that objectives orient the student more quickly to expectations, programs and schedules within the affiliating facility; assist student and therapist to identify the student's progress; assist the student and therapist in planning and sequencing the learning experience; encourage the students to assume responsibility for their own learning; form the basis for mutually refining objectives and setting priorities; and

provide a focus for communication between the student and the therapist. To ascertain whether such uses for objectives were evident in occupational therapy fieldwork experiences, objectives first had to be developed in one or more clinical facility.

The Process of Developing Objectives

In order to facilitate the development of objectives the Occupational Therapy Clinical Co-ordinator at the University of British Columbia (U.B.C.) conducted inservices for clinicians on the use of objectives, presented a model which showed the relationship of objectives to fieldwork evaluation (Figure 1) and provided resource material related to the formulation objectives. The intent was not to impose specific formats for objectives but to provide guidance to the therapists so that they could develop a "set" of objectives which would be meaningful in their agency and also meet undergraduate educational requirements.

Such a collaborative approach is supported by Perry (1977):

> The objectives of an experience are crucial to the planning of clinical education. The student, the centre and the educational program...should all have input into the clinical education program. When that input is in the form of objectives the whole program can be designed with more knowledge of the needs to be met (p. 58).

The process of developing objectives at Lion's Gate Hospital took place over a two year period and arose from a need to structure learning experiences for refresher interns. Following the inservice sessions from the U.B.C. Occupational Therapy Clinical Co-ordinator, all occupational therapy staff were actively involved in the development of the fieldwork objectives. Their input was solicited on content, format and specific requirements. The format of the final "set" of objectives was comprised of three sections which: (1) provided background information (intended as a guideline for orientation to the hospital), (2) indicated specific sessions which the student should attend for example, team meetings, inservice education, and (3) specified the requirements for performance. The headings in Section 3 were the same as those in the Performance Evaluation and Criteria for Occupational Therapy Students Manual (Burton & Ernest, 1980) in order to clearly relate the fieldwork objectives to the evaluation tool. These objectives formed the basis of the pilot study being discussed in this paper.

Bonnie Hawkes, B.A., O.T.R., O.T.(C), Occupational Therapist with the Medical Engineering Resource Unit, University of British Columbia, Vancouver, B.C. Formerly Director of Occupational Therapy at Lions Gate Hospital, North Vancouver, B.C.

Sue Ryan, Dip. O.T., B.S.R.(O.T.), O.T.(C), Occupational Therapy Clinical Co-ordinator, School of Rehabilitation Medicine, University of British Columbia, Vancouver, B.C.

Figure 1: Development of Criteria for Evaluation in Clinical Education – A Model. Ryan, S.J. February 1981, revised June 1983.

SECTION B.

Please check YES or NO, as applicable.

Did you find: Yes   No

(1) The objectives were useful as a worksheet to review your progress   _____   _____

(2) The objectives allowed you to become quickly oriented to this setting   _____   _____

(3) The objectives helped you in directing your own learning experience   _____   _____

(4) The objectives helped you to set realistic priorities for learning in relation to the length of your placement   _____   _____

(5) The objectives helped you to initiate meaningful discussion about your clinical experience with your supervising therapist   _____   _____

(6) The objectives *specifically* identified the expectations for your clinical experience   _____   _____

(7) The objectives selected for you were appropriate to:
    (a) your academic level
    (b) your current level of clinical experience   _____   _____

(8) Instructions for using the objectives as a learning tool were clearly explained to you at the beginning of the placement   _____   _____

(9) Your supervising therapist formally reviewed *all* the selected objectives at:
    (a) mid-term
    (b) final   _____   _____
                                                                                                                _____   _____

(10) Your supervising therapist referred to the objectives at periods other than at mid-term and final   _____   _____

    If YES, please indicate _____

(11) Further comments/explanations of your responses in Section B

Figure 2: Section B. of the Questionaire used by the Students in this Study.

Methods

Data Collection

In order to collect data relevant to the three research questions the authors devised two questionnaires. One was to be completed by students, the other by therapists. The questionnaires were divided into three sections. The first section included demographic data which differed on each questionnaire. In the second section questions focused on the possible uses of the objectives and with one exception required yes/no responses (Figure 2). These questions elicited the same information from both groups. The final section asked all respondents to indicate how frequently they referred to the objectives for guidance and also to list five objectives which were (a) most useful and (b) least useful.

Subject Selection

Students assigned to the Lions Gate Hospital Occupational Therapy Department between May 1st and August 31st, 1982 were asked to participate in the study. All agreed to participate giving a total 'n' of eight. Therapists who had a student assigned to them during that period were asked to complete the therapists' questionnaire. All of the therapists agreed to participate for an "n" of six. Therapists only responded once although they may have been assigned more than one student over the course of the summer.

Procedures

The normal "orientation" routine for all new students was followed on the first day of the fieldwork experience. This always included a thorough discussion of the objectives and recommendations for their use. By the middle of the first week the Director of the department met with each student and his/her supervising therapist and item by item selected those objectives which correlated with the competencies checked ($\sqrt{}$) in the "program" column of the "Performance Evaluation and Criteria Manual" (Burton and Ernest, 1980). Each student and therapist then decided independently how they would use the objectives during the remainder of the fieldwork experience.

Two days prior to completion of a placement both student and therapist were requested to participate in the study, given the questionnaires, and asked to return them to the Director of Occupational Therapy by the end of the placement.

Results

Section A: Demographic Data

Analysis of this section revealed that four of the six therapists involved in the study had more than 6.5 years of experience since graduation. The mean number of years for all therapists was 7.2 years. During the time in which data was collected four therapists worked in adult physical dysfunction areas and two in adult psychiatry.

All of the students who participated were from the University of British Columbia. Three were second year students (on four week full-time placements), four were third year students (on six week full-time placements) and one was a fourth year intern (on an eight week full-time internship). Three of the eight were assigned to placements in psychiatry, the remaining five to physical dysfunction areas.

Section B: Uses for Objectives

On all questions (refer to Figure 2) except for numbers 2, 3, 9 and 10 there was a 25% or less discrepancy between the responses of both groups. Both students and therapists answered 100% affirmatively on questions 3 and 9. Areas of substantial disagreement (greater than 25% discrepancy) existed on questions 2 and 10.

There were only two comments on question 11 which did not reiterate questions 1 to 10. In the first instance, one student and one therapist indicated they preferred the specifically stated objectives which indicated the minimum standard for performance, for example, "Following demonstration, conduct at *least* (3) (4) (6) (12) patient interviews, with close/moderate/minimal supervision". Secondly, one therapist stated that feedback to, and evaluation of the student improved because the use of the objectives ensured she was constantly reminded of the student's strengths and areas for improvement.

Section C: Usefulness of Objectives

Only the objectives which were listed twice or more as being most useful or least useful were considered in the data analysis of this section. Five students and three therapists indicated that they referred to their objectives throughout the fieldwork experience. One student and three therapists indicated mid-term and final evaluation periods only and two students indicated other combinations which were more than mid-term and final but less than weekly.

An analysis of the objectives that the students listed as *most useful* revealed that 75% were specifically stated; that is, the behaviour and the standards or criteria for performance were given. Similarly 71.4% of the objectives found to be most useful by therapists were specifically stated. Of the objectives most useful to the students 58.33% were also listed as most useful by the therapists; 50% of those selected by therapists were also chosen by the students.

The objectives given as least useful (by the students) included four which were only stated in general terms, three which were not relevant to the assigned clinical area and one which was considered inappropriate by two senior students. Of those least useful to the therapists, one was considered inappropriate and three were not relevant to the clinical area in which the student was assigned. Three out of four (75%) of those objectives therapists found to be least useful were also listed by the students. These represented 37.5% of the students' list.

190

Discussion

The results in Section B appear to suggest that both students and therapists perceived objectives to be valuable in fieldwork experiences at Lions Gate Hospital. Poor wording of the questions may account for the differences in questions 2 and 10. It is probable that the therapists' answers to question 2 were affected by comparisons made with previous students who had not used the objectives in their placements. Of the students, 37.5% (3) clearly perceived that they did *not* become quickly oriented to the setting; 62.5% (5) who responded positively could have been comparing their orientation in this setting to those in other settings without objectives. In question 10, 87.5% (7) of the students stated that their therapist referred to the objectives at periods other than mid-term and final evaluation, however only 50% (3) of the therapists agreed with the students. These therapists may not have considered the extra times or did not remember them because they were "outside" the formal evaluation periods and therefore blended with their regular client care and administrative duties.

The findings from Section C indicate that students and therapists found the objectives which were specifically stated most useful with two exceptions. Two of the objectives contained lists of types of evaluations and treatment methods and were rated by both groups as being most useful and least useful. Respondents comments suggested that they may be most useful because the lists served to cue and remind students and therapists of potentially suitable evaluations and intervention strategies. However, they were also considered least useful because not all of the items listed were relevant in every clinical area. It appears then, that these objectives were interpreted by some as general and by others as specific. In spite of these apparent exceptions a format which incorporates specific objectives may be more suitable at Lions Gate Hospital. Furthermore, one set of objectives does not seem to be desirable for all clinical areas; objectives perceived to be most useful included content specifically relevant to the students assigned clinical area.

Researchers persuing further studies in this area should consider increasing the sample size and revising the questionnaire, particularly Section B (Figure 2), to improve validity and reliability. Broader response alternatives such as a Lickert scale, may also be considered desirable. An evaluation of alternative formats for objectives may be useful to those in the process of developing fieldwork programs.

Conclusion

The findings appear to support previous empirical evidence from studies in the school system that objectives have a role to play in criterion-referenced evaluation. However they do not show that generally stated objectives are as useful as specific ones, at least in one occupational therapy setting. Even though the results provided feedback on all three research questions identified in the introduction, the findings should be interpreted with caution. Further research is necessary to validate the results from this pilot study.

REFERENCES

Boyle, P.G. 1981. *Planning better programs.* New York: McGraw Hill Book Company.

Burton, H. & Ernest, M. 1980. *Performance Evaluation and Criteria for Occupational Therapy Students.* Prepared for the Canadian Association of University Teachers of Occupational Therapy.

Caput, D.Z. 1976. Instructional Objectives. In Ford, C.W. and Morgan, M.K. (Eds.) *Teaching in the health professions.* Saint Louis: C.V. Mosby Co., 121-133.

Davies, I.K. 1976. *Objectives in curriculum design.* New York: McGraw Hill Book Company.

Gronlund, N.E. 1978. *Stating objectives for classroom instruction* (2nd ed.). New York: MacMillan Publishing Co. Inc.,

Mager, R.F. 1962. *Preparing instructional objectives.* Belmont, California: Fearon Publishers.

Perry, J.F. 1977. *Handbook of clinical faculty development.* Division of Physiotherapy, Department of Medical Allied Health Professions, School of Medicine, University of North Carolina at Chapel Hill.

Perry, J.F. 1981. A model for designing clinical education. *Physical Therapy, 61:* 1442-1446.

Reilly, D.E. 1980. *Behavioural objectives — Evaluation in nursing.* New York: Appleton-Century-Crofts.

Windom P.A. 1981. Developing a clinical education program from the clinician's perspective. *Physical Therapy, 61:* 1587-1593.

Résumé

Cet article présente une étude-témoin qui recherche les perceptions d'étudiants et de thérapeutes de la valeur d'objectifs en formant des expériences cliniques sur le terrain de travail. La méthode par laquelle les objectifs furent présentés, ainsi que leur contenu, est décrite. Le modèle utilisé pour guider les thérapeutes dans le développement des objectifs est tracé ainsi que les procécures d'étude. On discute aussi des résultats de cette étude et de leurs implications pour les éducateurs et thérapeutes qui planifient et organisent ces expériences cliniques.

Self-Directed Learning as a Post-Basic Educational Continuum

Vivien Hollis

The importance of applying theory to practice has always been a major consideration for occupational therapy training, especially at a pre-qualification level. The focus of this article is on continuing education at a post-basic level with the emphasis on self-assessment and reflective practice in clinical work. The educational process is related to self-directed learning, with recommendations for consideration for implementing a strategy to bridge the theory-practice divide and develop clinical excellence.

INTRODUCTION

'We shall not cease from exploration
And the end of our exploring
Will be to arrive where we started
And to know the place for the first time.'[1]

Clinicians and managers have given much consideration to the topic of making learning relevant to the work occupational therapists carry out. As an occupational therapy practitioner and a manager of occupational therapists the author has, over the years, been swept along on a tide of innovative approaches to reconcile the theory-practice divide. Job task analysis, job specification, standards for professional competence, quality standards, individual performance review and clinical supervision have all contributed to the need to identify average and superior performance so that proficiency and expertise could be developed.

Occupational therapists are well aware, if somewhat intuitively, that therapy is carried out at several levels of skill and competency. But how do we describe, quantify and measure the extraordinary energy, innovation and creativity exerted by those who embody and exemplify excellence?[2] More importantly, how do we motivate experienced occupational therapists to move to higher levels of clinical practice by increasing not only skills and knowledge but also, and especially, understanding and judgement? At present, there is no obligation for an occupational therapist to pursue post-basic education. An especial concern is that there is neither formal arrangement for updating knowledge, nor reassessment for practice following a prolonged absence from clinical work.

How, then, do we provide a forum for the identification, acquisition and application of progressive professional education, encourage occupational therapists to take part, and measure outcomes in relation to direct patient care? How do we make it meaningful for the individual, instead of using a broad brush approach?

THE EDUCATIONAL PROCESS

Anyone involved in formal education and training will be aware of the need to address the issues of identification of training needs, curriculum planning, setting aims and objectives, specifying content, selecting teaching media and assessing outcomes.

Self-directed learning is a particular educational approach which can be of immense value, by actively involving the occupational therapist in the whole process and integrating past experience and present needs.

'A self-directed learner is someone who, with or without the help of others, diagnoses her/his learning needs; sets relevant, feasible and measurable learning objectives; determines generally acceptable standards or criteria which will be applied to assess whether learning has in fact occurred as planned; and finally, formulates a coherent learning agreement or personal curriculum for the course.'[3]

Motivation

Motivation is a key concept in the learning process and deserves consideration in relation to self-directed learning. The early work of Maslow[4] still has something to offer the occupational therapist in that he identified higher and lower factors: the higher, such as security, are dependent on the lower, such as food and sleep, being achieved. This may be an initial step or a tool for identifying motivational factors.

The later work of Herzberg, McClelland and Lawler, as identified by Klyczek and Gordon,[5] who applied their studies to human work behaviour, has implications for self-directed learning. Herzberg, for instance, in dividing job factors into 'motivational/satisfiers' and 'maintenance/hygiene' factors,[5] gives us insight into factors which are not explicit motivators and not disincentives but which are responsible for dissatisfaction. Being able to identify factors which produce dissatisfaction (monotony, lack of challenge) is certainly important to establishing what direction should be taken. This theory, though, does not explain the relationship between these factors. The assumption that one set of factors, 'satisfiers' (job interest, responsibility, recognition), does not provide compensation for another set of factors, 'maintenance' (poor pay and conditions), could be challenged.[6]

McClelland's 'acquired needs theory', which identified the three basic needs, acquired as a result of life experience, of 'need for achievement', 'need for affiliation' (good interpersonal relationships) and 'need for power',[5] provides significant insight for the learner. Used in conjunction with a competency profile, it will be possible for the learner to identify his/her needs and the extent of these needs and to structure his/her learning programme to provide positive feedback and satisfaction.

Lawler's motivation model[7] has perhaps most to offer the self-directed learner. By identifying the three major components of effort, performance and reward, and viewing the whole as an interactive and therefore dynamic process, a deeper understanding can be gained of the individual's cogni-

Vivien Hollis, TDipCOT, SROT, District Head Occupational Therapist and Manager, Physical Handicap Services, West Dorset Health Authority, Dorset County Hospital, Princes Street, Dorchester, Dorset DT1 1TS.

tive process. For instance, a block to learning may exist in the effort component and be related to the understanding of how much work must be put into a task or the belief in being able to achieve the expected results, or indeed have much to do with how much the end result is valued. Performance may be impaired by these and also by the person's actual skills, ability and problem-solving techniques, together with environmental factors. Reward, of course, is not always immediate and the person's individual goals are not always achievable as a direct result of this process but, rather, affected by external variables. A working knowledge of the Lawler model enables us to analyse, isolate factors and adapt to changing circumstances.

Finally, the effect of assessment on motivation deserves comment. Evidence shows that students work harder during examination periods but, conversely, that some examinations produce stress and anxiety.[8] If the timing and type of assessment is negotiated by the self-directed learner, it would reduce stress, help the more able learner and be seen as part of the whole learning process and not just an end product.

Establishing motivational factors is perhaps the first step in the process of self-assessment, which underpins the self-directed learning approach. Although crucial to self-development, motivation cannot be imposed. A self-directed approach encourages motivation since it asks the learner to identify his/her needs, both now and as an ongoing process, and then to structure his/her learning appropriately.

Negotiated learning

Accepting the well argued concept that it is impossible to teach anyone anything, he/she can only be helped to learn,[9] and identifying a curriculum which is student-centred, aimed at learning not teaching, with negotiated aims and objectives, content, learning method and evaluation procedures, are the first steps to andragogy.*

Much work has been done in medical education by Engel[10] to show that this self-reliance is part of the whole philosophy of education for life. Problem-based learning allows complete and continuous integration of the basic and clinical sciences. The author's own experience of working within the pedagogy framework supports this approach. Trying to involve nurses in a learning programme when they had been told to attend but had not themselves felt the need, identified a result or, indeed, anticipated any personal achievement was impossible.

Again, the emphasis on negotiated learning is for self-assessment. The learner must be aware of his/her own needs, past experience, future expectations and pace of learning and incorporate this into the programme.

Reflective practice

Gibbs[12] has outlined a model for learning, based on research into learning styles, which identifies the learner's need to recognise his/her own learning style, be adaptable and develop new strategies. The four skills identified are the ability to use experience, reflection, conceptualisation and experimentation. This work would seem to be based on Kolb's experiential learning cycle,[13] itself a product of the work of Pounds, Simon, Wallas and Lewin. Learning is conceived as a holistic, adaptable process, integrating life experiences and providing

a bridge between theory and practice to lay foundations for a continuous process.

Learners able to use experience can recognise problems and sense opportunities; those able to reflect can define problems and create models; those able to use conceptualisation can develop theories and select from alternatives; and those with experimental ability are able to apply learning to new experiences by adapting and implementing. People vary in their ability to circumvent the learning cycle but the ability to assess their own styles and acquire new skills will certainly produce a more critical thinker.

Experience is, of itself, not a unique and separate entity. A person does not always learn from experience, but only learns from experience if that experience is reflected upon. Reflective practice, therefore, must surely be a most important skill in the occupational therapist's repertoire of competencies. In the absence, or indeed the plethora, of theories and concepts, the occupational therapist must be able to devise or select the most appropriate one for the referred client, given his needs at that particular time in his life.

Occupational therapists are justly proud of the fact that there is no recipe book from which to work. Problems do not fit neatly into categories and are not solved in a simplistic manner. The use of reflective practice, though, ensures that a critical approach has been developed to allow a move beyond merely applying technique towards clinical reasoning. It encourages a deep approach to learning, which Marton[14] found to be characterised by the learner using textbook content to complement previous learning and using knowledge in relation to the learner's own experience. In this way, understanding is linked to learning rather than concentrating on acquiring discrete facts.

While learners may adopt this technique on an independent basis, another person — a senior practitioner — may act as a 'facilitator of learning' to enable individuals to learn for themselves. Using this method of learning encourages people to look at all aspects of the learning process in relation to themselves. It helps learners to identify their learning styles[15] and acquire other learning strategies,[13] and encourages a deep as opposed to surface approach to learning.[14] The end product may be important but the whole learning experience is a valuable contribution to self-development.[16] Learners take responsibility for their own learning with regard to their understanding of their knowledge, learning how to learn and acquiring self-monitoring skills — metacognition. This in turn establishes self-efficacy and an internal locus of control.

Methods

Since the method of acquiring greater depth of knowledge is negotiable with a facilitator, the learner may choose from the whole range of teaching media: lectures, demonstrations, programmed learning, group work, practicals, projects, individualised instruction, reading and independent study. Items chosen for investigation should reflect the essence of self-directed learning, in that it is orientated towards work and social roles, learning is seen as performance centred rather than subject centred and, as already mentioned, it requires an independent approach and is based on a reservoir of previous experience.

Reflective practice is not an additional category, but part of each and every learning experience. Spencer[17] states that the best way of practising critical thinking is in repeated exposure to analytical case discussions of the type pioneered by Harvard's Law and Business Schools. Learners who are repeatedly asked to respond to questions, 'What's the problem? How could it be resolved? What is your supporting evidence?', rapidly gain the ability to draw critical distinctions and inferences from complex information.

---

*Andragogy is a term coined by Knowles[11] to describe an adult education learning culture, which is student orientated in a participative learning climate. This approach encourages responsibility for one's own learning and self-development and places the emphasis on education as an ongoing lifelong process.

Outcomes

Although assessment of outcome has been mentioned throughout this article, it is worthy of separate consideration.

Aims and objectives can be classified as cognitive (to do with thinking and intellectual processes), affective (to do with attitudes and feelings) and psychomotor (to do with muscular activity). Bloom[18,19] identified two taxonomies, one of cognitive and the other of affective objectives. The cognitive taxonomy has six main classes: the first is knowledge (to do with remembering, for example, facts, definitions and rules) and the remaining five are to do with intellectual abilities and skills — comprehension, application, analysis, synthesis and evaluation. These taxonomies may be useful in helping to establish logical analysis of the content and process of learning but cannot account for different levels of outcome.

APPLYING THEORIES TO CURRENT PRACTICE

The author's own experience has led her to believe that a one-to-one discussion with a facilitator, using a questioning technique, is the most effective method of integrating facts into concepts and adopting critical reasoning. This approach does, however, have its limitations. It is dependent on the effectiveness of the facilitator, although the learner will be quick to identify any shortfalls, and it is also dependent upon the environment being conducive to learning. Fear of learning about ourselves, fear of exposing our weaknesses and fear of 'authority' could inhibit a true and frank exchange between learner and facilitator.

In small groups, peer monitoring may be used, especially if it is guided along areas for constructive comment, such as technical quality, subject matter and ingenuity.[20] Rowntree states that Burke demonstrated how students were more 'realistic' when asked to assign grades to one another than when asked to grade themselves![20] Self-monitoring, while a useful tool, can be unrealistic and does not overcome the problem of learners needing the intellectual stimulus of others and acquiring subtle insights from peers.

Self-directed learning, used as described in an individual or peer group supervision session, not only helps occupational therapists to acquire clinical reasoning skills but, importantly, may also motivate them towards particular research areas. Additionally, at higher levels, research findings may be discussed to ensure complete and critical analysis of outcomes.

It should be noted that the actual implementation presumes that we have enough senior practitioners with these facilitating skills. It also assumes that all occupational therapists are articulate and have the same level of verbal and written skills. This method could in fact mediate against occupational therapists from a different cultural background, who may not have this level of communication.

A STRATEGY

It is not the purpose of this article to formulate a teaching programme, but rather to adapt the sequential approach to self-directed learning as used by Hammond and Collins[3] to provide a framework that may be used at a post-qualification level:

1. Learner and facilitator agree a learning period.
2. Learner completes a 'situation analysis' (identifies 'What are the occupational therapy needs of the population in my district? What occupational therapy services are not available? What occupational therapy services could be improved?')
3. Learner with facilitator completes a 'competency profile' ('What knowledge, skills, attitudes do I need to do my job? What skills do I lack? What skills am I particularly proficient in? What am I interested in?')

4. 'Learning objectives' are stated (these can be in cognitive or affective terms, but should identify the level of outcome).
5. A 'learning agreement' is drafted. (This is done in relation to objectives and agreed learning period. It consists of a teaching plan and agreed regular reviews.)
6. A self-assessment form is agreed (an individual assessment form compiled by learner and facilitator agrees items and levels for self-monitoring), for example:
   'In planning treatment I could:
   — discuss the method I have chosen with a medical practitioner
   — discuss the implications of using this method with a senior practitioner.'
7. Learner sees facilitator at regularly agreed times to discuss progress and, using reflective practice, integrates learning.

CONCLUSION

This article began by asking questions about getting a commitment from occupational therapists to pursue excellence. It is hoped that self-directed learning using reflective practice offers an opportunity to explore a qualitative approach to learning with the emphasis on not how much is learned but what is learned and how it is applied clinically.

The occupational therapy profession, now more than ever, faces increasing challenges from lack of qualified staff, increasing financial constraints, self-scrutiny and critical analysis from the public and professional bodies, the need to identify our 'product' and market it effectively, and devolved staff management. The ability of qualified practitioners consistently to improve professional competence will not only allow the therapist a greater repertoire of intervention for clients' needs, but will undoubtedly affect the ability to communicate occupational therapy skills, teach others and play an effective part in the future provision of health care.

Helping a practitioner improve practice must be the major theme for self-development and must not be forgotten in the rush to train increasing numbers of occupational therapy staff.

Acknowledgement

This article was presented as an assessed assignment for the MSc in Health Care: Professional Education, at Exeter University.

References

1. Eliot TS. Little Gidding. *Four quartets.* London: Faber & Faber, 1943.
2. Stoltzfus CL. Recognising and rewarding excellence. *J Nurs Admin* 1989; **19**(4): 11.
3. Hammond M, Collins R. Self-directed learning to educate medical educators, part 1: how do we use self-directed learning? *Med Teacher* 1987; **9**(3): 253-60.
4. Maslow AH. A theory of human motivation. *Psychol Rev* 1943; **50**: 370-96.
5. Klyczek JP, Gordon CY. Choosing a motivation construct. *Br J Occup Ther* 1988; **51**(9): 315-19.
6. Hubber D. Motivation in a clinical setting. *Comm Psychiatry* 1988; **1**(3): 38.
7. Lawler EE. *Pay and organisational effectiveness, a psychological view.* New York: McGraw Hill, 1971.
8. Bligh D, Jaques D, Piper DW. *Seven decisions when teaching students.* Exeter: Exeter University Teaching Services, 1981: 24-25.
9. Burnard P, Chapman CM. *Professional and ethical issues in nursing.* Chichester: John Wiley, 1988: 29-39.
10. Engel CE, Clarke RM. Medical education with a difference. *Programmed Learning Educ Technol* 1979; **16**(1): 70-87.
11. Knowles MS. *Using learning contracts.* San Francisco: Jossey Bass, 1986: 3-4.
12. Gibbs G. *Learning by doing.* London: Further Education Unit, 1988.
13. Kolb DA. *Experiential learning. Experience as the source of learning and development.* New Jersey: Prentice-Hall, 1984.

14. Marton F, Hounsell D, Entwistle N. *The experience of learning.* Edinburgh: Scottish Academic Press, 1984.

15. Mumford AL, et al. *Developing directors: the learning process.* Sheffield: Manpower Services Commission, 1987.

16. Usher RL, Bryant I. Re-examining a theory practice relationship in continuing professional education. *Stud Higher Educ* 1987; **12**(2): 201-12.

17. Spencer LM. *Soft skills competencies.* Edinburgh: Scottish Council for Research and Education, 1983.

18. Bloom BS. *Taxonomy of educational objectives, handbook 1: cognitive domain.* New York: McKay, 1956.

19. Bloom BS, Krathwohl D, Masier B. *Taxonomy of educational objectives, handbook II: affective domain.* New York: McKay, 1964.

20. Rowntree D. *Assessing students: how shall we know them?* London: Kogan Page, 1988: 146-49.

Learning in Context: Perceived Benefits of Fieldwork Education within Community Mental Health Settings

Michael Lyons

The emphasis on community-based services for people with psychiatric disorders requires a concerted response from occupational therapists, if we are to assist people to live meaningful lives in their own communities. This article draws on the fieldwork experiences of 16 Australian and American occupational therapy students, to reflect on fieldwork education and how it may be preparing students to meet the demands of proactive practice in psychiatry. Attention is drawn to the importance of fieldwork education in community contexts for occupational therapy students, if these future therapists are to be adequately prepared for the demands of community mental health practice.

Introduction

'I think [occupational therapy] is more practically orientated in the community. You're actually doing things to meet people's needs at that point, in a practical sense. Whereas in a hospital, to me a lot of it seems artificial. You're manufacturing things to be done. It seems a lot more diversional in a hospital than in the community' (Andrea).

This opinion, uttered by an Australian occupational therapy student completing her final year fieldwork in a community psychiatry setting, might not be uniformly endorsed by occupational therapists within psychiatric practice. It could be regarded as a naïve or ill-informed commentary by one too inexperienced to know any better. It cannot pretend to be based on a wealth of experience; nor, like any generalisation, should it be taken to represent fully the situation to which it refers. Nonetheless, it echoes a viewpoint aired in this journal by Joyce (1993) who questioned the relevance of much traditional occupational therapy practice in psychiatry, in the face of many people's 'real life' needs in community contexts.

This article draws upon some fieldwork experiences of a group of Australian and American occupational therapy students in psychiatric service settings. It is a by-product of some broad-based research into students' (primarily Australian) fieldwork experiences. Like the viewpoint of consumers of occupational therapy services, occupational therapy students' views are infrequently presented within literature analysing professional practices. Yet, perhaps there is something worthwhile to be learned from students' perspectives, as neophytes, about occupational therapy education.

The reader's attention is drawn to the interplay of the learning context with educational outcomes, in particular students' educational experiences in community mental health settings. This article reflects on the question: *Does fieldwork in community mental health settings provide students with unique learning experiences concerning the lives of people with psychiatric disorders?*

This question is predicated on the assumption that a richer understanding by professionals of the lives of people in context will enhance the effectiveness of occupational therapy responses to the daily life needs of people with psychiatric disorders. The research findings discussed are by no means definitive of the status of occupational therapy fieldwork education in North America, the United Kingdom or Australia. They are presented, rather, as an artefact of some research which, while bounded by time and place, can contribute to international debate about occupational therapy practice in psychiatry and the preparation of students for this.

Background
From institution to community

A major feature of psychiatric service systems in many industrialised countries has been a change in focus over the last three decades from institutionalised to community-based services (Thompson, 1990; Weir, 1991). As Shore (1992) has expressed the ideal:

'Community mental health is an organised, planned approach to mental health issues, built on an understanding of the structure and needs of a particular community, the acceptance by the community of responsibility for the mental health of all its residents, and the involvement of the community in the development and implementation of easily accessible preventive, curative, and rehabilitative mental health services.'

Hospitals, rather than providing long-term asylum, have moved towards admitting people only for short periods for the purposes of stabilisation of their condition, with the intent of early discharge to and follow-up within the community (Lamb, 1993).

The policy shift in favour of community services has been accompanied by the large-scale deinstitutionalisation of people in psychiatric hospitals in most Western countries (Weir, 1991). Supported in some quarters for its anticipated cost-cutting benefits and championed in others as representing a significant advance for the human rights of people with psychiatric disorders, the process has sparked considerable controversy (Burdekin, 1992; Lamb, 1993; Weinstein, 1990).

Deinstitutionalisation has been variously described as 'the most significant movement in the history of mental health

Michael Lyons, PhD, Lecturer, Department of Occupational Therapy, The University of Queensland, Queensland 4072, Australia.

care [in two hundred years]' (Eisen and Wolfenden, 1988) and 'a process by which responsibility for the care of large numbers of chronically disordered persons was abandoned by State mental health administrations' (Duckmanton R, unpublished report to National Health and Medical Research Council [Australia], 1987). As Lamb (1993) remarked: 'Care in the community has often been assumed almost by definition to be better than hospital care. In reality, poor care can be found in both hospital and community settings.'

The deinstitutionalisation movement has proceeded in the face of many inadequacies in community support structures. It is clear that the movement of people out of psychiatric institutions, along with reduced admissions and much briefer hospitalisations of newly diagnosed people, has in many cases not been accompanied by a corresponding transfer of funding (Brintnell, 1989; Lamb, 1993; Strong, 1994). Recent Australian data indicate that the 90-95% of people affected by psychiatric disorders, who are living in the community, manage to attract only 15-20% of the funds allocated to psychiatric services: the remainder is still tied up in downscaled institutional settings (Burdekin, 1992; Weir, 1991). Meanwhile, many people who have been deinstitutionalised and/or who are regarded as being severely mentally ill lack access to the basic amenities of adequate shelter, nutrition and health care (Deveson, 1991).

In Australia, a recent nationwide inquiry into psychiatric services, conducted by the Human Rights and Equal Opportunities Commission, revealed 'a story of neglect, abuse, discrimination, inefficiency and injustice, and that it is much more widespread than those localised examples which have had a great deal of media attention' (Burdekin, 1992). Despite the best efforts of many individuals, the psychiatric and social welfare systems in many countries are not responding effectively, it seems, to the needs of many people who have psychiatric disorders and their families (Deveson, 1991; Goldin, 1990; Pentland et al, 1992; Strong, 1994; Woodside, 1991).

Occupational therapy in the psychiatric system

One way in which occupational therapists commonly frame their practice in psychiatry is around models of medical treatment, which is a matter of concern for some within the field (Barris et al, 1983; Yerxa, 1993). As Kleinman (1992) has expressed it: 'In our tendency to cling to a medical model of service provision, we have allowed the scope and content of our services to be limited to what has been supported within this model.' For example, medical psychiatry's favouring of drug therapy over psychotherapeutic and social interventions has placed restrictions on the activities of occupational therapists and those other allied health personnel whose primary field of operation is the psychosocial domain.

Despite the large-scale movement of people with psychiatric disorders out of institutions and the change in focus towards the provision of psychiatric services within community settings, it appears that a disproportionate number of occupational therapists in many countries continue to be employed in hospital settings – a situation out of step with the times (Bonder, 1987; Kleinman, 1992; Sparling et al, 1992; Weir, 1991). In the interests of professional survival, Scott (1986) has warned: 'Only by recognising the external trends in the mental health system can occupational therapy personnel market their services effectively to those who use them.'

In psychiatry, along with other areas of practice, occupational therapists typically frame their intervention around a problem-solving process (Hagedorn, 1992; Rogers and Holm, 1991). In enacting this process, Kielhofner (1993) has cautioned occupational therapists to be aware both of the considerable power they may wield over a person's life and of the

bias they may unconsciously manifest. For example, 'Functional assessment is often used to determine what freedoms a person will and will not have, what roles he or she may take on, what activities he or she may do, and what benefits or resources he or she will receive' (Kielhofner, 1993). Our intervention involves making evaluative judgements to which the people being judged frequently have had little opportunity to contribute and which, not surprisingly, may not adequately reflect their viewpoint (Pentland et al, 1992; Polimeni-Walker et al, 1992; Skawski, 1987). As occupational therapists, 'our obligation is to provide services which are based on the values and vision of people with disabilities' (Law, 1991).

In summary, services for people with psychiatric disorders are shrouded in controversy associated with philosophical and structural changes that are occurring in the United Kingdom, North America and Australia. It appears that mental health systems are not yet responding adequately to the range of community support needs of their citizens with psychiatric disorders. The potential of occupational therapy to contribute to the wellbeing of people in community contexts appears to be under-exploited. Amongst other questions, this prompts consideration of how occupational therapy fieldwork education is preparing students to meet the demands of proactive practice in community mental health settings.

Method

This study employed a qualitative methodology to explore the psychiatric fieldwork experiences of 16 occupational therapy students. The study was conducted in two phases: a pilot study of three American students and a larger study of 13 Australian students. Data were collected over a 13-month period.

Informants

All informants in the study were female and were enrolled in either the third or the fourth year of an undergraduate programme. Twelve of the 16 informants were undertaking fieldwork in hospital settings, reflecting a situation where most of the psychiatric fieldwork places available to these students were within hospitals.

Sampling

Informants were selected by what Patton (1990) has termed 'stratified purposeful sampling'. The purpose of this strategy is to capture and describe the central themes or principal outcomes that cut across several major strata of participant or programme variation. Students were stratified on the basis of the type of setting in which they were undertaking their fieldwork. Setting types identified included: public versus private hospital, hospital versus community clinic, and short-stay versus medium-stay to long-stay psychiatric unit.

It was apparent that these facilities differed somewhat in their stated goals and anticipated outcomes for service users and, hence, differed in terms of their processes of intervention. It was reasoned that they might constitute substantially different learning environments for occupational therapy students. By including, within the sample, informants whom it was considered might have quite different fieldwork experiences, it was hoped to understand variations in experiences while at the same time identifying major shared elements of their experiences.

Data collection by interview

The primary technique used for collecting data on informants' experiences was unstructured (and later semi-structured) interviewing (Bogdan and Biklen, 1992). The aim of the interviewing was to have informants talk about the issues of most relevance to them and in a manner that allowed informants to use their own concepts and terms (Stainback and Stainback, 1989).

Typically, informants were interviewed on four or five occasions, each lasting approximately one hour. With the permission of informants, almost all interviews were audio-taped to provide for increased accuracy in capturing informants' words: the essence of what Maxwell (1992) has termed the 'descriptive validity' of their accounts. In attempting to maximise the *trustworthiness* of the data gathering, *member checking* (Krefting, 1991) was regularly engaged in; that is, questions were raised with informants about the interpretations of their fieldwork experiences discussed in prior interviews. Before the final interview with each student, all prior transcripts were reviewed in search of any gaps in the understanding of that student's perspectives. Within the context of the final interview, these were then addressed in what was usually the most structured of all the interviews conducted.

Supplementary data collection

In an effort to strengthen what Maxwell (1992) has termed 'interpretive validity' (or the accuracy of interpretation of informants' perceptions), this research drew on participant observation as an additional means of data gathering. Used in conjunction with interviewing, observation assisted to ascertain more of the meaning of what informants were saying in interviews, as well as the congruence between what they were saying in interviews and what they were doing in given situations (Tebes and Kraemer, 1991).

Most of the participant observations were conducted around groups of people with whom the informants were interacting on a regular basis during their fieldwork affiliations. They were typically groups of people using the services of the psychiatric facilities with which students were affiliated; for example, a social group at a neighbourhood centre, discussion groups on topics as diverse as self-esteem and leisure options, exercise and relaxation groups, and cooking groups where people prepared, ate and cleaned up after a meal. Typically, one participant observation session was undertaken with each informant. These lasted from 30 minutes to 3 hours, depending on the nature and duration of the activity being observed. Detailed field notes about the event observed were then prepared within 24 hours of leaving the setting.

Data analysis

The narrative data from interviews and observations were analysed inductively. 'Inductive analysis means that the patterns, themes, and categories of analysis come from the data; they emerge out of the data rather than being imposed on them prior to data collection and analysis' (Patton, 1990). Analysis began while the process of data collection was still under way. As data were being gathered through interviews and observations, they were being subjected to preliminary inspection and comparative analysis for the emergence of themes (Bogdan and Biklen, 1992; Henwood and Pidgeon, 1992). After data collection had been completed, a full thematic analysis was undertaken with the assistance of a computer package: the ethnograph (Seidel et al, 1988).

Results and discussion

Service systems and professions are created or arise in response to social needs (Reilly, 1962). Whether they, in fact, fulfil the needs they purport to is a complex issue. Within this study of occupational therapy students' fieldwork experiences, informants commented in various ways on their perceptions of the needs of people who have psychiatric disorders. How peo-

ple's needs were most commonly understood by informants appeared to be associated with the contexts (hospital or community) in which the people were encountered. This is hardly surprising for a variety of reasons. For example, in part it may reflect the state of mental health of people who have been hospitalised for treatment, as opposed to those discharged from hospital in what has been deemed a more stable mental state. It also accords with various understandings of the link between the context in which people are encountered and the meaning attributed to their behaviour by observers (Cuff et al, 1990; Rosenhan, 1973).

Identified problems

Within hospital settings, the students' basic reference point in relation to the task of serving patients with psychiatric disorders was usually *problems* rather than *needs*. This is understandable in the light of the problem orientation of medical services and the problem-solving approach commonly taught to occupational therapy students. Such an approach may fail to take account of the living circumstances and personal preferences of the person involved, to ascertain whether the problem is a need in the person's own view (Kielhofner, 1993). This suggests a discrepancy that can exist between professional and patient perspectives, and the dangers inherent in the former ascertaining what is best without regard for the latter's visions and values (Law, 1991).

Most potent were instances in hospital settings where a conflict arose between a person's expressed need and what staff members considered to be 'good' for them. For example:

'Well, they're here to get help and this shouldn't be a place for people just to come and relax. I've heard patients say like, "I want to stay longer. I need more time to sleep or more time to rest." Well, it's not supposed to be just like a vacation. It's supposed to be therapeutic, helping with their problems' (Paula).

In a similar vein, a student in another hospital setting reported that patients (all of whom were 60 years or older) were locked out of their rooms during the day to prevent them from spending too much time there. The student rationalised this with reference to her belief that it is unhealthy for people to stay in their rooms for long periods during the day. It is usually not a simple task for a helping professional (and hence for a student) to reconcile conflicts between personal or service values and service recipients' wishes. It is disturbingly easy, however, to discount the latter in favour of the former.

'So we're thinking of developing some kind of checklist so [recently arrived patients] can be given, by the doctor, what's offered on the unit. So they can say, "Well, this and this would be good for you." We can tell them what we think would be good for them and the doctor can reinforce it' (Paula).

Comments such as this are suggestive of a culture inclined to identify desirable outcomes for people on the basis of professional judgements about 'what is best' for them: the concept of professional *discretion* (Biklen, 1988; Jongbloed and Crichton, 1990). The assumption of a unity of concern or interest between those who bestow benevolence and those who receive it is, however, a questionable one (Pentland et al, 1992; Scheid-Cook, 1993; Vaughan, 1991). Such is the nature of some human service systems where people's rights to privacy and choice may be overlooked by well-meaning service workers intent on solving their problems: problems identified by workers drawing on values that may not accord with people's own sense of their best interests.

Desirable outcomes

From the perspective of hospital-based professionals, 'living in the community' may be glibly advocated as *the* desirable outcome for people with psychiatric disorders. Grave concerns have been expressed regarding the process of deinstitutionalisation. As Lamb (1993) has pointed out, it is foolish to assume that people are, by definition, better off merely by being out of hospital.

This was one issue where the impact of differences in service settings was apparent within students' experiences and, hence, their point of view. Those students in a community setting were generally more attuned to potential shortcomings of the system of psychiatric services, in responding to people's needs, than were their hospital-based counterparts. For example:

'People are being thrown out into the community and it all seems to be a money-saving measure. They've got all the ideals of normalisation but I'm not sure whether that's the real purpose [that] it's happened actually' (Andrea).

Andrea was involved with people who may not have had a permanent place to live; perhaps they were living on the streets. She and some of her peers in the community clinic recognised the significance of personal support. The majority of informants, however, were dealing with people being treated or maintained in hospital. In hospital, people have a roof over their heads, three meals a day, and supervision of their personal care. It is little wonder that the students in such different settings identified different needs for the people with whom they had contact. A student's responses will be influenced by particular fieldwork experiences which themselves are a function of the philosophy and goals of particular service settings.

Another example of how the fieldwork context seemed to enrich informants' insights into the lives (and possibly the needs) of the people whom they served concerns people's social affiliations. To students in a community clinic, the possibility of people's lack of friendships and social outlets was starkly revealed. For example:

'One lady brought in her birthday cake – it was her birthday – and we all sang "Happy Birthday" to her. I suppose [the weekly social group] is a sort of family. Like for them, it might be their idea of a family, which I thought was really nice; but then the reality hit me ... the reality of how lonely it might be that this might be the only contact' (Silla).

The social isolation and loneliness of many people with psychiatric disorders living in the community has been discussed (Deveson, 1991; Weir, 1991). A few of these students caught a glimpse of what a person's lifestyle might be like and the paucity of friendships therein. Again, this is something which is less evident in hospital where everyone is removed from their everyday surroundings; everyone is a visitor. People's lack of social intimacy is unlikely to be so apparent in a hospital.

Students sometimes were prompted to view a person's needs within the context of key people and roles in that person's life:

'I guess [the goal for the adolescents here] is just leading a meaningful life without ending up in some sort of institution or jail or on the streets or something like that. They have a more stable life or improved family relationships, getting a job or getting back to school and doing well: that sort of thing' (Jill).

This sense of individuals as part of a system – a family system and a network of normative community roles – seemed to be more within the grasp of those students in community placements. Perhaps the removal of a person to the hospital environment curbs the impetus for students to think globally (some would say holistically) about a patient's needs: in terms of a life lived with people, and engaged in normative roles and tasks such as school and work. Such a response would be understandable in the context of a hospital setting dedicated to acute medical care. However, it raises questions about the education of students for practice beyond acute hospital settings.

Also of concern are the indications from this research that many students' experiences of people with psychiatric disorders may occur only within the strictures of clinical contexts, as opposed to real life settings through which a more complete view of people might be obtained (Lyons, 1994). This was highlighted by several informants on placement in community clinics, who commented on how contact with people outside the clinical setting had influenced their perceptions markedly. For example, two students attended a week-long camp where they lived alongside some people with psychiatric diagnoses. From this experience and hearing these people's stories of their lives, the students reported a growing sense of respect for them as survivors against a backdrop of considerable trauma and hardship. It would appear that educational opportunities that arise from close engagement with service users (that is, prolonged personal contact with individuals) in naturalistic settings are more of a possibility within community mental health settings.

Conclusion

This article has reflected upon fieldwork education in psychiatry as a preparation for occupational therapy service in the community. A view has been advanced of community mental health settings as potentially 'rich' learning contexts for occupational therapy students. In support of this view, some experiences of a small group of students on fieldwork in psychiatric settings have been drawn upon.

It is apparent that, with the thrust in many countries towards more expansive community health services, occupational therapists are in short supply in community settings (Tissier, 1995), which in itself is problematic if students are to gain experience in community practice. Weir (1991) has exhorted Australian occupational therapists to take up more positions in community mental health and occupational therapy educators to ensure that fieldwork placements are relevant to changing work practices.

The preparation of students to be *effective* community practitioners is, of course, about more than just 'being there'. It is about being encouraged to question preconceptions and established modes of practice, in the light of fresh insights gained from clients about their daily life needs. For example, as one community-based informant in this study articulated:

'I had a talk to [a fellow student] today about the value of showing someone how to change a light bulb if they're not going to have to change it for another three months; and then, by then, they'll probably forget. And whether doing cooking skills with someone if they're not really interested in cooking; they're quite capable but it's easier to go to the shop' (Silla).

It is critical that students undertaking fieldwork in the community are challenged to recognise that quality services are driven by consumer priorities. As Joyce (1993) has suggested: 'Effective community care is not happy, smiling groups of occupational therapists performing in local community mental health centres.' If we are to be true to our heritage of 'giving meaningful life back to people whose lives have been taken from them' (Joyce, 1993), then our students must be learning from us about a service agenda that is client-orientated in the sense that it is personally relevant to the individuals whom we are paid to serve.

Acknowledgement

My thanks to my colleague, Merrill Crabtree, for her helpful comments on an earlier draft of this paper.

References

Barris R, Kielhofner G, Watts J (1983) *Psychosocial occupational therapy. Practice in a pluralistic arena.* Laurel, MD: Ramsco, 1983.

Biklen D (1988) The myth of clinical judgement. *Journal of Social Issues, 44,* 127-40.

Bogdan R, Biklen S (1992) *Qualitative research for education. An introduction to theory and methods.* 2nd ed. Boston: Allyn and Bacon.

Bonder B (1987) Occupational therapy in mental health: crisis or opportunity? *American Journal of Occupational Therapy, 41,* 495-99.

Brintnell S (1989) Occupational therapy in mental health: a growth industry. *Canadian Journal of Occupational Therapy, 56,* 7-9.

Burdekin B (1992) Mental health – your right. *Mental Health in Australia, 4(2),* 38-56.

Cuff E, Sharrock W, Francis D (1990) *Perspectives in sociology.* 3rd ed. London: Unwin Hyman.

Deveson A (1991) *Tell me I'm here.* Melbourne: Penguin.

Eisen P, Wolfenden K (1988) *A national mental health services policy.* Canberra: Department of Community Services and Health, 347.

Goldin C (1990) Stigma, biomedical efficacy, and institutional control. *Social Science and Medicine, 30,* 895-900.

Hagedorn R (1992) *Occupational therapy: foundations for practice.* London: Churchill Livingstone, 1992.

Henwood K, Pidgeon N (1992) Qualitative research and psychological theorising. *British Journal of Psychology, 83,* 97-111.

Jongbloed L, Crichton A (1990) A new definition of disability: implications for rehabilitation practice and social policy. *Canadian Journal of Occupational Therapy, 57,* 32-37.

Joyce L (1993) Occupational therapy: a cause without a rebel. *British Journal of Occupational Therapy, 56(12),* 447.

Kielhofner G (1993) Functional assessment: toward a dialectical view of person-environment relations. *American Journal of Occupational Therapy, 47,* 248-51.

Kleinman B (1992) The challenge of providing occupational therapy in mental health. *American Journal of Occupational Therapy, 46,* 555-57.

Krefting L (1991) Rigour in qualitative research: the assessment of trustworthiness. *American Journal of Occupational Therapy, 45,* 214-22.

Lamb H (1993) Lessons learned from deinstitutionalisation in the US. *British Journal of Psychiatry, 162,* 587-92.

Law M (1991) The environment: a focus for occupational therapy. *Canadian Journal of Occupational Therapy, 58,* 171-79.

Lyons M (1994) *Shadows and light: occupational therapy students' fieldwork experiences of people with psychiatric disorders.* Unpublished doctoral dissertation. Brisbane: University of Queensland.

Maxwell J (1992) Understanding and validity in qualitative research. *Harvard Educational Review, 62,* 279-300.

Patton M (1990) *Qualitative evaluation and research methods.* 2nd ed. Newbury Park, CA: Sage.

Pentland W, Krupa T, Lynch S, Clark C (1992) Community integration for persons with disabilities: working together to make it happen. *Canadian Journal of Occupational Therapy, 59,* 127-31.

Polimeni-Walker I, Wilson K, Jewers R (1992) Reasons for participating in occupational therapy groups: perceptions of adult psychi-atric inpatients and occupational therapists. *Canadian Journal of Occupational Therapy, 59,* 240-47.

Reilly M (1962) Occupational therapy can be one of the great ideas of 20th century medicine. *American Journal of Occupational Therapy, 16,* 1-9 .

Rogers J, Holm M (1991) Occupational therapy diagnostic reasoning: a component of clinical reasoning. *American Journal of Occupational Therapy, 45,* 1045-53.

Rosenhan D (1973) On being sane in insane places. *Science, 179,* 250-58.

Scheid-Cook T (1993) Controllers and controlled: an analysis of participant constructions of outpatient commitment. *Sociology of Health and Illness, 15,* 179-98.

Scott A (1986) Occupational therapy: the profession as a system. In: Robertson S, ed. *SCOPE: Strategies, concepts and opportunities for programme development. A curriculum for occupational therapy personnel.* Rockville, MD: American Occupational Therapy Association, 77-82.

Seidel J, Kjolseth R, Seymour E (1988) *The ethnograph.* Corvallis, OR: Qualis Research Associates.

Shore M (1992) Community mental health: corpse or phoenix? Personal reflections on an era. *Professional Psychology: Research and Practice, 23,* 257-62.

Skawski K (1987) Ethnic/racial considerations in occupational therapy: a survey of attitudes. *Occupational Therapy in Health Care, 4,* 37-48.

Sparling E, Clark N, Laidlaw J (1992) Assessment of the demands by general practitioners for a community psychiatric occupational therapy service. *British Journal of Occupational Therapy, 55,* 193-96.

Stainback W, Stainback S (1989) Using qualitative data collection procedures to investigate supported education issues. *Journal of the Association for Persons with Severe Handicaps, 14,* 271-77.

Strong S (1994) Action, not words! *Community Care,* 27 Oct/2 Nov, 14-15.

Tebes J, Kraemer D (1991) Quantitative and qualitative knowing in mutual support research: some lessons from the recent history of scientific psychology. *American Journal of Community Psychology, 19,* 739-56.

Thompson B (1990) Roles and settings. In: Creek J, ed. *Occupational therapy and mental health: principles, skills and practice.* London: Churchill Livingstone, 115-28.

Tissier G (1995) Occupational hazards. *Community Care,* 9-15 Feb, 28-29.

Vaughan C (1991) The social basis of conflict between blind people and agents of rehabilitation. *Disability, Handicap and Society, 6,* 203-17.

Weinstein R (1990) Mental hospitals and the institutionalisation of patients. *Research in Community Mental Health, 6,* 273-94.

Weir W (1991) Emerging from behind locked doors. *Australian Occupational Therapy Journal, 38,* 185-93.

Woodside H (1991) The participation of mental health consumers in health care issues. *Canadian Journal of Occupational Therapy, 58,* 3-5.

Yerxa E (1993) Occupational science: a new source of power for participants in occupational therapy. *Occupational Science: Australia, 1,* 3-9.

Factors Affecting a Clinician's Decision to Provide Fieldwork Education to Students

Margaret Tompson, Leonard F. Proctor

Key words:
- Fieldwork education,
- Qualitative research, occupational therapy

Margaret Tompson, M.C.Ed., O.T.Reg. (Sask.), O.T.(C) is Assistant Clinical Co-ordinator (Saskatchewan) in the School of Medical Rehabilitation, University of Manitoba, Winnipeg.
Mailing address: 736 University Drive, Saskatoon, Saskatchewan, S7N OJ4.

Leonard Proctor, B.A., B.Ed., M.Ed., M.L.S.,PhD. is an Associate Professor, in the Department of Communications, Continuing and Vocational Education, College of Education, University of Saskatchewan, Saskatoon.

This paper is based on a presentation made at the Annual CAOT conference in Kitchener, Ontario, June 1988.

ABSTRACT

Fieldwork represents an important component of the education of an occupational therapist. In this study thirteen occupational therapists in small Saskatchewan occupational therapy facilities were interviewed to determine the factors and the relationships among these factors that affected their involvement in the fieldwork process. The directors of the two large occupational therapy departments in Saskatchewan, together with eight Canadian university fieldwork co-ordinators were interviewed for comparison purposes. The findings of the study have shown that there were four major influences affecting Saskatchewan therapists' involvement in the fieldwork program of occupational therapy students. They were: workload; feelings of isolation; the parameters of a placement; and professionalism. This study is important because it has identified significant factors for university fieldwork co-ordinators to consider in their contact with therapists. It has also provided a model for other similar studies.

Fieldwork can be likened to a crucible. It is that part of the curriculum when a student's theoretical knowledge is melded with practical skills. Just as it would be impossible to produce steel without the smelting process, so it would be unthinkable to educate our students without fieldwork. Baines (1974), Coles (1985), and Ramsay (1974) have clearly described fieldwork as a bridging mechanism which supports the student in becoming a qualified professional. It has been considered a unique and important educational experience (Emery, 1981; Moore & Perry, 1976; Scully & Shepard, 1983) which involved a relationship between the faculty member, the therapist, the student, and the client (Snow & Mitchell, 1982). In Canada, fieldwork comprises approximately one-third of the curriculum.

One of the major issues facing Canadian educational occupational therapy programs is the lack of fieldwork placements for students ("S.O.S.", 1985; Tompson, 1987; Wilkins, 1986; Woodside, 1977). This shortage of fieldwork placements puts pressure on educational programs to use placements that might not be as appropriate as desired. This can have ramifications for the profession as the literature indicates that students' decisions, concerning areas of future employment are affected by the type of fieldwork experience that they had as a student (Christie et al., 1985; Clark & Schlackter, 1978; Harris & Ebbert, 1983;

Polatajko & Quintyn, 1986).

One of the key factors affecting the existence of a fieldwork placement is the decision of the therapist to become involved with working with a student as a clinical educator. This role has been described as primarily that of role model (Emery, 1981; Jacobson, 1974; Page, 1982), resource (Simon, 1976; Casbergue, 1978), designer of instruction and supervisor, change agent (Emery, 1981; Ramsden & Dervitz, 1972) and gatekeeper to the profession (Moeller, 1984). Several studies (May, 1983; Mayberry, 1973; Emery, 1984; Saarinen, 1982) have identified the skills necessary for individuals who are clinical educators. Usually the process of fieldwork has been described from the perspective of the faculty member or the student and rarely from the perspective of the clinical educator. Thus the purpose of this study was to identify and describe the factors affecting an occupational therapist's decision to become involved in the fieldwork process.

Method

A qualitative approach was chosen for this study because of the exploratory nature of the research (Miles & Huberman, 1984; Yerxa, 1981). Snow and Mitchell's (1982) model of the fieldwork process combined with Lewin's (1951) force field theory were used as the theoretical framework for this study. Snow and Mitchell based their model of fieldwork on the biological sciences in which "relationships between organisms can be identified as mutualistic, symbiotic or parasitic" (p.255). They described the ideal relationship between faculty member, clinical educator, and student as being "mutualistic". Lewin (1951) described how many forces act on an individual and cause him or her to behave in a certain way. Such forces can be positive or negative.

The theoretical framework was developed by superimposing Lewin's theory of force field anaylsis on an adapted version of Snow and Mitchell's (1982) model of fieldwork relationships. The fieldwork process is represented as a circle from which the segment representing the client and the therapist, who have a mandated relationship, have been separated (see Figure 1). The focus of the study was to identify and describe the factors which encouraged or

discouraged the therapist's involvement in fieldwork. This theoretical framework did not in anyway pre-determine what would be found.

A. Participants

Thirteen occupational therapists agreed to be involved in the study. They were therapists practicing in Saskatchewan, a Canadian prairie province with a population of approximately one million people. These therapists were predominantly female and Canadian. They were generally clinically experienced therapists with limited exposure to students. Nine of them had had virtually no contact with students while the other four had supervised some students outside Saskatchewan. All but two were functioning as sole-charge therapists.

B. Instrument

An interview format for a semi-structured interview was designed based on the following five guiding questions:

1. What were the perceived advantages and disadvantages of occupational therapists having students during their fieldwork placement?

2. What were the major concerns of occupational therapists involved in students' fieldwork placements?

3. Were there differences in perception between different categories of occupational therapists, based on size or location of the facility?

4. Were there differences in perceptions of occupational therapists who have

Figure 1

Lewin's (1951) force field theory superimposed on Snow and Mitchell's (1982) model of fieldwork relationships

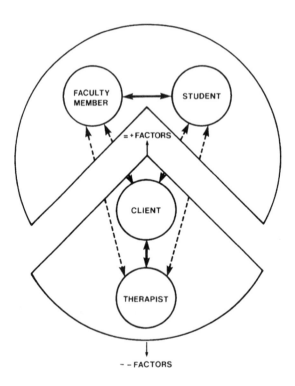

Note:
—— = voluntary relationship
- - - - = mandated relationship

had little or no experience with students, and those who were experienced?

5. Was the perspective of the occupational therapist in a small department in the role of a clinical educator different from that of the university fieldwork co-ordinator or the director of a large occupational therapy department?

One method for assessing the credibility of the findings of a study which uses qualitative research methods is through "triangulation" (Lincoln & Guba, 1985) of the data. This can be achieved by using different data sources or by using different data collection methods (Patton, 1980). In this study the directors of two large Saskatchewan occupational therapy departments and eight fieldwork co-ordinators from across Canada were interviewed and their responses compared to the responses of Saskatchewan therapists.

C. Analysis

In this study interview data were taped and verbatim transcripts made of all interviews. As this was a qualitative study, data analysis alternated throughout the study with data collection (Bogdan & Biklen, 1982; Miles, 1983). The data collected was sorted with the assistance of a computer program, the Ethnograph (Seidel, Jolseth, & Clark, 1985). This computer program

greatly facilitated the identification of the factors that affected Saskatchewan occupational therapists involvement in fieldwork. These factors were then studied further to develop patterns and themes to explain the relationship between these factors. Some factors were re-coded to show more detail and frequency counts were conducted of others in order to substantiate a linkage of these factors and the demographic characteristics of the participants.

Issues concerning the trustworthiness of the study were addressed through a variety of methodological approaches such as: the use of verbatim transcripts; double-coding; triangulation of data from the responses of the directors of large Saskatchewan occupational therapy departments and Canadian university fieldwork co-ordinators; and the provision of detailed descriptions of the decision processes carried out throughout the study.

Results

Saskatchewan therapists did want to work with students but many factors had to be considered before they felt they could offer a fieldwork placement. These factors could be divided into four major influences: workload; isolation; parameters of a placement; and professionalism. These four influences varied as to whether they encouraged or discouraged therapists from working with students. The therapists' descriptions of these influences was compared with the views of directors from two large Saskatchewan departments and Canadian university fieldwork co-ordinators. This comparison of perspectives highlighted similarities and differences.

1. Workload

a. Negative factors
Saskatchewan occupational therapists have extensive workloads. Several factors associated with these workloads contributed to having a negative influence on therapists (see Figure 2). The additional task of being responsible for a student had both direct and indirect effects on a therapist's workload. The direct effects of a student were related to: the preparation and planning for the student's arrival; the time required for supervision; and the slowing effect on the therapist's own productivity due to the explanations that were required. There was also resentment expressed by over a third of the therapists towards the extensive work required to apply for formal fieldwork accreditation by the national association.

Difficulties already present in a therapist's work environment which were exacerbated by the arrival of a student were considered indirect effects of the student on a therapist's workload. For example, three-quarters of the therapists perceived their administrative duties taking up a considerable amount of their time, time which was then not available to the student.

Then there were the therapist's personal needs. In a sole-charge position such factors as sickness, holidays and pressure at home all have to be taken into consideration before agreeing to provide a fieldwork placement. Staffing shortages were another difficulty which was affected by a student. As one therapist explained:

Do I have enough staff that I can afford the time? What would my staffing situation be at that time?

b. Positive factors
The student did however have some positive effects on workload. Nine of the therapists commented on the improvement a student made to the work capacity of a department. However, therapists did qualify this statement by indicating that it

Figure 2

Positive and negative factors related to the influence of workload on a Saskatchewan therapist

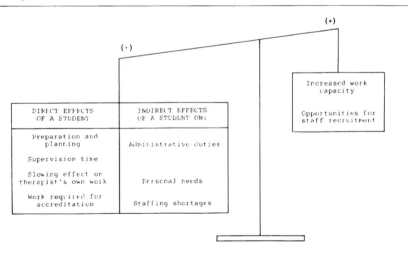

sometimes depended on the level of the student. There was also the recruitment benefits of having students which was commented on by a third of the therapists

It's the only way of getting out of this doldrum staffing business. I feel I can actually do something about it now....Finally I'm doing something that ten years down the road might have an effect.

The directors and fieldwork co-ordinators were in agreement with the therapists' concerns about the extra workload resulting from the presence of a student in a facility. Some of them also commented on the lengthy process of national accreditation. No comments were made about the administrative tasks of the sole-charge therapist.

2. Isolation

A major influence on the participant, of whom all but two were working alone, was the feeling of isolation. The effects of a therapist's feelings of isolation could be divided into four aspects: the effects of isolation on a therapist; the impact of the presence of a student on the facility; the effect of the student on the therapist; and the type of contact a therapist had with those in charge of the educational program. Each aspect had both positive and negative effects (see Figure 3)

a. The effect of isolation on the therapist

The feelings of isolation experienced by participants in this study were the same, whether they were in an urban or a rural area. This feeling of isolation had two outcomes on therapists. It produced a lack of confidence in therapists, which was slightly more pronounced in the rural rather than the urban areas, and it facilitated the development of misconceptions regarding fieldwork.

Participants expressed feelings of being out of date (11 respondents), of lacking experience (5 respondents), or simply not possessing the confidence to take students (8 respondents). This lack of confidence was exacerbated by a lack of any formal training or preparation for working with students. Most participants had had to acquire their knowledge by watching others or from personal experience. The misconceptions developed by therapists relating to fieldwork included: belief that sole-charge

therapists were not permitted to take students (3 respondents); and that there were sufficient fieldwork placements for all students (4 respondents).

b. Impact of the student on the facility

Secondly there was the impact of the student on the therapist. Overall therapists viewed the students in a very positive light as a "breath of fresh air". Over three-quarters of the therapists perceived the student as a catalyst who would in some way change the therapist's behaviour. Behaviour changes which were cited included: increased reflection; reorganisation; renewed enthusiasm; and a rekindling of the desire to learn. In addition all but two therapists commented on the two-way nature of the learning that occurs when there is a student in the department.

Therapists perceived only two negative aspects to the impact of the students presence. There was the difficulty of evaluating a student. Over a third of the therapists identified report writing or evaluation of staff or students as being the activity they disliked most in their work activities. Then

there were the problems of dealing with a difficult student. However this problem was only a concern of those therapists with recent experience of students and it was not the result of having had such a student. Rather it was the feeling of inevitability that one day they would get a student who would be difficult.

c. The effect of the student on the therapist

The third aspect affecting a therapist's feeling of isolation was the student's impact on the facility. Overall this was seen in a positive light. Students were perceived as being stimulating to the patients and three-quarters of the therapists commented on the increased status and profile a department received because it was considered suitable for a fieldwork placement. Having a student assigned to the department, also improved the quality of the work because therapists were aware someone was trying to learn by watching them. However there was some negativity expressed relating to the impact of the student on the facility in terms of the disruption to a patient's treatment program and the potential to overload

Figure 3
Positive and negative factors related to a therapist's feeling of isolation

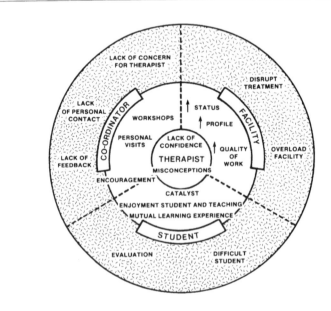

Note:

Postive factors

Negative factors

Figure 4
Positive and negative factors related to the parameters of a placement, shown on a continuum

	Positive factors	Negative factors
LENGTH OF A PLACEMENT	8 weeks	4 weeks
AMOUNT OF EXPERIENCE A STUDENT HAD	Senior	Junior
TIME OF THE YEAR	January - April Sept. - Nov.	May - August December
FREQUENCY WITH WHICH A FACILITY WAS USED FOR STUDENTS	Once or twice	Constantly (5 or more students a year)
SUPERVISOR-STUDENT RATIO	1 : 1	1 : 2

a clinical facility with students, as one therapist explained:

There tends to be more of a disruption in people's...normal programming. They tend not to be getting consistent active treatment. They get more assessments than treatments than they normally would get from a therapist.

d. Contact with the faculty of the educational program

The final aspect of the influence of isolation was seen as the impact of the contact with the educational program. At the time of the study this was a negative force. A great deal of frustration was expressed concerning the lack of contact with educational programs and the lack of support when difficulties arose.

Therapists complained that any contact was usually of an impersonal nature by mail or telephone. There was also a lack of feedback on how placements were viewed by the educational program, so therapists had no means of knowing if changes were necessary. Therapists expressed a need for more support in the form of: on-site visits by faculty; the provision of workshops on clinical supervision skills; and adequate feedback. If educational programs took such action, then therapists felt it would do much to encourage their involvement in the fieldwork process.

The directors but not the co-ordinators, recognised the problem Saskatchewan

therapists had with isolation. The co-ordinators identified lack of confidence as having an effect on therapists, but did not comment on the importance of adequate

feedback. However the therapists' concern with evaluation and problem students was recognised by the co-ordinators. The positive impact of the student on a facility was commented on by both the directors and co-ordinators. The majority of the co-ordinators agreed with the therapists on the degree and type of contact needed between therapists in the facilities and the university fieldwork co-ordinators from the educational programs.

3. Parameters of the placement

The third influence was related to the parameters of the fieldwork placement. These were viewed as being on a continuum between positive and negative effects (see Figure 4). Saskatchewan therapists felt four weeks was the minimum length for a placement with the ideal length being being between six and eight weeks. They preferred senior to junior students. Only three therapists stated they felt they could handle a ratio of two students per therapist and these therapists, though clinicallly experienced, had had limited experience with students. The other

Figure 5
The effect of different aspects of professionalism on a Saskatchewan therapist

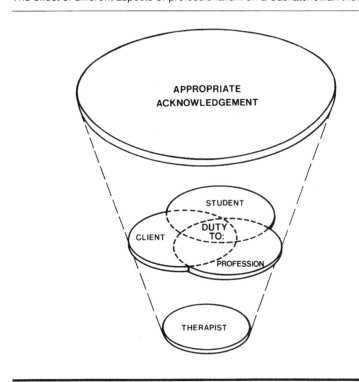

APPROPRIATE ACKNOWLEDGEMENT

STUDENT

CLIENT

DUTY TO:

PROFESSION

THERAPIST

therapists stated a preference for the 1:1 therapist-student ratio. The new year, spring and fall were the most popular times to offer fieldwork placements, with the summer months being least popular because of vacations. Unfortunately, summer is the time when the bulk of fieldwork placements are required across Canada. All therapists felt they needed a break from supervising students in their facilities. Generally there was consistency between the therapists, directors and co-ordinators on what were considered to be desirable parameters of a fieldwork placement.

4. Professionalism

The final influence on a therapist was identified as professionalism (see Figure 5). There were many facets to professionalism and all were closely interrelated and exerting conflicting forces on a therapist. On one level professionalism for a therapist within the context of the fieldwork process encompassed such factors as: duty to the client; duty to the student; and duty to the profession. There was conflict for a therapist between her duty to her client and her duty to the profession or the student. The dilemma for the therapist was that both types of professional involvement made extensive demands on her time. Therapists felt they were not in a position to do justice to both the client and the student.

On another level there was the therapist's own concept of what was an appropriate acknowledgement of her work with students. Inappropriate acknowledgement was seen as a reflection on her professionalism. For example, three-quarters of the therapists expressed negative feelings about any type of monetary reward.

The interrelated nature of these aspects of professionalsm made it impossible to delineate clearly it's overall effect on a therapist's involvement in the fieldwork process. What was clear was that all participants were very aware of their status as professionals with their corresponding professional obligations.

The dilemma of the therapist over duty to the client or the profession was commented on by one director and one co-ordinator. The majority of the co-ordinators recognised the importance of adequate acknowledgement of therapists' work with students.

Conclusions

Four major influences were identified as affecting a therapist's decision to become involved in the fieldwork process: workload; isolation; parameters of the fieldwork placement; and professionalism (see Figure 6). These influences consisted of a multitude of factors, many of which were interrelated. Three conclusions can be drawn from this study which have implications for those involved in the implementation of fieldwork education.

First, there was the effect of the distance between Saskatchewan therapists and the nearest educational program. The participants in this study were therapists in small departments, far away from any educational program who were just starting to become involved in the fieldwork process. The findings have pointed out the need and importance of adequate communication between therapists and fieldwork co-ordinators. In addition, interviews with fieldwork co-ordinators have illustrated for this researcher, together with her own experiences, the vital role played by the co-ordinator in bridging the gap between clinicians and the world of academia. Therapists welcomed the support the fieldwork co-ordinator provided and expressed a need for preparation in their role as clinical educators.

Secondly, the desirable parameters of a fieldwork placement that were identified, provide a framework within which university fieldwork co-ordinators can review the attitudes of their own pool of clinical educators. The effectiveness of encouragement from external sources points out the value of those involved with educational programs, and national and provincial professional associations to put more effort into encouraging the development of fieldwork placements.

Finally, research in fieldwork in

Figure 6

The four influences affecting Saskatchewan occupational therapists' involvement in fieldwork

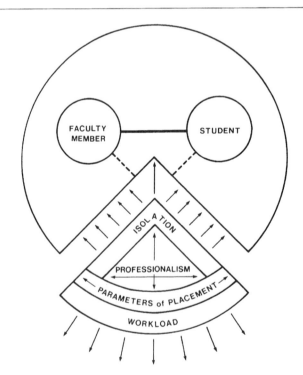

Note: Arrows indicate direction of influence. The small segment represents the therapist and client component of Snow and Mitchell's (1982) model of fieldwork relationships

occupational therapy in Canada is still in its infancy. This study has helped identify areas of future research which might make use of comparative, longitudinal, qualitative, and evaluative methodological approaches. This study has only scratched the surface in attempting to answer the question of why therapists choose or choose not to be active participants in the fieldwork education process.

Summary

The results of this study show that the question of whether or not to offer a fieldwork placement for a student is not a simple decision for a therapist to make. There are many factors that must be taken into consideration. The influences of workload, isolation, parameters of the placement and professionalism contain factors which have both negative and positive forces on clinicians. By focusing on the elimination of the negative factors and by enhancing the positive ones, everyone in the profession can work together toward reducing the shortage of fieldwork placements in Canada.

REFERENCES

Baines, T.R. (1974). The faculty supervisor. In J. Duley (Ed.), Implementing field experience education. *New Directions for Higher Education, 2*(2), 39-44.

Bogdan, R.C., & Biklen, S.K. (1982). *Qualitative research for education: An introduction to theory and methods*. Boston: Allyn and Bacon.

Casbergue, J. (1978). Role of faculty development in clinical education. In M.K. Morgan, & D.M. Irby (Eds.), *Evaluating Clinical Competence in the Health Professions* (pp.171-186). Saint Louis: C.V. Mosby.

Christie, B., Joyce, P., & Moeller, P.L. (1985). Fieldwork experience, Part 1: Impact on practice preference. *The American Journal of Occupational Therapy, 39*, 671-674.

Clark, S.L., & Schlachter, S. (1981). Development of clinical education sites in an area health education system. *Physical Therapy, 61*, 904-906.

Coles, M.A. (1985). Dialogue [Letter to the editor]. *Canadian Journal of Occupational Therapy, 52*, 38.

Emery, M.J. (1981). *Preparing clinical instructors: The consumer's perspective*. Unpublished master's thesis, University of Vermont.

Emery, M.J. (1984). Effectiveness of the clinical instructor. *Physical Therapy, 64*, 1079 - 1083.

Harris, D.L., & Ebbert, P.J. (1983). Effects of clinical preceptorship on career and practice site choices. *Western Journal of Medicine, 138*, 276-279.

Jacobson, B.F. (1974). Role Modeling in physical therapy. *Physical Therapy, 54*, 244-250.

Lewin, K. (1951). *Field theory in social sciences*. New York: Harper & Row.

Lincoln, Y.S., & Guba, E.G. (1985). *Naturalistic Inquiry*. Sage: London.

May, J. M. (1983). Teaching. A skill in clinical practice. *Physical Therapy, 63*, 1627 - 1633.

Mayberry, W.E. (1973). Some dimensions of clinical teaching. *Journal of Dental Education, 8* - 12.

Miles, M.D. (1983). Qualitative data as an attractive nuisance: the problem of analysis. In J.Van Maanen (Ed.) *Qualitative Methodology* (pp. 117 - 134). London: Sage.

Miles, M.B., & Huberman, A.M. (1984). *Qualitative data analysis*. Beverly Hills: Sage.

Moeller, P. (1984, August). Clinical supervision: Guidelines for managing the problem students. *Journal of Allied Health*, 205-211.

Moore, M.L., & Perry, J.F. (1976). *Clinical Education in Physical Therapy: Present status/future needs*. Washington, DC: American Physical Therapy Association.

Page, G. (1982, June). The clinical occupational therapist as an educator. Workshop conducted at the annual conference of the Canadian Association of Occupational Therapists, Vancouver.

Patton, M.Q. (1980). *Qualitative evaluation methods*. Beverly Hills, California: Sage.

Polatajoko, H., & Quintyn, M. (1986). Factors affecting occupational therapy job site selection in underserviced areas. *The Canadian Journal of Occupational Therapy, 53*, 151-158

Ramsay, W.R. (1974). Role of the agency supervisor. In J. Duley (Ed.), Implementing Field Experience Education. *New Directions for Higher Education, 2*, 45-54.

Ramsden, E.L., & Dervitz, H.L. (1972). Clinical education: Interpersonal foundations. *Physical Therapy, 52*(10), 1060- 1065.

Seidel, J.V., Jolseth, R., & Clark, J.A. (1985). *The Ethnograph - Version 2*. [Computer program]. Littleton, CO: Qualis Research Associates.

Scully, R.M., & Shepard, K.F. (1983). Clinical teaching in physical therapy education. *Physical Therapy, 63*, 349-358.

Simon, J.L. (1976). *A role guide and resource book for clinical preceptors*. (DHEW Publication No. HRA 77-14). Washington, DC: U.S. Government Printing Office.

Snow, T., & Mitchell, M.M. (1982). Administrative patterns in curriculum-clinic interactions. *American Journal of Occupational Therapy, 36*, 251-256.

"S.O.S.". (1985, January). *National, 2*(1), p.4.

Tompson, M.A.M. (1987). The evolution of standards for the fieldwork component of the curriculum. *Canadian Journal of Occupational Therapy, 54*, 237 - 243.

Wilkins, S. (1986). Presidential address. *National, 3*,(4), 4 and 20.

Woodside, H. (1977). Basic issues in occupational therapy today. *Canadian Journal of Occupational Therapy, 44*, 9-15.

Yerxa, E.J. (1981). Basic or applied? A "Developmental assessment" of occupational therapy research in 1981. *American Journal of Occupational Therapy, 35*, 820 - 821.

ACKNOWLEDGMENTS

This article is a synopsis of the first author's unpublished master's thesis (1986): *Factors affecting Saskatchewan Occupational Therapists' involvement in fieldwork*. University of Saskatchewan

The first author acknowledges the Canadian Occupational Therapy Foundation and the College of Graduate Studies and Research at the University of Saskatchewan for the financial support received while completing this research.

RÉSUMÉ

La formation clinique représente une partie importante de la formation de l'ergothérapeute. Dans cette étude, treize ergothérapeutes travaillant au sein de petits services d'ergothérapie du Saskatchewan, ont été interviewés pour déterminer les facteurs et les relations entre ces facteurs ayant des répercussions sur leur implication dans le processus de formation clinique. Afin d'établir une comparaison, les directeurs de deux grands services d'ergothérapie du Saskatchewan, de même que huit coordonnateurs de formation clinique d'universités canadiennes ont aussi été interviewés. Les résultats de l'étude démontrent qu'il y a quatre facteurs principaux qui influencent la participation des ergothérapeutes du Saskatchewan dans les programmes de formation clinique des étudiants en ergothérapie. Ce sont: la charge de travail; une impression d'isolement; les conditions du placement étudiant; et la compétence. Cette étude est importante parce qu'elle identifie des facteurs significatifs qui peuvent être repris par les coordonnateurs de formation clinique dans leurs contacts avec les ergothérapeutes. Cette étude sert aussi de modèle pour d'autres études semblables.

The Influence of Fieldwork on the Professional Socialisation of Occupational Therapy Students

Margaret-Ann Michelle Tompson and Alan G Ryan

This article describes a qualitative study which focused on the role played by fieldwork in the professional socialisation of four occupational therapy students. Data were collected through interviews, observational visits and a review of the students' daily journals. Four major themes relating to professional socialisation emerged during the study: the nature of professionalism; the concept of occupational therapy; learning the language of the professional; and the shifting focus of the different levels of placements. The results of this study have implications for the implementation of fieldwork experiences.

Introduction

Fieldwork is an integral part of the education of occupational therapists and can be said to be the crucible of the profession. It is during fieldwork that the theoretical knowledge that students acquire in the academic setting is mixed with practical experience to forge a sense of professional identity and ability. It is this sense of professional identity and the influence that fieldwork has on the professional socialisation of occupational therapy students which are the focus of this article.

Professional socialisation has been described as involving 'a complicated chain of perceptions, skills, values, and interactions. In this process, a professional identity is forged which is believable both to the individual and to others' (Lortie, 1966, p98). It is one of the purposes of the fieldwork process in occupational therapy (Nystrom, 1983). Although much has been written about professional socialisation, especially in the field of medicine (Becker et al, 1961; Coombs, 1978; Haas and Shaffir, 1987) and nursing (Olesen and Whittaker, 1968; Benner, 1984), there has been very little on this topic in occupational therapy (Sabari, 1985) or physical therapy (Schmoll, 1984).

Sabari (1985) described the professional socialisation of occupational therapists as involving sponsorship, selection/attrition, sequestration, sanctioning, didactic instruction, apprenticeship instruction, and certification. Sabari points out that occupational therapy students are influenced by a variety of individuals during the course of their educational programme. Of chief importance are academic staff, clinicians, other health care professionals, peers and clients.

Professional socialisation has been viewed as a process that extends over the lifetime of the professional (Houle, 1980; Benner, 1984). While agreeing with this viewpoint, others have pointed out that the professional school plays a key role in the process because it is the educational programme that is used 'to identify and screen individuals who are prospective deviants from the professional culture ... [and] provides test situations through initial and graduated exposures of the novice to the professional culture' (Greenwood, 1966, p18). Part of these test situations are the fieldwork placements, which have been likened to a bridge (Baines, 1974; Coles, 1985) between the academic world and the world of the practising professional.

Methodology

The main purpose of this study (Tompson, 1994) was to obtain the perceptions of four female occupational therapy students relating to their first 600 hours of fieldwork experiences. The curriculum of this Canadian occupational therapy educational programme was a traditional one, framed within a medical model in which there was a foundational year of basic sciences followed by applied courses and then advanced professional topics. All fieldwork placements were full-time ones and were interspersed throughout the curriculum.

All the placements in the study were of 4 weeks duration and consisted of two basic placements (the first 280 hours) and two placements at the intermediate level (the next 280 hours), for a total of 16 weeks. The two basic placements took place at the end of the first year and the beginning of the second year. The next two placements, the intermediate ones, took place at the end of the second year. The students' ages at the start of the study ranged from 19-22 and the students were all from the same cohort. Ten different sites were involved in providing the 16 placements of these students. These sites were predominantly institutional ones.

Two guiding questions within this study form the focus of this article. The first related to the patterns of change in students that occur over time during their early fieldwork experiences. The second was concerned with exploring how fieldwork affects students' concepts of occupational therapy and what it means to be an occupational therapist.

A naturalistic research methodology (Lincoln and Guba, 1985) was taken within an ethnographic framework (Fetterman, 1989). A variety of methods was used to collect data. Each student was interviewed at the beginning and the

Margaret-Ann Michelle Tompson, MCEd, PhD, OT(C), formerly a student in the doctoral programme at the Department of Curriculum Studies, College of Education, University of Saskatchewan, and now Education and Research Coordinator, Geriatric Medicine, Alberta Hospital Edmonton, Box 307, Edmonton, Alberta T5J 2J7, Canada.
Alan G Ryan, BA, MSc, PhD, Professor, Department of Curriculum Studies, College of Education, University of Saskatchewan, 28 Campus Drive, Saskatoon, Saskatchewan S7N 0X1, Canada.

end of the study and before and after each placement. These major interviews were approximately 60-90 minutes in duration. Weekly full-day observational visits were made to each student during her fieldwork placement and, during these visits, shorter (approximately half-hour) interviews were conducted at the beginning and the end of the day. These data were supplemented by the daily entries contained in a journal which each student was asked to keep. The topics covered during the interview process ranged over a wide area and were generated by observation of students in their placements and by points noted in their daily journals which seemed of key importance to the participants. An audio recording was made of all interview data which were later transcribed in full.

Data analysis was through the process of constant comparison (Glaser and Strauss, 1967), in which themes were identified as they emerged and compared with existing data. Thus, data collection and analysis become a recursive process rather than a linear one, with analysis of data revealing the direction of future data collection.

There were five phases to the data analysis process: initial exploration of the field or mapping (Schatzman and Strauss, 1973), analysis in the field, analysis away from the field, development of themes and patterns, and finally a comparison of the study with related literature. The trustworthiness of the study was ensured through a variety of strategies, such as prolonged exposure, time-sampling, reflexivity, peer examination, member checking, structural coherence, thick description, an audit trail and triangulation (Lincoln and Guba, 1985; Krefting, 1991).

Results

It became apparent in this study that learning to become a professional was a nebulous business. What was and what was not professional behaviour was hard to articulate for both therapists and students, possibly because of its complexity. Therefore, for the student, learning the attributes and roles of a professional came about more from a process of osmosis and modelling rather than through any explicit instruction. However, in observing these neophyte professionals, four key themes emerged: developing a concept of professionalism; learning the language of the professional; developing a concept of occupational therapy; and the shifting focus of the different levels of placement.

1. Developing a concept of professionalism

When the students entered the clinical setting, they grappled with what was appropriate behaviour for a professional. A large component of this process involved understanding the various boundaries that define their role and becoming responsible and independent.

Establishing internal boundaries

The students entered the clinical setting as adults who had been socialised into behaving in a manner that would not go against mainstream societal norms. When these students entered the world of clinical practice, they found themselves faced with behaving as neophyte 'professionals' in some ways which would have been considered inappropriate in the world of the lay person. One conflicting societal norm related to the right of the individual to privacy. This manifested itself in a number of ways.

There was the right to privacy of *personal information*, which conflicted with the need for the students to obtain personal histories:

'I'm still feeling a little bit uncomfortable, I'm digging into their lives when it's really none of my business but then, on the other hand, I've come to realise that it is my business in order

to do my job properly' (*Comment during first basic placement*).

There was the right to privacy of *physical space*, such as a client's room in a hospital, but then the students needed to contact clients:

'I don't know where I can go without interrupting but the other people walk into their [patients'] rooms with no problem, and to me that's invasion of privacy and I don't want to do the same to the patients' (*Comment during first basic placement*).

There was the right to privacy for *solitude*, yet the students needed to bring their clients into the treatment areas:

'I'm still not comfortable going to hunt the patients down. I don't want to disturb them when they're in their rooms. Everybody else does, so I guess it just takes a bit of getting used to it' (*Comment made in journal during first basic placement*).

Finally, there was the right to privacy of *the body*, which conflicted with the need for the students to deal with personal care and the physical handling of clients:

'She wanted to loosen his muscles because they were so stiff, which meant putting her hand under his clothes, close to his buttocks and sometimes on them. There didn't seem anything wrong with this, except again, I felt uncomfortable invading someone's privacy like that' (*Comment made in journal during a basic placement*).

The second major area of feelings of discomfort, when 'professional' behaviour seemed to conflict with societal norms for appropriate behaviour, occurred in the area of emotional expression. The students were told in the academic setting about the importance of keeping a professional distance but as one student commented:

'We were told not to get too friendly with the patients, it's hard not to, like I mean friendly, there's no defined line what friendly is, so it's hard to say' (*Comment made during first basic placement*).

The controlling of the emotional response was a hard one for the students. By virtue of wanting to be health care professionals, they had the inherent desire to help others, and yet this empathy and concern needed to be kept in check if the students were to be effective as professionals.

Establishing external boundaries

Part of the process of developing health care professionals is learning to understand their place within the system or within the team. First, the students had to learn the boundaries of their role as neophyte professionals. In the early basic placements, the students were particularly sensitive to being 'just students' and would interpret the behaviour of others towards themselves in terms of their student status rather than any other factor:

'You're a student, it's not like you're an OT, you're a student so if you get treated in any way, you know inferior or whatever, it's not because you're an OT, it's because you're a student (*Interview at end of basic placements*).

The students tended to feel more like therapists when others approached them for advice, asked for their assistance or behaved in a similar fashion to the way they did towards therapists. Second, the students had to learn the boundaries of their role as occupational therapists. The students' observations of how other team members worked together helped them in this process.

Not only were the students finding out how the roles of the various team members fitted together, they were also learning about the hierarchical nature of the clinical setting. Priority over clients' time, in accessing medical records or in speaking at team meetings were all indicators of a profession's status within the clinical setting:

'I don't think the nurses understand how important our role is, like when we're doing a group. I mean they had no second thoughts about coming and interrupting the groups and to me that really irritated me' (*Interview at end of first basic placement*).

The students felt that they were as essential to the rehabilitation process as was the air they breathed. Unfortunately, like the air around them, they became quickly conscious that other people were not so aware of it. The students' belief in the value of occupational therapy was impressive when they were constantly being faced with having to explain what occupational therapy was to clients and justify their role within the health care team but as one student indicated:

'I think to be a professional you have to be working towards making your profession a real profession in everyone else's minds' (*Interview at the end of the study*).

Accepting responsibility and becoming independent

A key concept of being a professional for the students was accepting responsibility. This was partly reflected in the extent to which the students worked independently. Indeed, there was some surprise at the amount of responsibility therapists were given and the speed with which they, as students, were expected to assume the mantle of responsibility:

'You put a tag on yourself, write occupational therapy student or whatever and they [the clients] automatically think you have a certain amount of knowledge and you're there to help them and that's a responsibility right there' (*Interview between basic placements*).

However, by the time of the intermediate placements, the students rarely commented on the responsibilities of the occupational therapist. They had come to expect and accept it.

This concept of professional responsibility was closely related to the extent to which students were encouraged and permitted to work independently. The dependence-independence aspect of a placement was a shifting one for students in two ways. First, it shifted over time from an unexpected surprise at being given independence to one of expecting it. Second, it shifted in terms of what students viewed as being independent activity. There was a shift from viewing independence as any activity done alone, however small or brief, to viewing independent activity in terms of the extent to which they were left entirely responsible for an activity.

2. Learning the language of the professional

The ability to communicate effectively, and in a professional manner, is an important skill for the developing professional and is a primary focus in the early placements. Learning to communicate professionally was akin to learning a foreign language, a point that was not lost on one student who commented enviously in the middle of her first placement:

'I hear the people around me talking, like they talk so fluently in this psychiatric setting, using medications and signs and symptoms' (*Comment during first basic placement*).

Communication skills were necessary in relating to clients and in written and verbal communication with other staff.

Communicating with clients

In the early days this was difficult because the students felt that they did not know anything and yet they were still meant to project an image of a person who was knowledgeable and who could provide help to her clients. Part of the difficulty for the students was knowing how to proceed once they had started the process:

'I think I got sort of the basics and then I didn't really know how to elaborate on any of the information I got. I didn't know what questions to ask next to get her to be a little more specific about things. So I kind of ran out of questions' (*Comment during intermediate placement*).

Written communication with other professionals

Written reports (charting) is used to both record and validate what the professional is doing. It is a visible and lasting record of the intervention of that professional. As one student indicated:

'Charting is probably the most relevant thing for the placement. The communication factor is so important' (*Interview between intermediate placements*).

The students got a feeling of accomplishment and excitement when they had completed their written reports in the early days. It was almost like a rite of passage when a student finally wrote her first report:

'DAY 6: Well today was very exciting. The biggest thing that happened to me today, was that I got to write my first ever chart note. It was so exciting! I was really nervous though. It was weird to think that others will be reading my notes' (*Comment made in journal during first basic placement*).

Unfortunately, the students' feelings of excitement about writing in the medical records soon gave way to feelings of frustration. Report writing was a particularly difficult activity for the students to practise because the medical record was a legal document. In this atmosphere of legalities, a student was faced with learning how to do something without the luxury of making mistakes. The solution for the students was to draft their report in rough form, have them corrected by the therapist and then rewrite them in the corrected form into the medical records. This process ended up making report writing one of the least preferred of the fieldwork placement activities.

The students soon learned that words which they used loosely as a layperson had to be scrutinised carefully before being used in a report. Awareness of the importance of the correct phrasing in report writing was reflected in the frequent comments made by the students on their record keeping techniques:

'The ideas are there but the technical terms aren't and the wording isn't maybe as clear ... Getting things concise and precise and in the terminology that's accepted and understandable and professional, it takes time. It's not going to be something that you can just go tush, tush and rip it off' (*Comment during an intermediate placement*).

All the students, without exception, judged their skill level in report writing in a fashion that was analogous to typing proficiency. In other words, there were two criteria: the extent to which therapists had to correct their reports, and the speed with which they accomplished the task.

Verbal communication with other professionals

The final form of professional communication that the students needed to learn involved meetings with other health care professionals. The students found that internal departmental meetings among only occupational therapy staff were not at all stressful. In fact, once the novelty had worn off, the students often found them boring and lacking in relevance. However, those meetings that involved health care professionals from other disciplines were viewed in a very different light from departmental meetings. In these situations, the students felt very much on stage and vulnerable:

'Trying to say what you want to say without saying something wrong, you want to be professional, you want to get across what you want to say, without disrupting or upsetting the situation' (*Comment during an intermediate placement*).

For the student, the situation was often one of speaking up in front of a room full of relative strangers. It meant trying to use the appropriate terminology. Part of the problem for the students in presenting was that team meetings were often conducted at relatively high speed. Again, using the analogy of learning a foreign language, the students felt awkward when they first spoke because of their unfamiliarity with the way in which to present their information. In addition, there was the uncertainty of when to speak up:

'Sometimes I was hesitant to speak up because I got the feeling that people were in a hurry ... I really didn't get my foot in the door ... It's hard to get a word in, it's intimidating too' (*Comment made during intermediate placement*).

3. Developing a concept of occupational therapy

Parallel with the students' developing concept of professionalism was their developing concept of their chosen profession, occupational therapy. The fieldwork experience did not seem to *change* the students' concepts of occupational therapy so much as help them to *operationalise* what it meant to work as an occupational therapist:

'Fieldwork has made our functioning clearer. I had an idea of what we did, but it just emphasised what we did more. It made it more concrete' (*Interview at end of first basic placement*).

Through fieldwork, the students gained an understanding of the breadth and depth of their role within the health care system. In addition, they became aware of some implicit assumptions that they held about the profession through experiencing the realities of working in the clinical setting. First, there was the hard work. Also, in some situations, far from being wanted and sought out by clients in need of care, the students would face rejection. One student commented:

'OTs are, like we fix them [clients]. We don't cause pain, we fix them. So it's like I'm shattering my own view, like this experience is kind of shattering. I mean although I know that we're not always doing that, it's not always fixing and that we can't fix everything. I want to in my heart as an OT be able to do that and it's kind of got to reality that it's not all fixing and a lot of it is assessing and doing things that patients don't want' (*Comment during intermediate placement*).

Finally, they learned that, no matter how well educated and prepared they might be, there would always be times when they would not know what to do:

'I would think as an occupational therapist you should know what to do right away and you should think beforehand so that if it comes up but you never know what's going to come up, when you're with a patient and learning that it's alright to be stumped' (*Interview during intermediate placements*).

One assumption that the students held, which seemed largely to have been fostered by the approaches that they had learned during their course work, was what constituted the occupational therapy intervention. During course work, the students had learned the full gamut of appropriate steps that needed to be taken. However, when the students arrived in the clinical setting, they often found a somewhat different picture. Different settings gave the various steps within the occupational therapy intervention different priorities:

'I don't think this is an area that's interesting to me. Just going there, do the assessment, see them once or twice and then discharge them. It's all ADLs [activities of daily living] and that type of thing. There's really no treatment going on' (*Comment made during intermediate placement*).

Another assumption was that occupational therapy would produce tangible results and it was apparent that students viewed an effective placement as one where they were very active and where they could obtain some feelings of accomplishment in their work with clients. Unfortunately, students found many psychosocial settings problematic in this regard, as one student commented:

'I didn't feel like I was really doing anything for them. I think psych. can be that way sometimes, like just supporting the person a lot of the time. At Placement C [physical medicine setting] I felt like I

was learning real skills and I think in psych. you rely a lot more on what you already have than the skills that you're learning' (*Comment made during an interview following the last intermediate placement*).

4. Shifting focus of the different levels of placements

The students' emerging sense of being a professional was reflected in the shifting focus for the two different levels of placement, the basic and the intermediate, which were encompassed by this study. The first two basic placements, especially the first one, should be viewed as a time when the students were learning how to be students in the clinical setting.

The time of the basic placement was a period when the students felt very positive towards everything. They felt that they were learning something from whatever they experienced. However, after several more placements, the students found it difficult to remember exactly what they had learned and were almost dismissive of these placements.

By the time the students started their intermediate fieldwork placements, they were feeling more confident of their role. There was a shift from learning to be students within clinical setting to learning to be occupational therapists. The students felt more competent in being able to handle the experience of going into a new placement:

'In the intermediate I got more the feeling like these last two placements, they wanted me to be more independent in my problem-solving and things like that. They were more willing to let me take the risk of finding out, maybe that wasn't such a good technique to use. Whereas in basic fieldwork they sort of baby you a little bit more. They don't want you to have a bad experience. They're really concerned about making you feel comfortable with people' (*Interview on completion of the last intermediate placement*).

Discussion

It must be remembered that this study focused on four students who were all female and who came from one particular occupational therapy educational programme. In addition, time constraints only allowed for study of these students' earlier fieldwork experiences. Therefore, the themes that emerged relating to the professional socialisation of occupational therapy students during their fieldwork experiences should be viewed as emergent ones and in need of further exploration.

Four aspects of these students' professional socialisation have implications for the way fieldwork experiences are organised and implemented: the technical-rational focus of their experiences, the implicit nature of the professional socialisation process, the importance of professional discourse, and issues of power.

Technical-rational focus

Fieldwork was equated with 'doing', so that students found more difficulties with placements which were not so focused on tangible 'doing', such as those in psychosocial settings. This finding has been highlighted in other studies (Coombs, 1978; Christie et al, 1985; Ezersky et al, 1989).

The difficulties that these students had with the more nebulous type of practice found in psychosocial settings could have implications for the profession. For example, there has been a steady decline in the numbers of occupational therapists working in psychosocial settings (Bonder, 1987; MacKinnon, 1987; Price, 1993). One cause may well be students' fieldwork experiences because one study found that 'Psychiatry was named three times more frequently than physical disabilities as a negative influence at the fieldwork level' (Christie et al, 1985).

Therefore, if the nebulousness of practice within such settings has tended to create problems, special attention needs to be paid to the way these placements are structured so as to give students a more tangible sense of accomplishment. This finding is similar to the Meyers (1989) study, in which her participants identified structure and supervision as being the key factors for an ideal environment in the psychosocial area so as to deal with 'some of the ambiguities of mental health practice' (p359). In addition, students and therapists need to become more explicit about what is and is not being accomplished. In settings where accomplishment may simply take the form of preventing a decline in social functioning, therapists need to help students appreciate the effects of their interventions.

Implicit nature of professional socialisation

The findings of this study show that professional socialisation is a process which is marked by its implicitness rather than its explicitness. This reflects Olesen and Whittaker's (1968) study of the professional socialisation of nurses which was entitled 'The Silent Dialogue'.

Interactions that did occur between therapist and student were very much focused on the here and now, and on the technicalities of therapeutic interventions. More studies need to be conducted to look at how therapists interact with students in various settings and the effect of these interactions within the setting. In the majority of cases, therapists were not in the position of taking time out explicitly to reflect on and discuss their role as therapists or their own feelings and experiences of being a professional. This led to professional socialisation through a process of osmosis. In other words, the underlying beliefs and values of the profession frequently went unaddressed and were left for the student to absorb unconsciously and interpret without questioning. Harris and Naylor (1992) had similar findings in their study of student physical therapists where they found 'there was little, if any, time available for critical reflection' (p125).

The importance of therapists taking time to talk with students has been pointed out in the literature (Cohn, 1989; McKay and Ryan, 1995). Cohn explained how 'through stories, fieldwork educators begin to share their reasoning process and the belief system that guides their practice. Students cannot learn clinical reasoning by watching our actions, because the thought behind the action is not self-evident' (1989, p243).

In the light of the findings of the study, therapists need to consider making the professional socialisation process of fieldwork much more explicit. They need to realise that talking with their students about their experiences as a professional fulfils a valuable educational role. In addition, by encouraging an exchange of views, beliefs and observations, therapists can promote the surfacing of the underlying assumptions that the student might be making based on their experiences and facilitate critical reflection by both therapists and students.

Another way to make the professional socialisation process more explicit would be to encourage students to write in a daily journal about their experiences. Such journal entries could be used for discussions when students met with their therapists (one recommended approach; Finlayson, 1993) or when they returned to the academic setting. Journal writing not only promotes reflection but also provides students with a written record that could help them identify any changes that might have occurred in themselves. In addition, it might help students to identify patterns of behaviour that might obstruct their learning.

The importance of professional discourse for occupational therapists

The uniqueness of any profession is reflected to some extent by the language it uses. A third important component of the professional socialisation of the students involved learning how to communicate within the health care setting. As has been outlined earlier in this article, such a communication process is not without its difficulties.

In this study, report writing seemed to create particular problems. Despite its obvious importance within the clinical setting, studies that focused on this aspect of an occupational therapist's activities could not be located. This situation is similar to the field of nursing where Sorrell (1991) reported: 'The assessment and decision-making processes involved in learning work-related writing have received little systematic study' (p162). As Fearing (1993) has pointed out, 'The absence of clear and practical guidelines for documenting on the health record often makes charting a disorganised and unsatisfying experience for occupational therapists' (p232).

The difficulty these participating students had with report writing (charting) is not surprising given that the faculty considered that they could learn it during their fieldwork experiences. However, Frisch and Coscarelli (1986) warn that this approach might be inappropriate because they have found that in the case of nursing:

'Charting is such a fundamental skill, and deficiencies in performance seemed to keep students from getting full benefit of their clinical rotation (and, incidentally, seemed to reinforce nurses' basic dislike of the task)' (p29).

It would seem, therefore, that students would benefit from more preparation in written communication prior to their fieldwork experiences if they are to maximise their fieldwork experiences. In addition, more needs to be known about factors that affect the development of professional discourse within the individual.

Issues of power

The final implication of the findings of this study in the area of professional socialisation relates to issues of power. Gutterman (1984) points out that 'students in professional schools tend to be marginal persons in the health care setting. They do not have a defined function in the hierarchy of a health care agency' (p146).

The students in this study were aware of their natural lowly position as neophyte professionals, but this position was compounded by their awareness of the low profile of the profession and its apparent invisibility. Part of the struggle for students was in dealing with the embedded hierarchy within the traditional health care institution of the physician as the key decision-maker.

Students come into placements with the layperson's concept of the overriding power of the physician. The majority of their fieldwork experiences did nothing very much to change this concept. The constant interchange and interactions between various members of the team working within health care institutions reinforce the hierarchical nature of the health care field in such settings. One student expressed her concern about this aspect of becoming a health care professional:

'At the beginning OT was a big light at the end of this tunnel and there was all good to it. But now there's not always good in it. You have to learn that there's boundaries that you don't cross. There's politics involved between other professionals as well as professionals in your own team' (Interview on completion of the last intermediate placement).

As can be seen, it would appear that far from empowering students, as educators from the critical-theorist paradigm would hope would happen (Bevis and Murray, 1990), some fieldwork experiences ensure, instead, that students are socialised into knowing their place within the medical hierarchy. Academic and fieldwork educators need to consider the ways in which they can demonstrate the empowerment of the profession while encouraging students to talk about the issues of power that they become aware of in some clinical settings. More needs to be known about which clinical settings lend themselves to empowering students and which ones would tend to reinforce the traditional hierarchy.

Conclusion

The socialisation of an individual into a profession is a complex process which involves many different factors. Fieldwork plays a crucial role in this process because it is during fieldwork that students both learn new behaviours and unlearn old ones and move from a state of passivity and dependency to one of becoming independent, active participants. However, much still needs to be learned about the various factors that affect this process. In addition, those involved in planning and implementing fieldwork experiences need to consider ways in which aspects relating to what it is to be a professional can be given as much attention as is currently paid to task-related activities. The future of the profession rests on the students of today. We need to share our experiences as professionals so that they can benefit from our mistakes and successes.

Acknowledgements

The senior author has received support through a doctoral fellowship from the Social Sciences and Humanities Research Council of Canada, a Graduate Scholarship from the University of Saskatchewan, and the Goldwin Howland Scholarship from the Canadian Occupational Therapy Foundation.

This article is based on work done for a doctoral dissertation entitled: 'The kaleidoscopic nature of student occupational therapists' fieldwork experiences'.

Highlights from this article were included in presentations made at the 1994 11th International Congress of the World Federation of Occupational Therapists held in London ('Fieldwork experiences: an opportunity to explore students' perspectives') and at the 1994 CAN-AM meeting in Boston ('Fieldwork: a glimpse into students' experiences').

References

Baines TR (1974) The faculty supervisor. In: J Duley, ed. Implementing field experience education. *New Directions for Higher Education, 2(2)*, 39-44.

Becker HS, Geer B, Hughes EC, Strauss A (1961) *Boys in white: student culture in medical school.* Chicago: University of Chicago.

Benner RN (1984) *From novice to expert: excellence and power in clinical nursing practice.* Don Mills, Ontario: Addison-Wesley.

Bevis EO, Murray JP (1990) The essence of the curriculum revolution: emancipatory teaching. *Journal of Nursing Education, 29(7)*, 326-31.

Bonder BR (1987) Occupational therapy in mental health: crisis or opportunity? *American Journal of Occupational Therapy, 41(8)*, 495-99.

Christie B, Joyce P, Moeller PL (1985) Fieldwork experience, part 1: impact on practice preference. *American Journal of Occupational Therapy, 39(10)*, 674.

Cohn ES (1989) Fieldwork education: shaping a foundation for clinical reasoning. *American Journal of Occupational Therapy, 43(4)*, 243.

Coles MA (1985) Dialogue (Letter). *Canadian Journal of Occupational Therapy, 52(1)*, 38.

Coombs RH (1978) *Mastering medicine: professional socialisation in medical school.* New York: Free Press.

Ezersky S, Havazelet L, Scott AH, Zettler CLB (1989) Specialty choice in occupational therapy. *American Journal of Occupational Therapy, 43(4)*, 227-33.

Fearing VG (1993) Occupational therapists chart a course through the health record. *Canadian Journal of Occupational Therapy, 60(5)*, 232.

Fetterman DM (1989) *Ethnography step by step* (Applied Social Research Methods Series, Vol. 17). London: Sage.

Finlayson M (1993) The consumer as educator: a fieldwork experience in health promotion. *Proceedings of the ACOTUP/ACPUE Conference: Innovations in occupational therapy education.* Halifax, Nova Scotia: ACOTUP/ACPUE, 109-114.

Frisch NA, Coscarelli W (1986) Systematic strategies in clinical teaching: outcomes in student charting. *Nurse Educator, 11(6)*, 29.

Glaser BG, Strauss AL (1967) *The discovery of grounded theory: strategies for qualitative research.* New York: Aldine.

Greenwood E (1966) The elements of professionalisation. In: HM Vollmer, DM Mills, eds. *Professionalisation.* Englewood Cliffs, NJ: Prentice-Hall, 18.

Gutterman SS (1984) A qualitative study of the physical therapy clinical affiliation (Doctoral dissertation, The Ohio State University, 1983). *Dissertations Abstracts International, 44/11A*, 3292, 146.

Haas J, Shaffir W (1987) *Becoming doctors: the adoption of a cloak of competence.* Greenwich, Connecticut: Jai.

Harris D, Naylor S (1992) Case study: learner physiotherapists' perceptions of clinical education. *Education and Training Technology International, 29(2)*, 125.

Houle CO (1980) *Continuing learning in the professions.* San Francisco: Jossey-Bass.

Krefting L (1991) Rigour in qualitative research: the assessment of trustworthiness. *American Journal of Occupational Therapy, 45(3)*, 214-22.

Lincoln YS, Guba EG (1985) *Naturalistic inquiry.* Newbury Park: Sage.

Lortie DC (1966) Professional socialisation. In: HM Vollmer, DM Mills, eds. *Professionalisation.* Englewood Cliffs, NJ: Prentice-Hall, 98-101.

MacKinnon JR (1987) National perspective: educating for the future. *Canadian Journal of Occupational Therapy, 54(4)*, 161-63.

McKay EA, Ryan S (1995) Clinical reasoning through story telling: examining a student's case story on a fieldwork placement. *British Journal of Occupational Therapy, 58(6)*, 234-38.

Meyers SK (1989) Programme evaluations of occupational therapy level II fieldwork environments: a naturalistic inquiry. *Occupational Therapy Journal of Research, 9(6)*, 359.

Nystrom EP (1983) A description and analysis of the educational purposes of occupational therapy clinical education (Doctoral dissertation, The Ohio State University, 1982). *Dissertations Abstracts International, 43/10A*, 3207.

Olesen VL, Whittaker EW (1968) *The silent dialogue: a study in the social psychology of professional socialisation.* San Francisco: Jossey-Bass.

Price S (1993) The issue is: new pathways for psychosocial occupational therapists. *American Journal of Occupational Therapy, 47(6)*, 577-59.

Sabari JS (1985) Professional socialisation: implications for occupational therapy education. *American Journal of Occupational Therapy, 39(2)*, 96-102.

Schatzman L, Strauss A (1973) *Field research: strategies for a natural sociology.* Englewood Cliffs, NJ: Prentice-Hall.

Schmoll B (1984) Clinical education as professional socialisation. In: *Planning for clinical education in 1990* (pp 25-29). A forum sponsored by the American Physical Therapy Association at Kansas City, Missouri.

Sorrell JM (1991) The composing processes of nursing students in writing nurses' notes. *Journal of Nursing Education, 30(4)*, 162.

Tompson MAM (1994) *The kaleidoscopic nature of student occupational therapists' fieldwork experiences.* Unpublished doctoral dissertation. University of Saskatchewan, Saskatoon.

Improving the links: fieldwork educators' conferences

Elizabeth M Walker

The change from diploma to degree courses in undergraduate physiotherapy education means that courses offered by schools of physiotherapy differ much more than in the past. This has increased the need for good communication between the academic (school) units and the fieldwork units where students gain their clinical experience. This article discusses the reasons why such communication is important and how communication may be facilitated by the introduction of fieldwork educators' conferences.

Ms Elizabeth M Walker is Lecturer in Physiotherapy, and is responsible for the organisation of fieldwork educators' courses, in the School of Occupational Therapy and Physiotherapy, University of East Anglia, Norwich NR4 7TJ

During the period when physiotherapy was a diploma-level course, students undertook the same national examination and schools of physiotherapy were similar, in that the content of the curriculum was that which was laid down in the Chartered Society of Physiotherapy's (CSP) curriculum of study. Since the implementation of honours degree programmes, however, the courses offered by schools of physiotherapy may differ considerably, not only in their content and philosophy but also in their methods of teaching and assessing students.

Good communication between the schools and the clinical placements has always been important. This has usually been conducted via the visiting school lecturers responsible for each clinical area and through correspondence between the school and the clinical educators. In recent years the introduction of fieldwork educators' courses has improved these links.

This article discusses the importance of communication between educators within the school and the clinical environment and how this process may be further facilitated by the implementation of fieldwork educators' conferences.

Importance of clinical education

Fieldwork (clinical) education is an essential component of undergraduate education in the health-care professions (Crist Hickerson, 1986). Fieldwork education allows the student to apply learned knowledge to clinical areas. Integration between theory and practice is considered to be vital. As Guilbert (1987) states:

'Without theory, practice becomes chaotic...without practice, theory becomes mere speculation.'

The transition of preregistration courses from diploma to degree status has necessitated the inclusion of behavioural sciences and research methodology into an already overloaded curriculum. Nevertheless the importance of clinical education continues to be recognised by the profession and the CSP which specifies that a minimum of 1000 hours of clinical education in the practice of physiotherapy be included in all undergraduate courses (CSP, 1984).

Increasing importance of communication

Changes in educational philosophy

The implementation of degree courses has resulted in many schools re-examining their course philosophy. The School of Occupational Therapy and Physiotherapy (OPT) at the University of East Anglia (UEA), for example, has decided to adopt the process model of curriculum (Stenhouse, 1975).

Since many clinical educators may have been educated using the behaviourist (product) approach, it is important that they are aware of the different methods implemented by other schools, the strengths and weaknesses of these different styles, and how they may affect both the students' approach to learning and the clinician's role as teacher during the clinical component of the course.

Locations of placements

Some schools have adopted an academic approach to supervision, as described by Bogo and Vayda (1987). Here clinical education takes the form of a block system which follows the learning of a particular area, e.g. neurology, in the school environment. The changing patterns of health care have resulted in some students being sent on 4–6 week 'block' clinical placements many miles away, instead of 'half-day' placements near the school. This has made day-to-day communication between school lecturers and clinical educators more difficult.

'Under the system of diploma courses, the main responsibility of lecturers was to teach and prepare their students for the national examinations organised by the CSP. The move to degree courses has resulted in internally assessed courses with additional work, including setting and marking examination papers and course work, preparing and submitting course documents, and implementing course evaluations.'

The changing role of physiotherapy lecturers

Demands on physiotherapy lecturers have increased. Under the system of diploma courses, the main responsibility of lecturers was to teach and prepare their students for the national examinations organised by the CSP. The move to degree courses has resulted in internally assessed courses with additional work, including setting and marking examination papers and course work, preparing and submitting course documents, and implementing course evaluations.

These factors have resulted in visits to clinical units by school lecturers taking place less frequently than before, and communication between lecturers and clinical educators occurring more often by telephone.

Increased demands on clinical educators

Clinical educators (supervisors) increasingly find they are responsible for the clinical education of students from a variety of schools throughout the academic year. Hence they need to be aware of changes in the curriculum that may occur in each school. Christie et al (1985) found that clinical educators of occupational therapy students required communication regarding curriculum changes in order to fulfil their teaching role.

Fieldwork educators' conferences

The UEA hold conferences once a year at the school of OPT in addition to their fieldwork educators' courses. All clinical educators of the school's physiotherapy and occupational therapy students are invited to attend. The morning is devoted to multiprofessional sessions. After the welcome, an update of developments at the school is given. This includes any changes that have occurred during the past year and new developments, e.g. the implementation of master's courses and other postgraduate opportunities. Last year an assessment session was included to introduce the honours degree classification for the clinical work carried out by students on their placement.

Fieldwork educators appear to appreciate input from students regarding their (students') needs (Walker and Openshaw, 1994). A uniprofessional session, which enables fieldwork educators and students to meet and discuss issues such as the students' expectations of their placement and the educators' expectations of the students, is included.

In the afternoon, concurrent workshops which favour an interactive approach in order to actively involve those who attend are organised. These may be uniprofessional or multiprofessional, recognising areas where there are benefits of shared learning and areas where there are uniprofessional needs. Last year, sessions focusing on specific units of teaching were included. Neville and Crossley (1993) and Walker and Openshaw (1994) found that clinical educators required more information regarding what the students had been taught and to what level. Such interactive sessions, led by the subject teachers, not only enables clinical educators to gain such knowledge, but also enables lecturers and clinical educators to discuss issues regarding current patient management. To assist clinical educators in their choice, agendas for each concurrent session are sent out with the day's programme to indicate their appropriateness to each profession and clinical specialty. *Figure 1* indicates some of the concurrent sessions offered at the last conference. Finally, an agenda-setting session for the next year's programme is always included.

Evaluation

Evaluation of the sessions is carried out by clinical educators, school teaching staff and, where appropriate, the students. For the purpose of this article, the content of four sessions is described and their evaluation is discussed.

Musculoskeletal

This session provides an opportunity for lecturers and clinical educators to explore various aspects of this module together. Issues such as content, type of learning, standards expected of students and how the learning occurring on the placement and that occurring in the school integrate and complement each other were covered.

Feedback indicated that the clinical educators valued this session:

> 'I needed input from the tutors regarding how and what the students are taught so that I can have realistic expectations of the students. The fact that we were asked about the various practical aspects of placements and current treatment practices made me feel that clinical physios were an important part of training'.

Neurology

This session was designed to provide the opportunity to discuss both what was presently covered within the physiotherapy neurology unit and what participants would like to see included in the future. During this session an outline of the neurological unit was provided and comments were invited regarding the content. Clinical educators were able to read the worksheets

---

Physiotherapy: neurology (uniprofessional)
This session will provide the opportunity to discuss both what is presently covered within the physiotherapy neurology unit and what participants would like to see included in the future.

Physiotherapy: musculoskeletal (uniprofessional)
This session will provide an opportunity for lecturers and clinicians to explore together various aspects of this module. Issues such as content and type of learning, standards expected of students, how the learning occurring on the placement and in the school integrates and complements each other will be covered.

Physiotherapy: cardiovascular and respiratory (uniprofessional)
The intention of this session is to discuss the standard and variety of experience gained by students in this area.

'The multisensory experience' (multiprofessional)
Participants will initially be given the opportunity to experience the multisensory environment, which is also known as Snoezelen. They will then be encouraged to reflect upon their experience and express their feelings about the use of such activities for themselves and people of all ages who have developmental disabilities.

Myth interpretation of students (multiprofessional)
This session will explore the strengths and weaknesses of occupational therapy and physiotherapy (OPT) students at the University of East Anglia while out on clinical placement. It will hope to establish the general themes associated with the preparation of students for placement (knowledge, skills — interpersonal and professional, awareness) and the performance of students during placement. Thus, at the end of the session it is hoped that a better awareness of the clinician's needs and the school's needs/beliefs may be gained. Any myths or misinterpretations can be explored and reviewed in the light of a better understanding of the preparation and student development at OPT.

How occupational therapists learn anatomy (uniprofessional)
This session will give occupational therapy clinicians the opportunity to experience how occupational therapy students in OPT are taught anatomy. They will take part in a practical session covering palpation and activity analysis. Occupational therapists who left their anatomy books behind a long time ago need not worry! This exercise will give the clinicians some insight into how the process approach can be used in practice.

Models of occupational therapy (uniprofessional)
This session will cover how models of OT are taught at OPT, what models are covered and also models in context.

Core skills (multiprofessional)
A multiprofessional discussion session to consider how core skills might be acquired and assessed and what might be expected at different stages of fieldwork experience. This session will reflect on whether students should be engaged in summative assessments which compare their performance with agreed standards or in 'value added' assessments which show their degree of progression.

Failure workshop (multiprofessional)
This multiprofessional workshop will begin to consider the problems associated with the identification of weak performance and giving fail grades. The session will encourage participants to review incidents which have highlighted dilemmas in this area.

Student research (multiprofessional)
This workshop will introduce participants to the structure and purpose of undergraduate research at OPT and how clinicians may be involved.

OT issues of community placements (uniprofessional)
This session will address the issues which arise from students doing community placements including supervision, working single-handedly, levels of student responsibility and any other issues which participants wish to raise.

Figure 1. Intentions of concurrent sessions at the fieldwork educators' conference held in 1994 at the University of East Anglia.

given to the students concerning their student-centred work. Teaching staff felt that it was a valuable experience. This was supported by the clinical educators:

> 'I always find that students are lost when first confronted with a neurological patient and I don't know where to begin. They then follow my system almost blindly in order to please me, the supervisor. It was useful to see just what methods (of treating patients) they have been taught. Free discussion enabled us to discuss the difference in experience offered and the different approaches to supervision used'.

Comments indicated that the session was well organised and that the format of the session was good.

Core skills

The group was presented with the results of a research project carried out to ascertain which qualities were considered to be important for physiotherapy and occupational therapy students to acquire in their first clinical placement. Whereas the facilitator had felt that physiotherapists (in the study) would be more concerned with psychomotor skills and occupational therapists more concerned with communication skills, it was found that both professional groups felt that communication skills were most important. The session then focused on identifying what the participants felt were the core skills required within their own clinical area, and discussing whether the acquisition of these skills should be school-based or fieldwork-based.

Failure

The purpose of this multiprofessional workshop was to consider the problems associated with the identification of weak performance and giving fail grades. The session was based on a research project in which lecturers, supervisors and students commented on what would constitute a fail grade on a clinical placement. This generated discussion on what would constitute a fail grade in their own placement, and how and when feedback would be given to the school and the student. Personal and professional implications of false-negative and false-positive grades were highlighted. Feedback from the supervisors included the following comments:

> '...was a very stimulating and informative session — research information given gave me food for thought...the common denominators of failure'.

'Very useful...helped me to deal with a recent potential failure with greater confidence'.

'Helpful to hear other peoples worries and difficulties...made you realise that you were not alone in feeling bad about failing a student'.

Other comments

These reflected the benefits of communication between clinical educators and lecturers and between the clinical educators themselves:

'It was very good to have an overall view of the placements throughout the training period, which I did not have before this day'.

'It was most important to discuss the honours degree classification as this is a new concept to most clinicians. The open discussion about the problems of assessment was helpful. I found the explanation of the assessment forms very helpful and felt that the school was taking positive steps towards linking theory and practice'.

'I thoroughly enjoyed the day and appreciated the opportunity for open discussion with both tutors and fellow fieldwork assessors...I left feeling very keen to attend a fieldwork educators' course as I felt this would be of great benefit. I think that conferences like this are a very important part of the student training to link the placements in with the school sessions and to maintain common aims and standards'.

Conclusion

Clinical education is a vital part of undergraduate education. Methods of improving communication and enabling joint collaboration between educators within the school and the clinical environment, such as fieldwork educators' conferences, are vital both for the students of today and for the future of our profession.

```
+----------------------------------------------+
|                 KEY POINTS                   |
|                                              |
|  ● There is an increased need for communi-   |
|    cation between clinical educators and     |
|    lecturers.                                |
|                                              |
|  ● Annual fieldwork educators' courses are   |
|    a useful means of communication between   |
|    the schools and clinical units.           |
|                                              |
|  ● Conferences involving both occupational   |
|    therapists and physiotherapists can       |
|    facilitate collaboration between the      |
|    two professions.                          |
+----------------------------------------------+
```

Bogo M, Vayda E (1987) *The Practice of Fieldwork Instruction in Social Work. Theory and Practice.* University of Toronto Press, Toronto

Chartered Society of Physiotherapy (1984) *Guidelines for the Approval of Courses Leading to Eligibility for Membership of the Chartered Society of Physiotherapy.* Chartered Society of Physiotherapy, London

Christie BA, Joyce PC, Moeller PL (1985) Fieldwork experience part II: the supervisors' dilemma. *Am J Occup Ther* 39(10): 675–81

Crist Hickerson PA (1986) *Contemporary Issues in Clinical Education Vol 1 No 3.* Slack Incorporated, New Jersey

Guilbert JJ (1987) *Educational Handbook for Health Personnel.* WHO Offset Publication, No 35. World Health Organisation, Geneva

Neville S, Crossley L (1993) Clinical education: perceptions of a clinical tutor's role. *Physiotherapy* 79(7): 459–64

Stenhouse L (1975) *An Introduction to Curriculum Research and Development.* Heinemann, London

Walker EM, Openshaw S (1994) Educational needs as perceived by clinical supervisors. *Physiotherapy* 80(7): 424–31

SECTION SEVEN

AOTA Fieldwork Task Force and Committee Reports and References

This section is devoted to major American Occupational Therapy Association (AOTA) task force, committee, and project reports on the subject of fieldwork. Those readers familiar with AOTA know such reports alone could fill an entire book. The documents selected represent only a few of the major discussions on the national level, including reports from committees who were charged by the AOTA Representative Assembly to study aspects of fieldwork. Some of the documents also arose out of national office activities to promote fieldwork to the general membership.

AOTA members may inquire to AOTA's Education Department about additional documents they may find useful for research.

Summary of Pilot Results: Project to Develop a Fieldwork Assessment Instrument

Jacquelyn A. Moore, MA, OTR
Project Coordinator

Janet Smith
Jim Vermillion
Consultants to Pilot Phase

The following document briefly summarizes the results of the pilot phase of the project to develop a fieldwork assessment instrument for Occupational Therapy Assistant students. A substantive report, which describes all phases of the project including the data analyses, is available through the Education Division of the American Occupational Therapy Association.

Summary of Findings and Recommendations

AOTA has undertaken to develop a standardized observation instrument for the assessment of the performance of the OTA student in the clinical setting. The Committee on Performance Assessment has drafted an instrument and a pilot study using that instrument has been completed. The pilot study of the Fieldwork Evaluation Form (FWEF) has been designed to assess the generalizability of the instrument, to obtain descriptive information on student performance and to obtain observer feedback on the use of the instrument. Seven schools participated in the pilot, including 60 students and 95 observers. The FWEF includes 24 observation items, assessing performance in evaluation, treatment, communication, and professionalism. Each item consists of 3–5 behavioral indicators which provide objective descriptions of levels of performance on the item. The final item is a summative assessment by the observer of whether the student is ready to enter clinical practice.

The analyses of pilot data have addressed two major substantive areas—generalizability of the instrument and descriptive, relational analyses. The research issues which the generalizability study has addressed include the extent to which the ratings of one observer correlate with those of another, the internal consistency of subscales and total scores, and norms for items included on the instrument. Thus, the design of generalizability study called for obtaining 2 or 3 independent observations of a student's performance. For analytic purposes, it was important that 3 or more schools provide observations by the same two observers of 10–15 students. School participation did not conform to this design; observations completed by different pairs of observers were obtained for 32 students in 6 schools. Two schools submitted 13 pairs each. Generalizablity coefficients were unusually low, suggesting that observer ratings were not completed independently. When an analysis of observer agreement was completed, substantial inter-observer agreement was found. Estimates of internal consistency were very satisfactory, both for the total score and subscales. Norms for the generalizability sample have been developed with which to interpret the future performance of individual students in relation to this study group.

The descriptive study has addressed research issues related to the major dimensions represented in the items, the relationship of particular assessments of performance (safety and readiness to enter practice) to performance overall and on subscales, and examinations of whether specific characteristics distinguish the top students in the sample, of scoring patterns within schools and of items not observed. Sixty students (including the generalizability sample) from seven schools made up the descriptive sample; 95 observers rated these students. Factor analysis of the pilot data provided weak evidence of two factors underlying the items: a responsiveness factor, including for example, considering client needs and responding in a therapeutic manner, and an instrumental factor, including data collection, safety, and budgeting time. Use of the safe practices and assessment of readiness to enter practice were related to total and subscale scores. Average total and subscale scores varied systematically by levels of performance on these two measures, with those scoring highest on the two criterion variables having higher mean scores. Four items on the instrument were not observed for at least a quarter of the sample: use of techniques of group process, administration of assigned evaluation procedures, development of a program based on long and short-term goals, and appropriate orientation of client and family. No patterns were found relating items not observed to students' performance, to school, or type of placement. Mean scores did not differ across schools.

The pilot FWEF contained three items soliciting observer feedback on the evaluation process. More than two-thirds of the raters felt the time to complete the instrument was reasonable, 81% felt the items and procedures used were reasonable and nearly 90% felt the process provided an accurate assessment of the instrument.

Based on the pilot experience recommendations may be made related to instrument modifications and to the process of OTA performance evaluation. With respect to instrument modification: the instrument should be set up with two items per page; the column *Description of Observed Instruments* would be dropped (the *not observed* option would be retained and placed under response categories); and the response options to assess readiness for practice should be expanded to include *yes, in a well supervised setting*, intermediate to the *yes* and *no* choices.

Fieldwork Evaluation: Revision of the FWPR

HISTORY

Field Work Performance Report (FWPR) in use since 1973. Purpose: "to assess the competence of student occupational therapists during their field work experience" (an evaluation and counseling tool).

Jane Slaymaker in Morgan & Irby's *Evaluating Clinical Competence in the Health Professions, 1978.* Lack of predictive validity and extensive rater error in FWPR.

"Report on Current Practices in Occupational Therapy Clinical Education Programs" by Tufts University-Boston School of Occupational Therapy. Comment section regarded as more useful than the graded section.

Resolution 584-82: Revise 1973 FWPR to reflect present entry-level requirements. Adopted by the Representative Assembly in 1982.

Committee of clinicians and educators met 1982–1986 in conjunction with a professional consultative service to design a new instrument.

Approved by Commission on Education in April, 1986 and Representative Assembly in September, 1986.

INSTRUMENT DEVELOPMENT

Purpose: "to be the assessment of student performance with related tasks." An evaluation tool; not a counseling tool.

Tasks as described in the following:

- The Entry-level Role Delineation of OTRs and COTAs (AOTA, 1981)

- The Uniform Terminology for Reporting Occupational Therapy Services (AOTA, 1979)

- The Essentials and Guidelines for an Accredited Educational Program for the Occupational Therapist (AOTA, 1983)

Committee developed pool of 500 items; these were screened and edited to 100.

Pilot study of 100 potential items by 56 clinicians and fieldwork educators reduced number to 53. (1984)

Field test of form with 53 items, assessing the significance (importance) to each site, establishing reliability, validity, and criterion scores. (Aug–Oct, 1985)

STATISTICAL ANALYSIS OF THE INSTRUMENT

69% of fieldwork educators agreed or strongly agreed that directions were clear and easy to use.

61% agreed or strongly agreed that there were no overlapping tasks.

75% agreed or strongly agreed that performance scale was easy to use.

44% agreed or strongly agreed that judgment scale was easy to use.

51% agreed or strongly agreed that attitude scale was easy to use.

88% felt all important tasks were included.

Student Profile:

1st fieldwork placement:	72%	Physical Disabilities:	42%
2nd fieldwork placement:	23%	Psychosocial:	54%
3rd fieldwork placement:	5%	Pediatrics:	3%

Of the 53 items rated all but two were found to be highly significant. "Determines the suitability of referrals" and "participates in quality assurance and program evaluation studies" were less than moderately significant (fewer than 50% of respondents scored the items as significant) and were dropped from the form.

Factor analysis rearranged the items into five subscores for Performance and single scores for Judgment and Attitude. Six items did not cluster into these subgroups and are indicated by the darkened boxes on the instrument. Their scoring potential is removed from the instrument to increase the reliability of the scores and the judgments based upon the scores.

Comparisons of mean scores with Recommend/Not Recommend and with Final Rankings were significant at $p < .0001$. Comparison with certification examination scores was positive. (validity)

USE OF THE INSTRUMENT

51 tasks are rated on the scales of performance, judgment and attitude.

Performance: The quality with which the student performs the task.

Judgment: Student demonstrates understanding of the rationale and justification for the performance of the task.

Attitude: Student exhibits professional behaviors and attitudes during the performance of the task.

A 5 point rating scale (1 = poor; 2 = fair; 3 = good; 4 = very good; 5 = excellent) is used for each task on the three scales.

Performance scale is scored in subscores of assessment, planning, treatment, problem solving and administrative/professionalism.

Judgment and attitude are scored in a total rating of each.

Items containing the darkened boxes are important and relevant to the assessment of student competency. For statistical reasons (reliability) they are not to be scored.

Criterion scores (minimally passing score) are given for the three scales.

AOTA recommends that the student pass all three scores. As fieldwork is a part of professional education, the individual school determines its own passing score(s) and grading system.

Each fieldwork facility is encouraged to develop its own behavioral objectives based on the items in the instrument and in keeping with the nature of the particular occupational therapy program.

The Final Report for the Field Work Performance Report Revision Committee, August, 1987

Submitted to: The Commission on Education.
Dr. H. Kav Grant OTR, FAOTA. Commission Chair.

By: The Fieldwork Revision Committee.
Richard G. Cooper, MOT, OTR, FAOTA. Committee Chair.
Dr. Kathleen Barker-Schwartz, OTR
Barbara Christie, OTR/L
Patricia Crist, MS, OTR, FAOTA
Diane Shapiro, MA, OTR, FAOTA
Bonnie Brooks, MEd, OTR, FAOTA

Introduction

The Committee presents this final report on our activities with a sense of accomplishment and appreciation. The committee believes that the charges presented to us (Resolution 584-82) have been achieved. The committee firmly believes that *The Fieldwork Evaluation* represents a solid step forward for the profession and for the students of Occupational Therapy. We are both proud and satisfied with this accomplishment. We also hold considerable appreciation for the support and assistance provided to us by The Commission on Education, The Division of Education, The National Office staff, and The Representative Assembly.

Activities Completed

The committee has completed the following activities since its last annual report:

1. The field test plan as described in *The proposed field test plan for vote,* (1985) was approved by The Commission on Education for implementation. A budget request was presented to, and accepted by, the Fiscal Advisory Board of The American Occupational Therapy Association.

2. The field test was initiated through Assessment Systems, Incorporated under the direction of Tom Samph, President. The field test was completed during July–September, 1986 with 597 field test forms being completed and submitted for data analysis.

3. The field test data was analyzed by Assessment Systems, Inc. and presented to the committee. The Committee reviewed the data with the assistance of Stephanie Pressler-Hoover and Madeline Gray. The Committee met with Tomas Samph and made the final decisions regarding the instrument to be recommended to the Commission on Education and the Representative Assembly.

4. The Committee constructed *The final summary report and recommendations of the committee for the revision of the fieldwork performance report (584-82).* This report was disseminated to the membership of The Commission on Education for vote at the National Conference of The American Occupational Therapy Association in Minneapolis (April, 1986). The instrument was presented to the small group sessions of COE by Richard Cooper and Kay Barker-Schwartz. Presentations were made to the program directors, student association, educators, and clinicians. Richard Cooper, committee chair, presented the results of the field test to the business meeting

of the Commission on Education. The presentation was followed by motions for vote. The motions included: acceptance of the report, acceptance of the recommended criterion scores, implementation of the instrument as of January, 1987, and review of the instrument on a five-year basis. The motions were presented to the voting members by H. Kay Grant. All of the motions passed by majority vote. The report and the COE recommendations were forwarded to the Representative Assembly and placed upon their agenda. The committee report was represented by the committee chair, Richard Cooper. The Representative Assembly reviewed the report and passed motions to accept the report on resolution 584-582, adopt the instrument for use as the measure of student performance in fieldwork experiences for the Occupational Therapist (pending review by the Standards Review Committee), and set the implementation date as January, 1987. The exact wording of these motions may be obtained through review of the minutes of The Commission on Education and The Representative Assembly.

5. The Committee was not disbanded at this time, as there were final decisions to be made on the printing of the instrument. Through the actions of the Division of Education, the final form of the instrument was moved through the Standards Review Committee and was printed in its final form (See Appendix B for final form).

6. The Committee is committed to the dissemination of the field test data and the use of the instrument to fieldwork educators. The committee felt that the data should not solely be included in Commission on Education and Representative Assembly minutes. Therefore, members of the committee have taken on the task of constructing, and submitting for publication, articles which relate to the history and use of the instrument, reliability of the instrument, and validity of the instrument. At the time of this final report, those publications are in the final review stages before submission to professional journals.

7. The Committee submitted a proposal to present the history and use of the adopted instrument to the National Conference at Indianapolis. That proposal was accepted by the conference committee and presented by Patricia Crist and Richard Cooper.

8. The Committee has continued to work with the National Office and the Division of Education (through Debbie Frum) to assist in the implementation of the instrument. The committee has reviewed

materials constructed by the National Office for the training of fieldwork educators in the use of the new form. The committee will continue to avail itself to The Association in the implementation phase of *The Fieldwork Evaluation.*

Summary of Critical Conclusions from the Field Test

The field test provided a large sample of completed and returned forms (N=597). The returns matched the pre-test estimated target populations in demographic characteristics for type of fieldwork placement and level of placement. The returns represented 42% from physical disabilities, 54% from psychosocial, and 3% from pediatrics. These were not statistically different from the pre-test estimates of equal splits in physical disabilities and psychosocial dysfunction with a smaller group in pediatrics. The majority of the students (72%) were on their first placement, 32% on their second placement, and 5% were on their third. This also matches the pretest estimates. The 32% on second placement represented a total of 120 students which was interpreted as an appropriate number for statistical analysis.

The distribution of the scores on the categories (and subcategories) of performance, judgement, and attitude indicate that the instrument differentiates levels of student performance with all probabilities falling at $p < .0000$. Reliability estimates (Cronbachs' coefficient alpha for internal consistency) for the scores and subscores of performance, judgement, and attitude demonstrate high stability in homogeneity and accuracy. All alphas fell between .924 and .961. The ability of the instrument to measure performance for recommending or not recommending entry to the profession was demonstrated through the comparison of mean scores on the three performance scales, and sub categories, to the fieldwork educators recommendations (to recommend or not recommend). The probabilities fell at the level of $p < .0000$. The accuracy of the instrument was also demonstrated through the comparison of all scores to the ranking of the students performance by the fieldwork educator (top 20% to lowest 20%). Again, the probabilities fell at the level of $p < .0000$. The analysis supports the ability of the instrument to discriminate different levels of student performance. The analysis also supports the homogeneity of the tasks, categories, and sub-categories within the instrument. The results of the field test support the use of this instrument as a measurement of performance for the Occupational Therapy Student.

Student evaluation of the field test form was completed through the return of 517 student evaluation forms. The form utilized a five point ranking scale on several specific questions. The students indicated a "very good" fit (mean = 3.81) between the performance scale items and the actual fieldwork demands. Ninety percent of the students indicated that the two scales of judgment and attitude represented a "good fit" (mean = 3.69) with their attitude and ability to use judgment. The average overall student reaction to the new form was "good" with only eight percent (7.8%) indicating that it was poor.

The fieldwork educators were also asked specific questions about the form. Sixty-nine percent agreed or strongly agreed that the directions were clear and easy to use. Sixty indicated that there were no overlapping tasks (mean = 3.47). The fieldwork educators clearly supported the use of the performance and judgement categories. The fieldwork educators were less supportive of the attitude scales, but this was seen as a reaction to the newness of the scales. The educators did not disagree with the use of the attitude scales, and therefore they are retained in the final form. In reviewing all of the categories and sub-categories of tasks, between 88% and 97% of the fieldwork educators thought that all of the important tasks were included on the form.

Criterion scores for successful completion of the fieldwork experience was addressed. The distribution of final recommendation by the supervisors was 94.8% recommended and 5.2% not recommended. To assure the protection of the profession from incompetent practitioners, the committee recommended the setting of the criterion scores at the level of two standard deviations below the means for the recommended group. This placed the criterion scores as follows: Performance 125, Judgement 132, and Attitude 146. These criterion scores capture the largest percentage of both the recommended and the not recommended groups with an expected ranking of 95% being recommended and 5% being not recommended. For a positive recommendation, the student should perform above the criterion score in all three categories of performance, judgement, and attitude. The criterion scores were adopted by the Association as recommendations to the academic institutions. The criterion scores are recommendations to the schools, with each academic institution then legislating its own academic standards.

Discussion and needs for further study

The major goals for the construction of the *Fieldwork Evaluation* were to produce an evaluation that:

represented current professional competencies (content validity), was reliable in measuring performance of individual students, and met the concern of the profession that student behaviors be included in the evaluation process. Additional committee goals included: that the evaluation be self-contained to reduce the need for rater training, represent the realities of fieldwork education, and reduce the "halo effect".

The three major goals have support through the construction process, pilot study, and field test. The new instrument was constructed from adopted professional documents which describe the current state of the profession and included student behavior. The individual tasks given in the instrument were reviewed by expert panels in both the pilot study and the field test. The final instrument included input and evaluation by a consumer group of students. The internal consistency measures demonstrated high homogeneity. The comparisons of all the mean scores to the final decisions to recommend and to the ranking of student performance demonstrated that the instrument has the ability to accurately discriminate levels of student performance.

The committee goal for a self-contained instrument was met in that the instrument has no separate raters manual or scorers manual. The field test produced very stable measures of student performance and accurately discriminated between levels of student performance. This was achieved without any rater training other than the directions given in the field test forms. The field test demonstrated that rater training on the new instrument was not necessary to achieve statistically robust measurements of student performance. The committees' concern with the realities of measuring student performance centered on the available time for the fieldwork educator to observe and record specific student actions which related to the performance tasks. Currently, the fieldwork educator tends to have very limited time for such direct observation and recording of specific data. From this concern came the use of clinical judgement by the fieldwork educator as to the level of student performance (excellent, very good, good, fair, and poor). The committee believed that having a self-contained, content valid, and reliable instrument which represented the realities of the fieldwork experience would reduce the "halo effect". The field test results supported the reduction of the "halo effect" through the comparisons of the mean scores (categories, sub-categories, and totals) to the final recommendations and rankings of the fieldwork educators ($p < .0000$).

While the field test provided considerable support for the adoption of the new instrument, concerns remain. The reliability estimates for the *Fieldwork Evaluation* were very high. The stability in these mean scores and criterion scores is expected after the instrument is implemented if used as it was during the field test. However, the form is currently being used for midterm evaluations in a modified manner (+, 0, −). This use of the instrument as a midterm measure could reintroduce both the "halo effect" and rater effort into the scores. If this occurs, then the mean scores will change as with the *Fieldwork Performance Report* (FWPR). Therefore, there exists a need for periodic recalculation of the mean scores and redefinition of the criterion scores. While the support for reliability is substantial there exists the need to test the new instrument for intra-rater reliability, inter-rater reliability, and test-retest reliability. Additional studies on predictive validity and construct validity are also important, although more difficult to achieve.

The field test results indicated no need for rater training to achieve statistically acceptable results. However, as with all new things, there appears to be a personal need for rater training within the fieldwork educators. This is seen as a natural occurrence. The Committee is supportive of any formal or informal efforts to facilitate a smooth implementation period. And, the committee members are available to participate in such activities as requested.

The significance scale was designed to indicate the importance of each item in the instrument. The scale was used to determine which items should be eliminated or retained. The significance scale could be incorporated, on a periodic basis, for the maintenance of content validity of the instrument.

Acknowledgements

The committee wishes to acknowledge several individuals who provided assistance, advice, and expertise to this project. We wish to acknowledge Dr. Stephanie Presseller-Hoover, Director, AOTA Division of Education, Dr. H. Kay Grant, Chair, AOTA Commission on Education (COE), Patricia Crist, COE Steering Committee Liaison, and Bonniee Brooks, AOTA Division of Education Liaison, for their combined efforts.

The committee wishes to acknowledge the consultive expertise of Drs. Mary Ann Bunda and James Sanders of *The Evaluation Center*, Kalamazoo and Dr. Tom Samph and Steve Nettles of *Assessment Systems, Inc.*, Philadelphia.

The committee also wishes to acknowledge the 56 participants of the pilot study, and the 597 students and clinical educators who participated in the field test. Without their combined involvement, this instrument would not be possible.

As committee chair, I wish to acknowledge the abilities and the dedication of the individual committee members, each of whom gave of their time, creativity, and expertise in completing this effort.

Lastly, we acknowledge the efforts of Debbie Frum, Division of Education Liaison to Fieldwork Education, who will be actively involved in the implementation of *The Fieldwork Evaluation*.

Prepared by,

Richard G. Cooper, MOT, OTR, FAOTA
Committee Chair
August, 1987

Appendices

The following documents are attached to provide a historical view of the process and critical events in the work of the revision committee. They have been sequenced in historical order with the most recent being last.

APPENDIX A
Historical Documents

Resolution 584-82.
Report to Commission on Education, January, 1983.
Report to Commission on Education, April, 1983.
Report to Commission on Education, August, 1983.
Minutes of Committee Meeting, Washington D.C., November, 1983.
Annual Committee Report to Commission on Education, November, 1983. Including:
> Minutes of Committee Meeting, Chicago.
> Rationale for Revision of the Fieldwork Performance Report.
> Minutes of Committee Meeting, Atlanta.

Pool of 499 Tasks, December, 1983.
Outline for Committee Meeting, February, 1984.
Cover Letter and Pool of 99 Tasks for Pilot Study.
Annual Report to Commission on Education, November, 1984. Including:
> Summary of Committee Meeting, February, 1984.
> Committee Report to Commission, July, 1984.
> Summary of Committee Meeting, October, 1984.

Report to Commission on Education, December, 1985.

APPENDIX B
Documents Published or Distributed by AOTA

Cooper, R., Barker-Schwartz, K., Brooks, B., Christie, B., Crist, P., & Shapiro, D. (1983). *The rationale for revision of the fieldwork performance report*. Rockville, MD: The American Occupational Therapy Association.

Proposed Field Test Plan For Commission on Education Vote. March, 1985.

Cooper, R., Barker-Schwartz, K., Brooks, B., Christie, B., Crist, P., & Shapiro, D. (1986). *The final summary report and recommendations of the committee for the revision of the fieldwork performance report (584-82)*. Rockville, MD: The American Occupational Therapy Association.

Report to the Standards Review Committee. September, 1986.

Cooper, R., Barker-Schwartz, K., Brooks, B., Christie, B., Crist, P., & Shapiro, D. (1987). *The fieldwork evaluation for the occupational therapist*. Rockville, MD: The American Occupational Therapy Association.

Additional Documents

The following are additional documents which are significant to the project, but are too bulky to be attached to this final report. These documents are available through the Division of Education, The American Occupational Therapy Association, or through the AOTA Library.

Background Literature Review Materials, (Notebook).

"The Report of the Pilot Study for the Fieldwork Evaluation."

"The Report of the Field Test of the Fieldwork Evaluation."

(*Editor's note:* Appendices A and B are not included in this anthology.)

Final Report of the Fieldwork Study Committee in Response to the Representative Assembly, The American Occupational Therapy Association

Submitted to H. Kay Grant, Ph.D., OTR/L, FAOTA Chairperson, Commission on Education

January, 1989

Origination

The Fieldwork Study Committee was charged by the Representative Assembly through the Commission on Education to explore alternative Level II fieldwork models. Concurrently the same task force was charged by Directions for the Future to study patterns of fieldwork including the locus of responsibility, coordination, and control. A list of committee members is attached and reflects the composition recommended in the RA charge. This report will address each article of the charge and related issues.

Introduction

The Fieldwork Study Committee first met in March of 1988. At that time, members were apprised of the foundational work of the previous committee, the Fieldwork Systems Task Force. It was the consensus of the Fieldwork Study Committee that beliefs and existing patterns of fieldwork must be illuminated before effective changes could be proposed and implemented. To provide a point of reference, the committee found it necessary to clarify the philosophy and intent of fieldwork. This statement is embodied in Appendix A, Perspectus-Fieldwork II. A memo was sent to the Essentials Committee of the Commission on Education recommending indicated changes.

To obtain as much information as possible about aspects of fieldwork nationally, two additional surveys were designed (Appendices B & C). Four hundred four responses were received from managers of clinical programs, twenty-seven from OTR program directors and from OTA program directors. Funds for detailed analysis were not available, however the trends indicate that opportunity for staff to develop and maintain clinical skills, supervisory and educational skills, visibility, and recruitment of staff are powerful incentives for clinical sites to conduct fieldwork education programs. The responsibility for data analysis will be assumed by two of the members of the committee who will also examine the relationship of the incentives to the activities most feasibly offered by the academic programs.

Additional perspectives pertaining to Level I Fieldwork and OTA Fieldwork have been generated by the committee to embody the beliefs, assumptions, and problems associated with fieldwork as perceived by the Fieldwork Study Committee. The committee offers these statements as springboards for future work. (Appendices D, E, F).

For a more accurate perspective of regional trends and fieldwork site utilization, the committee met with AOTA's Research, Information, and Evaluation Division. The Education Data Survey, annually published by AOTA, was targeted as a potentially valuable tool for routinely collecting regional data. It could help to more accurately delineate needs for alternative fieldwork sites by region. IT IS CONSIDERED ESSENTIAL TO DOCUMENT PATTERNS

OF AVAILABILITY AND UTILIZATION OF FIELDWORK SITES ANNUALLY.

Alternative Level II Fieldwork Models

The Fieldwork Study Committee reviewed the literature and documents relevant to the work of the previous committee the Fieldwork Systems Task Force. That committee compiled considerable information pertinent to other health professions' handling of the clinical component of professional preparation. It was felt that the needs of occupational therapy were not met by any one existing model due to differences in educational preparation, differences in fieldwork philosophy, sequencing of clinical experiences, and differences in relationships of the components contributing to fieldwork education. Divestiture did not seem to solve the problems inherent in fieldwork and was not seen as conducive to education quality, professional acculturation, or integrity of the field of occupational therapy.

Nevertheless, it is clear that the present system of occupational therapy fieldwork needs to be adapted to maximize the benefits of all contributing components while relieving the major burdens. In proposing changes, the committee first attempted to delineate the current system by task (Appendix G). Secondly, the committee tried to identify the interests of the contributing components (Appendix H).

Changes in the system have been proposed and diagrammed. These changes would entail the development of regional fieldwork systems under the auspices of the national office (AOTA). The model would require careful definition of relationships among academic programs, regional fieldwork systems, clinical sites, and students. The committee strongly felt that by rearranging the clerical burden of fieldwork, the relationship between academic programs and clinical sites could be enhanced by more appropriate activity. (Appendix I, Figure 1 and Figure 2) Essentially no changes are indicated which impact the current sequence of certification and entry into the field.

Determination of the financial implications for this model were seen to be beyond the scope of this committee. IT IS RECOMMENDED THAT A BUSINESS PLAN BE DEVELOPED WHICH FULLY REFLECTS FEASIBILITY, FISCAL IMPLICATIONS, AND FUNDING SOURCES RELATED TO IMPLEMENTATION. IT IS FURTHER RECOMMENDED THAT THIS MATTER BE REFERRED TO THE NATIONAL OFFICE AND THAT A DOCUMENT COMPARING THE CURRENT SYSTEM TO THE PROPOSED MODEL BE GENERATED REFLECTING ADVANTAGES AND DISADVANTAGES OF EACH. FURTHERMORE, UPON COMPLETION IT IS RECOMMENDED THAT THE MODEL AND COMPARATIVE ANALYSIS BE DISSEMINATED FOR REVIEW TO A) COE STEERING COMMITTEE B) SIS STEERING COMMITTEE C) REGIONAL FIELDWORK CONSULTANTS AND D) AOTA PROFESSIONAL SERVICES DIVISION. CONTINGENT UPON FEEDBACK FROM THIS REVIEW, IT IS RECOMMENDED THAT A PLAN FOR IMPLEMENTATION BE PRESENTED TO THE REPRESENTATIVE ASSEMBLY FOR VOTE IN 1991. THE FIELDWORK STUDY COMMITTEE EXPRESSES ITS WILLINGNESS TO ACCEPT CHARGES PERTINENT TO THE MODEL AS DEEMED APPROPRIATE.

Alternative Fieldwork Sites

At the 1988 Fieldwork Coordinators and Clinical Educators constituent group meeting of COE, several non-traditional fieldwork arrangements were discussed. This committee solicited help from program directors by mail to identify unique and creative fieldwork experiences. The response did not yield particularly surprising or extraordinary fieldwork arrangements. When SIS chairs were contacted, additional concerns, limitations, and potentialities arose. (See Appendix A - Parameters of Fieldwork) What becomes increasingly clear is that a strong linkage between the fieldwork center and the occupational therapy program benefits the fieldwork process. THE COMMITTEE HIGHLY SUPPORTS STRATEGIES WHICH STRENGTHEN COMMUNICATION AND PROBLEM-SOLVING BETWEEN CLINICAL AND ACADEMIC COMPONENTS OF FIELDWORK.

It is suggested that short papers be solicited for the constituent group meetings relevant to this topic. These selected papers should then be published in the Education Bulletin for broader dissemination.

Related Issues

Each of the papers, Appendices A, D, E, F, and I contain suggestions and recommendations pertinent to their respective content. It is hoped that those recommendations will be carefully considered. For example within Appendix A, a recommendation is made regarding Essentials and Guidelines for an

Accredited Educational Program for the Occupational Therapist. Appendix D emphasizes that it should not be assumed that fieldwork needs of OTA and OT students and programs are the same. Separate fieldwork learning activities should be designed for OT and OTA students.

To facilitate further study, it is recommended that all new articles, reports and documents pertaining to fieldwork be assembled, catalogued, and housed in the Wilma West Library in the AOTA National Office. A list of references used in the endeavors of this committee reflects the ongoing nature of fieldwork concerns.

The Fieldwork Study Committee strongly supports efforts of the AOTA and regional interest groups to effectively prepare clinicians to assume roles as fieldwork educators. THE COMMITTEE REITERATES AND ENDORSES A SYSTEMATIC PROCESS FOR CREDENTIALING FIELDWORK SUPERVISORS. Projects, such as Self-Instructional Package to Improve Clinical Education Supervision (SPICES), charged to a 1988–89 COE Committee, are deemed necessary to develop qualified, prepared fieldwork educators. Adequate preparation of supervisors was felt to directly impact the development of alternative fieldwork sites. The committee favors a uniform *process* sponsored by AOTA to provide foundations for further development. Continuing education efforts targeting fieldwork education coordinators could focus on program development and evaluation. It is recommended that we not lose sight of the importance and responsibility of the clinical site in providing appropriate learning opportunities.

FINALLY, IT IS STRONGLY RECOMMENDED BY THE FIELDWORK STUDY COMMITTEE THAT THE COMMISSION ON EDUCATION STEERING COMMITTEE DEVELOP AN ONGOING MECHANISM TO CONTINUALLY MONITOR AND RESPOND TO THE FULL SCOPE OF FIELDWORK ISSUES. THIS COMMITTEE SHOULD INCLUDE A REPRESENTATIVE FROM THE COMMISSION ON PRACTICE AND A REPRESENTATIVE FROM THE SIS STEERING COMMITTEE. SINCE FIELDWORK IS DEEMED CRITICAL TO OUR PROFESSIONAL DEVELOPMENT, IT IS THE RECOMMENDATION OF THE FIELDWORK STUDY COMMITTEE THAT IT BE ADDRESSED METHODICALLY AND CONSISTENTLY.

Respectfully submitted,

Karin J. Opacich, MHPE, OTR/L
Chairperson, Fieldwork Study Committee

Fieldwork Study Committee

Linda Florey, MA, OTR, FAOTA
Associate Chief of Rehabilitation Services and
Coordination of Training in Occupational Therapy
UCLA Neuropsychiatric Institute

Julie Halom, OTR, Director
Occupational Therapy Assistant Program
Duluth Technical Institute

Karin J. Opacich, MHPE, OTR/L
Assistant Professor
Department of Occupational Therapy
College of Health Sciences
Rush University

Shirley Peganoff O'Brien, MS, OTR
Assistant Professor
Department of Occupational Therapy
Kean College of New Jersey

Barbara Schell, MS, OTR/L
Director of Occupational Therapy
Harmarville Rehabilitation Center

Trudy LaGarde, OTR/L
Fieldwork Education Specialist
American Occupational Therapy Association, Inc.

List of Documents Generated by the Fieldwork Systems Task Force

1. Fieldwork Incentive Survey (targeted managers of clinical sites)

2. Fieldwork PERK Feasibility Survey (targeted academic program directors)

3. Perspectus Fieldwork II

4. Recommendations Regarding OTA Fieldwork Education

5. Guidelines for Fieldwork Level 1

6. Interim Reports - 4-88, 1-89

7. Current Major Tasks of Contributory Components Associated with Occupational Therapy Fieldwork as Perceived by the Fieldwork Study Committee

8. Primary Interests of Contributory Components of Occupational Therapy Fieldwork as Perceived by the Fieldwork Study Committee

9. Proposed Changes in Major Tasks of Contributory Components Associated with Occupational Therapy Fieldwork, Figure 1 & 2

References Utilized by the Fieldwork Study Committee

Books, Monographs:

Crist, P., & Hickerson A.,*Contemporary Issues in Clinical Education, 1*, Slack, 1986.

Occupational Therapy Education: Target 2000, proceedings, 1986. American Occupational Therapy Association.

Documents, Reports:

Report on Study of Level II Fieldwork at Basic Professional Level of Occupational Therapy, Kahepakaran et al, 1981.

Accreditation of Fieldwork Centers, Garibaldi, April, 1983.

Wiscouncil Guidelines for Establishing and Assessing Level II Fieldwork Sites, Schoening et al, 1981.

Report of Project to Study Certification of Fieldwork Supervisors/Centers, NEOTEC, 1981.

Literature Review Process: A Synthesis Through Formulation of Problem/Issue Statements, Sinott (Fieldwork Systems Task Force), 1987.

Report of the Fieldwork Systems Task Force, Susan Schwartz (Communication with Truby La-Garde), 1988.

Essentials and Guidelines of an Accredited Educational Program for the Occupational Therapist, AMA and AOTA, revised 1983.

Articles, Papers:

Nystrom, E. P., *A descriptive and analysis of the educational purposes of occupational therapy clinical education*, dissertation, Ohio State University, 1982.

Cohn & Frum, *Fieldwork: more education is warranted*, AJOT.

Shalik & Shalik, *The occupational therapy Level II fieldwork experience: Estimation of the fiscal benefit*, AJOT, 42, 1988.

Leonardelli & Caruso, *Level I fieldwork: issues and needs*, AJOT, 40, 1986.

APPENDIX A

Prospectus—Fieldwork II

Fieldwork Study Committee, COE, 1989

Purpose

Statements and recommendations about FW II have been collected from previous studies, from the recommendations of special task groups, and from the work of noted occupational therapy educators and scholars. The following statement reflects the consensus of the Fieldwork Study Committee and reiterates the themes consistently found in the literature.

It is the recommendation of the FWS Committee that the following be considered to be the official mission and purpose of occupational therapy fieldwork.

The purpose of the fieldwork component of occupational therapy education is to:

1. Promote clinical reasoning and reflective practice.

2. Transmit the values, beliefs, and ethical commitments of the field of occupational therapy.

3. Communicate and model professional behaviors attending to the developmental nature of career growth and responsibility.

4. Develop and expand a repertoire of occupational therapy assessments and treatment interventions related to human performance.

Literature reviewed by the FWS Committee and the preceding committee, the Fieldwork Systems Task Force repeatedly emphasized the role of fieldwork in providing opportunity to apply a core of knowledge pertaining to occupational therapy, to practice and refine clinical reasoning, to acculturate professionally, and to begin to assume responsibility for perpetuating the field of occupational therapy.

To support and encourage compliance with the mission and purpose of fieldwork, it is recommended that the language of the Essentials and Guidelines be more explicit as proposed below:

Section II.E6.C. Level II Fieldwork shall be required.

It shall:

1) Facilitate the continued development of innovative fieldwork arrangements, it is recommended that the period of time for fieldwork be designated in units equal to 26 weeks or the equivalent.

2) Emphasize the application of an academically acquired body of knowledge.

The purpose of Level II Fieldwork is to promote clinical reasoning and reflective practice; to transmit the values, beliefs and ethical commitments of the field of occupational therapy, to communicate and model professional behaviors attending to the developmental nature of career growth and responsibility; and to develop and expand a repertoire of occupational therapy assessments and treatment interventions related to human performance.

3) Include learning experiences designed to develop skills in the following areas:

    (a) Assessment/OTA Structural Assessment
    (b) Treatment Planning
    (c) Treatment Implementation
    (d) Documentation of Care
    (e) Service Management

4) The fieldwork objectives shall reflect such content.

Locus of Control

At this time a shift in responsibility rather than shift in locus of control of occupational therapy fieldwork is deemed an optimal solution to the scope of problems associated with fieldwork. A regional matching system to be conducted under the auspices of AOTA has been proposed by the Fieldwork Study Committee for further consideration. Nevertheless, occupational fieldwork education entails commitment and participation of all contributory components. By defining and strengthening those relationships, all parties are more likely to reap the benefits and to resolve the difficulties inherent in fieldwork.

Strategies to provide clinical sites with incentives for developing fieldwork programs are essential to the success of fieldwork. Likewise, the opportunity to provide students with quality practical experiences is critical to the academic programs. Collaborative planning can minimize polarization and best address the altruistic needs of the field of occupational therapy. By promoting an educator mindset, both clinicians and academicians can best serve the needs of aspiring occupational therapists. By clearly articulating entry level competencies and fieldwork learning objectives, clinical sites and academic programs establish a relationship which benefits the students and ultimately the field.

Parameters of Fieldwork

Fieldwork, designed as a medium for transition from student to practitioner, lends itself to the competency-based model. The competency model implies that the student is informed of outcome criteria and is provided with opportunities to master knowledge, skills, and attitudes necessary to achieve competence. Academic programs and clinical sites need to set realistic criteria and timelines for achieving entry level competency in various practice arenas. It seems likely that both sequence and duration of fieldwork experiences may differ. Based on a preliminary survey of SIS chairpersons, some sites may not be appropriate for professional level fieldwork education for the following reasons: ethical and litigous nature of the setting, range or scope of potential experiences, ratio of supervisor/supervisee, narrow focus of practice, etc.

Concerted effort is warranted to establish fieldwork programs in sites that are representative of the scope of the health care system. It may be advisable for contemporary sites to collaborate in developing fieldwork programs which would provide students with range and depth of clinical experience. The division of fieldwork into "physical dysfunction" and "psychosocial" categories may be artificial. If, in fact, the focus of fieldwork is to instill and practice a process of clinical problem-solving, particular classifications of settings and/or populations may be unnecessary. The fieldwork student should be able to apply occupational therapy theory to illuminate and intervene wherever human performance is jeopardized or dysfunctional. It is conceivable that preventive or wellness settings could provide valuable fieldwork perspectives.

Since the demographic characteristics of occupational therapy students are changing, it is important to consider the needs of these students if occupational therapy is to continue to be a viable choice of study and career. Some flexibility in fieldwork arrangements may be indicated for contemporary occupational therapy students, i.e. students who have dependent children and students who must work for renumeration due to financial need.

Fieldwork Supervision

Qualification and preparation of fieldwork supervisors have repeatedly been expressed as concerns of both clinical settings and academic programs. Certification of sites and/or supervisors has been proposed in the past but not implemented. Nevertheless, the need for more formalized preparation of fieldwork supervisors persists. The fact remains that fieldwork supervisors are clinical educators who must be apprised of educational content and technology to function competently. Clinical educators are indispensable in acculturating occupational therapy students and shaping clinical reasoning. Responsibility for preparing clinical educators for the role of fieldwork supervisor must be shared by academic programs, clinical settings, and the national association. Ideally AOTA sponsored, periodically presented regionalized programs uniformly addressing core content related to fieldwork supervision would provide some minimal quality assurance. Additional strategies could be developed to complement such a program. If we value competent fieldwork supervision, we must invest resources and recognize the accomplishment.

Karin J. Opacich, MHPE, OTR/L
Chairperson, Fieldwork Study Committee

ATTACHMENT A

Alternatives in Occupational Therapy

Facilities providing financial assistance - Facilities having difficulties recruiting occupational therapy staff may be encouraged to provide assistance to OT/OTA fieldwork students in return for a specified period of employment.

Faculty supervised Level II Fieldwork - Faculty contact an agency or facility and contract to provide occupational therapy for a specified period of time and provide supervision for fieldwork students. This situation in the past has resulted in a facility hiring an OT/OTA (graduate) and assists in maintaining and further developing the skills of the faculty member. This can be very beneficial to new programs with limited Level II Fieldwork centers or for new sites and inexperienced OT personnel interested in developing a fieldwork program.

Part-time Level II Fieldwork experience in conjunction with an academic course - The Level I Fieldwork model in which the clinical experience is part of an academic course is developed and expanded for Level II Fieldwork. Students are placed in a variety of fieldwork sites on a continuous basis and also attend class.

Classes can be presented on a seminar, panel discussion basis or organized by specialty area. Generic occupational therapy theory and principles can be discussed as they apply to the various areas of practice. Students can share a variety of fieldwork experiences. **Please note that this may require a change in the educational *Essentials* for OT and OTA programs.

*Residency (12 months) - A 12-month contract is developed with a facility to provide a rotation of fieldwork education experiences. Student may complete 3 months in psychiatry, 3 months in rehabilitation and then 6 months in area of their choice. Student is on salary and receives benefits. Facility may benefit by working with selecting students working on research projects and providing time for research studies.

*Rotation Fieldwork Experience - Therapists working at more than one facility may be able to develop fieldwork education programs. One example is a therapist who spends 1/2 time in a summer camp for handicapped children and 1/2 time in a general hospital. A six-month fieldwork program was developed. In the beginning most of the student's time would be at the summer camp and only 1–2 days at the hospital. As fall arrives, the student spends more time in the hospital and gradually makes a complete transition.

*Shared Fieldwork Education Program (3 months) - Several therapists who feel they cannot provide a full-time experience can collaborate to design a fieldwork experience, i.e., part-time therapists in a variety of settings, such as home health, hand clinic, private practice, etc.

———————

*As per conversation with P. Crist, December, 1988.

Fieldwork Study Committee Annual Report—Representative Assembly, February, 1989

A. Subject: Fieldwork Study Committee
                 Annual Report

B. To: Representative Assembly

C. From: Chair, Karin Opacich, MHPE,
                 OTR/L Committee: Linda Florey,
                 Julie Halom, Shirley Peganoff-
                 O'Brian, Barbara Schell, Truby La
                 Garde (N.O. Liaison)

D. Date: February, 1989

E. Report on Activities:

Exploration of Alternative Level II Fieldwork Models

The Fieldwork Study Committee was charged by the Representative Assembly through the Commission on Education to explore alternative Level II Fieldwork models. Concurrently the same task force was charged by Directions for the Future to study existing and alternative patterns of fieldwork including the locus of responsibility, method of scheduling, and control.

The Fieldwork Study Committee first met in March, 1988 and met for two additional meetings thereafter. The committee was fortunate to inherit voluminous information from the previous committee—The Fieldwork Systems Task Force, for analysis. The Fieldwork Study Committee itself generated several informational documents including its final report and recommendations to COE. Two surveys were designed and distributed, a memorandum was sent to the Essentials Review Committee, a perspectus was written regarding Level II Fieldwork and guidelines drafted for Level I Fieldwork. This report is the executive summary. Raw data and detailed information has been forwarded to COE for future consideration.

There are many various models of fieldwork in existence today. Some are arrangements derived from discussions at COE Fieldwork Coordinators and Clinical Educators Constituent Group meeting in 1988. Others are the results from solicitations of program directors and clinics themselves. They incorporate combinations of experiences, differing lengths of affiliations and utilization of contemporary delivery settings while meeting the *Essentials* for fieldwork. Continued identification and/or development of contemporary alternatives must be recognized as an on-going process. It is recommended that developing models be tracked by AOTA, Education Division, for further development, and broad dissemination.

SUMMARY ACTION ITEM FACE SHEET

A. Subject: 1. Title: Addendum to the Commission on Education Annual Report
                 2. Topic: Final Report of the Fieldwork Study Committee
                 3. Clarification: Exploration of Alternative Level II Fieldwork Models
                    INTENT—Many professional programs are under administrative pressure to divest from Level II Fieldwork due to financial but primarily curricular concerns. It is felt that in many cases fieldwork belongs outside the credit-bearing academic program.
                    The issue is a large one with many implications. Divestiture is only one model which must be explored. If a change is to be made, all models and their implications in all areas must be thoroughly considered.

B. To: Representative Assembly

C. From: H. Kay Grant, Ph.D., OTR/L, FAOTA, Chair

D. Date: February, 1989

E. <u>NO ACTION REQUESTED</u>

F. Fiscal Implications:

G. Relationship to the Long-Range Plan:

H. Index Tracking Code: II.B.1.

The following are suggested alternative models:

Facilities providing financial assistance - Facilities having difficulties recruiting occupational therapy staff may be encouraged to provide assistance to OT/OTA fieldwork students in return for a specified period of employment.

Faculty supervised Level II Fieldwork - Faculty contact an agency or facility and contract to provide occupational therapy for a specified period of time and provide supervision for fieldwork students. This situation in the past has resulted in a facility hiring an OT/OTA (graduate) and assists in maintaining and further developing the skills of the faculty member. This can be very beneficial to new programs with limited Level II Fieldwork centers or for new sites and inexperienced OT personnel interested in developing a fieldwork program.

Part-time Level II Fieldwork experience in conjunction with an academic course - The Level I Fieldwork model in which the clinical experience is part of an academic course is developed and expanded for Level II Fieldwork. Students are placed in a variety of fieldwork sites on a continuous basis and also attend class.

Classes can be presented on a seminar, panel discussion basis or organized by specialty area. Generic occupational therapy theory and principles can be discussed as they apply to the various areas of practice. Students can share a variety of fieldwork experiences. **Please note that this may require a change in the educational *Essentials* for OT and OTA programs.

* Residency (12 months) - A 12-month contract is developed with a facility to provide a rotation

of fieldwork education experiences. Student may complete 3 months in psychiatry, 3 months in rehabilitation and then 6 months in area of their choice. Student is on salary and receives benefits. Facility may benefit by working with selecting students working on research projects and providing time for research studies.

*Rotation Fieldwork Experience - Therapists working at more than one facility may be able to develop fieldwork education programs. One example is a therapist who spends 1/2 time in a summer camp for handicapped children and 1/2 time in a general hospital. A six-month fieldwork program was developed. In the beginning most of the student's time would be at the summer camp and only 1–2 days at the hospital. As fall arrives, the student spends more time in the hospital and gradually makes a complete transition.

*Shared Fieldwork Education Program (3 months) - Several therapists who feel they cannot provide a full-time experience can collaborate to design a fieldwork experience, i.e., part-time therapists in a variety of settings, such as home health, hand clinic, private practice, etc.

Some alternative models of fieldwork are being implemented in various geographic areas. All programs seem to require further study in order to evaluate their effectiveness and examine the quality of education.

Alternative models designed for the changing student populations need to be studied to determine their recruitment potential as well as their appropriate application to new and emerging roles and areas of practice for OT.

Locus of Control

The committee compiled considerable information pertinent to other health professions' administration of the clinical component of professional preparation. It was felt that the needs of occupational therapy would not be met by any other existing model. Major changes in the present system did not seem to be a viable solution and were not seen as conducive to maintaining or improving the quality of present occupational therapy education.

It seems possible that the present system of occupational therapy fieldwork may need to be adapted to maximize the benefits of all contributing compo-

---

*As per conversation with P. Crist, December, 1988.

nents while relieving the major administrative burdens.

Basically, the committee strongly felt that by regionalizing the clerical burden of fieldwork, the relationship between academic programs and clinical sites could be enhanced by more appropriate activity. The proposed model has been detailed in components and process and forwarded to COE for further consideration and development. All data and information compiled by this committee will also be forwarded to Directions for the Future for deliberation as they address fieldwork issues.

Final Report:
Fieldwork for the Future
Task Force

January, 1995

American Occupational Therapy Association, Inc.
Bethesda, Maryland

By

The Fieldwork for the Future Task Force

Barbara Townsend, MPH, OTR/L - Chairperson
Robin Bowen, EDD, OTR
Carole Hays, MA, OTR/L, FAOTA
Elizabeth Maruyama, MPH, OTR/L
Paula Young, BAS, COTA
Mary Ann Curtis, MBA, MA, OTR/L (AOTA Liaison)

For

Intercommission Council
Carol Clerico, OTR - Chairperson

INTRODUCTION/CHARGE

The Fieldwork For the Future Task Force was convened as the result of Resolution E, passed by the 1992 AOTA Representative Assembly. The original resolution was written by Sharon Nelson Sanderson, OTR/L, Toby Hamilton, OTR/L and Cyndy Robinson, OTR/L.

The Resolution asked that "The Intercommission Council (ICC) be charged to conduct a study of Level II Fieldwork by reviewing existing data and gathering new data, when indicated, to include, but not be limited to:

1. Whether the current way of conducting Level II Fieldwork is in the best interest of the student, the academic institutions, the clinical sites and the profession;

2. Feasibility and implications of fieldwork becoming a post-degree requirement;

3. Feasibility and implications of fieldwork becoming an internship (including stripend/salary) to be done following the completion of degree requirements;

4. Feasibility and implications of increasing the required time for Level II Fieldwork;

5. Feasibility and implication of central scheduling of all fieldwork by AOTA or other organization (profit or nonprofit);

6. Feasibility and implications of accrediting fieldwork sites;

7. Feasibility and implications of accrediting fieldwork instructors."

ACTIVITIES

The AOTA Fieldwork For the Future Task Force convened for the first time in Alexandria, Virginia, July 25–26, 1992. From that time until the completion of the final report, the Task Force was involved in the investigation of the history, current models, and possible future models of fieldwork education for occupational therapy students.

In order to complete the charge, the Task Force has engaged in a comprehensive review of historical documents written by members of the profession regarding fieldwork education. The Task Force also reviewed documents on fieldwork education written by those in other disciplines.

Through interview, survey, and document review, Task Force members gathered information that reflects the current fieldwork models most prevalent in the profession and studied models that are outside of what is considered "traditional." Members studied the fieldwork patterns and models of other health professions, including medicine, dietetics, and social work. Special emphasis was placed on the fieldwork models of the two professions that the Task Force felt have the most relevance and similarity to Occupational Therapy; namely, Physical Therapy and Speech/Language Pathology. The Task Force invited The American Speech/Language and Hearing Association (ASHA) and The American Physical Therapy Association (APTA) to meet with them.

Early in the process, the Task Force made a commitment to gather as much "grass roots" information as possible from occupational therapy practitioners and students and to give them numerous opportunities for input. A series of open hearings were held for occupational therapy practitioners and students as well as others who have a stake and an interest in the future of occupational therapy (consumers, deans of universities, etc.). These individuals were invited to present oral testimony directly to the Task Force concerning items included in the charge as well as any other information they felt was relevant. Those who were unable to appear in person were invited to send written testimony. A total of eight hearings were held in the following cities: San Antonio, TX; Seattle, WA; Detroit, MI; Charleston, WV; Bethesda, MD; Baltimore, MD; Boston, MA: Madison, WI; and Chicago, IL. Approximately 86 individuals presented testimony and approximately 400 attended the hearings and participated in discussions.

The Task Force invited a representative of the Canadian Occupational Therapy Association to testify at the hearing held in conjunction with the 1994 AOTA/CAOT joint Conference. Elaine Kuretsky, Liaison Officer, Credentialing and Standards, Canadian Association of Occupational Therapists, joined the Task Force and members from both Associations in the discussion of fieldwork models utilized in Canada. Members had the opportunity to share, compare, and contrast information related to clinical fieldwork.

Surveys were also utilized to solicit input from members and others. Targeted questions related to the project were added to the 1994 AOTA Education Data Survey. A general membership survey was included in *OT WEEK,* and surveys of recent OT graduates and academic fieldwork educators were completed.

At the end of the first two years of Task Force activity, preliminary recommendations and direction related to the charge began to emerge. The Task Force had great interest in presenting some of its preliminary thoughts to the membership prior to the completion of the charge, and prior to the submission of final recommendations. In early 1994, the Task Force wrote letters to major AOTA committees, commissions, and other groups, requesting that the Task Force be permitted to meet with them at the AOTA Conference in Boston to present draft recommendations and to have these groups comment and react to them with the understanding that the recommendations might be revised, based on these meetings and on experiences and activities of the Task Force's final year. This was an extremely valuable activity and was of significance in the formulation of the final recommendations that are presented in this report.

The recommendations presented in this report reflect activities engaged in by the Task Force over the three years it deliberated and are heavily reflective of the concerns and interests of the AOTA membership and other interested parties.

The complete minutes, supporting documents, and papers utilized by the Task Force are archived in the National Office of AOTA.

The Task Force would like to thank all who assisted in its deliberations, including those members who wrote historical documents, corresponded with the Task Force, testified at hearings, participated in surveys, and met informally and formally with the Task Force or individual Task Force members. Task Force members acknowledge and thank the members of The Intercommission Council (ICC) for their support and input throughout this process.

FIELDWORK FOR THE FUTURE TASK FORCE RECOMMENDATION SUMMARY SHEET

In reviewing existing and new data concerning occupational therapy Level II Fieldwork, the AOTA Fieldwork For the Future Task Force concludes that the current way of conducting Level II Fieldwork for occupational therapy students is inadequate, needs increased definition and clarity, and not meet the expanding and changing needs of the future, and as such, is not in the best interest of the students, the academic institutions, the clinical sites, or the profession. For that reason, the Task Force puts forth the following recommendations to the American Occupational Therapy Association:

RECOMMENDATION 1

Support and foster the creation of a statement that clearly articulates the purpose and value of occupational therapy fieldwork education.

RECOMMENDATION 2

Support the current COE project to identify terminal behavior objectives. These objectives should illustrate the expected performance of Level II Fieldwork students that will culminate in their ability to assume entry-level roles. Recommend that these objectives be included in the *Essentials* for Occupational Therapists and Occupational Therapy Assistants.

RECOMMENDATION 3

Initiate a voluntary credentializing process for clinical fieldwork educators by 1998. Consistent with Association policy, review the credentialing process, and phase in a plan for mandatory credentialing.

RECOMMENDATION 4

Do not increase the current requirements for the length of Level II Fieldwork clinical education.

RECOMMENDATION 5

Maintain the current model of linkage between academic institutions and fieldwork sites at this time.

RECOMMENDATION 6

Develop a fieldwork model of a paid clinical fellowship year for those institutions that have an interest in and the ability to utilize this model. Charge COE to solicit educational programs to work collaboratively with clinical sites to develop models for a clinical fellowship year.

RECOMMENDATION 7

Provide funding for demonstration projects that explore alternative fieldwork models as a means of improving the educational process, increasing the availability of fieldwork sites, and ultimately increasing the number of occupational therapy practitioners.

RECOMMENDATION 8

Initiate a voluntary computerized system that tracks fieldwork placement vacancies by 1997. Review the success of this system before considering an expanded system, including matching of students and fieldwork sites by 2000.

RECOMMENDATION 9

Utilize the Regional Fieldwork Consultants (RFWCs) to assist fieldwork educators in operationalizing new models. Support, publicize, and recognize the value of this role. The Task Force recommends that the RFWC become a Standing Committee in the reorganization of COE.

RECOMMENDATION 10

Support and expand current mechanisms for the broad and timely distribution of information related to innovative and emerging fieldwork models that successfully offer ideas for meeting the needs of a changing health care system, the growing number of academic programs, and a changing student body.

RECOMMENDATION 11

Support academic institutions that choose to make Fieldwork a postdegree requirement.

RECOMMENDATION 12

Create and publish an anthology that archives all works related to occupational therapy fieldwork education. The anthology will include journal articles and reports of Association Committees, Commissions and Task Forces, and will recognize those who have addressed this issue throughout the history of the profession. It will serve as a primary resource for future planning. The Task Force recommends the engagement of a single paid content editor to accomplish this task.

RECOMMENDATION 13

Utilize the established TriAlliance of Health and Rehabilitation Professions (AOTA, APTA, ASHA) to continue to discuss common concerns regarding clinical education. Establish and/or maintain relationships with other professional associations and consumer groups that affect the clinical education of occupational therapy practitioners.

ANALYSES OF RECOMMENDATIONS

RECOMMENDATION 1

Support and foster the creation of a statement that clearly articulates the purpose and value of occupational therapy fieldwork education. Inherent in this purpose statement is the recognition of the professional responsibility for all practitioners to assume the role of fieldwork educator.

In deliberations with Association members, during hearings and at informal and formal meetings, a concern was frequently expressed regarding the lack of a clearly identified statement expressing the value and purpose of clinical fieldwork education for occupational therapy practitioners. While the question arose from a broad contingent of individuals and groups, from practitioners to academicians, it was most clearly articulated at the June 18, 1993 meeting of the AOTA Academic Fieldwork Coordinators. Attendees at this meeting formed groups to study the issues identified in the Task Force's charge and to provide feedback to the Task Force to help guide its future activities. One of the groups at the meeting identified the following concerns and problems:

Although the purpose of fieldwork is stated in the *Essentials and Guidelines for Accredited Educational Programs for the Occupational Therapist* and *Essentials and Guidelines for Accredited Educational Programs for the Occupational Therapy Assistant* (1991), these statements are not widely known or utilized to direct our thinking about pragmatic issues.

From *Essentials* for the Occupational Therapist: "Level II Fieldwork shall be required and designed to promote clinical reasoning and reflective practice, to transmit the values and beliefs that enable the application of ethics related to the profession, to communicate and model professionalism as a developmental process and a career responsibility, and to develop and expand a repertoire of occupational therapy assessments and treatment interventions related to human performance."

From *Essentials* for Occupational Therapy Assistant:
"Level II Fieldwork shall be required and designed to provide in-depth experiences in delivering occupational therapy services and to develop and expand a repertoire of occupational therapy practice."

There is a dichotomy between the profession's espoused value of fieldwork education and current fieldwork practices. Research has documented that fieldwork experience and fieldwork supervisors have the greatest influence on socializing students to the profession, yet there is limited national support to prepare supervisors for this critical role.

Some students desire "economy of thought" and mechanistic/reductionist approaches that may be inconsistent with the profession's core values.

As a result of the many concerns voiced, the Task Force recommends that the Association develop and widely distribute a statement for Occupational Therapy fieldwork education that articulates the purpose of fieldwork education and that is congruent with the overreaching philosophy of the profession. This statement should help guide academic and clinical education.

Charge to: COE Steering Committee in Collaboration with Fieldwork Issues Committee

Financial Impact: - $0 - Done within existing budget

Timeline: 1 year (1995–1996)

RECOMMENDATION 2

Support the current COE project to identify terminal behavioral objectives. These objectives should illustrate the expected performance of Level II Fieldwork students that will culminate in their ability to assume entry-level roles. Recommend that these objectives be included in the *Essentials* for Occupational Therapists and Occupational Therapy Assistants.

Fieldwork content for occupational therapists is vaguely discussed in terms of clinical reasoning,

ethics, professionalism, and occupational therapy assessment and treatment interventions related to human performance (AOTA *Essentials* document, p. 7, section B, 7, c.). The content for the occupational therapy assistant is even less specific, stating that these fieldwork experiences should be "designed to provide in-depth experiences in delivering occupational therapy services and to develop and expand a repertoire of occupational therapy practice," (p.7, section B,4,b.) Both "Essentials" documents indicate that fieldwork experiences should vary, providing exposure across the life span, to various performance deficits (both physical and psychosocial), and different service delivery models. It is the feeling of the Task Force that while these criteria are critical, they alone do not provide adequate direction to the fieldwork site, the student, or the sponsoring academic institution. As changes are made to the *Essentials* in regard to fieldwork, this information should be reflected in Fieldwork Evaluation instruments.

While this recommendation was not part of the original mandate of Resolution E, it has become apparent that the open hearings and from input provided by fieldwork educators and academic faculty that revisions to the *Essentials* are needed to provide more specific direction. While the current *Essentials* describe specific content for academic course work, little direction is provided for fieldwork, instead they primarily address the structure and administrative issues surrounding fieldwork.

Charge to: COE committee to Executive Board (forward to ACOTE)

Financial Impact: $0, already budgeted - no additional costs

Timeline: 2 years

RECOMMENDATION 3

A. **Initiate a voluntary credentialing process for clinical fieldwork educators by 1998. Consistent with Association policy, review the credentialing process and phase in a plan for mandatory credentialing.**

The term "credentialing" has been chosen rather than the term "certification," which was originally used in Resolution E, as we feel it more accurately represents the criteria proposed herein for the designation of fieldwork educator.

Beyond the qualifications for a fieldwork educator as outlined in *Occupational Therapy Roles* document of the AOTA, requirements for credentialing could include a minimum length of experience in practice, specified training, and documentation of continuing education. Specific recommendations are addressed below and rationales are provided for each possibility.

(1) **For now, we recommend continuing to require one year of experience for a clinical supervisor.**

Rationale: A fieldwork educator needs to have adequate knowledge in the content area, the ability to impart that knowledge in an understandable manner, strong interpersonal skills, clinical reasoning skills, supervisory skills, and communication skills. (See AOTA's *Occupational Therapy Roles* document for a complete list of key performance areas.) Many have questioned whether one year of clinical practice prior to supervising Level II Fieldwork students is adequate, and some authors have suggested increasing the length of experience required.

It is also questionable whether a fieldwork educator with only one year of experience has developed clinical reasoning skills and the ability to navigate a student through the clinical reasoning process. The literature indicates that the more experience one has, the more clinical reasoning skills one develops, but there is no specific time passage associated with the development of clinical reasoning skills.

However, given the limited number of individuals and fieldwork sites willing to undertake the responsibilities associated with fieldwork education, to demand more clinical experience than is now required could be detrimental to the process. Therefore, we recommend that the current requirement of one year of experience remain.

In the future, as the supply of practitioners increases, and with the inauguration and stabilization of a system of preparing and credentialing fieldwork educators, we should be able to require more experience. Optimally, a period of three years of experience could be required, with this proposal being phased in once the training and credentialing systems are well established.

(2) **We recommend that all new fieldwork educators be trained using a common format (i.e., *SPICES*) and that this requirement be phased in gradually.**

Rationale: A common training experience would not only enhance the skills a fieldwork educator needs to competently supervise a fieldwork student, but may also result in greater interrater reliability between fieldwork educators when evaluating students and greater commonality of expectations and experiences for students.

SPICES appears to be an excellent training module and is already available. While it can be completed as an independent study, it seems it would be most beneficial to participate in a group training session where the participants could benefit from the knowledge and expertise of other participants and training leaders. Some educational facilities offer *SPICES* training as a graduate course. Current fieldwork educators should also be encouraged to participate in the training program.

Furthermore, we request that the training document (*SPICES* or another training document) be available "at cost," and that individuals be given the right to duplicate materials from within the document for training purposes. Finally, the training document should be routinely updated to meet the changing needs of the profession.

Another option that was mentioned in the nursing literature was to teach students about fieldwork supervision while in school (students commonly take courses in administration while in school, and it is likely that they will become fieldwork educators prior to becoming administrators). Students should also be taught the professional responsibility for lifelong learning, sharing knowledge, and the need to continually update one's skills in both established and new areas of practice.

It would also be ideal if prospective fieldwork educators could work under the supervision of an experienced fieldwork educator prior to working independently (a mentoring system).

(3) **To maintain credentials as a fieldwork educator, we recommend that a therapist attend a minimum of 12 hours of continuing education per year.**

Rationale: Continuing education is a professional responsibility and would help the practicing therapist maintain competency in the ever-changing health care environment. Continuing education activities should be related to practice, educational or administrative issues.

B. The foreseen implications of these recommendations are as follows:

One concern is whether administrators at fieldwork sites will be willing to provide support to have their staff obtain the training necessary to become credentialed as fieldwork educators. If a significant number of therapists obtain their jobs as a result of a fieldwork placement, this might be an incentive to comply with new standards. Also, if the role of fieldwork educator were seen as an honor, it might enhance compliance. Perhaps a special designation could be bestowed by AOTA or the credentialing agency (a set of initials that would identify the individual as a fieldwork educator and convey prestige), or perhaps this role could be incorporated as a higher step in the career ladder of an occupational therapy practitioner.

There are also financial implications to be considered. These costs would most likely be borne by the fieldwork educator or by the fieldwork site. If *SPICES* is used as the educational module, little or no expense would need to be incurred for educational materials development by the Association.

A registry of credentialed fieldwork educators would need to be developed, and ideally, a certificate or other proof of credentialing would be provided. AOTA or an independent entity could maintain such a list.

Regulation of continued credential maintenance of a fieldwork educator could be the responsibility of the contracting agency (the academic institution or the scheduling agency) or the entity that maintains the registry of credentialed fieldwork educators.

It is felt that this section of the charge is within the purview of AOTA for those fieldwork experiences taking place in the United States, and that this issue could be addressed in the *Essentials*. These criteria could be recommended for international affiliations, but enforcement would be difficult. If the affiliation were under the jurisdiction of a credentialing agency or AOTA, the criteria could be a prerequisite to being identified as a fieldwork site.

These recommendations, if instituted, will affect other AOTA documents (e.g., *Occupational Therapy Roles*, the *Essentials*, etc.). Appropriate bodies of AOTA would need to be charged to review existing documents and make necessary changes so that all documents would be in agreement and would incorporate the accepted recommendations.

Charge to: Executive Board (Recommended they charge Executive Director)

Financial Impact: Budget $15,000

Timeline: 2 years (1995–1997)

RECOMMENDATION 4

Do not increase the current requirements for the length of Level II Fieldwork clinical education.

The *Essentials and Guidelines for an Accredited Education Program for the Occupational Therapist* describe the intent of Level II Fieldwork as follows:

"The purpose of Level II Fieldwork is to provide an in-depth experience in delivering OT service to clients."

While the *Essentials* state that 6 months is the minimum requirement for Level II Fieldwork, a minimum of 940 hours is acceptable to meet the 6-month requirement.

The *Esssentials and Guidelines for an Accredited Educational Program for the Occupational Therapy Assistant* state that:

"Level II Fieldwork shall be required and designed to provide in-depth experiences in delivering OT services and to develop and expand a repertoire of OT practice."

The OTA *Essentials* state that 12 weeks is the minimum requirement for Level II Fieldwork, with 440 hours being acceptable to meet this 12-week requirement.

Information regarding the clinical education requirements of other health and service professions was collected to compare and contrast with the OT fieldwork requirements. (See Exhibit 2.) The Canadian Association of Occupational Therapists recently shortened their fieldwork requirements from 1200 hours to 1000 hours, effective March, 1993.

A review of the literature provided information on the costs and benefits to clinical sites providing student education. It was determined that clinical sites reaped significant benefits from student training for the last 8–9 weeks of fieldwork after experiencing losses in the initial 3–4 weeks of the experience.

Information from the Educational Data Survey of 1994 indicated that 79% of OT programs and 65% of OTA programs were not in favor of increasing the length of Level II Fieldwork. A survey published in the March 3, 1994, issue of *OT WEEK* that sampled general OT membership showed similar results, indicating that 68% of the respondents were not in favor of increasing Level II Fieldwork.

Discussion during the Open Hearings in San Antonio, Charleston, Seattle, and Chicago also reflected a negative reaction to increasing the length of Level II Fieldwork. Participants felt that increasing clinical education requirements placed a greater burden on the students in delaying their ability to earn an income. In addition, these delays could also affect the manpower needs of the profession.

While increasing the required length of Level II Fieldwork does not appear to be desirable at this time, the investigation and the design of innovative models of fieldwork and clinical education are warranted. We must be open to the changing needs of consumers and the needs of the nontraditional students who enter the OT educational process, and we must be willing to entertain and allow alternative models when considering the length of Level II Fieldwork.

RECOMMENDATION 5

Maintain the current model of linkage between academic institutions and fieldwork sites at this time.

Given the current system, the link between the academic institutions and the fieldwork sites must be maintained. The current *Essentials* allow Level II Fieldwork as a postdegree requirement, but allows the academic institutions to decide where, in the curriculum, Level II Fieldwork experiences should occur. If other mechanisms are in place in the future, the possibility of fieldwork becoming a postdegree requirement would warrant further investigation.

While the link between the academic institutions and clinical sites is felt by many to be beneficial, such a connection can pose legal complications for academic institutions. Clinical fieldwork supervisors are not actually employed by the academic institution, but are required to evaluate student performance. This places the academic institution in a precarious position if a student challenges a "grade" received on a Level II Fieldwork.

Other professions such as medicine and speech and hearing have adopted postdegree clinical models, but upon review of the literature, and in conversing with other health care professionals, it is evident that most professionals are struggling with clinical education issues. Also, the actual and anticipated changes in the health care delivery system are dramatic, and will drive the need to re-evaluate our current system.

While some programs could not embrace a postdegree model (their institutions' missions requiring that students be "job ready" upon graduation) others could adopt such a model. Also if several other recommendations included in this report are implemented, the transition to a postdegree model would be easier to implement. First, a refined and operational centralized fieldwork scheduling system that could be accessed by students independent of academic institutions would need to be in place. Second, fieldwork sites would no longer contract with academic institutions within such a model. Therefore, the credentialing of fieldwork supervisors would provide a level of quality assurance, compounded by the accreditation of the sites (such as CARF accreditation, not by AOTA). Finally, wide acceptance of the clinical fellowship year could facilitate the process of moving to a postdegree model.

Since these preliminary mechanisms would need to be in place before such a model could be functional, it would be premature to recommend such a change at this time. However, the possibility of Level II Fieldwork becoming a postdegree requirement should be reevaluated in the future. At this time it is not within the purview of the Association to mandate when Level II Fieldwork occurs, as this is the prerogative of the academic institutions.

RECOMMENDATION 6

Develop a fieldwork model of a paid clinical fellowship year for those institutions that have an interest in and the ability to utilize this model. Charge COE to solicit educational programs to work collaboratively with clinical sites to develop models for a clinical fellowship year.

The majority of respondents at the Open Hearings expressed concern about the financial burden that stipends would place on institutions that may already be experiencing financial constraints. However, respondents also noted that stipends could help ease the financial burden fieldwork places on students who are asked to relocate geographically. Survey results were mixed in regard to this issue, with students and educators primarily supportive of a paid internship, while department managers and administrators were not in favor of this model. In reviewing clinical education models being used by other professions, the idea of the clinical fellowship year (CFY) that speech pathology and audiology utilizes was closely investigated. In this model, students who have completed academic coursework and a 375 clock hours practicum arrange for a clinical placement and seek out a clinical supervisor for their 36 weeks of professional employment, with a minimum of 30 hours per week. The CFY amounts to 1080 hours of professional experience performed under the supervision of a individual who holds ASHA certificate of clinical competence. While the CFY is flexible to allow for part-time work to be done over a longer period (up to 72 weeks), the supervisory requirements and the clinical activity requirements are specific.

Through a literature review, it was discovered that there were other OT fieldwork models where long-term placements of 7, 9, or 12 months were utilized. These placements often allowed for rotation through several settings and provided the students with a wellrounded experience. Stipends were provided through special grant funding or through monies available for technicians' salaries. Larger institutions with a variety of practice settings are better suited for these experiences, but in some cases, interagency collaboration or a split placement arrangement can also provide this multisetting experience.

It is clear that innovative fieldwork models are necessary to meet the needs of the changing practice arenas that students will enter as new practitioners. While increasing the length of Level II Fieldwork may not be reasonable for all students, the idea of a paid clinical fellowship year may meet the needs of some students, institutions and consumers.

Charge to: COE to solicit educational programs to work collaboratively with clinical sites to develop models for a CFY.

Financial Impact: $20,000

$18,000 for stipends

$2,000 for administrative costs to implement

Recommend that RA provide seed money (matching funds) to support the development and implementation of the clinical fellowship year model. Funding will be for 2 OT and 2 OTA students.

(Matching Funds)

Stipends/OT Students - 1 Year
$6,000 × 2 = $12,000
Stipends/OTA Students - 6
Months $3,000 × 2 = $6,000
$18,000

Timeline: 2 years

RECOMMENDATION 7

Provide funding for demonstration projects that explore alternative fieldwork models as a means of improving the educational process, increasing the availability of fieldwork sites, and ultimately increasing the number of occupational therapy practitioners.

In the March, 1993 AOTA *Education Special Interest Section Newsletter,* Patricia Crist, Ph.D. OTR, FAOTA points out that "nontraditional" fieldwork education sites have become more prominent over the last several years for seven major reasons:

1. It was a strategy for increasing the number of fieldwork sites for a larger student population.

2. Emerging and existing practice areas such as pediatrics did not fit into the classic physical disabilities-mental health dichotomy.

3. Curriculum models were developing that necessitated congruent fieldwork processes.

4. The characteristics of the students and their financial resources changed.

5. The definitions of physical disability and mental health fieldwork changed as the practice of occupational therapy evolved.

6. The challenge of providing fieldwork, that is an ethical responsibility for every clinician,

had to be met in the presence of threats such as cost efficiency and revenue generation.

7. The *Essentials and Guidelines for an Accredited Educational Program for the Occupational Therapist and Occupational Therapy Assistant* (American Occupational Therapy Association (AOTA) and American Medical Association, 1991) further diversified fieldwork requirements to include a variety of groups across the life span that represent psychosocial and physical performance deficits and various service provision models. Practice areas such as home health, independent living, head injury, and worker training presented new opportunities for future and prominent practice and, as a result, became more frequent among fieldwork settings.

There continues to be a steady increase in the number of developing educational programs for occupational therapists and occupational therapy assistants. In the past 5 years, 40 programs for occupational therapists and 53 for occupational therapy assistants have been in various phases of development.

This reality has severely strained the ability of existing fieldwork sites to provide the necessary number of placements for students in developing and existing OT and OTA education programs. This is especially true given that the vast majority of fieldwork sites continue to use the "one supervisor/one student" and/or the "one facility/one student" models. Many academic programs must limit their enrollment because of the inability to secure the necessary number of fieldwork sites. This affects negatively the ability to provide an adequate number of practitioners to meet the needs of consumers. There continues to be a severe shortage of occupational therapy practitioners nationwide.

The Task Force recommends that since a shortage of occupational therapy practitioners is not in the best interests of those in need of OT services, the Association should provide funding for at least five proposals that are developed collaboratively between an academic and clinical fieldwork site. The models that are developed should demonstrate alternative fieldwork models that have the ability to improve the educational process, the availability of fieldwork sites, and the number of occupational therapy practitioners.

Charge to: - RA to provide funding
COE to develop the process and evaluation component.

Financial Impact: $10,000 (for 5 or more projects - maximum funding of $2,000 each)

Timeline: 3 years

Year 1 - plan and select sites (seek diverse models for OT and OTA students)
Year 2 - Implement
Year 3 - Evaluate

RECOMMENDATION 8

Initiate a voluntary computerized system that tracks fieldwork placement vacancies by 1997. Review the success of this system before considering an expanded system, including matching of students and fieldwork sites, by 2000.

The issue of a computerized, centralized scheduling system for fieldwork placement has been examined by the profession several times over the last 20 years (see Exhibit 1). Small demonstration projects have indicated the time-saving benefits as well as the ease with which a computer assisted scheduling program could be utilized. Other professions such as medicine, dietetics, speech pathology, and audiology use computer scheduling for clinical rotations with great success. In addition, the Canadian Association of Occupational Therapists arranges its students' fieldwork placements through a computer system. Although the CAOT arranges fewer than 1000 placements in a calendar year, students have an 85% chance of receiving one of their five designated choices.

There is a growing concern about the number of cancellations of fieldwork placements as well as the expanding need for more fieldwork sites as new OT and OTA education programs are developed with increased student enrollment. Fieldwork coordinators spend a great deal of their time tracking sites and searching for new sites when last-minute cancellations occur, or when students have individual or special needs. While participants in the Open Hearings were generally not in favor of a complete centralized scheduling program, they did express interest in a clearinghouse process that would allow schools to gain access to sites that were underutilized, and available, and thus help them better manage cancellations. In addition, this central clearinghouse would allow new sites to be identified and recognized by fieldwork coordinators. Students were especially favorable to the idea of a fieldwork clearinghouse system, as they felt this could expand their fieldwork options.

Survey questions regarding the use of centralized scheduling also produced initially negative responses from the majority of respondents. Educational programs expressed concern with an impersonal system placing students without taking into consideration individual needs and challenges. However, they did acknowledge the significant difficulties they have experienced with cancellations and with the shrinking number of available clinical sites. They were more favorable regarding a system that could help manage cancellations and explore underutilized sites.

Many educational programs are already using a computer database to place students in fieldwork. The use of a national system would expand their site pool while also encouraging a national informational link between educational programs and clinical sites. With the explosion of information networks, this national database could be used to best meet the needs of students while also easing the burden of the placement process for the educational programs.

Charge to: ICC in collaboration with the Executive Director to identify components, characteristics, and capabilities needed in the database.

Executive Board to initiate a voluntary computerized system for fieldwork placement/vacancies in most cost-efficient manner.

—Utilize AOTA resources

—Consider a representative to external agencies

Financial Impact: Year 1 - no additional costs
Year 2 - depending on decision of Executive Board, expect system to be financially self-sustaining by 1998 (offset by fees)

Timeline: 2 years (1995–1997)

RECOMMENDATION 9

Utilize the Regional Fieldwork Consultants (RFWC) to assist fieldwork educators in operationalizing new models. Support, publicize, and recognize the value of this role. The Task Force recom-mends that the RFWC become a Standing Committee in the reorganization of COE.

The Regional Fieldwork Consultants (RFWC) represent the nine regions of the United States and Puerto Rico. They are available on a daily basis to provide verbal or written guidance on fieldwork issues in their regions and to participate in regional fieldwork workshops. The consultants are current occupational therapy practitioners who have been selected for their demonstrated expertise in fieldwork issues. They serve in a voluntary capacity.

These consultants have been a vital link in disseminating information on innovative fieldwork. For the past year, each consultant has been responsible for presenting at least one workshop in his or her region on the topic of supervision in innovative fieldwork settings. In addition, the consultants have developed a workshop that focuses on innovation in fieldwork and dispels some of the myths associated with the word "innovative." Future plans include the development of a "traveling" fieldwork workshop on the fundamentals of supervision and fieldwork in a changing health care environment.

Increased funding support for the activities of the Regional Fieldwork Consultants is strongly recommended. This funding would enable the Regional Fieldwork Consultants to expand offerings for supervisory skills workshops and would enable them to assist fieldwork sites in operationalizing new fieldwork education models. Because these consultants are volunteers, and therefore a finite resource, it is important to identify all the major groups currently being employed to strengthen the skills of clinical educators, including the RFWC, the state and regional Fieldwork Councils, and the educational programs; to compare these resources against the overall need for training of a clinical educator population adequate to support the current population of entry-level students (17,523 as of calendar year 1993); and to plan for complementary systems to meet the needs of the profession.

Charge to: COE to have RFWC become a Standing Committee in the reorganization of COE.

Financial Impact: Increase funding from $3,600 to $9,000 ($1,000 per RFWC)

Timeline: Immediately (1995–1996 budget)

RECOMMENDATION 10

Support and expand current mechanisms for the broad and timely distribution of information related to innovative and emerging fieldwork models that successfully offer ideas for meeting the needs of a changing health care system, the growing number of academic programs, and a changing student body.

Traditionally, fieldwork has been an experience where an OT or OTA student spends 3 to 9 months in a physical disability or mental health setting, with further options for a specialized area of practice if the educational program requires it, or if the student wants to pursue a special interest. This fieldwork is often completed in hospitals or primary health care settings. There are currently many factors that contribute to the way occupational therapy practice and education are provided. These, in part, are: increased demand for OT services in expanding practice arenas, manpower shortages, increasing numbers of students needing fieldwork placements, and students with special needs. There seems to be a perception on the part of academic educators and others that fieldwork sites are "shrinking." It is not certain, however, if they are really "shrinking" or if they simply appear to be, due to increased competition for fieldwork sites from a growing student body. We do know that cancellations of fieldwork placements are increasing. An essential consideration in preparing students for entry-level practice is that fieldwork be reflective of current practice. This provides the impetus to expand and improve fieldwork education and to discuss innovations in fieldwork.

Mechanisms to distribute information regarding innovative or nontraditional fieldwork to the membership at large have been in place and active for the last 5 years:

The Fieldwork Issues Committee (FWIC), a subcommittee of the Commission on Education (COE), developed and compiled more than 40 innovative models of fieldwork nationwide. These models were categorized by the type of setting, the structure of the supervision, the intent of the objectives for fieldwork, and the geographic location of the fieldwork program. One of these models is highlighted each month in *OT Week* in the "News From the Fieldwork Corner" column.

The Regional Fieldwork Consultants (RFWCs) have been a vital link in disseminating information on innovative fieldwork in a broad and timely manner. There are nine consultants, representing nine regions of the United States and Puerto Rico.

There are strong fieldwork councils nationwide (e.g., MinnDak, Minnesota and Dakota(s) Fieldwork Council; NEOTEC, New England Occupational Therapy Educators Council; WISCouncil, Wisconsin Council on Education; and TREC, Therapist Education Resource Consortium in Kansas City), that meet routinely to discuss fieldwork issues and host mini-workshops for their area constituents. Participants in these councils are the academic fieldwork coordinators, faculty members, clinical educators and students.

The OT and OTA program directors receive the *OT Educator* newsletter, that also highlights all publications, packets, and the latest information from AOTA. This is distributed quarterly and serves as a medium for feedback from the educational programs to AOTA about desired new publications.

The entire February 1995 issue of *AJOT* is devoted to fieldwork, with the recurring theme of innovation. Plans are to continue with an annual fieldwork issue, including National Office perspectives on fieldwork.

Concurrently, the *Essentials and Guidelines for an Accredited Program for the Occupational Therapist and Occupational Therapy Assistant* will be revised in the very near future. The Accreditation Council for Occupational Therapy Education (ACOTE), with input from the Commission on Education (COE), will analyze the existing requirements in terms of their ability to reflect current practice.

As we have seen from the national perspective, there are many mechanisms already in place to promote the widespread distribution of innovative fieldwork models. We also envision more activity to support innovative fieldwork secondary to a changing health care environment with new service delivery models. The challenge is to seek more.

Charge to: Executive Director to plan and implement the following:

1. Identification of fieldwork as an AOTA conference theme/priority

2. One day of poster sessions (at AOTA conferences) dedicated to alternative fieldwork models

3. We further recommend that the Executive Board seek to have AOTF establish a funding priority for research projects associated with fieldwork education.

Financial Impact: No additional cost

Timeline: Immediately (1995–1996 Fiscal Year)

RECOMMENDATION 11

Support academic institutions that choose to make Fieldwork a postdegree requirement.

While a mandate related to this issue is not within the purview of AOTA, the Task Force recommends that AOTA support those institutions that create models that make fieldwork a postdegree requirement. Such models may provide valuable information and ideas for dealing with future fieldwork issues.

RECOMMENDATION 12

Create and publish an anthology that archives all works related to occupational therapy fieldwork education. The anthology will include journal articles and reports of Association Committees, Commissions and Task Forces, and will recognize those who have addressed this issue throughout the history of the profession. It will serve as a primary resource for future planning. The Task Force recommends the engagement of a single paid content editor to accomplish this task.

In the process of reviewing the history and development of the educational models employed by the profession, a rich foundation for the profession's clinical education evolution was located. It became clear during the search for resources that some studies, Task Force reports, consumer reports, and professional documents could not be easily retrieved or located. Scholars and planners in the future could have the same difficulties encountered by the Fieldwork for the Future Task Force in accessing the solid foundation of past and current research, the philosophy and models of clinical education, models of collaboration between academia and practice, and innovative and successful fieldwork models.

In the process of looking at the models of similar professions, The Task Force discovered that other professions have recognized this lack of a resource

for their clinical educators and scholars. As an example, the American Physical Therapy Association appointed a group of physical therapy scholars to review their clinical education literature, select significant material, and publish an anthology on clinical education. This publication, entitled *Clinical Education: An Anthology,* is now available for purchase from APTA.

The AOTA Fieldwork for the Future Task Force believes that a work of this magnitude for the occupational therapy profession would be an excellent addition to our body of knowledge. It would serve as a resource for academic and clinical educators. It would serve as a resource for the Association's decision-making bodies. It would serve as a resource for the therapists of the future.

After the initial development, the text could be updated on a 5-year cycle. This would allow future issues to have pertinent historical information and information while reflecting current thinking and research in the education of occupational therapy practitioners.

This publication would provide ongoing value in the development of the role of clinical educator for future practitioners.

Charge to: Executive Director

Financial Impact: $2,000 (Single, paid content editor)

Timeline: 1 year (1995–1996)

RECOMMENDATION 13

Utilize the established TriAlliance of Health and Rehabilitation Professions (AOTA, APTA, ASHA) to continue to expand common concerns regarding clinical education. Establish and/or maintain relationships with other professional associations and consumer groups that affect the clinical education of occupational therapy practitioners.

The TriAlliance was formed in 1988 when AOTA, the American Physical Therapy Association (APTA) and the American Speech-Language-Hearing Association (ASHA) joined together to form the TriAlliance of Health and Rehabilitation Professions. It represents a joint venture on the part of the three organizations to address issues of mutual concern and to initiate, as appropriate, collective action that will enhance their individual responses to major societal problems. The Steering Committee consists of the Presidents and Executive Directors of AOTA, APTA, and ASHA.

The Task Force met with key national office education staff members from APTA and ASHA to learn about their clinical education systems. These sessions provided a very useful forum for the exchange of ideas and a discussion of common concerns. The opportunity to meet with colleagues in ASHA and APTA to reflect on current education issues that affect our professions, to do mutual problem-solving on shared issues, and to exchange ideas for improvement of our respective education systems should be encouraged and supported.

The Task Force further recommends that relationships with other groups and professional associations be nurtured in order to improve occupational therapy and the education of professional and technical-level practitioners.

Charge to: Executive Board

Financial Impact: No additional cost

BIBLIOGRAPHY

Adelstein, L.A., Cohn, E.S., Baker, R.C., & Barnes, M.A. (1990). A part-time level II fieldwork program. *American Journal of Occupational Therapy, 44*(1), 60–65.

American Occupational Therapy Association. (1986). *Occupational Therapy Education: Target 2000.* Rockville, MD: Author.

American Occupational Therapy Association (1991). *Guide to Fieldwork Education.* Rockville, MD: Author.

American Physical Therapy Association. (1992). *Clinical Education: An Anthology.* Alexandria, VA: Author.

American Occupational Therapy Association. (1993). *Occupational Therapy Roles. American Journal of Occupational Therapy, 47*(12), 1087–1099.

Anderson, R.L. (1992). Level II Fieldwork: An Academic or Professional Responsibility? *Education Special Interest Section Newsletter, 2*(3), 2.

Anthony, A., & Gaiptman, B. (1989). Contracting in fieldwork education: The model of self-directed learning. *Canadian Journal of Occupational Therapy, 56*(1), 10–14.

Atwater, A.W., & Davis, C.G. (1990). The value of psychosocial level II fieldwork. *American Journal of Occupational Therapy, 44*(9), 792–795.

Balla, J.I. (1990). Insights into some aspects of clinical education—II: A theory for clinical education. *Postgraduate Medical Journal, 66*(774), 297–301.

Beck, S.J., Youngblood, P., & Stritter, F.T. (1988). Implementation and evaluation of a new approach to clinical instruction. *Journal of Allied Health, 17*(4), 331–340.

Bishop, K.F., & Masagatani, G.N. (1991). Fieldwork and academic education. *OT Week, 5*(9), 10–11.

Boyer, J.J. (1989). The ultimate in networking. *Administration & Management Special Interest Section Newsletter, 5*(1), 3.

Brunyate, R.W. (1962). The clinical center: An integral part of the education program. *The American Journal of Occupational Therapy, 16*(2), 61–65.

Brunyate, R.W. (1962). The student in pre-clinical education. *The American Journal of Occupational Therapy, 17*(5), 181–186.

Byrne, C., McKnight, J., Roberts, J., & Rankin, J. (1989). Learning clinical teaching skills at the baccalaureate level. *Journal of Advanced Nursing, 14*(8), 678–685.

Canadian Association of Occupational Therapy. (1993). *Standards of Occupational Therapy.*

Final Report: Fieldwork Supervision Focus Group

By

Phyllis F. Burchman
Research Program Manager
Research Information & Evaluation Department

Conducted at
AOTA National Office
4720 Montgomery Lane
Bethesda, MD

February 21 & February 23, 1995

TABLE OF CONTENTS

I. INTRODUCTION

This report summarizes the key findings from two focus groups conducted of AOTA members. The groups were held at the AOTA national office in Bethesda, MD on February 21 and February 23, 1995.

A. Purpose and Background

The purpose of the focus groups was to discover reasons why some occupational therapists and occupational therapy assistants supervise fieldwork students and why others do not. The idea to convene the focus groups grew out of the fieldwork "crisis" planning. Secondarily, innovative ideas for fieldwork were to be explored.

B. Methods and Procedures

The Fieldwork Program Manager (Education Department) decided that it would be necessary to convene two groups in order accomplish this task. One group consisted of current fieldwork supervisors and the other group consisted of therapists who were not currently supervisors.

The moderator was AOTA's Research Information & Evaluation Department Program Manager, who is not an occupational therapist. The panelists were told this and the moderator's role was described for them. The moderator characterized herself as a researcher and as a participant. Participants were asked to "give their honest feelings and opinions and not what they thought AOTA wanted to hear". The Discussion Guide was developed by the moderator, with input from the research department's director, the AOTA marketing department's director, and the education department's fieldwork program manager. The questions and their content were discussed with the education department's fieldwork program manager (client) so as to capture the correct intent of the questions. On the basis of those reviews, changes were made and additional items were added to the Discussion Guide. The sessions were audio taped for later review, thus freeing the moderator from taking notes during the proceedings.

C. Participants

Participants came from the Washington, D.C. metropolitan area as well as from Baltimore and Frederick, MD. The first group consisted of 10 participants, none of whom currently supervised fieldwork students. Of the 10, all were OTRs; 8 were female and 2 were male. Their number of years in OT practice ranged from 1 to 25 years (avg. 8.5 years) and their employment settings included hospitals (physical disabilities, psychiatric, VA), home health, rehab centers, skilled nursing facilities, and private practice (early intervention school-based). The second group (current supervisors) was made up of 14 participants. All were OTRs, however one had previously been a COTA (most of her career). There was one male in this group, the rest were female. Their years of OT experience ranged from 4 to 19 years (avg. 10 years). Work settings included hospitals (physical disabilities and psychiatric), skilled nursing facilities, home health, rehab centers and school-based OT.

II. IMPLICATIONS AND RECOMMENDATIONS

There were similarities in what both groups had to say. Supervisors typically had very specific thoughts. Many of them related to changes they were actually seeing in the environment. Basically, they supervise out of personal pride and to "give something back" to their profession. Non-supervisors had more broad-based ideas. They weren't altogether sure how the pieces of a fieldwork program fit together and generally felt less informed. That was attributed to the lack of any formal training for OTs to learn about becoming a fieldwork supervisor. The following statements attempt to encapsulate the

plethora of information which was gathered from the two groups.

It was generally understood and agreed upon that fieldwork supervision is extremely important.

Occupational therapists are not adequately trained to be fieldwork supervisors. Formal training in all aspects of supervision would alleviate a lot of the concerns surrounding fieldwork supervision.

OTs have a self-image problem which prevents them from teaching or mentoring other OTs or health professionals. OT students and new therapists need to be taught to see themselves as fieldwork supervisors and mentors. They must learn to envision themselves in these roles, as early as possible.

The health care environment is changing and many OTs presently work in multiple settings. Therefore, fieldwork affiliations must also take place in varied and multiple settings, not just the "old, medical model" approach. A variety of practice areas should be available for fieldwork affiliations. Mental health, pediatrics, and school-based settings should be used regularly. OT educational programs must keep pace with changes in the health care industry and must inform their students about such changes in the marketplace.

It takes a lot of additional work and stress to supervise a fieldwork student. Supervisors must be flexible and creative. That can be difficult, especially when employers place high productivity expectations on employees. Support from the facility's administration is vital.

Clinicians feel estranged from educational programs. A good relationship between the educational program and the clinical facility is invaluable. If fieldwork coordinators, and other school representatives were more visible and established regular communications with the supervisors, that would help promote successful affiliations. It would also set a good example for clinicians who might be considering becoming a supervisor.

A supportive network of current fieldwork supervisors would be helpful to those wishing to begin a program. It would provide informational resources which therapists need when making presentations to administrators (why reinvent the wheel?).

If mental health practitioners don't act as fieldwork supervisors, fieldwork in that practice area might disappear completely. The continuance of psychosocial fieldwork affiliations is considered to be of utmost importance.

Occupational therapy supervisors, take a lot of pride in their fieldwork program (probably many have had to fight for the program's very existence). They see themselves fitting into a supervisory role and they take the responsibility seriously (i.e. they are stable employees; don't change jobs often).

III. GENERAL SUMMARY OF FINDINGS

Predispositions

Participants in both groups attached a lot of emotions to fieldwork, especially supervision. The moderator kept the discussion narrowly focused on issues of supervision since the participants would have loved to have a "free for all discussion" of fieldwork. The overall mood of both groups was light-hearted but serious. They believed their opinions mattered and carried importance in the Association. An underlying assumption that seemed to be understood by all participants was that fieldwork is integral to OT practice and must continue.

The wisdom of convening two groups, was guided by the belief that there are probably differences in the way supervisors and non-supervisors feel about fieldwork supervision issues. If the groups were mixed, there might have been tension or anxiety on the part of the non-supervisors. They might have felt guilty, knowing how important fieldwork supervision is, yet they were not taking part. By separating the groups, the questions were less threatening to the non-supervisors and the answers were well-thought out, serious, and reasonable. After the supervisors group got underway, it became evident that two of the members worked together. One of that pair seemed to prod the other for responses similar to hers, as if to justify her own feelings and opinions. Nevertheless, the participation in that group progressed nicely and the fact that they worked together probably had only a minor effect, if any at all, on the group's interactions. Overwhelmingly, participants were happy to be "summoned" to the national office for their participation.

The participants were asked, at times, to place themselves in imaginary situations. Some people

inherently do that better than others. However, for an emotional topic such as fieldwork supervision, it seemed to work well and the creative results of the groups were useful.

The groups progressed through a series of events which are outlined below:

- General warm-up questions to move the group toward the topic of fieldwork supervision. Free-association type exercise to "get the juices flowing".

- Discussion of the necessity of OT supervision and the notion of incentives for fieldwork supervisors.

- Exposure to a series of scenarios in order to encourage them to be free-thinking and creative. Elements of successful fieldwork in real and "ideal" health care facilities. Advantages and disadvantages of fieldwork supervision. Top 3 negative and top 3 positive consequences to participants if the facilities where they work decided to take/not take students.

- Exploration of innovative ideas for fieldwork.

A. Both groups underwent warm-up exercises to get them thinking in the frame of fieldwork supervision.

Participants in both groups indicated that they were participating in the focus groups because fieldwork is important to their profession and they wanted to "help". Concern was expressed that fieldwork might be shortened or phased out (mental health fieldwork was especially worrisome). There seemed to be a general understanding that changes need to be made to fieldwork due to the changing health care environment. Basically that meant that OTs are working at more than one setting and there is a trend towards community-based OT and away from the traditional hospital setting. The notion that there is a shortage of fieldwork sites was also a reason for participating (some supervisors noted that they are "booked" through 1997!). Several non-supervisors mentioned that their facilities were considering beginning a fieldwork program. Many current fieldwork supervisors also expressed a selfish need to network with other fieldwork supervisors.

Words used to describe supervising fieldwork students did not differ much between the groups. Both groups used positive and negative words. Some of the words and phrases used were: rewarding, time consuming, extra work, self-learning, informative, mentoring, modeling, commitment, responsibility, stress, fun, frustrating, risk, "you learn something about yourself", and "makes you reason out loud what you're doing".

B. The groups discussed the necessity for fieldwork supervision and the growth potential or importance of incentives for fieldwork supervisors.

Neither group could imagine a world with practitioners who had not undergone fieldwork. "I learned more in 6 months of fieldwork than I learned during 4 years of college". Participants across the groups saw fieldwork as an opportunity for students to make mistakes, to put the theoretical they'd learned into practice, to see that there's a human component that goes along with the learned techniques, to "try-out" different practice areas, and to bridge the gap from classroom to practice. "It's an opportunity to be clumsy and be forgiven for it".

When asked why occupational therapists would want to supervise students and whether they should receive special incentives or recognition, the comments were somewhat varied. While participants in both groups felt that it was important and necessary for OTs to be supervisors, the group of current supervisors felt very responsible for their fieldwork supervision programs. That responsibility encompassed the maintenance of the program itself, as well as student welfare. They seemed to graciously accept the "sacrifices" that they made (like having less personal time and having to justify the program repeatedly to administrators). For some current supervisors, it was routine to have a student " . . . every spring, I'll have a student . . . it is very consistent . . . there is continuity". The supervisors group pointed out that teaching facilities typically take students from most of the medical professions, as if it was an expectation for any profession.

Interestingly, it was a non-supervisor who indicated that students oftentimes leave school with an attitude of being "entitled". There was an indication that some students want specific, custom-made arrangements for their fieldwork affiliations. Some students don't even want to be called students (possibly interns!).

The non-supervisors group recognized that a monetary incentive was not necessarily appropriate for a fieldwork supervisor, since supervising is a matter of "professional integrity" and wanting to "mentor folks in this profession". For this group,

the most essential element for supervising students would be having support from their facility or organization. They couldn't seem to fathom being a supervisor without such support. It is important to note here that facility support was important to both groups, but the supervisors were more flexible about the issue. The non-supervisors did give other examples of possible incentives: more CEUs, college credits given by the educational program (toward a master's degree) and job promotions ("supervising looks good on your resume").

Current supervisors emphasized less tangible perks such as having an established relationship with a local university, professional development and status (especially in a large OT department), personal satisfaction and growth. They said they would prefer having an extra hour a day to get supervisory duties done, instead of being offered additional money. Supervisor training was highly valued by this group, whether by university fieldwork coordinators, or others.

The groups were consistent in their ideas about incentives for facilities to maintain fieldwork supervision programs. Such programs were touted as great recruitment tools. Facilities gain staff from students who completed their fieldwork and already feel comfortable in the environment, with the patient population and with the other therapists. Apparently this argument is often used to justify the programs to administrators. It was also noted that facilities gain more prestige if they are viewed as a teaching facility ("they all want to come here to learn"). Some participants had heard of schools providing a lump sum of money to facilities who took students.

C. Participants were asked to imagine themselves as the head OT at the "ideal health care facility"—which does not currently have a fieldwork program. The scenario continued with the proposal of beginning such a program. Participants wrote down the advantages and disadvantages which they would consider in their decision-making process.

A definite advantage expressed by both groups was the energy and fresh ideas which students bring with them and the positive effect that can have on both the clinicians and the patients. "Students have some off the wall ideas because they don't have preconceived ideas about what will and will not work . . . sometimes their ideas are great and work well". "Patients respond well to students . . . they want to help them do well so they (the patients) work harder for them".

Disadvantages expressed by the non-supervisors included clinicians not feeling confident since they don't have any background or training in educating students. Also, mentioned were time consuming paperwork, understanding the legalities of being a supervisor (e.g. contracts, ethics, liability) and possibly having to mediate between the facility, the student and the university. Adding those responsibilities to their present caseload seemed untenable. However, they did think that having the support of their administrators would "solve" most of the problems and without that support, they would not even consider entering into such a program. The non-supervisors also felt that occupational therapists have a self-image problem as it relates to mentoring or teaching students. They did admit that beginning a fieldwork program might help to change that image. Selling the idea to administrators was also a concern, but recruitment (students who might eventually become employees) and increased productivity (requiring students to do a project) were mentioned as possible solutions. They also felt it would give the facility some clout to establish a link with a university. When asked to mark the "advantages grid" with an "x" to indicate their overall feeling about beginning such a program, it seemed that the advantages "outweighed" the disadvantages for this group. Some of the advantages they mentioned were the fresh outlook and information a student would bring to the facility and that a student would "keep them on their toes", since supervisors would need to constantly explain what they were doing and why.

The supervisors emphasized that the facility's name would become positively associated with employment. It was echoed that students would bring the latest information to the clinic and the additional responsibility of having to explain what they're doing and why would keep clinicians from getting complacent. Also, more creative work options would be available to staff clinicians. On the flip side, supervisors noted that if a student isn't "appropriate" for a particular setting, a lot of time and energy has been put in at a non-billable rate. Overall, this group seemed to say that when you get a student that is strong and the program is well-planned, it's a good situation which offers increased creativity and opportunities for staff and the morale is high. But if the student is weak and things aren't working well, it can be a bad situation for all concerned. Understandably, the concerns from this group were

very specific, but they were also fewer in comparison. The supervisors overwhelmingly placed their "x" marks on the grid indicating "a lot of advantages".

The fantasy scenario continued with the decision having been made to begin a fieldwork supervision program at this ideal health care facility. What would be the first thing they would do as the "head OT"?

Not surprisingly, the supervisors gave a concise accounting of what they felt would make a fieldwork supervision program successful. Their listing included educating themselves about beginning a program, outlining objectives and planning lessons, looking into supervisor training and a mention of some of the personality attributes which make up a "good" supervisor. They said they'd provide leadership to their newly-trained supervisors possibly beginning with Level I fieldwork students or even supervising a student themselves. They might also give their staff only brief experiences with students, so as not to overwhelm them.

The non-supervisors repeated the need for supervisor training and that they would be a role model for the new supervisors. In addition, they felt important attributes for a successful program would involve a diverse caseload, flexibility, supervisors who were interested in being teachers and had good organizational skills, and developing a plan for exactly how the supervision would be carried out. There was no consensus on whether they felt a "perfect" setting for a fieldwork program exists.

Participants were then asked how they would feel/act if just before they arrived that evening, they were told that their facility(s) would begin/ end a fieldwork supervision program. Participants were asked how this decision would affect them. They were instructed to write down the top 3 positive and top 3 negative consequences of the decision.

The supervisors, whose program would be ending, said they would be genuinely upset at the decision. Some indicated that they would feel personally responsible for the program's cessation. Some supervisors had drastic comments like "I would be so angry, I would feel like quitting". But others mentioned that even though they would take it as a personal and professional insult, they recognized that facilities oftentimes make similar changes, sometimes even abruptly. Several of the supervisors saw opportunities in this scenario. "How I would feel would depend on the reason. If we were trying to do something new in the facility like not take students, but do a research project instead, I'd go for that". As upsetting as this scenario sounded, it seemed to have legitimacy. (If it had really happened to them, it wouldn't have surprised them. Possibly because their program's existence is precarious anyway). It was also mentioned that the stress from supervising students would not be missed and the extra time would be valued. When considering the positive and negative consequences of the action, this group listed many more negatives than positives and betrayal (by the administration) came through their comments loud and clear. They indicated that although they would have more time to do other things, they wouldn't be doing the things they prefer!

There was an interesting side-bar to this scenario which concerned educational programs charging students for tuition during fieldwork (which they need to graduate) and the facilities not getting any of that money. Although the moderator kept this discussion to a minimum, it needs to be mentioned in the context of this issue, since the participants felt strongly about this connection.

Non-supervisors, who had a fieldwork supervision program suddenly thrust at them, were also defensive. They tried to decide exactly how a program would work; what components would be needed. Themes which emerged were the constancy of staff, space requirements, where the students would come from and the possibility of sharing students with other facilities. They also predicted that staff therapists might feel uncomfortable and overwhelmed, especially those who have been out of school for a long time, those who feel they're not up-to-date on the latest techniques and those who are uncomfortable as a teacher. Asking for volunteers would be the better way to choose supervisors, not forcing therapists into a supervisory role unwillingly.

When asked to list the top 3 positive and negative consequences of this action, things heard earlier were echoed once again. Positive: exciting possibilities were seen, teaching, challenge, professional development, growth for the facility and being forced to become more organized. Negative: less personal time, more stress, competency issues, weighty responsibility, confusion, unsure about possible decrease in productivity and generally not being prepared for a student.

FOCUS GROUP WRAP-UP: CONCLUDING TOPICS

Respondents were asked their opinions about the focus group and if there were any other questions they would have asked if they had been the moderator.

All of the participants from the non-supervisors group and many from the supervisors group thanked the moderator for allowing them to participate in the group. They were proud of their participation and felt appreciated by their professional association. They understood that the information provided would be considered carefully and used to help abate the fieldwork "crisis" situation. The groups were described as "a good brainstorming session". They also indicated that exciting ideas had been generated for them and confirmed to them that they are not "out there struggling, alone".

Several participants indicated that the group confirmed and validated their feelings on fieldwork issues. They seemed uplifted and motivated by AOTA's outreach. One supervisor indicated that she "appreciated the opportunity to collaborate with AOTA and (she) would like the opportunity to deal with AOTA on other practical matters".

Topics they would liked to have covered did not necessarily encompass supervision. They included, checking how fiscally sound a facility was before encouraging them to begin a fieldwork program and the fieldwork grading system. The latter topic seemed to be a serious bone of contention, not appropriate for this group, but one which was very emotional to the participants, and came up in both groups. The participants indicated that there is a lot of fluctuation from one facility to the next and also too much subjectivity in the grading of fieldwork students.

EXECUTIVE SUMMARY

Occupational therapists have long sought recognition by other health professionals, their patients and by the public. Now that much is known about what OTs do, and many facilities have established fieldwork supervision programs, therapists seem to be asking for help as to how they should go about managing their role as fieldwork supervisors. The constant flux of the health care arena only seems to complicate the issue. As clinicians move out of the traditional hospital settings and into community-based programs, so must the fieldwork affiliations shift.

Even though non-supervisors presented many issues which were indicative of their uncertainty about supervising, similarities existed between the two groups. It was felt that therapists should supervise students. If they currently are not supervisors, then they should begin to consider that role for themselves. That message should be taught to OT students and new therapists as soon as possible, so that being a mentor will become a part of their identity. It would be helpful to have formal training, outlining the proper duties of a supervisor, with an emphasis on flexibility, problem solving and creativity. Other ideas included a rational network to support clinicians who want to become fieldwork supervisors and fieldwork coordinators who would be visible or at least reachable. Affiliations need to be held at varied work settings and consist of numerous types of practice areas (especially in mental health, pediatrics and school-based practice). Plus, affiliations need to be lengthier (definitely not shorter!), allowing students to experience as many aspects of OT practice as possible. Successful affiliations depend upon serious commitments from the facility's administration. In addition, staff therapists have to want to be supervisors and they will need to make a 6–12 month time commitment.

INNOVATIVE IDEAS:

When pressed for innovative ideas regarding fieldwork, non-supervisors sent two messages: longer fieldwork affiliations and the affiliations should move away from a traditional, hospital environment. Affiliations need to be more flexible, with the student spending more hours in the facility and therefore maximizing the student's exposure to clinical practice. This will be especially advantageous for second career students who may be balancing school with other responsibilities. Varied work settings, especially home health, were stressed. Hospitals no longer keep patients for lengthy stays, so students aren't getting the benefit of seeing a varied patient population. "Nursing homes used to be a place where people went to die. Now they are a step away from the hospital and an interim (transitional) place. This setting should be emphasized for

fieldwork. The nursing home has become the hospital setting". "In hospitals today, you see a patient one day and evaluate them. They are discharged the next day. So you evaluate them and discharge them".

The supervisor's "innovative" ideas were concrete. Although they admitted that some of these things were being done currently, they are not considered to be the norm. Their ideas were:

- variety of patient populations

- 2 students to 1 supervisor

- multiple supervisors per student (even PTs!)

- more collaboration between OT (allied health professionals) and nursing when placing students

- pairing OT and OTA students (they learn about partnerships; indicates that facility promotes COTAs)

- supervise 2 students simultaneously from different schools

- have student affiliations dovetail (decreases orientation time; parting student gets a chance to shine; learn from each other)

- facilities share a student (student must still have primary supervisor; all supervisors must be in contact with one another)

- bring in Level 1 students at same time as Level II students . . . make it part of Level II student's responsibilities to be involved with the Level I student (e.g. a project)

- fieldwork coordinators should be more visible to facilities

- extended placements (especially for OTA students where 2 months is not enough to learn much at all . . . they have less knowledge anyway because their didactic part is less and they get less time to learn critical thinking skills)

- if facilities are willing to pay for student stipends/scholarships . . . why not pay for fieldwork? (the investment is in future practitioners)

SAMPLE MODERATOR'S GUIDE

MODERATOR'S GUIDE: FIELDWORK
SUPERVISION FOCUS GROUP
GROUP 1 - FEBRUARY 21, 1995
MODERATOR: PHYLLIS F. BURCHMAN

GOAL: To determine why OT practitioners do not supervise fieldwork students and what factors affect that decision-making process.

LOCATION: SAMMONS CONF CENTER ROOM "A"
AOTA NATIONAL OFFICE
4720 MONTGOMERY LANE
BETHESDA, MD

Let's all finish getting food and drink and let's sit down. Please sit behind the tent card with your name. WELCOME THEM. THANK THEM FOR COMING. INTRODUCE SELF.

We are gathered here tonight to discuss why OT practitioners do not supervise fieldwork students. This is called a Focus Group. Has anyone taken part in a focus group before? (RECORD NUMBER OF RAISED HANDS). It's obvious that the organization sponsoring this focus group is AOTA. This group was convened because the OT profession is facing specific challenges regarding fieldwork. The number of OT educational programs continues to increase at a fast pace and therefore the number of students needing placements has risen and will continue to do so. Also, the places where fieldwork occurs is changing. Health care environments are changing rapidly in the U.S. and so fieldwork issues are involved with that too. Basically, focus groups are a qualitative research method which measures the mood or climate of a group of individuals and will in turn, hopefully generate ideas (programmatic changes) which can be expanded to a broader population (namely, AOTA members). Focus groups were first held in people's living rooms. They are now a widely recognized marketing tool which AOTA is using to get member input (ideas and thoughts) toward a targeted or focused topic. You should all feel good that you are participating in something which, hopefully will help your profession to grow.

I am not an OT. I am a researcher—STATE MY POSITION AT AOTA. Therefore, I have not personally gone through fieldwork. I have no stake in these discussions other than the fact that I am a national office employee. I have no axe to grind regarding fieldwork supervision. I am the facilitator of the discussion, but I'm still a part of this group. In order for me to be part of the discussion tonight, I will need to audiotape the proceedings. I don't have a photographic memory and focus group notes or tapes must later be transcribed into a meaningful report. That is how we'll learn and benefit from tonight's discussion. By the way, focus groups are oftentimes videotaped and in more sophisticated settings even viewed behind a one-way mirror. Please view the tape recorder only as an aid to me.

Feel free to respond to anything that will be said here tonight. Just wait until the person who is speaking is finished. That way, everyone can be heard. You don't have to agree with everything that is said. Your experiences with fieldwork (supervision) are probably quite varied and therefore, I'm sure you have a lot to say. If someone says something and everyone nods their heads in agreement, I'll assume that everyone agreed totally (remember the tape recorder won't pick up head nodding!). Don't send me away misinformed. If you don't agree with something which was said, speak up. Please don't talk over each other. If you do, the tape recording will sound like a strange foreign language and I won't be able to make heads or tails out of what was said when I review the tape. If you have a thought and someone else is speaking, keep track of it. Focus groups depend on only having one conversation instead of concurrent ones.

Remember, nothing you say is wrong or unimportant. I am only one part of this group, but there are (###) of us here tonight. Your colleagues or neighbors aren't here tonight. We want to know YOUR THOUGHTS AND FEELINGS. We are not looking for consensus. We are not looking for you to agree on any particular thing. Don't tell us what you think AOTA wants to hear. Be honest. Be blunt.

For the sake of tonight's discussion, fieldwork means Fieldwork Level II. But if it helps you to relate to our discussion to consider Fieldwork Level I or any other experience you've had, go ahead.

You may be asked to write something down and then talk about it.

LOGISTICAL THINGS: Point out the rest rooms. You don't need to ask permission to go, just try to hurry back. The same goes for getting a drink. There's coffee, tea, soft drinks, etc. The incentive payment for coming tonight will be mailed to you. But for now, let's get down to work.

WARM-UP EXERCISE: (HAND OUT BLANK SHEETS OF PAPER)

On the blank sheet of paper, briefly jot down the following information:

Your name, where you're from (city, state), whether you're an OTR or COTA, how many years in profession, the kind of facility you work in (primarily), what you like to do in your spare time and why you wanted to participate in tonight's group.

(START TAPE PLAYER)

(HAVE THEM INTRODUCE THEMSELVES AND TELL ANY OF THE BITS OF INFO THEY JOTTED DOWN THEN COLLECT SHEETS)

QUESTION 1: (HAND OUT BLANK PIECES OF PAPER) On the blank sheet of paper, jot down words that come to mind to describe supervising fieldwork students. Sort of a free-association exercise.

(HAVE THEM READ THEIR WORDS ALOUD) Did anyone use different words which haven't already been mentioned? (COLLECT SHEETS)

QUESTION 2: Why does fieldwork supervision exist? What's the point of supervising fieldwork students? How does it help the profession/the student? What does it accomplish? Is it effective? Does the supervising of students still have a function in 1995?

What is the growth potential for OTs who are fieldwork supervisors? How does it help their careers as OTs to be fieldwork supervisors? Should fieldwork supervisors get special incentives or perks? If so, what should they be awards, recognition, money, what else?)

Should OTs get special recognition if they supervise FW students or should professional pride or altruistic reasons be their reasons for doing it? Should it be part of every OTs job description (i.e. required)?

QUESTION 3: Let's pretend that you are the head of the OT dept. for the ideal health care facility—which by the way *does not take fieldwork students currently.*

(HAND OUT "ADVANTAGES ATTITUDINAL GRID")

Okay, you are the head honcho of the OT dept. This is an ideal health care environment. There are no real-world constraints. Let's say the idea that your facility should begin supervising FW students was presented to you, the decision-maker. Jot down on the grid, what distinct advantages and disadvantages you believe there are re: fieldwork students being supervised (at your ideal facility).

(WAIT A FEW MINUTES FOR THEM TO DO THIS).

Now, place an "X" on the part of the grid which describes your overall feeling about this issue. Maybe where you think your final decision would be.

(HAVE THEM READ THE ADVANTAGES AND DISADVANTAGES FROM THEIR PAPERS).

Now, let's say you decided to accept fieldwork students at this ideal facility. Why do you think it may have been important to you to decide to accept FW students?

What would be the first thing you would need to do to insure a good experience for both the student, your facility, and the supervising OT? (policies, physical things, attitudes)

Type of facility, type of person (characteristics) for ideal FW supervisor, type of person would not make a good fieldwork supervisor. What would make that supervisor successful or unsuccessful?

Any special equipment needed at FW site?

As head of the OT dept. do you foresee any situations whereby OTs at your facility would not or could not supervise students? I.e. are there any work settings which are inherently not conducive to the supervision of fieldwork students?

(COLLECT THEIR PAPERS).

QUESTION 4: Back to reality: poof! It's Feb. 21, 1995 again! If your facility suddenly decided that starting today, OT fieldwork students would be accepted and supervised how do you feel about that?

(HAND OUT A PIECE OF PAPER WITH "TOP 3 GOOD AND TOP 3 BAD" ON THE PAGE).

Remember, this is not the ideal facility, anymore . . . this is your current employer! The real world applies! Write down the top 3 positive and top 3 negative consequences which would impact you in your job, if this were to happen today. What changes would need to be made either policies or specifically in your job, etc.

What would turn you on and off about supervising students on fieldwork?

(HAVE THEM SHARE THEIR TOP 3'S, THEN CONTINUE DISCUSSION)

Any specific support needed for a successful program to begin?

How do you think supervisors would be chosen from among the current staff?

How much say would you (or the staff therapists) have in whether you/they would want to supervise students . . . or would it be thrust upon you as a job requirement?

How far is your facility from taking fieldwork students? Do you see it happening anytime soon? Do you ever see yourselves being a fieldwork supervisor? When? In a year from now? . . . In 5 years? . . . In 10 years?

QUESTION 5: I'd like you to think about your own fieldwork experiences throughout your career (not just currently).

Imagine now that I have a device which can overhear your thoughts! Scary, thought, isn't it?

If someone could overhear your *true thoughts* about supervising fieldwork students, what would they hear?

What I really think and feel about supervising fieldwork students is: _____.

QUESTION 6: Let's go on one more little fantasy-trip! I'd like you to think about what innovative ideas you have regarding fieldwork supervision or fieldwork in general. Basically I mean any ideas which you have besides the typical one-on-one model.

This can be anything under the sun . . . no matter how fantastic! This can be a wish-list or even a nebulous concept without details.

If struggling, maybe it would help to think about FW in its infancy—what design would make sense to you? Or . . . ask about different supervision models or unique or different work settings for fieldwork that they either know of or can envision.

If there is extra time, miscellaneous questions:

—When did you first learn about supervising fieldwork students—during the time you were a student?

—Is fieldwork supervision like mentoring? How else could fieldwork supervision be described?

—Do you have any feelings or experiences about whether managed care has had or is expected to have an effect on fieldwork? (i.e. is fieldwork supervision a viable option for facilities under managed care, capitation, etc? or does that not matter?)

—What are the legal issues surrounding supervising fieldwork students?

WRAP UP:

If you were sitting here instead of me, what would *you* have asked about fieldwork supervision? Do you think the answers would have been different?

If you had to summarize how this group felt about the things we discussed, what would *you* say? [or] if you were asked to describe to someone what happened this afternoon, what could you say? . . .

How would you describe what the group decided as a whole?

Thank them—if they want to add anything later give out your business card

Remind them that incentive will be mailed as long as they signed in with Chris . . . in the lobby at the before the group began.

Thank you and have a good evening.

ADDITIONAL PROBES

Why do you feel the way you do?

Can anybody support that?

Good point, do others feel that way too (or agree/ disagree)?

If someone could overhear your TRUE thoughts about . . . what would they hear?

Do you agonize over . . . Why?

What would you tell a co-worker about . . .
new just-out-of-school co-worker about . . .
stranger . . .

What kind of person is a supervisor
what kind is not?

What words would you use to describe . . .

The American Occupational Therapy Association's Professional Development Programs

Say Yes to Fieldwork

On-line Training for Clinical Educators

■ Oct. 23 – Nov. 27, 1995

(Registration deadline Oct. 20, 1995)

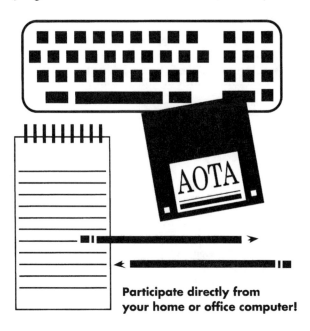

Participate directly from your home or office computer!

Learn How to Develop a Top-notch <u>OT/OTA</u> Student Fieldwork Program

S tudent supervision is a critical part of the fieldwork experience. Students depend on fieldwork supervisors and academic advisors to guide them through this learning experience so that they can make a smooth transition to professional practice. In order for students to get the most out of their fieldwork experience, practitioners and faculty must work together to address fieldwork needs and supervision issues in an ever changing health care environment.

Say Yes to Fieldwork is the fourth AOTA on-line workshop and an ideal training aid for the new as well as experienced fieldwork supervisor. This on-line workshop will use the text from Self Paced Instruction for Clinical Education and Supervision (SPICES), which has been a popular and widely used text by clinical educators. The workshop will also include a supplemental packet of SPICES worksheets.

From your home or office computer, you can have the opportunity to participate in an in-depth discussion on preparing to become a fieldwork educator, managing the fieldwork experience, developing your program, and coordinating supervision with academia.

Sign up for **Say Yes to Fieldwork** today and you'll gain the focused training in fieldwork supervision that you'll need to ensure that your program meets the needs of your students, and keeps pace with health care reform and other changes that affect occupational therapy professionals today.

Here's How It Works

From the convenience of your home or office, you'll use a special toll-free number to access the workshop through The Reliable SOURCE, AOTA's computer bulletin board system (BBS). If you do not subscribe to the SOURCE, you'll receive a temporary logon ID and password; if you're a subscriber, you'll use your current logon ID and password.

Once you log on, you'll have access to the special **Say Yes to Fieldwork** conference area, and to the lesson files from SPICES that await you. An on-screen menu will guide you through the various topics. Download the lessons into your own computer for review at your convenience.

You may interact with the workshop faculty by asking questions and making comments through the electronic mail (E-mail) function of The Reliable SOURCE. You'll also see the questions and comments made by other participants so that you can benefit and learn from others.

What You'll Need to Participate

To participate in the on-line workshop, you'll need the following:

- Computer (IBM, IBM-compatible, or Apple)
- Modem (speeds supported: 300 bps to 14,400 bps)
- Basic knowledge of file transfer procedures (downloading)
- Printer

A user-friendly guidebook/tutorial will show you how to get on-line with The Reliable SOURCE, download lecture files, and send and receive E-mail. Communications software will be provided for IBM or compatible users.

Workshop Access Dates and Times

The **Say Yes to Fieldwork** on-line workshop will begin at 9:00 a.m. EST on Monday, October 23, and end at 9:00 a.m. EST on Monday, November 27, 1995. Throughout this four-week period, you will have 20 minutes of daily connect time to download the lessons, pose questions to the faculty, and review E-mail responses. For current subscribers to The Reliable SOURCE, this 20-minute daily access will be in addition to the normal connect time.

From the first day of the workshop, all lesson material will be available to you for downloading from The Reliable SOURCE. You may work at your own pace!

Who Should Participate?

Occupational therapists and certified occupational therapy assistants who work in hospitals, rehabilitation centers, school systems, home health agencies, outpatient clinics, mental health settings, and work programs who are considering student supervision or who are currently student supervisors.

Workshop Objectives

Participate in **Say Yes to Fieldwork** on-line workshop and you'll be able to:

- Provide your workplace with a rationale to establish a fieldwork program
- Assess your workplace's readiness to accept students for a fieldwork program
- Assess your readiness for fieldwork supervision
- Develop a fieldwork philosophy and investigate resources (including staff and materials)
- Develop fieldwork objectives and learning activities
- Establish communication with OT/OTA academic programs
- Understand the developmental and learning needs of students
- Facilitate a foundation for clinical reasoning skills
- Structure the learning experience for OT/AOTA students
- Assess your students by using the AOTA OT/OTA fieldwork evaluation

Workshop Registration Fees

- $115 AOTA member
- $155 nonmember

The Rewards of Your Efforts

Upon completion of the workshop, you'll be awarded 8 contact hours which may be applied toward your state's annual continuing education requirements.

The Faculty

Learn how to develop a top-notch fieldwork program from these workshop faculty members:

Chris Bird, OTR, Education Coordinator, National Rehabilitation Hospital, Washington, D.C.

Michelle Fisher, OTR, Academic Fieldwork Coordinator and Instructor, University of Kansas Medical Center

Michelle Krohn, OTR/L, Staff Occupational Therapist, Wake Rehabilitation Institute Outpatient Services, Raleigh, NC

Brenda Taubman, OTR/L, OTA Program Coordinator, Apollo College, Phoenix, AZ

Deborah Walens, MHPE, OTR/L, FAOTA, Academic Fieldwork Coordinator, University of Illinois at Chicago

Say Yes To Fieldwork!

Occupational Therapy Clinical Education Is For You!

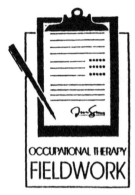

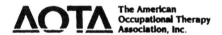
FIELDWORK

Look inside for helpful tips from colleagues on how you can become a first-rate fieldwork supervisor. . .

AOTA The American Occupational Therapy Association, Inc.

Am I Eligible To Be A Student Supervisor?

The AOTA Essentials for an Accredited Educational Program for the Occupational Therapist and Occupational Therapy Assistant state:

Level I: OT/OTA student supervision shall be provided by qualified personnel including, but not limited to, certified occupational therapists, certified occupational therapy assistants, teachers, social workers, nurses, and physical therapists.

Level II: OT student supervision shall be provided by a certified occupational therapist with a minimum of 1 year experience in a practice setting.

OTA student supervision shall be provided by a certified occupational therapist or a certified occupational therapy assistant with a minimum of 1 year experience in a practice setting.

AOTA and OT/OTA Education Programs have fieldwork supervision training resources available for further development of your role as a student supervisor.

The Facts About Supervising Students

Colleagues who supervise fieldwork students say that their experience:

◆ *Provides a sense of personal pride*
◆ *Enhances personal and professional development*
◆ *Offers an opportunity to give back to the profession*
◆ *Brings new ideas to the clinic*
◆ *Provides an opportunity to be part of a mentoring facility*
◆ *Exposes clients and staff to the latest techniques and theories in the field*
◆ *Fosters a beneficial relationship with academia*
◆ *Offers them an opportunity to see that clients respond well to students*

What Does It Take To Be A Fieldwork Supervisor?

- *Patience*   - *Tolerance*
- *Creativity*   - *Open-mindedness*

All those characteristics that led you to the profession in the first place!

Why Does An Organization Participate in OT Fieldwork?

Testimonials from administrators and clinical managers

We know we have a responsibility to pass our skills and knowledge on to others in an effort to produce quality professionals, just as it's our responsibility to provide quality health care. One does not exist without the other.
John Austin, OTR/L, CHT

Participation in student fieldwork is the best recruitment technique. It is good public relations with universities and communities and it provides educational opportunities for staff.
Nancy Thomas, OTR/L

Student fieldwork programs are an important aspect of professional growth and development for both clinicians and students.
Sandy Oleson, OTR/L

Teaching students creates enthusiasm for patient care with new projects and activities that are appreciated by staff.
Simon H. Pincus, MD

Student fieldwork programs contribute to the education of health care providers
Diana Lee Ramsay, OTR

Before and After Supervising Students I Felt. . .

Uncertain and inexperienced but as my first student and I pieced things together it became a positive and enlightening experience.
Barbara Harrington, OTR

Nervous before and proud after seeing their growth.
Mary Ann Byrd, OTR

Before, I felt anxious. After, I was more sure of my clinical skills.
Sandy Oleson, OTR/L

Before? Nervous! Wondering if I would be able to transfer the essential information in the time allotted. After? I knew I could see the world through students' eyes and guide them through the learning process. Now after many students, I know the experience is as unique and individual as they are.
John Austin, OTR/L, CHT

To learn more about how you can become a student supervisor, call the AOTA Education Department at 1-800-SAY-AOTA, or contact:

Why Do We Supervise Students?

Testimony from the field on why you should become a student supervisor

I know from my own experience how fieldwork can play a critical role in shaping professional development and choices regarding a career path.
Barbara Thompson, OTR

I feel an OTA student being supervised by an experienced COTA will have a much better understanding of the COTA's job and relationship with OTRs.
Diane Goss, COTA/L

Both therapist and student have numerous opportunities to develop skills, make professional contacts, and build friendships and support systems.
Rebecca Welch, OTR/L

Teaching someone else helps clarify things in your own mind.
James Swett, OTR

I enjoy getting to know students and keeping aware of the knowledge base they get from their school curriculum.
David Brick, OTR/L

The pleasure of watching the development of the next generation of therapists.
Fred Snively, OTR

Report on Fieldwork
AOTA Fieldwork Promotion Campaign
November 30, 1995

A. SUBJECT:
1. TITLE/ORIGINATOR: Report on Fieldwork
2. TOPIC: AOTA Fieldwork Promotion Campaign
3. CLARIFICATION/INTENT: Review of National Office Fieldwork Activities

B. TO: Executive Board

C. FROM: Jeanette Bair, MBA, OTR, FAOTA (Prepared by Christine Rogers, MA, OTR/L Fieldwork Education Program Manager)

D. DATE: November 30, 1995

E. REPORT ON ACTIVITIES:

The following is a summary of the Fieldwork Promotion Campaign which began Spring, 1994 and continues as of this report:

1) Marketing:

   a) AOTA currently distributes neon stickers that read "Just Say Yes To Fieldwork Students" at annual conferences, fieldwork councils, staff/volunteer speaking engagements, and upon member request. The stickers are also offered in the AOTA products catalog.

   b) The theme of "Just Say Yes To Fieldwork Students" is apparent in all new fieldwork projects and products and will continue through 1996.

   c) AOTA held two Fieldwork Focus Groups (February, 1995) as a marketing strategy to determine why OTs do/do not supervise students. The participants of the first group were individuals who were fieldwork supervisors and the second group were individuals who had never supervised fieldwork students. The average number of years the supervisors had practiced OT was 10 years, and the average number of years as fieldwork supervisors was 8 years. The average number of years the non-supervisors practiced OT was 8.5 years. The practice areas of both groups included home health, skilled nursing facilities, pediatrics, mental health, and rehabilitation. Please refer to the Focus Group attachments for a summary of the data.

   d) AOTA developed a brochure "Say Yes To Fieldwork: Occupational Therapy Clinical Education Is For You!" This brochure targets potential new supervisors and could facilitate the recruitment of new fieldwork educators. The brochure was just completed in October, 1995 and will be disseminated to the following: Program Directors and Academic Fieldwork Coordinators in regular Education Department mailings: members who inquire about starting a fieldwork program and are sent a packet; the Regional Fieldwork Consultants; fieldwork constituents at staff and volunteer speaking engagements; AOTA's annual conference and the SIS practice conference; and publicized in the RA/CSAP voice mail, *OT Week* and the *OT Practice* magazine. Please see sample included with this report.

2) Mailings

The Education Department has revised the packet of information that is mailed to members seeking information on how to start a fieldwork program (approximately 25 inquiries per month). The new packet is less cumbersome and more interesting to attract fieldwork educators.

3) AOTA Database Options on *The Reliable SOURCE*

a) AOTA currently offers the on-line workshop "Say Yes To Fieldwork: On-Line Training For Clinical Educators" and the disc of the workshop will soon be available.

b) The fieldwork database on *The Reliable SOURCE* is continuously updated by national office staff. A pilot project to have schools input their sites directly to *The Reliable SOURCE* resulted in poor outcomes. The pilot project was a result of fieldwork constituents requesting that AOTA keep an accurate national listing of fieldwork centers. AOTA currently has a national listing of fieldwork centers on *The Reliable SOURCE* that is difficult to maintain for accuracy. A survey was sent (Fall, 1994) to all education programs in the accreditation system requesting information and seeking their cooperation for entering their fieldwork center data directly to *The Reliable SOURCE* on a regular basis. The pilot project commenced with 10 schools participating and only three schools remained at the completion of the pilot project. The primary reasons the schools withdrew from the project were the perceived inability and refusal of the schools to share fieldwork center information. The Education department plans to consider the feasibility of a second pilot study.

4) Certificate Program

The Education Department has explored and researched the possibility of offering AOTA certificates of achievement to fieldwork supervisors. The project is in the first phase and sample certificates have been collected, fieldwork constituents and volunteers have been informally contacted for consultation, and design and logo ideas have been discussed. The certificates could be awarded to any OT practitioner who participates in fieldwork supervision. The certificates could be sold to the schools at cost, who could then offer them to the fieldwork centers. The

next step will involve surveying the schools for feedback and selecting and designing the certificate. A sample certificate is attached.

5) The Regional Fieldwork Consultants (RFWC) currently represent nine regions of the United States and are selected based on their demonstrated expertise in fieldwork. Currently, the RFWC Network is managed by the Fieldwork Education Program Manager. However, the proposed reorganization of COE would restructure the RFWC as a standing committee under the COE beginning fiscal year 1996–1997. The RFWC serve three-year terms and they are responsible for two written reports each year to the Fieldwork Education Program Manager, AOTA. According to their reports of November 15, which represent the period of time May 15– November 15, 1995, the RFWC have presented a total of thirteen workshops, seminars, or presentations. These have occurred at the Mountain Central Conference, the California, Florida, Illinois, and North Carolina state conferences, two OT University fieldwork councils, one OTA program fieldwork council, one hospital inservice, one meeting for area OT directors, and the AOTA on-line workshop. The presentation topics included general supervision guidelines, innovative and collaborative fieldwork models, *SPICES*, and clinical reasoning.

The RFWC fielded a total of thirty phone calls from academic programs and fieldwork supervisors and students. Primary topics of conversation were supervision guidelines, the difficult or failing student, interpretation of off-site supervision, and statistics on the cancellation of fieldwork sites. These phone calls also included the time/effort to plan for the workshops.

One other function of the RFWC is to correspond within their regions by letter, fax, e-mail, etc. The new RFWC sent introductions to the faculty in their regions and have been active in utilizing e-mail with fieldwork constituents. One RFWC currently authors a fieldwork column for a state newsletter.

The RFWC report three re-emerging and/ or new issues with fieldwork. The first issue relates to developing objectives and how the objectives match the Fieldwork Evaluation Form. The second issue concerns off-site supervision and the interpretation of how much and what kind of supervision can be provided off-site during fieldwork. The third issue is the impact of managed care on clinical education. The practitioners have questions about how to balance productivity pressures and a student fieldwork program simultaneously.

6) On-Going Dissemination of Innovative Models and Fieldwork in *OT Week/OT Practice/AJOT/JOTS/OT Line* (ASCOTA), etc.

a) Monthly column in *OT Week* for fieldwork and innovative fieldwork models (began January, 1994).

b) Bi-monthly column for fieldwork in the Practice File section of the *OT Practice* magazine (beginning November, 1995).

c) *AJOT* Fieldwork Issue (February, 1995).

d) ASCOTA Strategic Plan 1994–1998—on-going Delegate Task Force on fieldwork.

e) Regional Fieldwork Consultant institute, workshop, or roundtable at the AOTA annual conference (Seattle, 1993; Boston, 1994; Denver, 1995; Chicago, 1996) on the topic of innovative fieldwork.

Attachments: "Say Yes to Fieldwork: Occupational Therapy Clinical Education If For You" Brochure
Focus Group Charts (3)
Sample Certificate

Bibliography

Crepeau, E.B., & La Garde, T. (1991). *Self-Paced Instruction for Clinical Education and Supervision (SPICES)*. Bethesda, MD: American Occupational Therapy Association.

Curtis, K.A. (1988). How to handle personality and style clashes: A training program for clinical instructors. Los Angeles: Health Directions Educational Services for the Health Professions.

Gaiptman, B., & Anthony, A. (1993). *Fundamentals of supervision: Reaching your potential as a supervisor.* Canada: Endorsed by the Canadian Occupational Therapy Foundation and the Ontario Ministry of Health.

Mattingly, C., & Fleming, M.H. (1994). *Clinical reasoning: Forms of inquiry in a therapeutic practice.* Philadelphia: F.A. Davis Company.

Meyers, S.K., & Swinehart, S. (1995). *Creating a positive level I fieldwork experience.* Bethesda, MD: American Occupational Therapy Association.

Neistadt, M.E. (1990). *An independent living skills model for level I fieldwork.* Bethesda, MD: American Occupational Therapy Association.

Opacich, K.J., & Frum, D.C. (1987). *Supervision: Development of therapeutic competence.* Bethesda, MD: American Occupational Therapy Association.

Smith, V. (1994). *Occupational therapy: Transition from classroom to clinic—Physical disability fieldwork applications.* Bethesda, MD: American Occupational Therapy Association.

Guide to fieldwork education. (1994). Bethesda, MD: American Occupational Therapy Association.

OT roles and career exploration and development. (1994). Bethesda, MD: American Occupational Therapy Association.

Index

Guilford's Inventory of Factors ST-DCR, occupational therapy student, 157–162

H

Hermeneutic dialectic process
administrator, fieldwork benefits identification, 91–95
occupational therapy student, fieldwork benefits identification, 91–95
patient, fieldwork benefits identification, 91–95
student supervisor, fieldwork benefits identification, 91–95
Home care
fieldwork, 346
resource list, 346
Level II fieldwork, 301
Hospital, psychosocial Level II fieldwork, 83
Hospital occupational therapy training
distribution of time, 135–143
hospital type, 137–143
length of time, 135–143
Hypothetical reasoning, 12–13
hypothesis-testing strategy, 12

I

Identity, 225
Implementation skills, evaluation, 238
In-class evaluation, clinical reasoning, 39–44
Independent study, 204–208
Independent thought, 215–216
Individualization, Clinical Reasoning Study, 16
Individualized education program, 24–25
Information chunking, 6
Information peer, 284
Information processing, 15
Integrity, evaluation, 237
Intelligence
clinical reasoning, 61–62
new ideas on intelligence, 62–64
interactive mode, 61
logical mode, 61
multiple aspects, 61–62
occupational therapy student, 157
Piaget model, 61
projective mode, 61
Interactive reasoning, 30, 40
community aspect of practice, 30
teaching strategies, 33–34

Intermediate school district
fieldwork, 358
mental retardation, 299
International occupational therapy, 360
Interpersonal skills, supervisor, 171

J

Jargon, professionalism, 394–395
Job performance
Certification Examination for Occupational Therapists Registered, 91–101
certification examination score, 96–101
college grades, 229–233
Field Work Performance Report, 91–101
fieldwork experience rating, 96–101
occupational therapy student, relationship, 229–233
Job satisfaction
Certification Examination for Occupational Therapists Registered, 91–101
certification examination score, 96–101
Field Work Performance Report, 91–101
fieldwork experience rating, 96–101
Job satisfaction questionnaire, 91–101
Judgment
defined, 11
evaluation, 237

K

Knowledge
hierarchical structure, 15
structure, 15
Kohlberg model of moral development, 209
Kolb's LSI, 185
Kuder Preference Record, occupational therapy student, 157–162

L

Labeling theory, 262
Lawton's hierarchy of behavioral areas, evaluation, 33

Learning capacity, evaluation, 237
Learning contract, self-directed learning, 363–365
evidence, 364
learning resources and strategies, 364
objectives, 364
validation, 364–365
Learning process, motivation, 376–377
Learning style
Canada, 367–371
Canfield-Lafferty Learning Styles Inventory, 259–261
achievement, 259
affiliation, 259
content, 259
direct experience, 260
eminence, 259
expectation, 260
inanimate, 259
listening, 260
mode, 259–260
qualitative, 259
reading, 260
structure, 259
clinic performance, relationship, 66–71
defined, 367
field dependence, 367–371
field independence, 367–371
Fieldwork Performance Reports, 66–71
interpersonal competencies, 367–371
Learning Style Inventory, 66–71
literature review, 368–369
occupational therapy student, 219, 220
focus discussion group, 184–189
preferences, 258–261
supervisor perceptions, 184–189
student performance
academic course work, 8–9
clinical course work, 8–9
supervision, 367–371
Your Style of Learning and Thinking, 66–71
Learning Style Inventory, 8–9
learning style, 66–71
Mental Health Fieldwork Performance Report, correlation, 66–71
Physical Disabilities Fieldwork Performance Report, correlation, 66–71
Least restrictive environment, 21

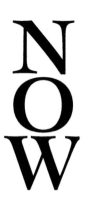

FROM **AOTA** The American
Occupational Therapy
Association, Inc.

Educating Students with Disabilities:
What OT Educators and Fieldwork Supervisors Need to Know

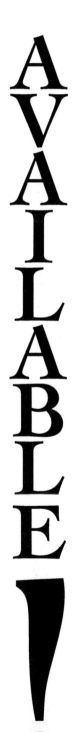

On July 29, 1990, the Americans with Disabilities Act was signed into law. This Act, along with its precursor, the Rehabilitation Act of 1973, prohibit colleges, universities, and other public entities from discriminating against individuals with disabilities.

But what do these statutes mean for college admissions personnel, occupational therapy program managers, and fieldwork sites and supervisors?

This book addresses the *critical issues* that educators and fieldwork supervisors must know about:

- what exactly the laws say and *don't* say, and what it means

- what resources and supports should or do exist to assist in the successful development and implementation of policies pertaining to students with disabilities

- how to disseminate the new policies and work with individual students, both in the classroom and the fieldwork setting

- what strategies are most successful in helping to empower a student with a disability

- how to define and understand what the phrase "reasonable accommodation" means for the student, the program, the school, and the clinic.

The book also contains a detailed list of resources for more information on educating students with disabilities.

For more information on Educating Students with Disabilities: What OT Educators and Fieldwork Supervisors Need to Know, *product #1169, call 301-652-AOTA (2682), ext. 2739. Visa and MasterCard orders only. $13 AOTA member, $17 nonmember*

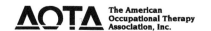

AOTA The American
Occupational Therapy
Association, Inc.

FROM **AOTA** The American Occupational Therapy Association, Inc.

A Guide to Reasonable Accommodation for OT Practitioners with Disabilities: Fieldwork to Employment

Shirley A. Wells, OT, MPH – Sandy Hannebrink, OTS
Editors

Approximately 150 pages

The information presented in this book focuses on the steps needed to ensure compliance with the ADA. The information and resources contained in it will help to maximize the employment of occupational therapy practitioners with disabilities, ensure fieldwork opportunities for students with disabilities, and fulfill the goal of making occupational therapy a diverse and inclusive profession. This publication provides information for making informed decisions about reasonable accommodations in the clinical environment. It offers guidelines on where to begin and how to find the resources to effectively include practitioners and students with disabilities in all areas of the profession.

To order **A Guide to Reasonable Accommodation for OT Practitioners with Disabilities: Fieldwork to Employment,** *product#1104, call 310-652-AOTA (2682), ext. 2739. Visa and Mastercard orders only. $20 AOTA member, $25 nonmember*

NOW AVAILABLE!